Statistical Testing Strategies in the Health Sciences

Chapman & Hall/CRC Biostatistics Series

Published Titles

Adaptive Design Methods in Clinical Trials, Second Edition
Shein-Chung Chow and Mark Chang

Adaptive Designs for Sequential Treatment Allocation
Alessandro Baldi Antognini and Alessandra Giovagnoli

Adaptive Design Theory and Implementation Using SAS and R, Second Edition
Mark Chang

Advanced Bayesian Methods for Medical Test Accuracy
Lyle D. Broemeling

Advances in Clinical Trial Biostatistics
Nancy L. Geller

Applied Meta-Analysis with R
Ding-Geng (Din) Chen and Karl E. Peace

Basic Statistics and Pharmaceutical Statistical Applications, Second Edition
James E. De Muth

Bayesian Adaptive Methods for Clinical Trials
Scott M. Berry, Bradley P. Carlin, J. Jack Lee, and Peter Muller

Bayesian Analysis Made Simple: An Excel GUI for WinBUGS
Phil Woodward

Bayesian Methods for Measures of Agreement
Lyle D. Broemeling

Bayesian Methods for Repeated Measures
Lyle D. Broemeling

Bayesian Methods in Epidemiology
Lyle D. Broemeling

Bayesian Methods in Health Economics
Gianluca Baio

Bayesian Missing Data Problems: EM, Data Augmentation and Noniterative Computation
Ming T. Tan, Guo-Liang Tian, and Kai Wang Ng

Bayesian Modeling in Bioinformatics
Dipak K. Dey, Samiran Ghosh, and Bani K. Mallick

Benefit-Risk Assessment in Pharmaceutical Research and Development
Andreas Sashegyi, James Felli, and Rebecca Noel

Biosimilars: Design and Analysis of Follow-on Biologics
Shein-Chung Chow

Biostatistics: A Computing Approach
Stewart J. Anderson

Published Titles

Causal Analysis in Biomedicine and Epidemiology: Based on Minimal Sufficient Causation
Mikel Aickin

Clinical and Statistical Considerations in Personalized Medicine
Claudio Carini, Sandeep Menon, and Mark Chang

Clinical Trial Data Analysis using R
Ding-Geng (Din) Chen and Karl E. Peace

Clinical Trial Methodology
Karl E. Peace and Ding-Geng (Din) Chen

Computational Methods in Biomedical Research
Ravindra Khattree and Dayanand N. Naik

Computational Pharmacokinetics
Anders Källén

Confidence Intervals for Proportions and Related Measures of Effect Size
Robert G. Newcombe

Controversial Statistical Issues in Clinical Trials
Shein-Chung Chow

Data Analysis with Competing Risks and Intermediate States
Ronald B. Geskus

Data and Safety Monitoring Committees in Clinical Trials
Jay Herson

Design and Analysis of Animal Studies in Pharmaceutical Development
Shein-Chung Chow and Jen-pei Liu

Design and Analysis of Bioavailability and Bioequivalence Studies, Third Edition
Shein-Chung Chow and Jen-pei Liu

Design and Analysis of Bridging Studies
Jen-pei Liu, Shein-Chung Chow, and Chin-Fu Hsiao

Design & Analysis of Clinical Trials for Economic Evaluation & Reimbursement: An Applied Approach Using SAS & STATA
Iftekhar Khan

Design and Analysis of Clinical Trials for Predictive Medicine
Shigeyuki Matsui, Marc Buyse, and Richard Simon

Design and Analysis of Clinical Trials with Time-to-Event Endpoints
Karl E. Peace

Design and Analysis of Non-Inferiority Trials
Mark D. Rothmann, Brian L. Wiens, and Ivan S. F. Chan

Difference Equations with Public Health Applications
Lemuel A. Moyé and Asha Seth Kapadia

DNA Methylation Microarrays: Experimental Design and Statistical Analysis
Sun-Chong Wang and Arturas Petronis

DNA Microarrays and Related Genomics Techniques: Design, Analysis, and Interpretation of Experiments
David B. Allison, Grier P. Page, T. Mark Beasley, and Jode W. Edwards

Dose Finding by the Continual Reassessment Method
Ying Kuen Cheung

Dynamical Biostatistical Models
Daniel Commenges and Hélène Jacqmin-Gadda

Elementary Bayesian Biostatistics
Lemuel A. Moyé

Empirical Likelihood Method in Survival Analysis
Mai Zhou

Exposure–Response Modeling: Methods and Practical Implementation
Jixian Wang

Frailty Models in Survival Analysis
Andreas Wienke

Fundamental Concepts for New Clinical Trialists
Scott Evans and Naitee Ting

Generalized Linear Models: A Bayesian Perspective
Dipak K. Dey, Sujit K. Ghosh, and Bani K. Mallick

Handbook of Regression and Modeling: Applications for the Clinical and Pharmaceutical Industries
Daryl S. Paulson

Published Titles

Inference Principles for Biostatisticians
Ian C. Marschner

Interval-Censored Time-to-Event Data: Methods and Applications
Ding-Geng (Din) Chen, Jianguo Sun, and Karl E. Peace

Introductory Adaptive Trial Designs: A Practical Guide with R
Mark Chang

Joint Models for Longitudinal and Time-to-Event Data: With Applications in R
Dimitris Rizopoulos

Measures of Interobserver Agreement and Reliability, Second Edition
Mohamed M. Shoukri

Medical Biostatistics, Third Edition
A. Indrayan

Meta-Analysis in Medicine and Health Policy
Dalene Stangl and Donald A. Berry

Mixed Effects Models for the Population Approach: Models, Tasks, Methods and Tools
Marc Lavielle

Modeling to Inform Infectious Disease Control
Niels G. Becker

Modern Adaptive Randomized Clinical Trials: Statistical and Practical Aspects
Oleksandr Sverdlov

Monte Carlo Simulation for the Pharmaceutical Industry: Concepts, Algorithms, and Case Studies
Mark Chang

Multiregional Clinical Trials for Simultaneous Global New Drug Development
Joshua Chen and Hui Quan

Multiple Testing Problems in Pharmaceutical Statistics
Alex Dmitrienko, Ajit C. Tamhane, and Frank Bretz

Noninferiority Testing in Clinical Trials: Issues and Challenges
Tie-Hua Ng

Optimal Design for Nonlinear Response Models
Valerii V. Fedorov and Sergei L. Leonov

Patient-Reported Outcomes: Measurement, Implementation and Interpretation
Joseph C. Cappelleri, Kelly H. Zou, Andrew G. Bushmakin, Jose Ma. J. Alvir, Demissie Alemayehu, and Tara Symonds

Quantitative Evaluation of Safety in Drug Development: Design, Analysis and Reporting
Qi Jiang and H. Amy Xia

Quantitative Methods for Traditional Chinese Medicine Development
Shein-Chung Chow

Randomized Clinical Trials of Nonpharmacological Treatments
Isabelle Boutron, Philippe Ravaud, and David Moher

Randomized Phase II Cancer Clinical Trials
Sin-Ho Jung

Sample Size Calculations for Clustered and Longitudinal Outcomes in Clinical Research
Chul Ahn, Moonseong Heo, and Song Zhang

Sample Size Calculations in Clinical Research, Second Edition
Shein-Chung Chow, Jun Shao, and Hansheng Wang

Statistical Analysis of Human Growth and Development
Yin Bun Cheung

Statistical Design and Analysis of Clinical Trials: Principles and Methods
Weichung Joe Shih and Joseph Aisner

Statistical Design and Analysis of Stability Studies
Shein-Chung Chow

Statistical Evaluation of Diagnostic Performance: Topics in ROC Analysis
Kelly H. Zou, Aiyi Liu, Andriy Bandos, Lucila Ohno-Machado, and Howard Rockette

Statistical Methods for Clinical Trials
Mark X. Norleans

Published Titles

Statistical Methods for Drug Safety
Robert D. Gibbons and Anup K. Amatya

Statistical Methods for Immunogenicity Assessment
Harry Yang, Jianchun Zhang, Binbing Yu, and Wei Zhao

Statistical Methods in Drug Combination Studies
Wei Zhao and Harry Yang

Statistical Testing Strategies in the Health Sciences
Albert Vexler, Alan D. Hutson, and Xiwei Chen

Statistics in Drug Research: Methodologies and Recent Developments
Shein-Chung Chow and Jun Shao

Statistics in the Pharmaceutical Industry, Third Edition
Ralph Buncher and Jia-Yeong Tsay

Survival Analysis in Medicine and Genetics
Jialiang Li and Shuangge Ma

Theory of Drug Development
Eric B. Holmgren

Translational Medicine: Strategies and Statistical Methods
Dennis Cosmatos and Shein-Chung Chow

Chapman & Hall/CRC Biostatistics Series

Statistical Testing Strategies in the Health Sciences

Albert Vexler

The State University of New York at Buffalo, USA

Alan D. Hutson

The State University of New York at Buffalo, USA

Xiwei Chen

The State University of New York at Buffalo, USA

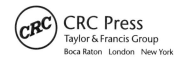

CRC Press
Taylor & Francis Group
Boca Raton   London   New York

CRC Press is an imprint of the
Taylor & Francis Group, an **informa** business

A CHAPMAN & HALL BOOK

CRC Press
Taylor & Francis Group
6000 Broken Sound Parkway NW, Suite 300
Boca Raton, FL 33487-2742

© 2016 by Taylor & Francis Group, LLC
CRC Press is an imprint of Taylor & Francis Group, an Informa business

No claim to original U.S. Government works

Printed on acid-free paper
Version Date: 20160321

International Standard Book Number-13: 978-1-4987-3081-5 (Hardback)

Visit the Taylor & Francis Web site at
http://www.taylorandfrancis.com

and the CRC Press Web site at
http://www.crcpress.com

To my parents, Octyabrina and Alexander, and my son, David

Albert Vexler

To my wife, Brenda, and three kids, Nick, Chance, Trey

Alan D. Hutson

To my parents, Dongsheng Chen and Xuemei Pei

Xiwei Chen

Contents

Foreword xix
Preface.. xxi
Authors xxv

1. **Preliminaries: Welcome to the Statistical Inference Club. Some Basic
   Concepts in Experimental Decision Making**..1
   1.1   Overview: Essential Elements of Defining Statistical Hypotheses and
         Constructing Statistical Tests 1
         1.1.1   Data...2
                 1.1.1.1   Data Collection 2
                 1.1.1.2   Types of Data 3
                 1.1.1.3   Data Preparation..3
                 1.1.1.4   Data Cleaning 3
         1.1.2   Statistical Hypotheses 4
   1.2   Errors Related to the Statistical Testing Mechanism 5
         1.2.1   Rationality and Unbiasedness in Hypothesis Testing 7
   1.3 p-Values..8
         1.3.1   Expected p-Values 10
   1.4   Components for Constructing Test Procedures 11
   1.5   Parametric Approach and Modeling 12
         1.5.1   Example of Pretest Procedures Pertaining to Model Assumptions.......14
   1.6   Warning and Advice: Limitations of Parametric Approaches. Detour to
         Nonparametric Approaches 15
   1.7   Large Sample Approximate Tests 16
   1.8   Confidence Intervals..16
   1.9   When All Else Fails: Bootstrap? 17
         1.9.1   Statistical Functional Is the Parameter of Interest 17
         1.9.2   Bootstrap Confidence Intervals 19
   1.10 Permutation Testing versus Bootstrap Methodology 20
   1.11 Remarks...22
   1.12 Atlas of the Book 23

2. **Statistical Software: R and SAS** 25
   2.1   Introduction 25
   2.2   R Software..25
         2.2.1   Rules for Names of Variables and R Data Sets 25
         2.2.2   Comments in R...26
         2.2.3   Inputting Data in R...26
         2.2.4   Manipulating Data in R 27
         2.2.5   Printing Data in R...29
   2.3   SAS Software 30
         2.3.1   Rules for Names of Variables and SAS Data Sets...............................31
         2.3.2   Comments in SAS 31
         2.3.3   Inputting Data in SAS...32

	2.3.4	Manipulating Data in SAS	33
	2.3.5	Printing Data in SAS	35
	2.3.6	Summarizing Data in SAS	36
2.4	Supplement		37

3. Statistical Graphics ... 39
3.1	Introduction		39
3.2	Descriptive Plots of Raw Data		40
	3.2.1	Boxplots	40
	3.2.2	Scatterplots	42
	3.2.3	High-Dimensional Plots	43
		3.2.3.1 Perspective Plots	43
		3.2.3.2 Contour Plots	43
3.3	Empirical Distribution Function Plot		45
3.4	Two-Sample Comparisons		50
	3.4.1	Quantile–Quantile Plots (Q–Q Plots)	50
	3.4.2	Probability–Probability Plots (P–P plots)	52
	3.4.3	Modifications, Extensions, and Hybrids of Q–Q and P–P Plots	54
	3.4.4	Derivatives of Probability Plots	55
3.5	Probability Plots as Informal Auxiliary Information to Inference		57
	3.5.1	Specific Internal Comparison Probability Plotting Techniques	58
	3.5.2	Residuals in Regression Analysis	60
	3.5.3	Other Applications	61
3.6	Heat Maps		62
	3.6.1	Visualization of Data in the Heat Map Manner	62
	3.6.2	Graphical Comparisons of Statistical Tests	64
3.7	Concluding Remarks		66
3.8	Supplement		67

4. A Brief Ode to Parametric Likelihood ... 71
4.1	Introduction		71
4.2	Likelihood Ratio Test and Its Optimality		73
4.3	Likelihood Ratio Based on the Likelihood Ratio Test Statistic Is the Likelihood Ratio Test Statistic		74
4.4	Maximum Likelihood: Is It the Likelihood?		75
	4.4.1	Reconsideration of Data Example	76
4.5	Supplement		78
	4.5.1	One-Sided Likelihood	86
4.6	Appendix		90
	4.6.1	The Most Powerful Test	90
	4.6.2	The Likelihood Ratio Property $f_{H_1}^L(u) = f_{H_0}^L(u)u$	92
	4.6.3	Wilks' Theorem	93

5. Tests on Means of Continuous Data ... 95
5.1	Introduction		95
5.2	Univariate and p-Dimensional Likelihood Ratio Tests of Location Given Normally Distributed Data		95
5.3	t-Type Tests		96
	5.3.1	One-Sample t-Test	96

5.3.2 Two-Sample *t*-Test 97
  5.3.2.1 Equal Variances 97
  5.3.2.2 Unequal Variances (Welch's *t*-Test) 97
5.3.3 Paired *t*-Test 97
5.3.4 Multivariate *t*-Test 99
5.4 Exact Likelihood Ratio Test for Equality of Two Normal Populations 101
5.5 Supplement 102

6. Empirical Likelihood 105
6.1 Introduction 105
6.2 Classical Empirical Likelihood Methods 106
6.3 Techniques for Analyzing Empirical Likelihoods 108
6.4 Density-Based Empirical Likelihood Methods 112
6.5 Combining Likelihoods to Construct Composite Tests and Incorporate
    the Maximum Data-Driven Information 115
6.6 Bayesians and Empirical Likelihood: Are They Mutually Exclusive? 116
  6.6.1 Bayesian Empirical Likelihood 117
  6.6.2 Empirical Likelihood–Based Empirical Bayesian Posterior 118
    6.6.2.1 Nonparametric Posterior Expectations of
            Simple Functionals 118
    6.6.2.2 Nonparametric Analogue of James–Stein Estimation 120
6.7 Three Key Arguments That Support the Empirical Likelihood
    Methodology as a Practical Statistical Analysis Tool 121
6.8 Supplement 122
6.9 Appendix 140
  6.9.1 Several Results That Are Similar to Those Related to
        the Evaluations of *ELR* (θ) 140
  6.9.2 R Procedures for Executing the Two-Sample Density-Based ELR Test 141

7. Bayes Factor–Based Test Statistics 143
7.1 Introduction 143
7.2 Representative Values 144
7.3 Integrated Most Powerful Tests 145
7.4 Bayes Factor 146
  7.4.1 Computation of Bayes Factors 147
    7.4.1.1 Asymptotic Approximations 153
    7.4.1.2 Simple Monte Carlo Evaluations, Importance Sampling,
            and Gaussian Quadrature 156
    7.4.1.3 Simulating from the Posterior 156
    7.4.1.4 Combining Simulation and Asymptotic Approximations 157
  7.4.2 Choice of Prior Probability Distributions 157
  7.4.3 Decision-Making Rules Based on the Bayes Factor 161
  7.4.4 Data Example: Application of Bayes Factor 168
7.5 Remarks 171
7.6 Supplement 171
7.7 Appendix 183
  7.7.1 Optimality of Likelihood Ratio Test in the Simple Hypothesis
        Testing Case 183

7.7.2 Most Powerful Test in the Hypothesis Testing H_0: $X \sim f_0$ versus H_1: $X \sim f_0 \exp(\theta_1 x + \theta_2)$ 184

7.7.3 Bayes Factor Test is an Integrated Most Powerful Decision Rule 185

8. Fundamentals of Receiver Operating Characteristic Curve Analyses 187
8.1 Introduction 187
8.2 ROC Curve Inference 188
8.3 Area under the ROC Curve 191
    8.3.1 Parametric Approach 191
    8.3.2 Nonparametric Approach 192
    8.3.3 Nonparametric Comparison of Two ROC Curves 193
8.4 ROC Analysis and Logistic Regression: Comparison and Overestimation 194
    8.4.1 Retrospective and Prospective ROC 196
    8.4.2 Expected Bias of the ROC Curve and Overestimation of the AUC 196
    8.4.3 Remark 203
8.5 Best Combinations Based on Values of Multiple Biomarkers 203
    8.5.1 Parametric Method 204
    8.5.2 Nonparametric Method 205
8.6 Notes Regarding Treatment Effects 206
    8.6.1 Best Linear Combination of Markers 206
    8.6.2 Maximum Likelihood Ratio Tests 208
        8.6.2.1 Remark Regarding Numerical Calculations 210
8.7 Supplement 210
    8.7.1 ROC 210
    8.7.2 AUC 216
    8.7.3 Combinations of Markers 222
8.8 Appendix 227
    8.8.1 General Form of the AUC 227
    8.8.2 Form of the AUC under the Normal Data Distribution Assumption 227
    8.8.3 Form of the Function h Associating μ_{11} with, μ_{21}, μ_{31}, μ_{41}, μ_2, Σ_1, Σ_2 under H_0 227

9. Nonparametric Comparisons of Distributions 229
9.1 Introduction 229
9.2 Wilcoxon Rank-Sum Test 229
9.3 Kolmogorov–Smirnov Two-Sample Test 231
9.4 Density-Based Empirical Likelihood Ratio Tests 231
    9.4.1 Hypothesis Setting and Test Statistics 232
        9.4.1.1 Test 1: H_0 versus H_{A1} 232
        9.4.1.2 Test 2: H_0 versus H_{A2} 236
        9.4.1.3 Test 3: H_0 versus H_{A3} 237
    9.4.2 Asymptotic Consistency and Null Distributions of the Tests 238
9.5 Density-Based Empirical Likelihood Ratio Based on Paired Data 239
    9.5.1 Significance Level of the Proposed Test 242
9.6 Multiple-Group Comparison 244
    9.6.1 Kruskal–Wallis One-Way Analysis of Variance 244
    9.6.2 Density-Based Empirical Likelihood Procedures for K-Sample Comparisons 245

9.7 Supplement 246

    9.7.1 *K*-Sample Comparison 250

9.8 Appendix 252

    9.8.1 R Code to Conduct Two-Sample Density-Based Empirical
Likelihood Ratio Test 260

10. Dependence and Independence: Structures, Testing, and Measuring 263

10.1 Introduction 263

10.2 Tests of Independence 265

    10.2.1 Classical Methods 265

        10.2.1.1 Pearson Correlation Coefficient 266

        10.2.1.2 Spearman's Rank Correlation Coefficient 266

        10.2.1.3 Kendall's Rank Correlation Coefficient 267

    10.2.2 Data-Driven Rank Tests 267

    10.2.3 Empirical Likelihood–Based Method 270

    10.2.4 Density-Based Empirical Likelihood Ratio Test 271

10.3 Indices of Dependence 272

    10.3.1 Classical Measures of Dependence 272

    10.3.2 Maximal Information Coefficient 273

    10.3.3 Area under the Kendall Plot 274

10.4 Structures of Dependence 277

    10.4.1 Basic Structures 277

    10.4.2 Random Effects–Type Dependence 279

10.5 Monte Carlo Comparisons of Tests of Independence 284

10.6 Data Examples 312

    10.6.1 TBARS 312

    10.6.2 Periodontal Disease 315

    10.6.3 VEGF Expression 315

10.7 Discussion 317

10.8 Supplement 318

11. Goodness-of-Fit Tests (Tests for Normality) 327

11.1 Introduction 327

11.2 Shapiro–Wilk Test for Normality 327

11.3 Supplement 329

    11.3.1 Tests for Normality 329

    11.3.2 Tests for Normality Based on Characteristic Functions 332

    11.3.3 Test for Normality Based on Sample Entropy 332

    11.3.4 Tests for Multivariate Normality 333

12. Statistical Change-Point Analysis 337

12.1 Introduction 337

12.2 Common Change-Point Models 339

12.3 Simple Change-Point Model 342

    12.3.1 Parametric Approaches 342

        12.3.1.1 CUSUM-Based Techniques 342

        12.3.1.2 Shiryayev–Roberts Statistic-Based Techniques 346

12.3.2 Nonparametric Approaches...350
    12.3.2.1 Change in Location...350
    12.3.2.2 U-Statistics-Based Approaches...353
    12.3.2.3 Empirical Likelihood–Based Approach..............................356
    12.3.2.4 Density-Based Empirical Likelihood Approaches.................357
12.3.3 Semiparametric Approaches..360
12.4 Epidemic Change Point Problems..362
  12.4.1 Parametric Approaches..363
    12.4.1.1 Simple Case of the Problem...363
    12.4.1.2 General Case of the Problem...369
  12.4.2 Nonparametric Approaches..372
  12.4.3 Semiparametric Approaches..374
12.5 Problems in Regression Models...376
  12.5.1 Linear Regression...377
  12.5.2 Segmented Linear Regression..378
    12.5.2.1 Simple Case of the Problem...379
    12.5.2.2 General Case of the Problem...379
12.6 Supplement...380
  12.6.1 Simple Change Point..380
    12.6.1.1 Parametric Methods...380
    12.6.1.2 Nonparametric Methods..382
  12.6.2 Multiple Change Points..383
    12.6.2.1 Parametric Methods...383
    12.6.2.2 Nonparametric Methods..385
  12.6.3 Problems in Regression Models...386
    12.6.3.1 Linear Regression...386
    12.6.3.2 Threshold Effects..388
    12.6.3.3 Segmented Regression..389
    12.6.3.4 Structural Change...391
    12.6.3.5 Change Points on Phylogenetic Trees..................................392
    12.6.3.6 Statistical Quality Control Schemes.....................................393
12.7 Appendix..394

13. A Brief Review of Sequential Testing Methods..395
13.1 Introduction..395
13.2 Two-Stage Designs...397
13.3 Sequential Probability Ratio Test..398
  13.3.1 SPRT Stopping Boundaries..400
  13.3.2 Wald Approximation to the Average Sample Number.....................400
  13.3.3 Asymptotic Properties of the Stopping Time N 401
13.4 Group-Sequential Tests..404
13.5 Adaptive Sequential Designs...406
13.6 Futility Analysis...407
13.7 Postsequential Analysis...407
13.8 Supplement...408
13.9 Appendix: Determination of Sample Sizes Based on the Errors'
    Control of SPRT..420

14. A Brief Review of Multiple Testing Problems in Clinical Experiments 421
    14.1 Introduction 421
    14.2 Definitions of Error Rates 422
         14.2.1 Family-Wise Error Rates 422
         14.2.2 False Discovery Rate and False Discovery Proportion 426
    14.3 Power Evaluation 427
    14.4 Remarks 427
    14.5 Supplement 428

15. Some Statistical Procedures for Biomarker Measurements Subject to Instrumental Limitations 429
    15.1 Introduction 429
    15.2 Methods 432
         15.2.1 Additive Errors 432
               15.2.1.1 Repeated Measurements 432
               15.2.1.2 Bayesian-Type Method 434
               15.2.1.3 Hybrid Pooled–Unpooled Design 434
         15.2.2 Limit of Detection 436
               15.2.2.1 Methods Based on the Maximum Likelihood Methodology 436
               15.2.2.2 Bayesian-Type Methods 437
               15.2.2.3 Single and Multiple Imputation Methods 437
               15.2.2.4 Hybrid Pooled–Unpooled Design 438
    15.3 Monte Carlo Experiments 439
    15.4 Concluding Remarks 441
    15.5 Supplement 442

16. Calculating Critical Values and p-Values for Exact Tests 451
    16.1 Introduction 451
    16.2 Methods of Calculating Critical Values of Exact Tests 452
         16.2.1 Monte Carlo–Based Method 452
         16.2.2 Interpolation Method 453
         16.2.3 Hybrid Method 455
               16.2.3.1 Introduction of the Method 455
               16.2.3.2 Method 457
    16.3 Available Software Packages 462
    16.4 Supplement 463
    16.5 Appendix 465

17. Bootstrap and Permutation Methods 471
    17.1 Introduction 471
    17.2 Resampling Data with Replacement in SAS 477
    17.3 Theoretical Quantities of Interest 485
         17.3.1 Bias Estimation 488
         17.3.2 Variance Estimation, MSE Estimation, and the Double Bootstrap 491
    17.4 Bootstrap Confidence Intervals 501
         17.4.1 Percentile Method 502
         17.4.2 Bootstrap-*t* Method 507

17.4.3 Variance-Stabilized Bootstrap-*t* Method 514
17.4.4 Bootstrap-*t* Method via Double Bootstrapping 519
17.4.5 Bias-Corrected Method 522
17.4.6 Bias-Corrected and Accelerated Method 527
17.4.7 Calibration of the Intervals 534
17.5 Simple Two-Group Comparisons 537
17.5.1 Summary Statistics 538
17.5.2 Bootstrap p-Values 540
17.5.3 Using the SAS Macro Language for Calculating
Percentile Intervals 543
17.5.4 Using the SAS Macro Language for Calculating
Bootstrap-*t* Intervals 545
17.5.5 Repeated Measures and Clustered Data 549
17.5.6 Censored Data 556
17.6 Simple Regression Modeling 559
17.7 Relationship between Empirical Likelihood
and Bootstrap Methodologies 570
17.8 Permutation Tests 571
17.8.1 Outline of Permutation Theory 572
17.8.2 Two-Sample Methods 574
17.8.3 Correlation and Regression 582
17.9 Supplement 586
17.10 Appendix: Bootstrap-*t* Example Macro 587

References 591

Author Index 633

Subject Index 645

Foreword

This comprehensive book takes the reader from the underpinnings of statistical inference through to cutting-edge modern analytical techniques. Along the way, the authors explore graphical representations of data, a key component of any data analysis; standard procedures such as the *t*-test and tests for independence; and modern methods, including the bootstrap and empirical likelihood methods. The presentation focuses on practical applications interwoven with theoretical rationale, with an emphasis on how to carry out procedures and interpret the results. Numerous software examples (R and SAS) are provided, such that readers should be able to reproduce plots and other analyses on their own. A wealth of examples from real data sets, web resources, supplemental notes, and plentiful references are provided, which round out the materials.

Nicole Lazar
Department of Statistics, University of Georgia
Athens, Georgia

Preface

SUMMARY: In all likelihood, the universe of statistical science is relatively or privately infinite, and it is expanding in a similar manner as our universe, satisfying the property of a science that is alive. Hence, it would be an absolute impossibility to include everything in one book written by humans, even around a statistical topic such as statistical testing strategies. One of our major goals is to provide readers a road map of where and what to look for, corresponding to their interests, while steering them away from improper or suboptimal approaches.

Modern studies in health sciences require formal comparisons and evaluations based on correct and appropriate statistical decision-making mechanisms. In many scenarios, the statistical design and analysis of a health-related study are carried forth under strict federal guidelines and review; for example, the Food and Drug Administration (FDA) reviews and approves the safety and efficacy of new drugs and medical devices based on rigorous statistical approaches. The cost of these types of investigations is enormous and time-consuming. Thus, the use of cost-effective and appropriate statistical methods is a high priority. In addition to federal reviews, scientific journals have become much more rigorous as well, in terms of making sure an appropriate analysis plan was applied, usually employing statisticians as reviewers.

The primary objective of this book is to provide a compendium of statistical approaches for decision-making policies ranging from graphical methods and classical procedures through computational-intensive bootstrap strategies to newly advanced empirical likelihood techniques. Historically, many of the approaches that we present in this book were not feasible due to the computational requirements. In the past, this meant relying on approximations that may or may not be accurate in the finite sample setting. However, in the modern age, we are generally no longer constrained by computational issues and have a greater flexibility in terms of the statistical approaches that we may employ to data analysis problems. In some sense, the computational power of modern computers has spurred a renaissance in new and modern statistical methods, which is the thrust of what we wish to accomplish. These methodologies may be applied to various problems encountered in medical and epidemiological studies, including clinical trials.

Theoretical aspects of various decision-making procedures, including those based on parametric and nonparametric likelihood methods, have been extensively discussed in the literature. We introduce correct and efficient testing mechanisms with the aim of making these techniques accessible to a wide variety of data analysts at different skill levels by providing the accompanying software routines. In terms of the book's content, we cannot cover every statistical testing scenario and strategy. For example, we do not include tests based on survival data or topics such as regression models. In general, the techniques covered in this book span robust statistical methods to more computationally intensive approaches.

Our intent is that this book provides material that will bridge the gap between highly relevant theoretical statistical methods and practical procedures applied to the planning and analysis of health-related experiments. The theoretical underpinnings of the methods presented in this book are introduced with a substantial amount of chapter notes to point readers to additional references. We work from a theoretical framework and move toward the practical application for each concept, providing real-world examples that are made easily implementable by providing the corresponding statistical software code. We also show the basic ingredients and methods for constructing correct and powerful statistical decision-making processes to be adapted toward complex statistical applications.

We start the book by laying the foundation for properly framing health-related experiments in terms of formal statistical decision rules. We also include novel theoretical and applied results, which have been published in high-impact biostatistical and statistical journals, including those developed by the authors. In order to help transfer statistical theory into practice, we provide easily accessible software routines for a majority of the methods described in the book based on both the R and SAS statistical software packages. Descriptions of the R and SAS languages at an introductory level are also presented in our book.

Generally speaking, we try to balance presenting the materials in a manner that is useful to medical researchers who have some training in statistics and statistical computing and need only a reminder of some of the basic statistical tools and concepts with the interests of research-oriented statisticians who are concerned with the theoretical aspects of the methods we present. In the book, the reader will find new theoretical methods, open problems, and new procedures across a variety of topics for their scholarly investigations. We present results that are novel to the current set of books on the market and results that are even new with respect to the recent scientific literature. Our aim is to draw the attention of theoretical statisticians and practitioners in epidemiology and clinical research to the necessity of new developments, extensions, and investigations related to statistical testing and its applications. In the context of focusing this book on applied work, we emphasize the following topics:

- Correctly formulating statistical hypotheses with respect to the aims of medical and epidemiological studies
- Constructing and providing statistical decision-making test rules corresponding to practical experiments
- Using simple but efficient graphical methods, including the receiver operating characteristic (ROC) curve analysis and Kendall-type plots
- Using basic test procedures and their components in practical decision-making problems
- Employing parametric and nonparametric likelihood testing techniques in applied research
- Understanding the basic properties of likelihood ratio-type tests in parametric and nonparametric settings
- Using Bayesian concepts to develop decision-making procedures
- Applying goodness-of-fit tests and tests for independence
- Understanding the concepts of retrospective and sequential decision-making mechanisms
- Solving multiple testing problems in clinical experiments
- Defining and solving change point detection problems
- Comparing statistical tests and evaluating their properties
- Understanding and employing bootstrap and permutation methods
- Implementing the statistical software at a beginning level
- Learning modern techniques and their applications presented in the recent statistical literature

For the more research-oriented statistician, our book describes important properties and new as well as classical theoretical results of testing statistical hypotheses. We introduce several methodological tools to evaluate different theoretical characteristics of statistical procedures, for example, Chapters 4, 6, and 7. We present higher-level theoretical developments relative to parametric and empirical likelihood functions and Bayesian approaches to statistical inference, which may be extended, modified, and investigated using asymptotic and finite sample size propositions. We lay the foundation for new dependence measures based on Kendall plots in terms of both summary statistical measures and graphical displays. New methods for combining biomarkers based on ROC methods are presented. Learning the book material, one can easily find interesting open problems. For example, in Chapter 1 we introduce the approach of expected p-values. The reader can recognize that the formal notation for expected p-values has a form of the area under the ROC curve (AUC). Then the problem to obtain the best combinations of different test statistics (Chapter 14) can be stated in a manner related to the maximization of AUCs, mentioned in Chapter 8. The introduced bootstrap-type techniques (e.g., Chapter 17) are very attractive to be employed in this context. In a similar mode, the areas under the Kendall plot (Chapter 10) can be considered. The software code mentioned in this book can certainly be improved, optimized, and extended.

This book describes statistical strategies for handling multiplicity issues arising in hypothesis testing across medical and epidemiological studies. We cover a variety of bootstrap methods from a practical point of view, making sure the limitations of the approach are understood in the finite sample setting, and develop strategies for scenarios when the most basic bootstrap approach may fail. We also introduce the concept of permutation—or so-called exact tests—which under certain conditions is a very desirable and robust testing strategy. We display traditional statistical testing techniques as well as present novel testing approaches. The book shows efficient methods for constructing powerful procedures to test for composite hypotheses based on data that can be subject to different issues related to problematic data, for example, data with observations containing measurement errors or limit of detection issues. We introduce several strategies to evaluate and compare treatment effects based on multiple biomarkers. Our book offers tools that help the reader to fully understand statistical approaches for decision making. This book points out comparisons between different statistical methods based on real medical data.

The organization of the material within the book is primarily based on the type of questions to be answered by inference procedures or according to the general type of mathematical derivation. We consider a wide class of decision-making mechanisms, starting from probability plotting techniques via the receiver operating characteristic curve analysis, which is widely applied in diagnostic studies, and moving to modern nonparametric likelihood approaches. The arrangement of chapters makes the book attractive to scientists who are new to the biostatistical research area, including those who may not have a strong statistical background. It can help attract statisticians interested in learning more about advanced topics. We explain step-by-step procedures and present a practical opportunity for trainees not only to acquaint themselves with statistics in the health sciences and understand statistical analysis in the medical literature, but also to be guided in the application of planning and analysis in their own studies.

The book is also intended for graduate students majoring in biostatistics, epidemiology, health-related sciences, or in a field where a statistics concentration is desirable, particularly for those who are interested in formal decision-making mechanisms. This book can be used as a textbook for a one- or two-semester advanced graduate course. The material in the book should be appropriate for use as both a text and a reference. We hope that the mathematical level and breadth of examples will recruit students and teachers not only from statistics and biostatistics, but also from a broad range of fields. We anticipate that the book will induce readers to learn a variety of new and current statistical techniques, and that by employing these new and efficient methods, they will change the practice of data analysis in clinical research.

A very important reason for writing this book was to refocus the scientist toward a better understanding of the underpinnings of appropriate statistical inference in a well-rounded fashion. It is our experience that applied statisticians or users often neglect the underlying postulates when implementing formal test procedures and interpreting their results. Consider, for example, the following telling quote:

> *P* values are widely used in science to test null hypotheses. For example, in a medical study looking at smoking and cancer, the null hypothesis could be that there is no link between the two. Many researchers interpret a lower *P* value as stronger evidence that the null hypothesis is false. Many also accept findings as 'significant' if the *P* value comes in at less than 0.05. But *P* values are slippery, and sometimes, significant *P* values vanish when experiments and statistical analyses are repeated. (*Nature* 506, 150–152, 2014.)

In this book, we provide the definition of a p-value and describe its formal role in decision-making mechanisms (e.g., see Chapter 1). Under the null hypothesis, p-values are uniformly [0,1] distributed random variables. At this rate, it is difficult to use p-values as the measurement. Oftentimes, practitioners misinterpret the notion of a p-value relative to a given statistical test. Without considering the statistical design of a given experiment and other information, careless interpretations of p-values can yield to absurd and unrealistic conclusions. This has resulted in different cases when practitioners try to avoid applications of statistical tools. For example, in 2015, the editors of *Basic and Applied Social Psychology* (*BASP*) announced that the journal would no longer publish papers containing p-values because the statistics were too often used to support low-quality research.

Finally, we would like to note that this book attempts to represent a part of our lives that consists of mistakes, stereotypes, puzzles, and so forth—all that we love. Thus, our book cannot be perfect. We truly thank readers for their participation in our lives. We hope that the presented material can play a role as prior information for various research outputs.

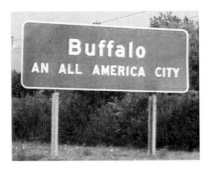

Albert Vexler
Alan D. Hutson
Xiwei Chen

Authors

Albert Vexler earned his PhD in statistics and probability theory from the Hebrew University of Jerusalem in 2003. His PhD advisors were Moshe Pollak, fellow of the American Statistical Association, and Marcy Bogen, professor of statistics at Hebrew University. He was a postdoctoral research fellow in the biometry and mathematical statistics branch at the National Institute of Child Health and Human Development (National Institutes of Health, Bethesda, Maryland). Currently, Dr. Vexler is a tenured associate professor in the Department of Biostatistics, The State University of New York at Buffalo. Dr. Vexler has authored and coauthored various publications that contribute to both the theoretical and applied aspects of statistics in medical research. Many of his papers and statistical software developments have appeared in statistical and biostatistical journals that have top-rated impact factors and are historically recognized as leading scientific journals, including *Biometrics, Biometrika, Journal of Statistical Software, American Statistician, Annals of Applied Statistics, Statistical Methods in Medical Research, Biostatistics, Journal of Computational Biology, Statistics in Medicine, Statistics and Computing, Computational Statistics and Data Analysis, Scandinavian Journal of Statistics, Biometrical Journal, Statistics in Biopharmaceutical Research, Stochastic Processes and Their Applications, Journal of Statistical Planning and Inference, Annals of the Institute of Statistical Mathematics, Canadian Journal of Statistics, Metrika, Statistics, Journal of Applied Statistics, Journal of Nonparametric Statistics, Communications in Statistics, Sequential Analysis, STATA Journal, American Journal of Epidemiology, Epidemiology, Paediatric and Perinatal Epidemiology, Academic Radiology, Journal of Clinical Endocrinology and Metabolism, Journal of Addiction Medicine,* and *Reproductive Toxicology and Human Reproduction.*

Dr. Vexler was awarded a National Institutes of Health grant to develop novel nonparametric data analysis and statistical methodology. His research interests include receiver operating characteristic curve analysis, measurement error, optimal designs, regression models, censored data, change point problems, sequential analysis, statistical epidemiology, Bayesian decision-making mechanisms, asymptotic methods of statistics, forecasting, sampling, optimal testing, nonparametric tests, empirical likelihoods, renewal theory, Tauberian theorems, time series, categorical analysis, multivariate analysis, multivariate testing of complex hypotheses, factor and principal component analysis, statistical biomarker evaluations, and best combinations of biomarkers. Dr. Vexler is the associate editor for *BMC Medical Research Methodology*, a peer-reviewed journal that considers articles on methodological approaches to healthcare research. In 2015, he was appointed the associate editor for *Biometrics*. These journals belong to the first cohort of academic literature related to the methodology of biostatistical and epidemiological research and clinical trials.

Alan D. Hutson earned his BA in 1988 and MA in 1990 in statistics from the State University of New York (SUNY) at Buffalo. He then worked for Otsuka America Pharmaceuticals, Rockville, Maryland, for two years as a biostatistician. He then earned his MA in 1993 and PhD in 1996 in statistics from the University of Rochester, Rochester, New York. His PhD advisor was Professor Govind Mudholkar, a world-renowned researcher in statistics and biostatistics. Dr. Hutson was hired as a biostatistician at the University of Florida, Gainesville, in 1996, as a research assistant professor and worked his way to a tenured associate professor. He had several roles at the University of Florida, including interim director of the Division of Biostatistics and director of the General Clinical Research Informatics Core. Dr. Hutson moved to SUNY at Buffalo in 2002 as an associate professor and chief of the Division of Biostatistics. He was the founding chair of the new Department of Biostatistics in 2003 and became a full professor in 2007. Dr. Hutson's accomplishments as chair included the implementation of several new undergraduate and graduate degree programs and a substantial growth in the size and quality of the department faculty and students. In 2005, Dr. Hutson also became chair of biostatistics (now biostatistics and bioinformatics) at Roswell Park Cancer Institute (RPCI), Buffalo, New York, was appointed professor of oncology, and was the director of the Core Cancer Center Biostatistics Core. He helped implement the new bioinformatics core at RPCI. He is currently chair of biostatistics and bioinformatics at RPCI. Dr. Hutson recently became the biostatistical, epidemiological, and research design director for SUNY's recently awarded National Institutes of Health– funded Clinical and Translational Research Award. Dr. Hutson is a fellow of the American Statistical Association. He is the associate editor of *Communications in Statistics*, the associate editor of the *Sri Lankan Journal of Applied Statistics*, and a New York State NYSTAR Distinguished Professor. Dr. Hutson has membership on several data safety and monitoring boards and has served on several high-level scientific review panels. He has more than 200 peer-reviewed publications. In 2013, Dr. Hutson was inducted into the Delta Omega Public Health Honor Society, Gamma Lambda Chapter. Dr. Hutson's methodological work focuses on nonparametric methods for biostatistical applications as they pertain to statistical functionals. He has several years of experience in the design and analysis of clinical trials.

Xiwei Chen earned her bachelor's degree in mathematics from Peking University, Beijing, China, in 2008, and her MS degree in applied statistics from the Rochester Institute of Technology, Henrietta, New York, in 2010. In 2016, Dr. Chen earned her PhD in biostatistics from the State University of New York at Buffalo. Her adviser was Dr. Albert Vexler. Between 2011 and 2015, she worked as a research assistant at the Roswell Park Cancer Institute, Buffalo, New York. Currently, Dr. Chen is employed as a biostatistician at Johnson & Johnson Vision Care, Inc. Her areas of specialty are the empirical likelihood methods, the receiver operating characteristic curve methodology, and statistical diagnosis and its applications. Dr. Chen has authored or coauthored more than 10 papers and several book chapters in biostatistical areas concerning statistical approaches related to disease diagnoses. She is also very active as a reviewer for statistical journals.

1

Preliminaries: Welcome to the Statistical Inference Club. Some Basic Concepts in Experimental Decision Making

"I'm just one hundred and one, five months and a day."

"I can't believe that!" said Alice.

"Can't you?" the Queen said in a pitying tone. "Try again: draw a long breath, and shut your eyes."

Alice laughed. "There's no use trying," she said: "one can't believe impossible things."

"I daresay you haven't had much practice," said the Queen. "When I was your age, I always did it for half-an-hour a day. Why, sometimes I've believed as many as six impossible things before breakfast."

Lewis Carroll (Charles Lutwidge Dodgson), 1871*

1.1 Overview: Essential Elements of Defining Statistical Hypotheses and Constructing Statistical Tests

The majority of experiments in biomedicine and other health-related sciences involve mathematically formalized tests. The common goal in testing is to employ appropriate and efficient statistical procedures to make informed decisions based on data. Mathematical strategies for constructing formal decision rules play an important role in medical and epidemiological discovery, policy formulation, and clinical practice. In order to draw conclusions about populations on the basis of samples from populations, clinical experiments commonly require the application of the mathematical statistics discipline. It is often said that statistics is the language of applied science.

The aim of the scientific method in decision theory is to simultaneously maximize quantified gains and minimize losses when reaching a conclusion. For example, clinical experiments can have stated goals of maximizing factors (gains), such as the accuracy of diagnosis of a medical condition, faster healing, and greater patient satisfaction, while minimizing factors (losses), such as misdiagnoses, human resource expenditures, employed efforts, duration of screening for a disease, side effects, and costs of an experiment.

In order to correctly define statistical testing procedures and interpret the corresponding results, practitioners should research the nature of clinical data, experimental limitations, and instrumental sensitivities, as well as appropriate state objectives and their corresponding hypotheses.

---

* *Through the Looking-Glass, and What Alice Found There*, 1871. Lewis Carroll is a writer, mathematician, and logician.

1.1.1 Data

In clinical studies, researchers collect and analyze data with the goal of soliciting useful information. One of the first critical components of the data analysis procedure is data collection and entry. This is the process where the raw data are checked for accuracy and subsequently cleaned. Once the data are deemed relatively accurate, then data modeling and decision-making mechanisms are carried forth based on a set of underlying assumptions regarding the stochastic and deterministic components of the data.

A reliable data management process has several distinct stages:

- The first stage consists of data capture and entry. There are several techniques for ensuring the accuracy of the data entry, such as built range checks and double data entry.

- The next stage involves data cleansing, where date entry errors are documented and corrected. In this stage, records are reviewed regarding consistency and completeness.

- Once the data have been cleansed, they can then be summarized descriptively and again checked for accuracy; that is, oftentimes data entry errors are caught via graphical methods or summary statistical checks.

- Once the data are deemed accurate relative to scientific standards, it is generally "frozen" as the source for inferential statistical analysis that can be performed using hypothesis testing, confidence interval generation, or Bayesian approaches. It is at this point that the analyst verifies the underlying model assumptions based on his or her understanding of the limitations of the model and then draws scientific conclusions based on formal statistical procedures. This stage also involves properly interpreting the results from the scientific evaluations, which requires considerations of unmeasured factors that may have influenced subject selections, measurements, and risks, as well as issues in statistical inference.

1.1.1.1 Data Collection

To succeed in its objectives and goals, every study requires rigorous designs, appropriate and sensible analysis, and careful execution of the study or field work, guided by a simple principle that the strongest bridge between the design and the analysis should be created. To ensure the quality of the study or the field work, researchers should oversee and test the design of the data collection instruments, incorporating quality control methods in every phase of the study.

Data can be collected with standard instruments, such as paper or web-based forms, designed to increase the validity of the study comparisons. A variety of instruments are available. For example, in epidemiology or health-related research, we can consider in-person telephone interview questionnaires, self-administered questionnaires, paper and electronic medical records, physical examinations, biospecimen collections, and environmental samples. Other types of studies, such as clinical trials, have very rigorous data collection guidelines, oftentimes dictated by regulatory agencies such as the Food and Drug Administration. Information from various sources is generally compiled into a single study-related database. Exceptions to this may be genomics data, which require specialized and sometimes distributed storage systems.

1.1.1.2 Types of Data

The data collected may be categorized into two major types: (1) categorical (also called nominal) and (2) numerical or measurement data. Qualitative data generally describe an attribute or feature and are called categorical data, for example, species (lion, tiger, bear) or gender (male, female). Numerical or measurement data are represented by variables measured on either a discrete ordinal or continuous scale; for example, a pain rating from 0 to 10 would be considered a discrete ordinal measure, while temperature measurements, using a fine instrument, would be considered continuous. Examples of other forms of data would include things such as medical images, videos, handwriting samples, and free text.

1.1.1.3 Data Preparation

Data collected in the field should be transcribed into clean tables of "data sets" to be used for data analysis. The post–data collection step is receipt of data by the study center (hardcopy forms or electronic files), followed by coding (if applicable), data entry (if applicable), and computer editing. Regardless of whether the questionnaires or other data collection instruments are involved, quantification and coding of data elements are required either during or after data collection. For example, occupational data obtained from interviews need to be quantified using formatted coding, as do drug information, medical history, and many other types of data. Furthermore, coding should be restricted to judgmental tasks. For example, age at interview can be coded, but it can also be calculated analytically from the recorded date of birth and recorded date of interview. Allowing age to be calculated analytically, rather than by coding, will reduce errors in the data set (Rothman et al. 2008). Oftentimes, various ontologies for coding data are based on national standards.

1.1.1.4 Data Cleaning

Raw data should be inspected carefully for errors. Correction of such errors must be made whenever possible. Errors find their way into data in a variety of ways; some errors are detectable during entry or editing, for example, values out of range or misaligned with logic checks, and some are not, for example, transposed numbers in an age such as 45 for 54.

Checking the quality of the data involves scrutinizing each variable for impossible or unusual values. For example, gender may be coded 1 for male and 2 for female, in which case any other recorded value for gender will represent an error or an unknown value. Any inadmissible values should be examined against the source data forms. Unusual values such as unknown gender or unusual age should also be inspected. A good data entry program will provide for the detection of such values via logical checks and cross-checking against other data entry fields; for example, date of death cannot come before date of birth. The distribution of each variable in the database should also be examined both graphically and through descriptive statistics in order to detect unexpected observations and other anomalies. All data entry errors and their subsequent resolutions should be documented in a separate log file.

The distribution of each measurable variable in the database should also be examined both graphically and through descriptive statistics in order to detect unexpected observations and other anomalies. Sophisticated data entry software usually provides features for checking the consistency between variables and can flag potential errors, for example, dates and ages. The use of a redundant second question can also provide a good error checking device. However, even the most meticulous data collection efforts can suffer from errors that are undetectable during data cleaning. If quality checks for data are planned as a routine part of the data handling, such errors may not cause serious problems. However, lack of quality control processes may lead to data errors that will likely bias subsequent analyses. For more details, we refer the reader to Rothman et al. (2008).

Appropriate data preparation and thorough data cleansing are pieces of data accuracy. Measurements of data need to be precise and as consistent as possible; for example, different laboratory technicians or evaluators may measure a process differently, but should be within some degree of an acceptable range. Accuracy, commonly associated with systematic error (sometimes called statistical bias), refers to the extent of the closeness of an average of a statistical measure to its true population value; for example, systematically adding 1 pound to a series of weight measures by mistake would bias the average of all of the weights by 1 pound. Precision, usually related to random error due to a set of uncontrolled factors, refers to the degree to which repeated measurements under unchanged conditions show the same results, that is, reproducibility and repeatability (Taylor and Thompson 1998). If measurement error is anticipated in advance of the experiment, for example, processing differences between batches, oftentimes a good statistical design can overcome these challenges.

Both systematic error and random error contribute to measurement error (ME), which is common in many empirical studies (Fuller 2009). Measurement error may arise from assay or instrumental error, biological variation, or errors in questionnaire-based self-report data (Guo and Little 2011). Furthermore, measurements may be subject to limits of detection (LODs), especially in epidemiologic or health-related studies, where values of a process below certain detection thresholds are not measurable with any degree of accuracy. In these instances, partial information needs to be incorporated as part of the analysis (Schisterman and Little 2010). Ignoring the presence of ME or LOD effects in problematic data can result in biased estimates and invalid decision-making procedures (Perkins et al. 2011). In Chapter 15, we outline several statistical strategies to tackle measurement error and instrument limitation problems. We provide some statistical decision-making mechanisms that can account for these issues.

1.1.2 Statistical Hypotheses

There are many constraints and formalisms to deal with while constructing statistical hypothesis tests. An essential part of the test construction process is that statistical hypotheses should be clearly formulated with respect to the measurable objectives of the clinical study. Statistical hypotheses are not to be confused with the clinical hypotheses or specific aims of a research study. Note that there is a distinction between how statistical hypotheses and clinical hypotheses are formalized and evaluated. Commonly, statistical hypotheses and the corresponding clinical hypotheses are stated in different forms and orders.

In most clinical experiments, we are interested in tests regarding characteristics or distributions of one or more populations. In such cases, the statistical hypotheses must be very carefully formulated and clearly stated in terms of a feature of a population that can be measured, for example, the nature of associations between characteristics or distributions of populations. For example, suppose that the clinical hypothesis is that the population mean time for a wound to heal following antibiotic treatment is improved compared to the mean time for a wound to heal without antibiotic treatment. In this case, the corresponding main (null) statistical hypothesis is stated that the population mean time to heal for the antibiotic treatment group equals the mean time to heal for the nonantibiotic treatment group. This hypothesis is either rejected or not rejected. In this example, we will test for the treatment equivalence through the mean parameters corresponding to the two populations. One could also test whether the overall distributions for time to heal are equivalent.

The term *null hypothesis*, formally symbolized as H_0, is commonly used to define our primary statistical hypothesis. For example, when the clinical hypothesis is that a biomarker of oxidative stress has different circulating levels with respect to patients with and without atherosclerosis, a null hypothesis can be proposed corresponding to the assumption that levels of the biomarker in individuals with and without atherosclerosis are distributed equally. Note that the clinical hypothesis points out that we want to indicate the discriminating power of the biomarker, whereas H_0 says there are no significant associations between the disease and the respective biomarker levels. In general, the reason for this lies in the ability to formulate H_0 clearly and unambiguously. This in turn allows us to readily quantify and calculate the expected errors in decision making. Decisions about H_0 take the form "reject" or "do not reject." If the null hypothesis were formed in a similar manner to the clinical hypothesis, perhaps it would not be possible to unambiguously determine for which sort of links between the disease and biomarker levels we should test. There are exceptions and more complex statements within hypothesis test procedures, but the common testing problems are formulated as above. Roughly speaking, the Bayesian methodologies discussed later have the framework that there are many hypotheses, such that a probability distribution on the set of hypotheses may be generated as a function of the data, where more likely and least likely hypotheses may be inferred. Other variants of frequentist testing do include complex composite null hypotheses or sequential tests, but are outside the scope of this book.

The term *alternative hypothesis*, formally symbolized as H_1, is defined as all possibilities not contained in H_0 and factors into the statistical design of an experiment; for example, the treatment is effective at some level different from H_0. The alternative hypothesis aligns more with the clinical hypothesis; for example, a new treatment is effective. In several situations, assumptions regarding data distributions may be incorporated into statements of hypotheses or may be considered as circumstances in which the hypotheses are denoted. For example, observing biomarker levels, say X, one can define the following statements: (1) H_0: X has a distribution function F and the mean of X is 0 versus H_1: X is not distributed as F or the mean of X is not 0. (2) Assume a probability distribution function F fits a distribution of X and we are interested in testing for H_0: the mean of X is 0 versus H_1: the mean of X is not 0.

1.2 Errors Related to the Statistical Testing Mechanism

There are two types of errors that can be made in terms of statistical decision making within the hypothesis testing framework described above. One could state that H_0 is false when in fact it is true, a Type I error, or one could state that H_1 is false when in fact it is true, a Type II error. In order to provide a formal test procedure, as well as compare mathematical strategies for making decisions, algorithms for monitoring test characteristics associated with the probability to reject a correct hypothesis should be considered. The two probability quantities of interest, in terms of false decisions and statistical design considerations, are the Type I error and Type II error rates. In addition, we will discuss statistical power, which is a Type II error rate.

In practice, the Type I error rate (α) is strongly recommended by the statistician to be under control at some pre-defined level, for example, $\alpha = 0.05$. The Type I error rate is also referred to as the significance level of the test. A 0.05 Type I error rate implies theoretically that if the null hypothesis was true and we repeated the experiment an infinite number of times, 5% of the time we would falsely reject H_0. Whether a statistical test "maintains" the Type I error rate, either approximately or exactly, depends on how well the underlying assumptions of the statistical test at hand are maintained. In terms of a general construction, assume for clarity of explanation that L is the test statistic based on the observed data, C is a threshold, and the decision rule is to reject H_0 for large values of L, that is, when $L > C$; then, the threshold should be defined such that $\Pr(L > C|H_0) = \alpha$, where α is a presumed significance level, that is, the probability of committing a Type I error. (The probability of rejecting a hypothesis H, conditional when H is true, $\Pr(\text{reject } H|H)$, can also be notionally displayed as $\Pr_H(\text{reject } H)$.) This approach aids in clearly defining properties of statistical tests. For example, we can denote an unbiased statistical test when the probability of committing a Type I error is less than the significance level, $\Pr(\text{reject } H_0|H_0) \le \alpha$, and that of getting the power, $\Pr(\text{reject } H_0|H_0 \text{ is not true}) \le \alpha$.

We can also compare the efficiency of statistical tests having the same endpoint by fixing their respective Type I error rates at the same level and ordering them by their statistical power. When choosing between different statistical tests, which can achieve the same objectives, the goal is to choose the test that is unbiased and more powerful, that is, a test that is more efficient than its competitors given an underlying set of assumptions, where higher power implies greater efficiency. A test that is most powerful over all possible alternatives included in H_1 given a set of underlying assumptions is termed uniformly most powerful.

As noted above, classical statistical methodology is directed toward the use of decision-making mechanisms with fixed significant levels. Classic inference requires special and careful attention of practitioners relative to Type I error control since it can be defined by different functional forms. For example, we assume that uncertainties under the null hypotheses can be considered to be an unknown nuisance quantity, represented by θ. Then, for any presumed significance level, α, the Type I error control may take the following forms:

1. $\sup_\theta \Pr_{H_0}(\text{reject } H_0) = \alpha$

2. $\sup_\theta \lim_{n \to \infty} \Pr_{H_0}\left(\text{reject } H_0 \text{ based on observations} \{X_1,...,X_n\}\right) = \alpha$

3. $\lim_{n \to \infty} \sup_\theta \Pr_{H_0}\left(\text{reject } H_0 \text{ based on observations} \{X_1,...,X_n\}\right) = \alpha$

4. $\int \Pr_{H_0}\left(\text{reject } H_0\right) \pi(\theta) d\theta = \alpha$

where θ is an unknown nuisance parameter. Note that form 1 is the classical definition (e.g., Lehmann and Romano 2006). However, in some situations, it may occur that $\sup_\theta \Pr_{H_0}\left(\text{reject } H_0\right) = 1$. If this is the case, the Type I error is not controlled appropriately. In addition, the formal notation of the supremum is mathematically complicated in terms of derivations and calculations, either analytically or via Monte Carlo approximations (regarding Monte Carlo methods to control the Type I error rate, we refer the reader to Chapter 16 of this book). Form 2 is commonly applied when we deal with maximum likelihood ratio tests, as it related to Wilks's theorem (Wilks 1938). However, since form 2 is an asymptotical large sample consideration, the actual Type I error rate $\text{Pr}_{H_0}\left(\text{reject } H_0\right)$ cannot be close to the expected level α given small or moderate fixed sample sizes n. Form 3 is rarely applied in practice. Form 4 is also introduced in Lehmann and Romano (2006). This definition of the Type I error control depends on the choice of the function $\pi(\theta)$ in general.

The Type II error rate (β) is defined as $\beta = \text{Pr}(L < C | H_1)$ given that we assume that L is the test statistic based on the observed data, C is a threshold, and the decision rule is to reject H_0 when $L > C$. Type II errors may occur when the sample size is relatively small compared to the design objectives; that is, the signal-to-noise ratio is small or the test is biased (Freiman et al. 1978). Essentially, it is the dichotomization of the study results into the categories "significant" or "not significant" that leads to Type I and Type II errors. Although errors resulting from an incorrect classification of the study results would seem to be unnecessary and avoidable, the Neyman–Pearson (dichotomous) hypothesis testing approach is ingrained in scientific research due to the apparent objectivity and definitiveness of the pronouncement of significance (Rothman et al. 2008). The Type II error rate may be reduced by increasing the sample size. However, it is not practical to have large sample sizes in many settings. Hence, in statistical design there is a trade-off between error control and feasibility. In some scientific disciplines, hypothesis testing has been virtually eliminated in exchange for a confidence interval approach. However, like all scientific methods, the strengths and limitations of the methodology need to be understood well by the end user.

It is clear that in order to construct efficient statistical tests, we must formalize objectives of the experiments in terms of measurable quantities and make assumptions regarding the underlying stochastic and deterministic processes. A violation of the underlying statistical assumptions for a given test may lead to inflated Type I error rates or a reduction in power and an increased likelihood of an erroneous conclusion.

1.2.1 Rationality and Unbiasedness in Hypothesis Testing

In several hypothesis testing situations, the "optimality" or "reasonability" criterion of a testing procedure may vary according to the aims of clinical experiments.

In a classical hypothesis testing scheme, where a uniformly most powerful unbiased (UMPU) test exists, unbiasedness is a widely accepted property, because it merely requires that one be at least as likely to accept (reject) the null hypothesis under every situation in which the null hypothesis is correct (false) than under every situation for which it fails (holds). Thus, it is rational that when a UMPU size α test (the significance level is α) exists, it should always be used as the optimal testing procedure. Sackrowitz and Samuel-Cahn (1994) discussed in great detail the concepts of unbiasedness and what we shall call rationality as these terms relate to testing statistical hypotheses, especially regarding situations when one has incomplete data.

As an example, consider the observations X_1 and X_2, which are independently and exponentially distributed with parameters θ_i, $i = 1, 2$, where θ_i is the reciprocal of the expected value (see Section 1.5 for details). Now we focus on testing $H_0 : \theta_1 = \theta_2$ against $H_1 : \theta_1 < \theta_2$ or against $H_2 : \theta_1 \neq \theta_2$. Let $I\{\cdot\}$ denote the indicator function, where $I\{A\} = 1$ when event A is true and $I\{A\} = 0$ otherwise. It is well known that UMPU size α tests exist for both of the following test scenarios given by $\phi_1(X_1, X_2) = I\{X_2 \leq \alpha/(1 - \alpha)X_1\}$ and $\phi_2(X_1, X_2) = I\{X_2 < \gamma X_1 \text{ or } X_1 < \gamma X_2\}$, respectively, where $\gamma = \alpha/(2 - \alpha)$, such that we reject H_0 if $\phi_1 = 1$ (or $\phi_2 = 1$);

see Chapter 4 of Lehmann (1986) for more details. In this case, these tests would be well acceptable as optimal test procedures.

For incomplete data, Sackrowitz and Samuel-Cahn (1994) defined the notion of a "rationality criterion" to reflect a desirable character of a given statistical procedure. Let M denote a statistical procedure, which can accommodate censored data (partial information), and let R be an optimal or otherwise preferred procedure when complete or uncensored data are available. If the data were not censored, then R would be the procedure of choice. If M takes the same action as R whenever the action of R can be determined from the censored data, then M is a *rational* choice relative to R.

As an illustrative example of the rationality principle, suppose that based on two observations X_1 and X_2, the procedure R rejects the null hypothesis if and only if $X_1 + X_2 \geq 100$. Now suppose that the data are right-censored at 75 so we observe only $Y_i = \min(X_i, 75)$, $i = 1, 2$. In this case, a procedure M based on Y_1 and Y_2 that is rational relative to R must reject the null hypothesis if $X_1 + X_2 \geq Y_1 + Y_2 \geq 100$, for example, $Y_1 = 30$ and $Y_2 = .75$. Though X_2 is unknown, it can be inferred that the decision-making rule based on R would reject the null hypothesis. If instead $Y_1 = 20$ and $Y_2 = 75$ were observed, then it is uncertain whether or not $X_1 + X_2 \geq 100$. In this case, rationality implies nothing about the procedure M.

When adapting the rationality criterion to a UMPU test, it is possible that only in certain instances we can determine if a test is unbiased. An open question for further investigation is whether the rationality criterion or unbiasedness is more rational? We refer the reader to Berger and Wolpert (1988), Pratt (1961, 1962), and Sackrowitz and Samuel-Cahn (1994) for more detailed discussions of these important concepts.

1.3 *p*-Values

A majority of traditional testing procedures are designed to draw a conclusion (or make an action) with respect to the binary decision of rejecting or not rejecting H_0, depending on locations of the corresponding values of the observed test statistics, that is, detecting whether test statistics' values belong to a fixed sphere or interval. In simple cases, test procedures require us to compare corresponding test statistics values based on observed data with test thresholds. p-Values can serve as an alternative data-driven approach for testing statistical hypotheses based on using the observed values of test statistics as the thresholds in the theoretical probability of the Type I error. p-Values can themselves also serve as a summary type result in that they provide meaningful evidence about the null hypothesis.

As a continuous data-based measure of the compatibility between a hypothesis and data, a p-value is defined as the probability of obtaining a test statistic (a corresponding quantity computed as a function of the data, e.g., a *t*-statistic or sample median) at least as extreme as or close to the one that was actually observed, assuming that H_0 is true (Goodman 1999a). p-Values can be divided into two major types: one-sided (upper and lower) and two-sided. Assuming there are no biases in the data collection or the data analysis procedure, an upper one-sided p-value is the conditional on the data probability under the null hypothesis that the test statistic will be no less than the observed value. Similarly, a lower one-sided p-value is the probability under the null hypothesis that the test statistic will be no greater than the observed value. The two-sided p-value is defined as twice the smaller of the upper and lower p-values (Berger and Delampady 1987; Rothman et al. 2008).

If the p-value is small, it can be interpreted that the sample produced a very rare result under H_0; that is, the sample result is inconsistent with the null hypothesis as stated. On the other hand, a large p-value indicates the consistency of the sample result with the null hypothesis. At the pre-specified α significance level (Type I error rate), the decision is to reject H_0 when the p-value is less than or equal to α; otherwise, the decision is to not reject H_0. In addition to providing a decision-making mechanism, the p-value also sheds some data-based light on the strength of the evidence against H_0 (Berger and Delampady 1987). It should be emphasized that regardless of the size of the p-value, the decision is to either reject or not reject H_0 at a fixed Type I error rate; for example, we would not reject H_0 more or less strongly given the magnitude of the observed p-value.

In many situations, the probability of the null hypothesis being true given the observed data can be computed, but it will almost always be far from a two-sided p-value (Rothman et al. 2008). As noted above, p-values can be viewed as a random variable since they are a function of random data values. p-Values are uniformly distributed between 0 and 1 if the null hypothesis is true. For example, suppose that the test statistic L has a cumulative distribution function (CDF) F under H_0. Under a one-sided upper-tailed alternative H_1, the p-value is the random variable $1 - F(L)$, which is uniformly distributed under H_0 (Sackrowitz and Samuel-Cahn 1999).

Misinterpreting the magnitude of the p-value as strength for or against the null hypothesis or as a probability statement about the null hypothesis can lead to a misinterpretation of the results of a statistical test. Several common weaknesses or misinterpretations of the p-value are as follows: (1) employing the p-value as the probability that the null hypothesis is true can be wrong or even far from reasonable; the p-value strongly depends on current data in use; (2) the p-value is not very useful for large sample sizes, because almost no null hypothesis is exactly true when examined using real data, and when the sample size is relatively large, almost any null hypothesis will have a tiny p-value, leading to the rejection of the null at conventional significance levels; and (3) model selection is difficult; for example, simply choosing the wrong model among a class of models or using a model that is not robust to statistical assumptions will lead to an incorrect p-value or inflated Type I error rates.

Instead of having just two hypotheses to choose from, one may have several models under consideration; for example, in a regression model, when a collection of potential explanatory variables are available, several potential models may be under consideration. Classical hypothesis testing is often used as part of the model selection procedure, for example, forwards, backwards, and stepwise algorithms. Not only are the resulting significance levels suspect, but the methods for comparing nonnested models are not widely used. Alternatively, the Bayesian approach to hypothesis testing can be considered, which answers aforementioned complaints, at the cost of requiring a prior distribution on the parameter; that is, Bayesian methods are constructed such that one can consider the probability distribution of a set of hypotheses or parameters of interest. For more details, we refer the reader to Marden (2000).

Misinterpretations of p-values are common in clinical trials and epidemiology. For example, p-values are often erroneously displayed as the error probability for rejection of the hypothesis or, even worse, as the posterior probability that the null hypothesis is true. Sellke et al. (2001) investigated the fact that these interpretations can be completely misleading for testing precise hypotheses via simulations. The authors developed two methods of calibrating p-values so that they can be interpreted in a Bayesian or in a frequentist way. From the Bayesian perspective, the calibration of the p-value, p, is simply $B(p) = -ep\log(p)$, when $p < 1/e$, which is interpretable as a lower bound on the odds provided by the data (or Bayes factor', which will be introduced in Chapter 7) for H_0 to H_1. In terms of the frequentist significance level, α, the second method of calibration of the p-value p is $\alpha(p) = (1 + (-ep\log(p))^{-1})^{-1}$, which can be interpreted as either a (conditional) frequentist error probability or the posterior probability of the hypothesis. More details can be found in Sellke et al. (2001).

1.3.1 Expected p-Values

As noted above, p-values are random variables whose distributional forms depend on H_0 or H_1 being true. The stochastic characteristics of p-values are often ignored; for example, see the entries for p-values in the *Encyclopedia of Statistical Sciences* (Gibbons 1986) or Gibbons and Pratt (1975), as well as Deming (1943) and David (1998); however, these stochastic properties provide important information in their own right.

The pioneering work of Dempster and Schatzoff (1965), as well as Schatzoff (1966) and Sackrowitz and Samuel-Cahn (1999), investigated the great potential relative to the usefulness of understanding the stochastic aspect of p-values. They primarily concentrated on the expected p-value (EPV) under the alternative hypothesis. The EPV is also denoted as the expected significance level (see, e.g., Dempster and Schatzoff 1965).

In terms of examining the distributional properties of a p-value, let us start first with defining L to be the test statistic. Denote the distribution function of L as a function of θ under H_0 and under some specific alternative as given by $F_0(u) = \Pr(L < u | H_0)$ and $F_\theta(u) = \Pr(L < u | H_1$ given a quantity $\theta)$, respectively, where F_0 is assumed to be absolutely continuous. For example, F_0 and F_θ can correspond to the test of H_0 that the mean θ equals 0 against H_1 that the mean is θ (not 0).

Then the p-value is the random variable $X = 1 - F_0(L)$, uniformly distributed over the interval $[0, 1]$ under H_0. For a specified alternative θ (i.e., F_θ), the power at the significance level α based on L can be expressed as

$$\Pr_\theta(X \le \alpha) = 1 - F_\theta\left(F_0^{-1}(1-\alpha)\right), \quad 0 < \alpha < 1,$$

where $F_0^{-1}(\cdot)$ represents the inverse (quantile) function, such that $F_0\left(F_0^{-1}(\gamma)\right) = \gamma$ for $0 < \gamma < 1$. Accordingly, the expected value of X under the alternative θ, to be denoted EPV(θ), can be computed given the distribution $\Pr_\theta(X \le \alpha)$. In a simpler and more useful way for both direct evaluation and simulation, EPV(θ) can be expressed in the form

$$EPV(\theta) = \Pr(L^* \ge L),$$

where L^*, independent of L, is distributed according to $F_0(\cdot)$ and L is distributed as $F_\theta(\cdot)$. For more details about the computation and explanation of the EPV, we refer the reader to Sackrowitz and Samuel-Cahn (1999). As a practical example, we assume that $L^* \sim N\left(\mu_1, \sigma_1^2\right)$ and $L \sim N\left(\mu_2, \sigma_2^2\right)$. Then we have $EPV = \Pr\left(L - L^* \le 0\right) = \Phi\left((\mu_1 - \mu_2)/\left(\sigma_1^2 + \sigma_2^2\right)^{1/2}\right)$, where Φ is the cumulative standard normal distribution (regarding this parametric assumption, see Section 1.5 for details). Note that the formal notation $EPV(\theta) = \Pr(L^* \ge L)$ is similar to that introduced in Chapter 8. In this context, one can reconsider the expected p-value in terms of the area under a receiver operating curve (ROC). The reader can use the ROC curve methodology to develop new concepts regarding the EPV, including graphical visualizations.

For fixed Type I and Type II error rates, the EPV is almost constant over distributions and test statistics in the case where the test statistic has a limiting distribution that is normal (Sackrowitz and Samuel-Cahn 1999). The EPV has many utilities, including the following:

1. *A measure of the performance of a test:* In many testing situations, power functions are used to compare different test procedures. Such a practice may be problematic, due to (a) the dependence of power functions on the choice of the significance level and (b) the difficulty to obtain a specific fixed significance value without resorting to randomization when a test statistic is a discrete random variable, for example, Fisher's exact test. In such instances, comparison of test procedures can be conducted on equal footing by employing the EPV, where the matching of significance levels and randomization is not required.

2. *Understanding of the effectiveness of a chosen test:* When dealing with hypothesis testing, it is often neglected that a separate power function must be evaluated for each value of a significance level, even when a specified alternative is considered. On the contrary, the EPV depends on the alternative, but not the significance level. Therefore, for a particular alternative, the global effectiveness of a test can be judged by one value alone, the EPV for that given alternative. A smaller value of the EPV implies a more powerful test.

3. *Interpretation of obtained p-values:* Knowledge of EPVs provides an intuitive idea of which alternative the observed value is most representative of in terms of the underlying distribution, as a function of the parameter(s) of interest.

4. *Determination of the sample size:* Usually, the sample size determination requires the specification of the alternative hypothesis at a fixed point and a fixed significance level and power value. A study of the EPV for varying sample sizes for the same test of interest would be simpler and potentially more useful.

Sackrowitz and Samuel-Cahn (1999) discussed in detail the comparison of different tests for the equality of two distribution functions, including the Mann–Whitney–Wilcoxon two-sample test, the Kolmogorov–Smirnov test, and the corresponding t-test, for a variety of underlying distributions. The comparison is conducted by means of the EPV instead of the commonly used criteria of asymptotic relative efficiency (either Pitman or Bahadur; see Lehmann [1998] for details). The EPV allows for small- and medium-sized comparisons, while the asymptotic relative efficiency only speaks to the large sample behavior.

In conclusion, the EPV, which can be easily computed or simulated, provides a useful tool in judging the strength of a test for a specified alternative, enables comparisons of tests through a single number, and enhances the interpretation of the obtained p-value. For additional details, see, for example, Dempster and Schatzoff (1965), Schatzoff (1966), Hung et al. (1997), and Sackrowitz and Samuel-Cahn (1999).

1.4 Components for Constructing Test Procedures

In order to translate clinical hypotheses into a statistical decision-making procedure, a clinician needs to express clinical outcomes in terms of events that can be measured and collected in sample data, as well as define statistical hypotheses. Two additional pieces of information can be incorporated to develop or select an efficient statistical decision-making process. The first is a defined function that consists of the explicit, quantified gains and losses in reaching a conclusion, and their relative weights. Frequently, this function determines the loss that can be expected corresponding to each possible decision. This type of information can incorporate a loss function into the statistical decision-making process. For example, a treatment may be more effective, but it also may be more costly or have a worsened quality of life. These additional aspects can be modeled as part of the decision-making process.

The second source reflects prior information. Commonly, in order to derive prior information, researchers should consider past experiences in similar situations. The Bayesian methodology formally provides clear technique manuals on how to construct efficient statistical decision rules for various complex problems related to clinical experiments, employing prior information (Berger 1985; Vexler et al. 2014d). The use of prior information in the clinical setting is also a key part of frequentist methodology; for example, sample size determination and model building based on past experience are keys to good experimental design. In addition, weighted likelihoods may be incorporated as well in frequentist approaches based on prior information; however, within the frequentist context, this tends to inflate the Type I error rate if not done carefully. There are relative merits of both Bayesian and frequentist approaches, which go beyond the framework of this book. For a nice essay on the matter, see Bland and Altman (1998).

1.5 Parametric Approach and Modeling

A clinical statistician may use technical statements related to the observed data, while constructing or selecting the corresponding decision rules. Broadly speaking, these statements are termed assumptions regarding the distribution of data. The assumptions often correspond to a fit of the data distribution to a functional form that is completely known, or known up to a set of parameters, since complete knowledge of the data distribution will provide all the information investigators need for efficient application of a statistical technique.

Parametric modeling refers to a class of models to fit data distributions and deterministic components of a clinical study for which the distribution function and its related quantities can fully be defined as a mathematical function and a set of parameters (usually 1 to 5 in number). When these models are implemented, it is assumed that the observed data were sampled from the assumed model, which is a representation of some theoretical population. When parametric assumptions are close to reality, this type of modeling provides very simple, efficient, and powerful statistical tests. However, when the model assumptions are not met, the resulting tests will be biased and Type I error control will be compromised. In many scenarios, parametric assumptions are presumed and are very difficult to validate. For example, in the case when data consist of partial information due to the limit of detection of a measuring device, there can be not enough information to test goodness of fit. Oftentimes, statistical tests about assumptions are underpowered relative to the overall hypothesis testing goals of the study.

Common parametric distribution functions employed in clinical experiments include, but are not limited to, normal or Gaussian, lognormal, t, χ^2, gamma, F, binomial, uniform, Wishart, and Poisson distributions. In reality, there have been thousands of models that have been published, studied, and available for use via software packages.

As noted before, parametric distribution functions can be defined up to finite set of parameters (Lindsey 1996). For example, in the one-dimensional case, the normal (Gaussian) distribution has the notation $N(\mu, \sigma^2)$, which corresponds to density function defined as $f(x) = \left(\sigma\sqrt{2\pi}\right)^{-1}\exp\left(-(x-\mu)^2/(2\sigma^2)\right)$, where the parameters μ and σ^2 represent the mean and variance of the population and the value of x is over the entire real line. The shape of the density has been described famously as the bell-shaped curve. The values of the parameters μ and σ^2 may be assumed to be unknown. If the random variable X has a normal distribution, then $Y = \exp(X)$ has a lognormal distribution. Other examples include the gamma distribution, denoted Gamma(α, β), with shape parameter α and rate parameter β. The density function for the gamma distribution is given as $(\beta^\alpha/\Gamma(\alpha))x^{\alpha-1}\exp(-\beta x)$, $x > 0$. The exponential distribution, denoted $\exp(\lambda)$, has rate parameter λ with the corresponding density function given as $\lambda\exp(-\lambda x)$, $x > 0$. Note that the exponential distribution is a special case of the gamma distribution with $\alpha = 1$. It is often the case that simpler, well-known models are nested within more complex models with additional parameters. While the more complex models may fit the data better, there is a trade-off in terms of efficiency when a simpler model also fits the data well.

In order to plot these distributions as examples of the various shapes that might occur, we used the R (R Development Core Team 2014) statistical software package. R will be introduced at a beginning level in Chapter 2. The R code given below produced the plots of the density function of the standard normal distribution $N(0,1)$, as shown in Figure 1.1a; the density function of the Gamma(2,1) distribution, as shown in Figure 1.1b; and the density function of the exp(1) distribution, as shown in Figure 1.1c.

Note that oftentimes measurements related to biological processes follow a lognormal distribution (Koch 1966). For example, exponential growth is combined with further symmetrical variation: with a mean concentration of, say, 10^6 bacteria, one cell division more or less will result in 2×10^6 or 5×10^5 cells. Therefore, the range will be multiplied or divided by 2 around the mean; that is, the density is asymmetrical. Such skewed distributions of

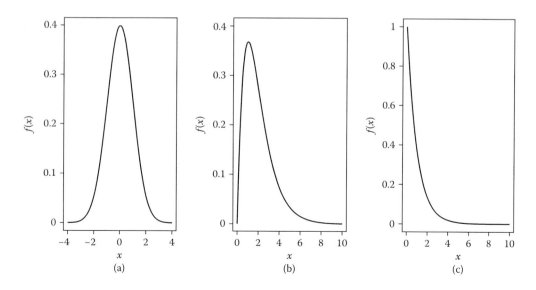

FIGURE 1.1
Density plots display the density functions of the (a) standard normal distribution, (b) Gamma(2,1) distribution, and (c) exp(1) distribution.

these types of biological processes have long been known to fit the lognormal distribution function (Powers 1936; Sinnot 1937). Skewed distributions that often closely fit the lognormal distribution are particularly common when mean values are low, variances are large, and values cannot be negative, as is the case, for instance, with species abundance and lengths of latent periods of infectious diseases (Balakrishnan et al. 1994; Lee and Wang 2013). Limpert et al. (2001) discussed various applications of lognormal distributions in different fields of science, including geology, human medicine, environment, atmospheric sciences, microbiology, plant physiology, and the social sciences.

1.5.1 Example of Pretest Procedures Pertaining to Model Assumptions

In hypothesis testing applications, oftentimes a preliminary test is necessary to validate the assumptions on a relevant nuisance parameter or the data distribution. To illustrate this issue, we consider the two-sample t-test for equality of the means in two normal samples (see Chapter 5 for the relevant material), in which the variances are assumed to be equal (Hoel 1984). Commonly, a preliminary F-test for testing equality of the variances in the two samples should be conducted, according to the main two sample t-test. In fact, the combined procedure is a two-step procedure, consisting of a preliminary F-test, followed by the t-test when the null hypothesis of equality of variances is accepted, and testing via, for example, Welch's t-test in the case of rejection. Such a combined procedure can be termed a pretest procedure. A pretest procedure consists of a preliminary test on a nuisance parameter, investigating whether it equals a given value or not, followed by the main testing problem on the parameter of interest.

Formally, let $X_1, ..., X_n$ be independent and identically distributed (i.i.d.) data points with density $f(x; \theta, \tau)$ with respect to some measure μ. Define the main testing problem as $H_0: \theta = \theta_0$ versus $H_1: \theta = \theta_1$. If the nuisance parameter is known, say $\tau = \tau_0$, we would like to test $\theta = \theta_0$ in the family $f(x; \theta, \tau_0)$. To see whether this information is useful, we perform a pretest of $\bar{H}_0: \tau = \tau_0$ against $\bar{H}_1: \tau \neq \tau_0$. This strategy leads to the following procedure: if H_0 is accepted, test H_0 in the restricted family $f(x; \theta, \tau_0)$; otherwise, test H_0 against H_1 in the complete family $f(x; \theta, \tau)$. This procedure is the pretest procedure. The idea is that practitioners prefer a simpler test as long as possible, due to the convenience of greater simplicity and the possibility of higher statistical power arising from the knowledge of the nuisance parameter.

In the special case of normal distributions, a χ^2 pretest and the Gaussian (or t) test are (almost) independent. However, in general, independence between the preliminary test and the main tests does not necessarily hold. For large values of correlations of the test statistic applied for the preliminary test and the main tests, the size (significance level) of the pretest procedure may greatly differ from the presumed level, leading to unacceptable and unavoidable violations of the underlying assumptions. Hence, pretest procedures are only of interest if the correlations of the test statistic applied for the preliminary test and the main tests are small.

In the analysis of pretest procedures, the correlation of the test statistic applied for the preliminary test and the main tests plays an important role. Let ρ denote this correlation. For an appropriate class of tests, containing all standard first-order optimal tests, Albers et al. (2000) derived an approximation for the differences in size and power between the pretest procedure and the one-stage test in the complete family using second-order asymptotic results. (See Section 1.7 for material related to large sample size evaluations.) The accuracy of the approximation is $O(\rho^3 + \rho n^{-1/2}) + o(n^{-1/2})$, where n is the sample size and the big O and small o notations correspond to boundedness and convergence rates, respectively.

This means that there exist a constant C and a sequence $\{a_n\}$ with $\lim_{n\to\infty} a_n = 0$ such that the error terms due to the approximations are bounded by $C(p^3 + pn^{-1/2}) + a_n n^{-1/2}$ for all p and n. Therefore, Albers et al.'s approximations are *uniformly* valid in p and n, but are only meaningful for $n \to \infty$ and $p \to 0$; for more details, we refer the reader to the paper of Albers et al. (1997).

1.6 Warning and Advice: Limitations of Parametric Approaches. Detour to Nonparametric Approaches

The statistical literature has widely addressed the issue that parametric methods are often very sensitive to moderate violations of their underlying assumptions, that is, nonrobust (Freedman 2009). Parametric assumptions can be tested in certain scenarios in order to reduce the risk of applying an ill-fitting parametric model (see, e.g., Section 1.5.1); however, these tests are oftentimes underpowered. Graphical methods are also useful in assessing parametric assumptions (e.g., see Chapter 3 for details). Note that in order to test for parametric assumptions, a goodness-of-fit test, introduced in Chapter 11, can be applied. In this case, statisticians can try to verify the assumptions, while making decisions with respect to main objectives of the clinical study. This leads to very complicated topics relative to multiple hypothesis testing (we refer the reader to see Chapter 14 for details). For example, it turns out that a computation of the expected risk of making a wrong decision strongly depends on the errors that can be made by not rejecting the parametric assumptions. The complexity of this problem can increase when researchers examine various functional forms to fit the data distribution relative to applying parametric methods. A substantial body of theoretical and experimental literature discusses the pitfalls of multiple testing in this aspect, placing blame squarely on the shoulders of the many clinical investigators who examine their data before deciding how to analyze them, or neglect to report the statistical tests that may not have supported their objectives (Austin et al. 2006). We give the corresponding aphorism of George Box: "Since all models are wrong the scientist cannot obtain a 'correct' one by excessive elaboration. On the contrary following William of Occam he should seek an economical description of natural phenomena. Just as the ability to devise simple but evocative models is the signature of a great scientist so overelaboration and overparameterization is often the mark of mediocrity" (Box 1976).

In the context of examining the robustness of given parametric models, one can present different examples, both hypothetical and actual, to get to the heart of these issues, especially as they pertain to parametric models used in the health-related sciences. Note also that in many situations, due to the wide variety and complex nature of problematic real data (e.g., incomplete data subject to instrumental limitations of studies), statistical parametric assumptions are hardly satisfied, and their relevant formal tests are complicated or not readily available (Vexler et al. 2015b).

Unfortunately, even clinical investigators trained in statistical methods do not always verify the corresponding parametric assumptions, or attend to probabilistic errors of the corresponding verification, when they use well-known elementary parametric statistical methods, for example, Student's t-tests. This is especially problematic with data coming from small samples. Thus, it is known that when the key assumptions are not met, the parametric approach may be extremely biased and inefficient when compared to its robust *nonparametric* counterparts.

Nonparametric methods, broadly defined, make use of the empirical distribution function defined as $\hat{F}(x) = \sum_{i=1}^{n} I(X_i \leq x)/n$, where $I(\cdot)$ denotes the indicator function, to model the data. Rank-based methods are a special class of nonparametric methods. The key idea is that the empirical distribution function converges to the true population distribution function in the limit. The empirical distribution function can be defined under both the null and the alternative hypothesis such that accurate, robust, and efficient inferential procedures can be constructed. Statistical inference under the nonparametric regime offers decision-making procedures, avoiding or minimizing the use of the assumptions regarding functional forms of the data distributions.

In general, the balance between parametric and nonparametric approaches boils down to expected efficiency versus robustness to assumptions. One very important issue is preserving the efficiency of statistical techniques through the use of robust nonparametric likelihood methods, minimizing required assumptions about data distributions (Gibbons and Chakraborti 2010; Wilcox 2012).

1.7 Large Sample Approximate Tests

The development of the statistical decision-making theory has historically been supported by extensive use of the mathematical asymptotic arguments. Asymptotic analysis is shown to be beneficial in testing statistical hypotheses when the exact distributions of test statistics are unavailable or very complicated to be computed. Prior to the advent of high-performance computing and statistical software, many statistical tests were based on large sample approximations and tables of normal and χ^2-distributed variables. Many of these so-called large sample tests are still quite commonly employed in statistical software today.

Fundamental to a majority of these tests is the fact that averages of various forms tend to have an approximate normal distribution regardless of the parametric distribution from which the data were sampled. This is the basic tenet of the various formal central limit theorems in that, as the sample size grows, the approximate distribution of a test statistic constructed as an average or sum should get closer and closer to normal. Similarly, quadratic functions of averages tend to have approximate χ^2-distributions. Examples of such tests are using a normal approximation to model a sample proportion (which is an average of 0's and 1's) and the large sample distribution of the sample correlation coefficient (which is a function of sums). These tests provide approximate and biased Type I error control that improves for larger and larger sample sizes. The pitfalls of such tests are that when they are used in small finite sample settings, they may have substantial bias. Statistical software packages that utilize such tests do not warn the end user of such issues. We refer the reader to Reid (2003) for more details regarding asymptotic arguments applied into statistical inference.

1.8 Confidence Intervals

An alternative approach to inference that has a one-to-one mapping to hypothesis testing about a parameter, set of parameters, or functions is the generation of confidence intervals or regions. For a single parameter, for example, the population mean, one can construct a confidence interval based on manipulating the probability statement that a parameter lies between a lower and an upper bound, which are functions of the data. In many instances, the concept of a pivot can be used to manipulate the terms of the probability statement in order to obtain a confidence interval. Confidence intervals can be based on both parametric and nonparametric approaches, as well as large sample approximations. A two-sided $1 - \alpha$-level confidence interval for a single parameter, which consists of a lower and a upper bound, is not the probability that the parameter lies within the lower and upper bounds. The frequentist interpretation is that if an experiment was repeated many times, the true population parameter would lie within the lower and upper bounds $100 \times (1 - \alpha)$ percent of the time. In terms of confidence intervals and their relationship to hypothesis tests, we would reject H_0 for a two-sided test if the parameter under H_0 fell outside the confidence interval bounds. A parallel development in Bayesian methodologies is the highest posterior density region, where one defines the probability of a parameter (considered random in this framework) being within an interval.

Two recent references in which core material, in the tradition of statistical confidence interval inference stemming from R. A. Fisher and J. Neman, were presented in detail are Schweder and Hjort (2002) and Singh et al. (2005).

1.9 When All Else Fails: Bootstrap?

The bootstrap statistical method, as popularized by Efron (1979), is a powerful tool that can oftentimes be misapplied and misunderstood due to the relative simplicity and power of its Monte Carlo–based resampling approximations. It is of key importance that data analysts who apply bootstrap resampling methodologies have a clear understanding of the actual parameter of interest and the corresponding estimator. For "well-behaved" and "smooth" statistics, bootstrap methods tend to perform well. An example of a smooth statistic would be the arithmetic mean. An example of a nonsmooth statistic would be the sample median. However, even in the well-behaved cases, there may be poor performance in terms of inferential properties as a function of small sample sizes. When applied properly, bootstrap methodologies provide nonparametric, semiparametric, and parametric solutions to problems that are otherwise intractable and provide robust and powerful alternatives to problems where standard approaches rely heavily on parametric assumptions. The focus in this book is on nonparametric methods. Generally, bootstrap methods are utilized to estimate standard errors of a statistic and to generate confidence intervals in a nonparametric fashion. We also discuss bootstrap hypothesis testing in Chapter 17 as it relates to permutation testing. It should be noted that the bootstrap methodology literature spans several decades and is ever expanding. Our focus within this section is on the basic principles toward applying the bootstrap method.

1.9.1 Statistical Functional Is the Parameter of Interest

When applying bootstrap resampling methodologies, it is of vital importance to link a statistic to the parameter of interest, say θ. It is irresponsible from a scientific and inferential point of view to apply bootstrap methodologies starting only with the observed statistic without knowing what the statistic is estimating. This is oftentimes the biggest mistake practitioners make: not understanding what the procedure is actually estimating. In the context of using bootstrap methods, the parameter of interest takes the form $\theta = T(F)$, where $T(F)$ is what is termed a *statistical functional* and $F(\cdot)$ is the cumulative distribution function assumed to be absolutely continuous. Departures from these assumptions are valid in certain settings, but require a more specific understanding of the problem. If we have an i.i.d. sample of size n, given as $x_1, \ldots, x_n$ from F, then the corresponding estimator of $\theta = T(F)$ is given as $\hat{\theta} = T(\hat{F})$, where $\hat{F}(x) = \sum_{i=1}^{n} I(x_i \le x)/n$ is the empirical distribution function and $I(\cdot)$ denotes the indicator function. In this setting, $\hat{\theta} = T(\hat{F})$ would be the non-parametric estimator of $\theta = T(F)$. It should be noted that for many statistics, $(\hat{\theta}) = \theta + o(n^{-1})$, where the small o notation is a technical device to quantify how fast the statistic converges to the true value ($o(n^{-1})n \to 0$ as $o(n^{-1})n \to 0$), in this case as a function of the sample size n. Hence, greater care needs to be taken when using bootstrap settings for small samples relative to larger samples when interpreting results due to a finite sample bias. Below are some common examples of statistical functionals and their corresponding estimators.

Example 1.1: The Mean

In this case, $\theta = T(F) = \int x \, dF$. Efron uses the term *plugging in $\hat{F}$ for F* in order to obtain the statistic, which in this case is given as $\hat{\theta} = T(\hat{F}) = \sum_{i=1}^{n} x_i/n = \bar{x}$, that is, the sample mean. The result follows by noting that $\hat{F}$ is constant in the interval $[x_{(i)}, x_{(i+1)}]$, where $x_{(i)}$ denotes the ith order statistic. The sample average then follows from the integration of $\int x \, d\hat{F}$. It should be noted that the bootstrap estimator of the standard deviation of the mean is essentially the sample standard error. Hence, Monte Carlo methods are not required.

Example 1.2: Median and Quantiles

The classic introductory textbook estimator of the median $F^{-1}(1/2)$ is given as $\hat{\theta} = T(\hat{F}) = x(m)$, where $m = (n+1)/2$ for an odd sample size, and $\hat{\theta} = T(\hat{F}) = (x_{(m)} + x_{(m+1)})/2$, where $m = n/2$ for an even sample size. In terms of a statistical functional formulation, $T(F) = \min_{\theta} \int |x - \theta| \, dF$. Technically speaking, there is not a unique solution for $T(F)$ given an even sample size: any solution in the interval $[x_{(m)}, x_{(m+1)}]$ satisfies the mini-mization criteria above for even sample sizes. More generally, the statistical func-tional corresponding to the uth quantile, $0 < u < 1$, is given as $T(F) = \min_{\theta} \int |x - \theta| + (2u - 1)(x - \theta)df$, with the estimator given by the value of θ that satisfies $T(\hat{F}) = \min_{\theta} \sum_{i=1}^{n} \frac{\{|x_i - \theta| + (2u-1)(x_i - \theta)\}}{n} = \min_{\theta} \sum_{i=1}^{n} |x_i - \theta| + (2u-1)(x_i - \theta)$. The boot-strap standard deviations of these statistics can also be calculated directly without Monte Carlo resampling; for example, see Hutson and Ernst (2000).

In more complex multidimensional cases, the same ideas above may be extended via substituting in the p-dimensional empirical distribution function estimator for the p-dimensional cumulative distribution function in the statistical functional of interest. In the p = two-dimensional case, with i.i.d. samples of size n given as $(x_1, y_1), (x_2, y_2), \ldots, (x_n, y_n)$ the empirical distribution function has the form $\hat{F}(x, y) = \sum_{i=1}^{n} I(x_i \le x, y_i \le y)/n$.

Parametric and semiparametric bootstrap approaches have the same underlying features as the nonparametric approach described above. The difference now is that the choice of $\hat{F}$ applied to $\hat{\theta} = T(\hat{F})$ may be a semiparametric or fully parametric estimator of F; for example, we could use a cumulative distribution function assuming normality with the classic maximum likelihood estimators for location and scale employed.

1.9.2 Bootstrap Confidence Intervals

Historically, bootstrap methodology has been used primarily as a way to generate confidence intervals for the parameter given as the statistical functional $\theta = T(F)$. The most well-known and straightforward approach is the percentile interval method. As a rule of thumb, the percentile method will always have good large sample statistical properties; given $\hat{\theta} = T(\hat{F})$ may be shown to be asymptotically normal with variance that shrinks as a function of n and $E(\hat{\theta}) = \theta + o(n^{-1})$. Most statistics that are in the form of a weighted average meet these criteria. Examples of statistics that do not fall into this category given support over the real line are the minimum $x_{(1)}$ and maximum $x_{(n)}$ order statistics. In the scenario of using the minimum or maximum statistic in bootstrap procedures, one needs to take care in understanding the given statistical functional of interest in terms of what is being estimated and any potential pitfalls. More complex methods, such as the bootstrap-t and bias-corrected accelerated methods, were developed to improve the coverage probabilities in small samples. With the exception of a few special cases, such as a simple quantile function estimator, calculating confidence intervals for most statistical functionals requires Monte Carlo resampling approximations.

The basic bootstrap confidence interval was developed using classic *pivotal* methods. When constructing a confidence interval, it is desired to have a statistic whose distribution is free of the parameter of interest, which in this case our parameter of interest is $\theta = T(F)$. The goal of confidence interval estimation in general is to find upper and lower values as a function of the data such that $\Pr(\theta_L(x) < \theta < \theta_U(x)) = 1 - \alpha$, where α denotes the Type I error. For example, the classic interval for the population mean given normality yields $\theta_L(x) = \bar{x} - z_{1-\frac{\alpha}{2}} \frac{s}{\sqrt{n}}$ and $\theta_U(x) = \bar{x} - z_{\frac{\alpha}{2}} \frac{s}{\sqrt{n}}$, where z_α is the αth percentile of a standard normal distribution. Using bootstrap resampling, we can approximate these pivotal quantities in a nonparametric fashion.

If we have B bootstrap replicates of the statistic via resampling and given as $T(\hat{F}_1^*), T(\hat{F}_2^*), ..., T(\hat{F}_B^*)$ this provides an empirical approximation to the true distribution of $\hat{\theta} = T(\hat{F})$. If we center the observations as $(\hat{F}_1^*) - T(\hat{F}), (\hat{F}_2^*) - T(\hat{F}), ..., (\hat{F}_B^*) - T(\hat{F})$, it is assumed that these centered observations approximate a distribution that is parameter-free, that is, a pivot about a location parameter. A key assumption under this formulation is that the variance and other aspects of the centered distribution are also parameter-free. This assumption can also be examined and corrected approximately using bootstrap variance stabilization techniques described later in the book. An example where this assumption is not met is in the case of the Pearson correlation coefficient used as an estimator of the population correlation.

Now assuming that the centered observations represent a parameter-free distribution, we can utilize the percentile points of this bootstrap distribution to obtain an approximate pivotal quantity and construct an approximate bootstrap confidence interval. We start with the classic representation for a $1 - \alpha$-level confidence interval, which has the form $1-\alpha = \Pr\left(a < T\left(\hat{F}\right) - T(F) < b\right)$, and this interval can be approximated by $\Pr\left(a < T\left(\hat{F}^*\right) - T\left(\hat{F}\right) < b\right)$. This yields $\Pr\left(T\left(\hat{F}^*\right) - b < T\left(\hat{F}\right) < T\left(\hat{F}^*\right) - a\right)$, where technically a and b can be any two quantiles of the distribution of $T\left(\hat{F}_1^*\right) - T\left(\hat{F}\right)$, $T\left(\hat{F}_2^*\right) - T\left(\hat{F}\right)$, ..., $T\left(\hat{F}_B^*\right) - T\left(\hat{F}\right)$ such that $a < b$ and $1-\alpha = \Pr\left(a < T\left(\hat{F}^*\right) - T\left(\hat{F}\right) < b\right)$. Practically speaking, we can utilize a to be the lower $\alpha/2$th quantile and b to be the upper $1-\alpha/2$th quantile of the distribution of the centered resampled values $\left(\hat{F}_1^*\right) - T\left(\hat{F}\right)$, $T\left(\hat{F}_2^*\right) - T\left(\hat{F}\right)$, ..., $T\left(\hat{F}_B^*\right) - T\left(\hat{F}\right)$. Using these two quantile estimates, there is a general assumption that this approach will provide the shortest-length confidence interval, at least asymptotically, for statistics that have large sample normal approximation. Let us denote the uth quantile of the noncentered resampled values $T\left(\hat{F}_1^*\right)$, $T\left(\hat{F}_2^*\right)$, ..., $T\left(\hat{F}_B^*\right)$ as z_u^*. Then the $1-\alpha$-level approximate bootstrap-level confidence interval is given as $\left(T\left(\hat{F}\right) - \left(z_{1-\frac{\alpha}{2}}^* - T\left(\hat{F}\right)\right), T\left(\hat{F}\right) - \left(z_{\frac{\alpha}{2}}^* - T\left(\hat{F}\right)\right)\right)$.

Similar to classic normal-based confidence interval estimation under an assumption of symmetry, this process can be simplified to the interval given as $\left(z_{\frac{\alpha}{2}}^*, z_{1-\frac{\alpha}{2}}^*\right)$. This interval is termed the *bootstrap percentile interval* and is likely the most utilized bootstrap confidence interval by practitioners. For moderate to large samples, this approach is very reasonable. Theoretically, $\Pr\left(z_{\frac{\alpha}{2}}^* < T(F) < z_{1-\frac{\alpha}{2}}^*\right) = 1-\alpha + O\left(n^{-1/2}\right)$ (e.g., see Carpenter and Bithell 2000). Specific examples of more complex procedures with more accurate finite sample coverage probabilities are provided in later sections of this book.

1.10 Permutation Testing versus Bootstrap Methodology

We outline permutation theory, also referred to as rerandomization tests, in Chapter 17. The general perception in practice is that permutation methods are for testing hypotheses and generating p-values, while bootstrap methods are related to confidence interval estimation. While it is true that this is how these procedures are used the majority of the time, in practice it is not an absolute given; that is, bootstrap methods can be used to test hypotheses, and permutation tests can be used to generate confidence intervals. Each methodology has its own sets of assumptions. Using permutation methods to generate confidence intervals and bootstrap methods to test hypotheses is oftentimes much more computationally intensive than their more popular uses. Hence, it is important to know when it is better to use one approach over the other either for testing or confidence interval generation. Heuristically, one can think of permutation methods as using a sampling without replacement approach, while bootstrap methods utilize a sampling with replacement approach.

When interest is in a single parameter $\theta = T(F)$, in terms of either a hypothesis test or generating a confidence interval, there are permutation and bootstrap approaches available for both inferential approaches. In general terms and in a univariate setting, a permutation test requires very strong assumptions compared to bootstrap methods regarding the underlying distribution, if, for example, testing H_0: $\theta = \theta_0$ about a location parameter is of interest.

However, if the permutation test assumptions are met, the test is considered *exact* in terms of maintaining the desired Type I error control. If the permutation test assumptions are not met, there can be an inflation of the Type I error rate in certain scenarios, that is, an increased likelihood of a false positive result. For both the permutation and bootstrap methods, the key idea is to approximate the null distribution of the test statistic $\hat{\theta} = T(\hat{F})$ given $H_0: \theta = \theta_0$ is true. In order for the permutation test to control the Type I error correctly in this simple case, the key assumption is symmetry of the underlying distribution about $\theta = \theta_0$. Under a symmetry assumption of the null distribution of the test statistic, we can additionally carry out a two-sided test.

In general, most test statistics have symmetric distributions, particularly for large sample sizes. Classic tests in the one-sample setting are the permutation one-sample *t*-test, the sign test, and Wilcoxon's sign rank test. In terms of a confidence interval, one can invert the permutation-based hypothesis test by varying the values of θ_0 and numerically finding the values for which the permutation p-value is equal to the desired lower and upper percentiles relative to the confidence level of interest; for example, p-values of 0.025 and 0.975 would provide upper and lower bounds for a 95% confidence interval for θ. The inversion-based permutation interval is exact as well under the symmetry assumption. In permutation parlance, the observed values $x_i - \theta_0$, $i = 1, 2, \ldots, n$, are *exchangeable* with respect to the $\pm$ sign under $H_0: \theta = \theta_0$.

Bootstrap confidence intervals and hypothesis tests in general provide p-values with approximate Type I error control and confidence intervals with approximate coverage probabilities such that the accuracy of the approximations improves with an increase in sample size. The trade-off with permutation tests is that the major assumption in the i.i.d. nonparametric setting is $\hat{\theta} = T(\hat{F}) \to \theta = T(F)$ for large sample sizes. In terms of hypothesis testing, in this simple univariate setting one can simply assume a location-shift model relative to the most basic bootstrap approaches or use more complex bootstrap tilting methods (e.g., Davison and Hinkley 1997). These methods and their relative accuracies are described in more detail in Chapter 17. In general, for small samples exact methods are available for permutation tests, while in general the bootstrap method requires Monte Carlo approximations. For large samples, both methods rely on Monte Carlo methods relative to being computationally feasible.

In the two-sample independent group setting there is not much that changes with respect to the nonparametric bootstrap methodology compared to the univariate setting as above. In terms of the permutation setting, the assumptions are slightly relaxed compared to the univariate case. Now say we have the following $X \sim F$ and $Y \sim G$ such that the parameters of interest are $\theta = T(F)$ and $\tau = T(G)$. Now suppose we are interested in testing $H_0: \theta = \tau$. In order for a permutation test to have exact Type I error control (exact meaning bounded), an exchangeability assumption has to hold as before under the null hypothesis. In this case, exchangeability implies $F(t) = G(t)$, $\forall t$ under H_0 being true. Inversion of the hypothesis test can be done under a shift alternative assumption; for example, test $H_0: \theta = \tau + \delta$ across various values of δ and given a one-sided alternative (e.g., p-values of 0.025 and 0.975) would provide upper and lower bounds for a 95% confidence interval for $\theta - \tau$ as a function of δ. If exchangeability assumptions hold, the best approach would be to use a permutation test. If the exchangeability assumption may not hold, then calculation bootstrap confidence intervals for $\theta - \tau$ would be the recommended approach, or alternatively, one could use more complex bootstrap tilting methods.

In the paired data setting, $(X, Y) \sim F_{xy}$, tests about location generally reduce to the one-sample setting described above, for example, a paired *t*-test. However, if the association between X and Y is of interest, for example, correlation, again, bootstrap and permutation methods may be considered. Speaking in general terms, permutation tests are most readily utilized to test whether there is any association between X and Y, for example, testing H_0: $\rho(X,Y) = 0$, where $\rho(X,Y)$ denotes the correlation between X and Y. In general, permutation tests of the form H_0: $\rho(X,Y) = \rho_0$ ($\neq 0$) are not easily carried out using a permutation test due to the lack of an exchangeability mechanism under H_0. In the case H_0: $\rho(X,Y) - 0$, exchangeability implies $F_{xy} = F_x F_y$. Examples of procedures of this type are given in Chapter 17. For the bootstrap methodology, focus in these settings is mainly on confidence interval generation with the assumption that the bivariate functional $\hat{\rho} = T\left(\hat{F}_{xy}\right) \to \rho = T\left(F_{xy}\right)$.

1.11 Remarks

The primary objective of this book is to provide a compendium of wide fields of statistical testing techniques, from classical methods to newly advanced empirical likelihood techniques, as well as nonparametric bootstrap and semiparametric permutation methodologies, applied to various problems encountered in the medical and epidemiological studies. Theoretical aspects of various decision-making procedures based on these approaches will be presented throughout the book. We will provide the corresponding statistical R and SAS software codes. Note that we focus on the straightforward and useful application of the theoretically derived aspects of statistical decision-making mechanisms as they pertain to statistical practice. We represent accurate R and SAS programming, which in some sense may not be perfectly optimal but is always functional. The readers can improve upon our coding methods as interested.

Furthermore, the intent of the book is not to cover every statistical testing scenario and strategy. For example, we do not include tests based on survival data. In this instance, we refer the reader to Klein and Moeschberger (2003), as well as Kleinbaum and Klein (2005), for methods and techniques involved in different aspects of survival analysis.

Due to the page limitation and the dynamic nature of statistical theory development, we cannot cover all relevant issues pertaining to decision-making mechanisms given problematic data. For example, we do not consider the topic of misclassification in multinomial cell entries in a contingency table, which may lead to problems of identifiability categorized into two types: (1) the permutation-type nonidentifiabilities that may be handled with constraints that are suggested by the structure of the problem and (2) the identifiability that can be addressed with informative prior information via Dirichlet distributions. We refer the reader to Swartz et al. (2004) for details.

In this book, we aim to display a rigorous and systematic presentation of selected important classical and novel parametric and nonparametric approaches. We emphasize their practical applications, providing practitioners with a road map for correctly and efficiently using the presented classical and novel statistical tools. Theoretical statisticians may also find new focus areas for their research stemming from the material presented in this book.

In addition to what we present, a never-ending wealth of additional applied and theoretical materials related to statistical decision-making procedures may be found in a variety of scientific publications, for example, Rothman et al. (2008), Gibbons and Chakraborti (2010), Sackrowitz and Samuel-Cahn (1999), Freedman (2009), Wilcox (2012), Lehmann and Romano (2006), and Riffenburgh (2012).

1.12 Atlas of the Book

This book is organized as follows: In Chapter 2, the R and SAS statistical software packages are outlined at a beginning level. Chapter 3 introduces simple and efficient statistical procedures to analyze data in a graphical manner. The parametric likelihood methodology is described in Chapter 4. In Chapter 5, we show different tests for means of continuous data and review the exact likelihood ratio test for equality of two normal populations. Chapter 6 focuses on distribution function– and density function–based empirical likelihood methodology. Chapter 7 presents principles for developing and analyzing Bayesian-type decision-making policies. In Chapter 8, we introduce common strategies based on the receiver operating characteristic (ROC) curves used in biomedical and epidemiological researches to make statistical decisions (e.g., Pepe 2003; Vexler et al. 2008b). In Chapter 9, we review distribution-free tests for comparing data distributions, including the classical Wilcoxon two-sample test, a nonparametric analogy to the two-sample *t*-test, as well as new statistical test algorithms. Different well-known and new measures and tests for independence are shown in Chapter 10. In this chapter, we propose novel concepts to visualize and measure dependency. Goodness-of-fit tests are reviewed in Chapter 11 to show several methods regarding how to decide that assumed distributions are appropriate for modeling observed data. Various change-point detection problems, their definitions, and applications of corresponding change-point detection policies are considered in Chapter 12. Chapter 13 shows basic concepts of sequential principles for designing experiments based on data with unfixed sample sizes. Chapter 14 outlines multiple testing problems and their solutions in clinical experiments. Statistical procedures based on problematic data are presented in Chapter 15. Chapter 16 depicts several methods for calculating critical values of statistical tests. Chapter 17 covers the fundamentals of bootstrap and permutation testing.

All chapters are supported with supplemental materials that present classical and modern results published in journals and books that are highly recognized in science.

2

Statistical Software: R and SAS

2.1 Introduction

In this chapter, we outline the elementary components of the R (R Development Core Team 2014) and SAS (Delwiche and Slaughter 2012) statistical software packages. Both packages allow the user to implement powerful built-in routines or employ programming features for customization. For example, Desquilbet and Mariotti (2010) presented the use of a SAS macro (customized SAS code) using the third National Health and Nutrition Examination Survey data to investigate adjusted dose–response associations (with different models) between calcium intake and bone mineral density (linear regression), folate intake and hyperhomocysteinemia (logistic regression), and serum high-density lipoprotein cholesterol and cardiovascular mortality (Cox model). Similarly, Wason and Seaman (2013) illustrated the use of R to fit a linear model of the mean logarithm of the tumor shrinkage using generalized least squares based on baseline tumor size and the time of the observation. Examples of R and SAS programs are employed throughout the book.

2.2 R Software

R is an open-source, case-sensitive, command line–driven software for statistical computing and graphics. The R program can be installed using the directions found at www.r-project.org.

Once R has been loaded, the main input window appears, showing a short introductory message (Gardener 2012). There may be slight differences in appearance depending on the operating system. For example, Figure 2.1 shows the main input window in the Windows operating system, which has menu options available at the top of the page. Below the header is a screen prompt symbol > in the left-hand margin indicating the command line.

2.2.1 Rules for Names of Variables and R Data Sets

A syntactically valid R name consists of letters, numbers, and the dot or underline characters and starts with either a letter or the dot not followed by a number. Reserved words are not syntactic names.

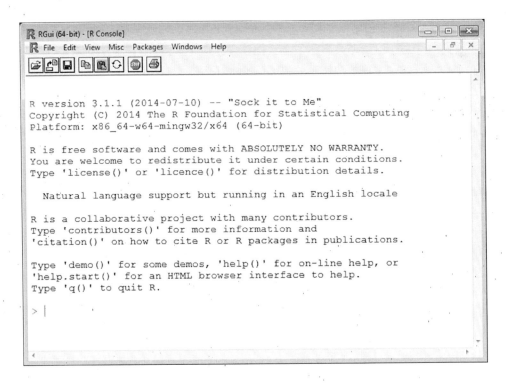

FIGURE 2.1
Main input window of R in Windows.

2.2.2 Comments in R

Comments can be inserted starting with a pound (#) throughout the R code without disrupting the program flow.

2.2.3 Inputting Data in R

R operates on named data structures. The simplest form is the numeric vector, which is a single entity consisting of an ordered collection of numbers. One way to input data is through the use of the function c(), which takes an arbitrary number of vector arguments and whose value is a vector obtained by concatenating its arguments end to end. For example, to set up a vector *x*, consisting of four numbers, namely, 3, 5, 10, and 7, the assignment can be done with

```
> x<-c(3,5,10,7)
```

Notice that the assignment operator (<–), which consists of the two characters less than (<) and minus (–) occurring strictly side by side, "points" to the object receiving the value of the expression. In most contexts, the equal operator (=) can be used as an alternative.

In order to display the value of *x*, we simply type in its name after the prompt symbol > and press the Return key

```
> x
```

As a result, R provides the following output:

```
[1]  3  5  10  7
```

Assignment can also be made using the function `assign()`. An equivalent way of making the same assignment as above is with

```
> assign("x", c(3,5,10,7))
```

The usual assignment operator (<–) can be thought of as a syntactic shortcut to this.

In some cases, the elements of a vector may not be completely known and the vector is *incomplete*. When an element or value is "not available" or a "missing value" in the statistical sense, a place within a vector may be reserved for it by assigning it the special value NA. In general, without further suboption specification, any operation on an NA becomes an NA.

Note that there is a second kind of missing value, which is produced by numerical computation, the so-called Not a Number (NaN) value. The following examples give NaN since the result cannot be defined sensibly:

```
> 0/0
> Inf - Inf
```

The function `is.na(x)` gives a logical vector of the same size as x with value TRUE if and only if the corresponding element in x is NA or NaN. The function `is.nan(x)` is only TRUE when the corresponding element in x is NaNs.

Missing values are sometimes printed as <NA> when character vectors are printed without quotes.

2.2.4 Manipulating Data in R

In R, vectors can be used in arithmetic expressions, in which case the operations are performed element by element. The elementary arithmetic operators are the usual: + (addition), – (subtraction), * (multiplication), / (division), and ^ (exponentiation). The following example illustrates the assignment of y, which equals $x^2 + 3$:

```
> y <- x^2 + 3
```

R can be programmed to perform simple statistical calculations as well as complex computations. Table 2.1 shows some simple commands that produce descriptive statistics of a vector x given a sample of measurements $x_1, \ldots, x_n$. The setting `na.rm = FALSE` is set to indicate a missing statistic value is returned if there are missing values in the data vector.

TABLE 2.1

Selected R Commands That Produce the Descriptive Statistics of a Numerical Vector x

Syntax	Definition
mean(x, na.rm = FALSE)	Gives the arithmetic mean
sd(x, na.rm = FALSE)	Gives the standard deviation
var(x, na.rm = FALSE)	Gives the variance
sum(x, na.rm = FALSE)	Gives the sum of the vector elements

Instead of using the built-in functions contained in R, such as those shown in Table 2.1, customized functions can be created to carry out additional specific tasks. For this purpose, the function() command can be used. The following example shows a simple function mymean that determines the running mean of the first i, $i = 1, \ldots, n$ elements of a vector x, where n is the number of elements in x. Results are shown for x, our toy data set from above, by applying the customized function mymean.

```
> # to define the function
> mymean <- function(x) {
+       tmp <- c()
+       for(i in 1:length(x)) tmp[i] < - mean(x[1:i])
+       return(tmp)
+ }
> # execute the function using the data defined above
> mymean(x)
[1] 3.00 4.00 6.00 6.25
```

Note that the symbol plus (+) is shown at the left-hand side of the screen instead of the symbol greater than (>) to indicate the function commands are being input. The built-in R functions length, return, and mean are used within the new function mymean. For more details about R functions and data structures, we refer the reader to Crawley (2012).

In addition to vectors, R allows manipulation of *logical* quantities. The elements of a logical vector can be values TRUE (abbreviated as T), FALSE (abbreviated as F), and NA (in the case of "not available"). Note, however, that T and F are just variables that are set to TRUE and FALSE by default, but are not reserved words and hence can be overwritten by the user. Therefore, it would be better to use TRUE and FALSE.

Logical vectors are generated by conditions. For example,

```
> cond <- x > y
```

sets cond as a vector of the same length as x and y, with values FALSE corresponding to elements of x and y if the condition is not met and TRUE where it is. Table 2.2 shows some basic comparison operators in R.

A group of logical expressions, say cond1 and cond2, can be combined with the symbol & (and) or |(or), where cond1 & cond2 is their intersection and c1|c2 is their union (or). And !cond1 is the negation of cond1.

Often, the user may want to make choices and take action dependent on a certain value. In this case, an if statement can be very useful, which takes the following form:

```
if (cond) {statements}
```

TABLE 2.2

Selected R Comparison Operators

Symbol	Meaning
==	Equals
!=	Not equal
>	Greater than
<	Less than
>=	Greater than or equal
<=	Less than or equal
%in%	Determines whether specific elements are in a longer vector

Three components are contained in the `if` statement: `if`, the keyword; `(cond)`, a single logical value between parentheses (or an expression that leads to a single logical value); and `{statements}`, a block of codes between braces (`{}`) that has to be executed when the logical value is TRUE. When there is only one statement, the braces can be omitted. For example, the following statement set the variable `y` equal to 10 if the variable `Gender` equals `"F"`:

```
if (Gender == "F") y <- 10
```

To execute repetitive code statements for a particular number of times, a `for` loop in R can be used. For loops are controlled by a looping vector. In each iteration of the loop, one value in the looping vector is assigned to a variable that can be used in the statements of the body of the loop. Usually, the number of loop iterations is defined by the number of values stored in the looping vector, and they are processed in the same order as they are stored in the looping vector. Generally, `for` loop construction takes the following form:

```
for (variable in seq) {
    statements
}
```

If the goal is to create a new vector, a vector to store member variables should be set up before creating a loop. For example,

```
x <- NULL
for (j in 1:50) {
    x[j] <- j^2
}
```

The program creates a vector of 50 observations $x = j^2$, where j ranges from 1 to 50.

2.2.5 Printing Data in R

In order to display the data or the variable, we can simply type in its name after the prompt symbol > and press the Return key.

There are many routines in R developed by researchers around the world that can be downloaded and installed from CRAN-like repositories or local files using the command `install.packages("packagename")`, where `packagename` is the name of the package to be installed and must be in quotes; single or double quotes are both fine as long as they are not mixed. Once the package is installed, it can be loaded by issuing the command `library(packagename)`, after which commands specific to the package can be accessed. Through an extensive help system built into R, a help entry for a specified command can be brought up via the `help(commandname)` command. As a simple example, we introduce the command `EL.means` in the EL library.

```
> install.packages("EL")
Installing package into 'C:/Users/xiwei/Documents/R/win-library/3.1'
(as 'lib' is unspecified)
trying URL 'http://cran.rstudio.com/bin/windows/contrib/3.1/EL_1.0.zip'
Content type 'application/zip' length 53774 bytes (52 Kb)
opened URL
downloaded 52 Kb

package 'EL' successfully unpacked and MD5 sums checked
```

```
The downloaded binary packages are in
        C:\Users\xiwei\AppData\Local\Temp\Rtmp4uRCPS\downloaded_packages
> library(EL)
> help(EL.means)
```

The EL.means function provides the software tool for implementing the empirical like-lihood tests that we will introduce in detail in Chapter 6.

As another concrete example, we show the mvrnorm command in the MASS library.

```
> install.packages("MASS")
Installing package into 'C:/Users/xiwei/Documents/R/win-library/3.1'
(as 'lib' is unspecified)
trying URL 'http://cran.rstudio.com/bin/windows/contrib/3.1/MASS _ 7.3-34.zip'
Content type 'application/zip' length 1083003 bytes (1.0 Mb)
opened URL
downloaded 1.0 Mb

package 'MASS' successfully unpacked and MD5 sums checked

The downloaded binary packages are in
        C:\Users\xiwei\AppData\Local\Temp\Rtmp4uRCPS\downloaded_packages
> library(MASS)
> help(mvrnorm)
```

The mvrnorm command is very useful for simulating data from a multivariate normal distribution. To illustrate, we simulate bivariate normal data with mean $(0, 0)^T$ and an identity covariance matrix, where the sample size $n = 5$.

```
> n <- 5  # define the sample size
> mu <- c(0,0)  # define the mean vector
> Sigma <- matrix(c(1,0,0,1), byrow=TRUE, ncol=2) # define covariance matrix
> set.seed(123)  # define the seed to fix the sample
> X <- mvrnorm (n, mu=mu, Sigma=Sigma) # generate data
> X
            [,1]        [,2]
[1,] -1.7150650 -0.56047565
[2,] -0.4609162 -0.23017749
[3,]  1.2650612  1.55870831
[4,]  0.6868529  0.07050839
[5,]  0.4456620  0.12928774
```

For more details about the implementation of R, we refer the reader to Gardener (2012), Crawley (2012), Kleinman and Horton (2009), Bretz et al. (2010), Wickham (2009), and Murrell (2005).

2.3 SAS Software

SAS software is widely used to analyze data from various clinical trials and manage large data sets. SAS runs on a wide range of operating systems. More information about SAS can be found at the website http://www.sas.com/.

SAS can be run in both an interactive and a batch mode. To run SAS interactively, type SAS at your system prompt (UNIX/LINUX) or click the SAS icon (PC). Figure 2.2 shows the SAS interface in Microsoft Windows.

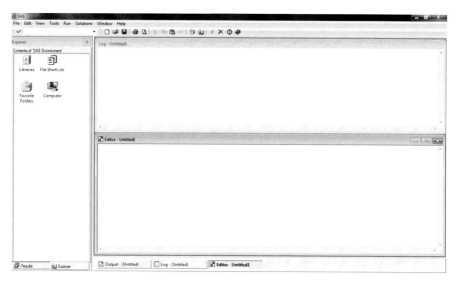

FIGURE 2.2
Interface of SAS.

In the interactive SAS environment, one can write, edit, and submit programs for processing, as well as view and print the results.

A SAS program is a sequence of statements executed in order. A statement provides instructions for SAS to execute and must be appropriately placed in the program. Statements can consist of SAS keywords, SAS names, special characters, and operators. SAS is a free format language in that SAS statements

1. Are not case sensitive, except those inside of quoted strings
2. Can start in any column
3. Can continue on the next line or be on the same line as other statements

The most important rule is that every SAS statement ends with a semicolon (;).

2.3.1 Rules for Names of Variables and SAS Data Sets

When making up names for variables and data sets (data set names follow similar rules as variables, but they have a different namespace), the following rules should be followed:

1. Names must be 32 characters or less in length, containing only letters, digits, or the underscore character (_).
2. Names must start with a letter or an underscore; however, it is a good idea to avoid starting variable names with an underscore, because special system variables are named that way.

In SAS, there are virtually no reserved words; it differentiates user-defined names with keywords or special system variable names by context.

2.3.2 Comments in SAS

Note that there are two styles of comments in SAS: one starts with an asterisk (*) and ends with a semicolon (;), as shown in the example. The other style starts with a backslash asterisk (/*) and ends with an asterisk backslash (*/). In the case of unmatched comments, SAS cannot read the entire program and will stop in the middle of a program, much like unmatched quotation marks. The solution, in batch mode, is to insert the missing part of the comment and resubmit the program.

2.3.3 Inputting Data in SAS

In SAS, DATA steps are used to read and modify data, and can also be used to simulate data. The DATA step is flexible relative to the various data formats. DATA steps have an underlying matrix structure such that programming statements will be executed for each row of the data matrix. There are multiple ways to import data into SAS. Either way, you must type raw data directly in the SAS program, link SAS to a database, or direct SAS to the data file. Other more complex methods for reading data into SAS, such as using PROC SQL, go beyond the scope of this book.

The following SAS program illustrates how to type raw data and use the INPUT and DATALINES statement:

```
* Read internal data into SAS data set Namelists;
DATA Namelists;
        INPUT Name $ Gender $ Age;
        DATALINES;
Lincoln M 46
Sara F 32
Catherine F 18
Mike M 35
        ;
RUN;
```

The keywords, for example, DATA, INPUT, DATALINES, and RUN, identify the type of statement and instruct the execution in SAS. For example, the INPUT statement, a part of the DATA step, indicates to SAS the variable names and their formats. To write an INPUT statement using list input, simply list the variable names after the INPUT keyword in the order they appear in the data file. If the variable is a character, then leave a space and place a dollar sign ($) after the corresponding variable name.

Separating the data from the program avoids the possibility that data will accidentally be altered when editing the SAS program. For data contained in external files, the INFILE statement can be used to direct SAS to the data from ASCII files. The INFILE statement follows the DATA statement and must precede the INPUT statement. After the INFILE keyword, the file path and the filename are enclosed in quotation marks.

By default, the DATA step starts reading with the first data line, and if SAS runs out of data on a line, it automatically goes to the next line to read values for the rest of the variables. Most of the time this works fine, but sometimes data files cannot be read using the default settings. In the INFILE statement, the options placed after the filename can change the way SAS reads raw data files. For instance, the FIRSTOBS= option tells SAS at what line to begin reading data; the OBS= option can be used anytime you want to read only a part of your data file; the MISSOVER option tells SAS that if it runs out of data, do not go to the next data line but assign missing values to any remaining variables instead; the DELIMITER=, or DLM=, option allows SAS to read data files with other delimiters (the default is a blank space).

Moreover, SAS assumes that the number of characters, including spaces, in a data line (termed as a record length) of external files is no more than 256 in some operating environments, for example, the Windows operating system. If the data contain records that are longer than 256 characters, the LRECL= option in the INFILE statement specifies a record length at least as long as the longest record in the data file. For more details about the INFILE options, we refer the reader to Delwiche and Slaughter (2012). More complex data import and export features are available in SAS, but go beyond the scope of our applications.

To illustrate, the following program reads data from a tab-separated external file into a SAS data set using the INFILE statement:

```
* Read internal data into SAS data set Namelists;
DATA Namelists;
      INFILE 'c:\MyRawData\Namelists.dat' DLM = '09'X;
      INPUT Name $ Gender $ Age;
RUN;
```

With SAS, there is commonly more than one way to accomplish the same result, including the input of data. For more details about other ways of inputting data, for example, the IMPORT procedure, we refer the reader to Delwiche and Slaughter (2012).

When a variable exists in SAS but does not have a value, the value is said to be *missing*. SAS assigns a period (.) for numeric data and a blank for character data. By the MISSING statement, the user may specify other characters instead of a period or a blank to be treated as missing data. To illustrate, the following example declares that the characters u are to be treated as missing values for the character variable `Gender` whenever they are encountered in a record.

```
DATA two;
      MISSING u;
      INPUT $ Gender;
CARDS;
RUN;
```

Missing values have a value of false when used with logical operators such as AND or OR (see the subsequent paragraphs for more details).

2.3.4 Manipulating Data in SAS

In SAS, the users can create and redefine variables with assignment statements using the following basic form:

```
variable = expression;
```

On the left side of the equal sign is a variable name, either new or old. On the right side of the equal sign can be a constant, another variable, or a mathematical expression. The basic types of assignment statements may use operators such as + (addition), − (subtraction), * (multiplication), / (division), and ** (exponentiation). The following example illustrates the assignment of `Newvar`, which equals the square of `OldVar` plus 3:

```
NewVar = OldVar ** 2 + 3;
```

In the case where a simple expression using only arithmetic operators is not enough, SAS provides a set of numerous useful and built-in functions. Table 2.3 shows selected SAS numeric functions; see Delwiche and Slaughter (2012) for more numeric functions and character functions.

There are a variety of *control statements* that control the flow of execution of statements in the data step.

If the user wants to conditionally execute a SAS statement based on certain conditional logic, that is, to conduct computations under certain conditions, in this scenario, the IF–THEN statement can be used, which takes the general form

```
IF condition THEN action;
```

The condition is an expression comparing arguments, and the action is what SAS will execute when the expression is true, often an assignment statement. For example,

```
IF Gender = 'F' THEN y=10;
```

This statement tells SAS to set the variable y equal to 10 whenever the variable Gender equals 'F'. The terms on either side of the comparison, separated by a comparison operator, may be constants, variables, or expressions. The comparison operator may be either symbolic or mnemonic, depending on the user's preference. Table 2.4 shows some basic comparison operators.

A single IF–THEN statement can only have one action. To specify multiple conditions, we can combine the condition with the keywords AND (&) or OR (|). For example,

```
IF condition AND condition THEN action;
```

TABLE 2.3

Selected SAS Numeric Functions

Syntax	Definition
MEAN(arg-1,arg-2,…arg-n)	Arithmetic mean of nonmissing values
STD(arg-1,arg-2,…arg-n)	Standard deviation of nonmissing values
VAR(arg-1,arg-2,…arg-n)	Variance of nonmissing values
SUM(arg-1,arg-2,…arg-n)	Sum of nonmissing values

TABLE 2.4

Selected SAS Comparison Operators

Symbolic	Mnemonic	Meaning
=	EQ	Equals
¬ =, ^ =, or ~ =	NE	Not equal
>	GT	Greater than
<	LT	Less than
>=	GE	Greater than or equal
<=	LE	Less than or equal
	IN	Determine whether a variable's value is among a list of values

A group of actions can be executed by adding keywords DO and END:

```
IF condition THEN DO;
      action;
      action;
END;
```

The DO statement designates a group of statements to be executed as a unit until a matching END statement appears. The DO statement, the matching END statement, and all the statements between them define a do-loop. There are several variations of the DO-END statement. The following example presents an iterative DO statement that executes a group of SAS statements repetitively between the DO and END statements:

```
DO index = start TO stop BY increment;
      statements;
END;
```

The number of times statements are executed is determined as follows. Initially, the variable index is set at the value of start and statements are executed. Next, the value of increment is added to the index and the new value is compared to the value of stop. The statements are executed again only if the new value of index is less than or equal to stop. If no increment is specified, the default is 1. The process continues iteratively until the value of index is greater than the value of stop. We illustrate with a simple example:

```
DATA one;
      DO j = 1 TO 50;
      x = j**2;
      OUTPUT one;
END;
DROP j;
CARDS;
RUN;
```

The program creates a SAS data set with 50 observations and a variable $x = j^2$, where the index variable j ranges from 1 to 50. The DROP statement helps get rid of the index variable j. The OUTPUT statement tells SAS to write the current observation to the output data set before returning to the beginning of the DATA step to process the next observation.

2.3.5 Printing Data in SAS

The PROC PRINT procedure lists data in a SAS data set as a table of observations by variables. The following statements can be used with PROC PRINT:

```
PROC PRINT DATA = SASdataset;
      VAR variables;
      ID variable;
      BY variables;
      TITLE 'Print SAS Data Set';
RUN;
```

where `SASdataset` is the name of the data set printed. If none is specified, then the last SAS data set created will be printed. If no VAR statement is included, then all variables in the data set are printed; otherwise, only those listed, and in the order in which they are listed, are printed. When an ID statement is used, SAS prints each observation with the values of the ID variables first instead of the observation number, the default setting. The BY statement specifies the variable that the procedure uses to form BY groups; the observations in the data set must either be sorted by all the variables specified (e.g., use the PROC SORT procedure) or be indexed appropriately, unless the NOTSORTED option in the BY statement is used. For more details, we refer the read to Delwiche and Slaughter (2012).

2.3.6 Summarizing Data in SAS

After reading the data and making sure they are correct, one may summarize and analyze the data using built-in SAS procedures or PROCs. For example, PROC MEANS provides a set of descriptive statistics for numeric variables. Virtually all SAS PROCs have additional options or features, which can be accessed with subcommands; for example, one can use PROC MEANS to carry out a one-sample *t*-test.

As another example, the following program sorts the SAS data set Namelists by gender using PROC SORT, and then summarizes the Age by Gender using PROC MEANS with a BY statement (the MAXDEC option is set to zero, so no decimal places will be printed):

```
* Sort the data by Gender;
PROC SORT DATA = Namelists;
      BY Gender;
* Calculate means by Gender for Age;
PROC MEANS DATA = Namelists MAXDEC = 0;
      BY Gender;
      VAR Age;
      TITLE 'Summary of Age by Gender';
RUN;
```

Here are the results of the PROC MEANS by gender:

Summary of Age by Gender

The MEANS Procedure

Gender = F

		Analysis Variable: Age		
N	Mean	Standard Deviation	Minimum	Maximum
2	25	10	18	32

Gender = M

		Analysis Variable: Age		
N	Mean	Standard Deviation	Minimum	Maximum
2	41	8	35	46

For more details about the data summarization by descriptive statistics or graphs, we refer the reader to Delwiche and Slaughter (2012).

For a majority of the examples in later chapters, the reader is expected to understand the basic commands of the DATA step, such as do-loops and the OUTPUT statement, and be familiar with the various statistical PROCs that he or she might use generally given parametric assumptions. Some knowledge of the basic SAS macro language and PROC IML (a separate way to program in SAS) will also be helpful. It is our goal that most of the code provided in this book will be easily modified to handle a variety of problems found in practice. It should be noted that R routines can be implemented within SAS PROC IML.

SAS programming can be quite complex, and careers around SAS programming are numerous and require several years of experience. Our goal is to demonstrate how to use SAS at a more basic level in order to perform interesting data analyses. For more details about the implementation of SAS, we refer the reader to Westfall et al. (2011), Kleinman and Horton (2009), Dmitrienko et al. (2007), and Littell (2006).

2.4 Supplement

1. Murrell (2005) described the graphics system in R. There are many pictures that demonstrate the variety and complexity of plots and diagrams that can be produced using R. The book presents the different output formats that R graphics can produce and the overall organization of the R graphics facilities, giving the reader some idea of where to find a function for a particular purpose.

2. Dmitrienko et al. (2007) provided a well-organized overview of important statistical topics applied in pharmaceutical drug development, from drug discovery to late-stage clinical studies. The book exhibits a good balance between explanation of the statistical theory and solutions to examples of practical problems. The statistical methodology is covered in depth and is well explained, but requires an advanced knowledge of SAS programming in pharmaceutical drug development. The solutions are up-to-date and well illustrated by down-to-earth examples using SAS code and SAS output.

3. Cody (2007) introduced major SAS concepts and procedures with extensive use of examples and liberal annotation. The book provides approaches to perform data manipulation and basic statistical analyses in SAS.

4. Kleinman and Horton (2009) presented a range of commonly used data management, statistical procedures, and graphing techniques available in both SAS and R. This book provides a very useful bridge between the two packages, which are very different in how they are structured and the code needed to run them.

5. Wickham (2009) described ggplot2, a new data visualization package for R that uses graphics to create a powerful and flexible scheme for constructing data graphics. The ggplot2 package produces publication-quality plots virtually hassle-free; for example, details such as drawing legends are easily carried forth.

6. Lawson (2010) demonstrated a comprehensive treatment of the design and analysis of experiments, linking concepts to practice illustrated with the SAS program. The book includes examples from a wide range of areas, including pharmaceutical science and industrial manufacturing.

7. Bretz et al. (2010) depicted the applications of multiple comparison procedures, with discussion and analysis of many examples implemented in R.

8. Westfall et al. (2011) provided cutting-edge methods, specialized SAS macros, and procedures for a broad variety of problems that call for multiple inferences, illustrated with real-world examples and solutions. The book also discusses the pitfalls and advantages of various methods, thereby helping the reader decide the most appropriate approach to deal with multiple inferences. The book includes specialized code and explanations throughout. It discusses in detail pairwise comparisons and comparisons with a control. Additional topics include general linear contrasts, multiple comparisons of multivariate means, and multiple inferences with mixed models, discrete data, and survival analysis.

9. Gardener (2012) introduced the R language using simple statistical examples. The book presents the use of R for simple summary statistics, hypothesis testing, creating graphs, regression, and much more. It covers formula notation, complex statistics, manipulating data and extracting components, and elementary programming.

10. Crawley (2012) introduced the riches of the R environment, aimed at beginners and intermediate users in the fields ranging from science to economics and from medicine to engineering. The book covers data handling, graphics, mathematical functions, and a wide range of statistical techniques, for example, regression, analysis of variance, generalized linear modeling, Bayesian analysis, spatial statistics, and multivariate methods.

3

Statistical Graphics

A picture is worth a thousand words.

Barnard (1927)

Graphs are essential to good statistical analysis.

Anscombe (1973)

The greatest value of a graph is when it forces us to see what we never expected.

Tukey (1977)

A picture may be worth a thousand words, but it may take a hundred words to do it.

Tukey (1986)

Visualization is critical to data analysis.

Cleveland (1993)

3.1 Introduction

In this chapter, we introduce graphical statistical methods both as a powerful stand-alone exploratory data analysis and summary tool to complement and provide visual insight into more complex and formal statistical testing procedures. Statistical graphs have various purposes, including but not limited to (1) providing a descriptive summary of the data, (2) providing a visualization tool to examine associations between variables, (3) providing insight for model selection based on the data under scrutiny, (4) graphically checking model assumptions about the behavior of the data as it pertains to a given statistical test, and (5) helping to determine if more complicated modeling is necessary. With increased computing speed and user-friendly graphics packages, implementation of graphical visualization as an exploratory data analysis tool is ever expanding, for example, heat maps for microarray data and various three-dimensional (3D) plots.

For the purpose of this book, we focus on some commonly used statistical graphics displays, such as scatterplots and boxplots, as well as the implementation of probability plotting methods, including quantile–quantile (Q–Q) plots, probability–probability (P–P) plots, and modifications and hybrids of these. Heat maps commonly used in microarray data analysis are also introduced. Suggestions as to what may form the basis for the development of a general probability plotting procedure are also given. In general, graphical methods can be applied to the following areas: the comparison of samples, graphical estimates, and displays of distributions and summary measures; the presentation of results on sensitivity and specificity trade-offs of diagnostic methods; checking model assumptions; the analysis of collections of contrasts and sample variances; the assessment of multivariate contrasts; and the structuring of analysis of variance mean squares. Many of the objectives and techniques presented in this chapter are illustrated with examples. In addition, graphical methods may be useful in detecting data entry errors not easily seen when the data are in tabular form.

We start with the basic visualization of the raw data. We then proceed to the description of the use of the empirical cumulative distribution function in the visualization of data, including two basic illustrative examples. Probability plots and other graphical transforms, stimulated by the probability plotting method, and the use of probability plots are described as informal aids to inference. Applications of probability plotting, such as the comparison of distributions and analysis of variance, are also presented. We then introduce the use of heat maps and close with a brief conclusion pertaining to the utility of graphical methods.

Note that in the context of the probability plots, Chapter 8 will introduce the receiver operating characteristic curves and Chapter 10 will introduce the Kendall plot.

3.2 Descriptive Plots of Raw Data

Graphical representations can often exhibit subtleties that are not apparent from summary statistics or simply provide a quick visual overview of the data. Various types of graphical displays of data are available and can be used for exploratory and summary purposes. When employing graphical methods, consideration should be given as to how data can best be presented to the human eye and how they will be perceived by the human mind.

3.2.1 Boxplots

A boxplot (also termed a box-and-whisker plot) is a commonly used five-number graphical summary of the data consisting of the maximum, upper-quartile, median, lower-quartile, and minimum values. The boxplot was developed by the well-known statistician John Tukey. Some boxplot-generating programs define outliers as well, given as a certain distance from the central mass of the data. Figure 3.1 illustrates a boxplot of the death rate on the log scale that was abstracted from the Surgeon General's report *Smoking and Health* (U.S. Department of Health, Education, and Welfare 1964). The construction of the boxplot was generated by the following R code:

```
> smoker<-c(3.4,4.1,4.6,5.1,5.4,5.8,6.2,6.8,7.1)
> nonsmoker<-c(2.9,3.3,3.7,4.35,4.7,5.2,5.7,6.1,6.6,6.5)
> death.rate<-c(smoker, nonsmoker, ylab="Death rate (log scale)")
> boxplot(death.rate)
```

The lines extending from the box, called whiskers, indicate variability outside the upper and lower quartiles. It clearly shows that the death rate is approximately symmetric and has short tails. Though there is no outlier shown in Figure 3.1, outliers may be plotted as individual points.

Examining group differences is facilitated by plotting boxplots side by side, for example, smokers versus nonsmokers. Figure 3.2 presents the comparative boxplot of the death rate

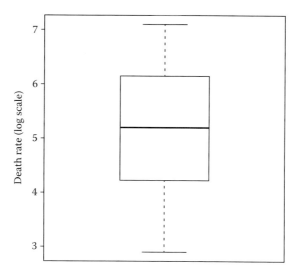

FIGURE 3.1
Boxplot of the death rate (log scale) in a prospective study of mortality in U.S. veterans.

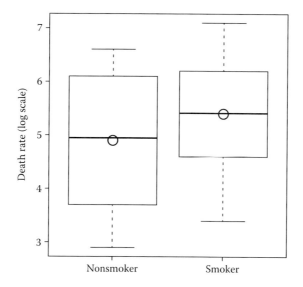

FIGURE 3.2
Comparative boxplot of the death rate (log scale) in a prospective study of mortality in U.S. veterans, where the circles represent the mean in each group.

(log scale) by a group variable identifying whether the person is a smoker or nonsmoker. The construction of the boxplot was generated by the following R code:

```
> group<-c(rep("Smoker",length(smoker)),rep("Nonsmoker",length(nonsmoker)))
> boxplot(death.rate~group,ylab="Death rate (log scale)")
> means <- tapply(death.rate,group,mean) # obtain the mean for each group
> points(means,pch=18,cex=2) # add the means to the boxplot
```

The circles represent the sample mean of the death rate in each group. The vertical line in the box displays the estimated median. This side-by-side boxplot clearly demonstrates that smokers have a higher death rate than nonsmokers.

3.2.2 Scatterplots

Suppose we have measurements on a pair of variables, for example, the death rate and age; then it may be of interest to explore how the data behave in two dimensions in order to graphically examine any potential dependence or correlation structure between the two variables. A standard graphical tool for this purpose is the so-called scatterplot, which displays values for two paired variables for a set of data using Cartesian coordinates. Through the scatterplot, we can see whether points appear to be randomly scattered, have a functional relationship, or cluster in groups. If clustered, we can visualize the locations and shape of these clusters. We may also check via the scatterplot if two variables are dependent. If dependent, we can roughly see the nature of the dependence. Furthermore, a good legend can help identify the pattern and extract information from the data. For example, Figure 3.3 provides a rough duplicate of a plot of death rate in log scale versus age that was shown in the 1964 Surgeon General's report *Smoking and Health*, given by the following R code:

```
> age.smoker<-c(42,47,52,57,62,67,72,77,81)
> age.nonsmoker<-c(42,47,52,57,62,67,72,75,77,81)
> smoker<-c(3.4,4.1,4.6,5.1,5.4,5.8,6.2,6.8,7.1)
> nonsmoker<-c(2.9,3.3,3.7,4.35,4.7,5.2,5.7,6.1,6.6,6.5)
> plot(age.smoker, smoker,ylim=c(2,7),xlim=c(40,80),pch=16,cex=1.3,xlab=
  "Age",ylab="ln(Death Rate per 10000 man-years)")
> points(age.nonsmoker, nonsmoker,pch=1,cex=1.3)
> legend("bottomright",c("Smokers","Non-Smokers"),pch=c(16,1))
```

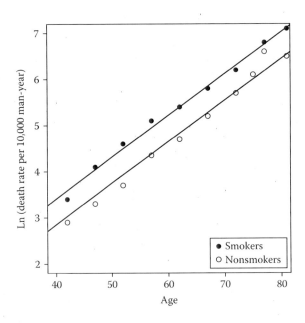

FIGURE 3.3

Scatterplot of death rate (log scale) versus age in a prospective study of mortality in U.S. veterans.

The death rates are plotted on the vertical axis, and age is plotted on the horizontal axis. It appears graphically that the death rate tends to increase as the age increases. In addition, it clearly displays that smokers, shown in solid dots, die sooner than nonsmokers, shown in circles, and that smoking appears to subtract approximately 7 years from life expectancy. Note that color is oftentimes used to assist in emphasizing features or group differences in graphs. However, details may be lost if a colored graph is transferred to a black-and-white setting. In addition, the use of colors may sometimes yield visual miscues regarding the true associations between variables.

3.2.3 High-Dimensional Plots

A $d + 1$-dimensional graph is the plot of a set of points $(\mathbf{x}, f(\mathbf{x}))$ in the $d + 1$-dimensional Euclidean space, where $\mathbf{x} \in \mathbf{R}^d$ and the function $f: \mathbf{R}^d \to \mathbf{R}$. When $d = 2$, that is, in the case of a two-dimensional (2D) function $z = f(x, y)$, $x, y \in \mathbf{R}$, we can visualize the relationship among the 3D set $g(x, y, z)$ by drawing a perspective plot of the function or a contour plot showing the level curves of the function.

3.2.3.1 Perspective Plots

A perspective plot (also termed surface plot, mesh plot, or wire mesh surface) is a wireframe plot, with hidden lines removed. The 3D effect is depicted by the perspective and by hiding the background features. The function is evaluated on a grid, and the wireframe plot shows the lines that connect the points.

To illustrate, Figure 3.4 demonstrates a perspective plot of a surface over the x-y plane, where $x = y$ is equally spaced ranging from -10 to 10, $z = \sin(r)/r$ and $r = \sqrt{x^2 + y^2}$. The plot is generated by the following R code:

```
> x <- seq(-10, 10, length= 30)
> y <- x
> # define the function z=f(x,y)
> f <- function(x,y){
+   r <- sqrt(x^2+y^2)
+   z <- sin(r)/r
+   return(z)
+ }
> z <- outer(x, y, f)
> z[is.na(z)] <- 1
> op <- par(bg = "white")    # set up plotting parameters
> par(mar=c(.5,.5,.5,.5))
> persp(x, y, z, theta = 30, phi = 30, expand = 0.5, col = "grey")
```

The box around the plot heightens the perception of depth.

3.2.3.2 Contour Plots

A contour plot is a graphical technique for representing a 3D surface by plotting contours, that is, constant z slices where $z = f(x, y)$, $x, y \in \mathbf{R}$, on a 2D x-y plane. The z-level curve of function $f: \mathbf{R}^d \to \mathbf{R}$ is defined by $\Gamma(f, \lambda) = \{x \in \mathbf{R}^d : f(x) = \lambda\}$, where $z \in \mathbf{R}$. Given a value for z, lines are drawn for connecting the (x, y) coordinates where that z value occurs.

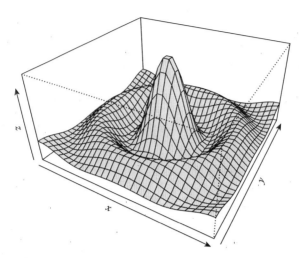

FIGURE 3.4

Perspective plot of a surface over the *x-y* plane, where $x = y$ is equally spaced ranging from –10 to 10 and $z = \sin\left(\sqrt{x^2 + y^2}\right)\Big/\sqrt{x^2 + y^2}$.

As an example, Figure 3.5 presents a contour plot corresponding to the perspective plot of Figure 3.4. The numbers in the contour plot show the levels of the level curves. The contour plot is generated by the following R code:

```
> x <- seq(-10, 10, length= 30)
> y <- x
> # define the function z=f(x,y)
> f <- function(x,y){
+    r <- sqrt(x^2+y^2)
+    z <- sin(r)/r
+    return(z)
+ }
> z <- outer(x, y, f)
> op <- par(bg = "white")   # set up plotting parameters
> par(mar=c(.5,.5,.5,.5))
> persp(x, y, z, theta = 30, phi = 30, expand = 0.5, col = "grey")
```

Contour plots do not suffer from hiding structure, as is the case in perspective plots, of the function. A contour plot is suitable for smooth functions, but for piecewise constant functions, a perspective plot is usually preferred. One may have difficulty visualizing functions that have flat regions and sharp jumps with contour plots. Moreover, difficulties may occur when one visualizes heavy-tailed densities by means of contour plots. In addition, contour plots do not visually differentiate between local minima and local maxima. The information as to whether a local extreme is a minimum or a maximum and whether the function is increasing or decreasing in a region is described by the level numbers attached to the contour lines. In support of the contour plot, it is also useful to draw a perspective plot for better visualization (Klemelä 2009). As a general point, these two plots used in conjunction with each other are a powerful representation of 3D data.

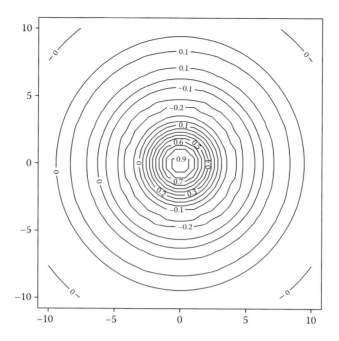

FIGURE 3.5

Contour plot, where $x = y$ is equally spaced ranging from –10 to 10 and $z = \sin\left(\sqrt{x^2 + y^2}\right)\Big/\sqrt{x^2 + y^2}$.

A 3D function may be visualized by drawing a perspective plot of level surfaces. For a high-dimensional function, one has to reduce the dimension of the function in order to use perspective plots and contour plots. The use of slices and projections is classical. For example, four-dimensional (4D) functions may be pictured by visualizing 3D-level curves of a series of slices as the fourth variable changes over its range. For more details about plotting high-dimensional functions, we refer the reader to Klemelä (2009).

3.3 Empirical Distribution Function Plot

The statistical literature addresses well the empirical distribution function (EDF) (e.g., Barton and Mallows 1965). The present discussion focuses on the descriptive uses of the EDF rather than formal tests as applied directly to the case of univariate samples.

In many phases of data analysis, one-dimensional (1D) characterizations of complex data are often appreciated and involved. For instance, in a study of the energies in a spoken word associated with a cross-classification according to time and frequency, the data were treated as a 1D sample, ignoring the associated structure among the observations (Wilk and Gnanadesikan 1968). The visual EDF displays provided a summary measure of energy as a measure of speech recognition.

For an independent and identically distributed (i.i.d.) 1D sample $X_1, \ldots, X_n$ from an unknown cumulative distribution function (CDF) $F(x)$, the EDF is $F_n(x) = n^{-1} \sum_{i=1}^{n} I\{X_i \leq x\}$, where $I\{\cdot\}$ is the indicator function. It is a natural estimator of the true CDF, and it is essentially the CDF associated with the empirical measure of the sample, which puts mass

$1/n$ on each data point. Tukey (1962) noted that the EDF is the empirical counterpart of the CDF and suggested the term *empirical representing function* to describe this function. The EDF graphical display is a plot of the ith ordered value on the ordinate against the $(i - 1/2)/n$ value on the abscissa. This graphical summary provides a concise description of the data under the following assumptions: (1) the order of the observations is immaterial; (2) there is no classification of the observations, based on extraneous considerations, that one wishes to employ; and (3) if the sample is nonrandom, then appropriate weights are specified (Wilk and Gnanadesikan 1968). The EDF has an approximate normal distribution, estimates the true underlying CDF of the data, and converges with probability 1 to the CDF according to the Glivenko–Cantelli theorem (Tucker 1959). The EDF is in essence a sample proportion given a fixed x.

The use of the EDF does not depend on any parametric distributional assumption. It is useful in describing data even when the data are not i.i.d., for example, time series data. The use of the EDF has many advantages, such as the following:

1. It is invariant to monotone transformations.

2. The complexity of the graph is independent of the sample size.

3. It lends itself to graphical representation as a summary measure, and it can be modified based on interpolation and smoothing techniques.

4. It is a robust and informative relative to the location, shape, and dispersion of a distribution and does not involve the grouping difficulties arising in histogram bin size selections.

5. It can be extended to accommodate censored data.

6. It is directly associated with probability plotting procedures.

The EDF plays a key role in the statistical treatment of 1D samples. Some useful features of the EDF are now illustrated by two examples.

We first illustrate data from a case-control study evaluating biomarkers related to atherosclerotic coronary heart disease. A cross-sectional population-based sample of randomly selected residents (ages 35–79) of Erie and Niagara Counties of the State of New York was the focus of this study. The New York State Department of Motor Vehicles driver's license rolls were employed as the sampling frame for adults between the ages of 35 and 65, whereas the elderly sample (ages >65–75) was randomly selected from the Health Care Financing Administration database. The study sample consists of 542 individuals, including 105 individuals with myocardial infarction and 437 controls. Participants provided a 12-hour fasting blood specimen for biochemical analysis at baseline, and a number of characteristics were evaluated from fresh blood samples, including measurements of thiobarbituric acid reactive substances (TBARS) and high-density lipoprotein (HDL) cholesterol, biomarkers of oxidative stress and antioxidant status.

Summary statistics of all 542 measurements of TBARS in the form of sample mean and sample standard deviation are 1.3808 and 0.4166, respectively. The sample mean and sample standard deviation of all 542 HDL cholesterol measurements (mg/dl) are 49.9384 and 11.7765, respectively. Another clear and useful statistical presentation of the entire body of the data is provided in Figure 3.6, which is the EDF. Figure 3.6 plots the EDF of

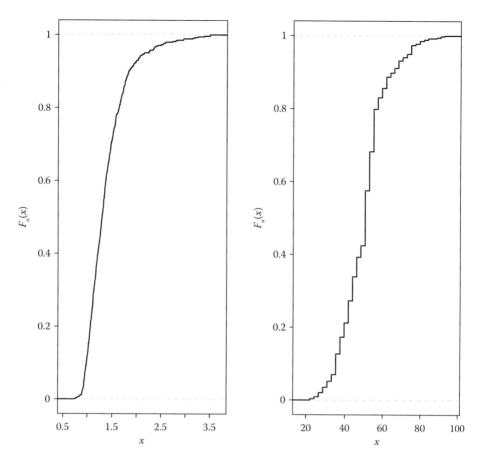

FIGURE 3.6
EDF of the data of TBARS measurements (left) and HDL measurements (right).

measurements of TBARS in the left and the EDF of measurements of HDL cholesterol in the right, produced by the following R code:

```
> tbars<-c(tbars.x,tbars.y)
> Fn.tbars<-ecdf(tbars)     # ECDF of TBARS
> hdl<-c(hdl.x,hdl.y)
> Fn.hdl<-ecdf(hdl) # ECDF of HDL
> par(mfrow=c(1,2))
> plot(Fn.tbars, verticals = TRUE, do.points = FALSE,main="TBARS",lwd=2)
> plot(Fn.hdl, verticals = TRUE, do.points = FALSE,main="HDL",lwd=2)
```

The depicted EDFs of the TBARS measurements and the HDL cholesterol have stable behavior and provide quick indications of location and scale.

As shown in the left panel of Figure 3.6, the TBARS measurements seem to be reasonably smooth with no indication of extreme observations. The corresponding distribution is skewed to the right, where the values above the mean occur relatively more often.

The plot of the EDF of HDL cholesterol measurements, shown in the right panel of Figure 3.6, appears to be not as smooth as the one of the TBARS measurements. This is mainly due to the fact that the TBARS measurements are measured with three-decimal precision, while the HDL cholesterol measurements are rounded to the nearest even decimal. In addition, the plot of the EDF of the HDL cholesterol measurement indicates a slight bimodal pattern, implying that the biomarker HDL cholesterol has a potentially better discriminant ability than the biomarker TBARS. To further investigate this, we plot the EDF of TBARS measurements in the left panel of Figure 3.7 and HDL cholesterol measurements in the right panel of Figure 3.7 for the diseased and nondiseased groups separately.

The plots indicate slight differences in the EDFs of TBARS measurements between the diseased and nondiseased groups, especially for lower values of TBARS. On the contrary, the differences in the EDFs of HDL cholesterol measurements between the diseased and nondiseased groups are obvious, suggesting that the HDL cholesterol biomarker has a strong discriminatory ability for myocardial infarction. Moreover, comparing Figure 3.6 with Figure 3.7, it can be noted that the complexity of the plot of EDF of data may not be increased when a large sample size is involved.

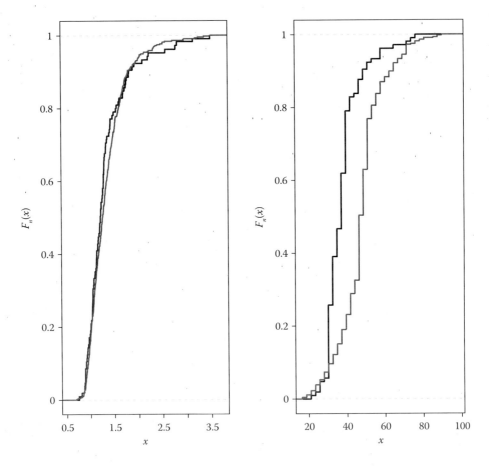

FIGURE 3.7
(See color insert.) EDF of the data of TBARS measurements (left) and HDL measurements (right) for the diseased (black) and nondiseased (red) groups, respectively.

A second example consists of 299 observations and 2 variables, including the eruption time (in minutes) and the waiting time for this eruption (in minutes) for the Old Faithful geyser in Yellowstone National Park from August 1 to August 15, 1985 (Azzalini and Bowman 1990).

Figure 3.8 presents the EDF for the waiting time for eruptions, produced by the following R code:

```
> library(MASS)
> wait<-geyser$waiting
> Fn.wait<-ecdf(wait)
> plot(Fn.wait, verticals = TRUE,do.points = FALSE)
```

The EDF of the geyser data clearly displays the degree and location of quantization of the waiting time. Given the inflection points, it is apparent from Figure 3.8 that the data are bimodal, with a major mode at around the point of 80 minutes and a minor mode around the point of 55 minutes. The plot suggests a test for homogeneity of the sample. In addition to providing location and scale information, the EDF plot provides a robust basis for choosing descriptive summary statistics by demonstrating skewness, bimodality, and outliers, among other distributional properties of interest.

The EDF is just one tool for the graphing and conceptualization of data. Alternate statistical summary approaches can be used, such as a simple tabulation, a histogram, or a list of moment statistics or quantiles. However, in general, especially in a preliminary investigation of data, the EDF is a convenient tool for summarizing and exploring data and can avoid some ambiguities found in other approaches, such as grouping difficulties that arise in the use of a histogram.

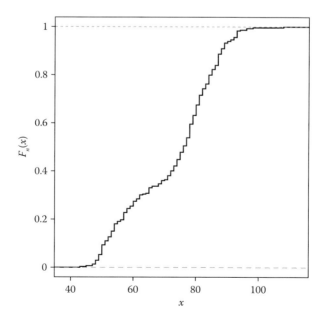

FIGURE 3.8
EDF of the waiting time for eruptions for the Old Faithful geyser data.

3.4 Two-Sample Comparisons

In this section, we discuss the comparison of two probability distributions, in terms of basic probability plots such as quantile–quantile plots (Q–Q plots), probability–probability plots (P–P plots), and various hybrids and extensions in terms of the CDFs of the two samples. For the purposes of our preliminary discussion pertaining to graphical methods, we avoid the technical discussion regarding the differences between EDFs and CDFs in terms of the differences between finite and infinite samples since the underlying graphics are similar.

For any ordinate value, $p \in [0,1]$, there are two quantile values $q_X(p)$ and $q_Y(p)$ corresponding to the random variables X and Y. A Q–Q plot is a scatterplot of $q_Y(p)$ versus $q_X(p)$ for across values of $p \in [0,1]$. Corresponding to any abscissa value q, there are two CDF values $p_X(q)$ and $p_Y(q)$. Plotting $p_Y(q)$ versus $p_X(q)$ based on the samples of X and Y for various values of q gives the P–P plot. Figure 3.9 illustrates the definition of Q–Q plots and P–P plots via two CDFs.

In a special case when the two random variables X and Y are both uniform on $[0,1]$, Q–Q plots and P–P plots are identical. This may occur, for example, when both the X and Y variables are functions of probability integral transforms. Furthermore, extensions and mixtures of basic Q–Q plots and P–P plots will be discussed and illustrated with examples.

3.4.1 Quantile–Quantile Plots (Q–Q Plots)

If distributions of X and Y are identical, then the points in the plot of $q_Y(p)$ versus $q_X(p)$ will fall in a straight 45° line. If the distributions being compared have a linear Q–Q plot, then there may be location differences between the two distributions. This elementary linear invariance property has made the use of Q–Q plots valuable and appealing. The reason for this is that linearity can be perceived most sensitively in geometric configurations, and departures from linearity can be easily ascertained.

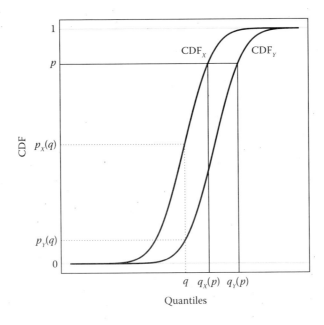

FIGURE 3.9
Definition of Q–Q and P–P plots.

The Q–Q plot tends to emphasize the comparative structure in the tails and blur the distinctions in the middle of the distributions for variables with long tails (unlimited range). This is due to the fact that as p changes, the quantile changes rapidly in the tails where the densities are sparse, while changing slowly in the middle where the densities are compact.

As a concrete example, Figure 3.10 illustrates a plot of the quantiles of a double exponential distribution with median 0 and scale 1 against those of a standard normal distribution. The plot shows a smooth nonlinearity across the range of quantiles. The plot demonstrates the distinctions between a double exponential distribution and a standard normal distribution. The slope being less than 1 in the central region illustrates the greater probability mass at the center of the double exponential distribution relative to the normal distribution. The slope of the curve exceeds 1, increasing at large absolute quantile values, which indicates heavier tails of the double exponential distribution.

Q–Q plots can serve as a graphical indicator of differences between distributions and can provide a useful basis for gauging the adequacy of composite hypotheses about location or scale parameters.

Figure 3.11 presents the use of a Q–Q plot as one way of examining the adequacy of the approximation of the distribution of the $\log(\chi^2(\text{degree of freedom} = 8))$ variable by a standard normal variable and was produced using the following R code:

```
> n=4000
> dd=seq(0.000001,.999999,length.out=n)
> x=log(qchisq(dd,df=8))
> y=qnorm(dd)
> qqplot((x-mean(x))/sd(x),(y-mean(y))/sd(y), xlim=c(-4,4),ylim=c(-4,4),
+       xlab=expression(paste("Quantiles of the standardized
          log(",{chi^2},"(8))")),
+       ylab="Quantiles of the standard normal")
> abline(a=0,b=1)
```

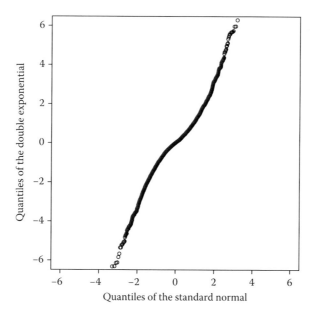

FIGURE 3.10
Q–Q plot of the double exponential distribution versus the standard normal distribution.

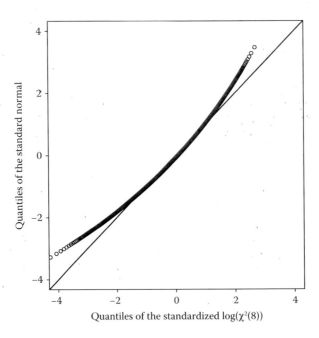

FIGURE 3.11
Q–Q plot of the standardized $\log(\chi^2(8))$ against the standard normal distribution.

The comparison of the plotted points with the 45° line indicates the systematic error in the tails and shows a small but definite asymmetry in the approximation. This plot suggests the region over which the quantile approximation may be regarded as adequate or inadequate.

To illustrate an empirical Q–Q plot, we revisit the data of TBARS measurements and the HDL measurements shown in Figure 3.7. Figure 3.12 shows the empirical Q–Q plot of the data of TBARS measurements in the left panel and HDL measurements in the right panel, which was produced by the following R code:

```
> par(mfrow=c(1,2))
> qqplot(tbars.x,tbars.y,xlim=c(0.5,3.7),ylim=c(0.5,3.7),main="TBARS")
> abline(a=0,b=1)
> qqplot(hdl.x,hdl.y,xlim=c(25,100),ylim=c(25,100),main="HDL")
> abline(a=0,b=1)
```

The empirical Q–Q plot of the TBARS data, shown in the left panel of Figure 3.12, basically falls on the 45° line configuration. This indicates a slight difference between distributions between the case and control data. The Q–Q plot of the HDL data, shown in the right panel of Figure 3.12, indicates a better discriminant ability of the biomarker HDL cholesterol than of the TBARS biomarker.

3.4.2 Probability–Probability Plots (P–P plots)

If the random variables X and Y are distributed identically, then a P–P plot for $p_Y(q)$ versus $p_X(q)$ will be a straight 45° line going from (0,0) to (1,1). The P–P plot is not location or scale invariant; for example, if we change one variable for meters to inches, the P–P plot will not remain linear.

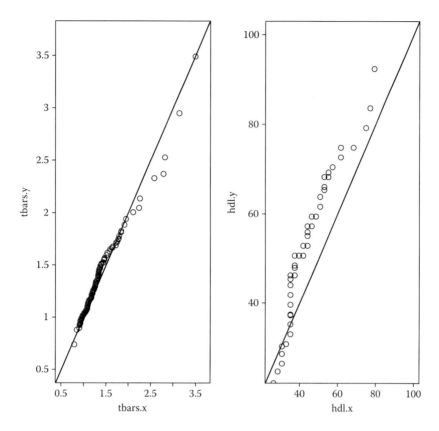

FIGURE 3.12

Q–Q plot of the data of TBARS measurements (left) and HDL measurements (right).

This is not true for the Q–Q plot. Hence, Q–Q and P–P plots need to be interpreted differently. In particular, P–P plots are especially sensitive to discrepancies in the middle of a distribution rather than in the tails for reasons complementary to those in the case of Q–Q plots. Moreover, the basic idea of P–P plots can be extended to the multivariate case, unlike the Q–Q plot, which does not have a multivariate analogue; that is, we cannot invert a multivariate distribution function around a single quantile. Approaches for employing, generalizing, and interpreting the general P–P plot require further investigation, including developing estimation procedures and examining robustness properties found in data standardization methods.

Figure 3.13 exemplifies the use of a P–P plot, showing the results for the normal approximation to the distribution of the $\log(\chi^2(8))$ variable. It was generated by the following R code:

```
> install.packages("StatDA") # install the packages for the first time
> library(StatDA)
> x<-log(rchisq(n,df=8))
> ppplot.das((x-mean(x))/sd(x), pdist = pnorm,cex.lab=1, xlab=expression
  (paste("Probabilities of the standardized log(",{chi^2},"(8))")),ylab=
  "Probabilities of the standard normal distribution")
```

The results of the P–P plot are similar to those of the Q–Q plot given in Figure 3.11 and clearly show that the distributions differ not only in the tails but also in the middle.

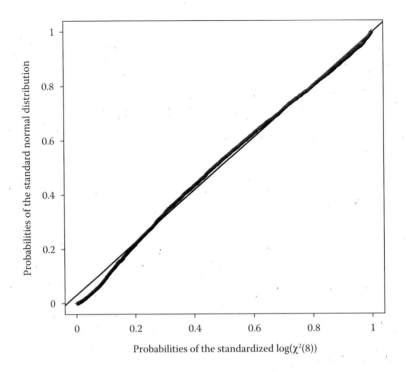

FIGURE 3.13
P–P plot of the standardized $\log(\chi^2(8))$ against the standard normal distribution.

Another particular useful application of P–P plots is in the presentation of the statistical power of a hypothesis test as a function of the significance level. In fact, the power function is the CDF of the p-value, p, which is a random variable. Thus, the x-coordinate is the p-value under the null distribution, while the y-coordinate is the p-value under the alternative. To illustrate this property, we present the comparison of the empirical power of seven tests for the equality of population means given samples of size 25 for $X \sim N(1, \sqrt{5})$, $Y \sim N(2,1)$ in Figure 3.14. We included the two-sample t-test with unpooled variances and pooled variances, the paired two-sample t-test, the Mann–Whitney U-test, the Wilcoxon signed-rank test, the Kolmogorov–Smirnov test, and the empirical likelihood test. We will further discuss the comparison of these tests and the presentation of statistical power in Section 3.5.2.

3.4.3 Modifications, Extensions, and Hybrids of Q–Q and P–P Plots

In this section, we discuss some direct modifications and immediate extensions of P–P and Q–Q plots. A Q–Q plot has been described as a plot of $q_X(p)$ against $q_Y(p)$ for any $p \in [0,1]$, which can be viewed as a special case of the plot of $g(q_X, q_Y)$ versus $h(q_X, q_Y)$. Similarly, the concept of P–P plots can be extended in the same way.

In some circumstances, it is very useful to employ mixtures of Q–Q and P–P plots, for instance, to plot $g(q_X(p), q_Y(p))$ versus $p \in [0,1]$, or, more generally, $g(q_X(p), q_Y(p))$ versus $h(p)$. Similarly, a plot of $g(p_X(q), p_Y(q))$ versus $h(q)$ can be considered.

Figures 3.15 and 3.16 show examples of hybrid plots, which summarize the adequacy of a normal approximation to the distribution of $\log(\chi^2(v))$, for various degrees of freedom $v = 5, 8,$ and 25. These plots show the difference $q_X(p) - q_Y(p)$ versus $p \in [0,1]$, and the

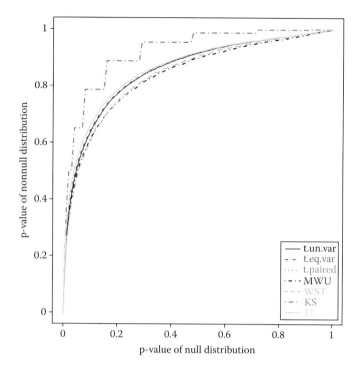

FIGURE 3.14
(See color insert.) P–P plot for comparisons among empirical power of seven tests for equality of means where $X \sim N(1, \sqrt{5})$, $Y \sim N(2,1)$ and the sample size is 25. The tests considered include the two-sample t-test with unpooled variances (t.un.var) or pooled variances (t.eq.var), the paired two-sample t-test (t.paired), the Mann–Whitney U-test (MWU), the Wilcoxon signed-rank test (WST), the Kolmogorov–Smirnov test (KS), and the empirical likelihood test (EL).

difference $p_X(q) - p_Y(q)$ versus q, respectively, where X corresponds to the standardized $\log \chi^2(v)$ variables and Y corresponds to the standard normal distribution. As the degrees of freedom of the chi-square distribution increase, it can be noted from both plots that the approximation improves.

Other modifications or extensions can be employed and chosen appropriately in terms of different circumstances. For example, in the verification of a normal assumption of data distribution, a P–P plot may be plotted in terms of an equivalent normal deviate, or instead of the difference $p_X(q) - p_Y(q)$ shown in Figure 3.16, one might plot the difference of two angle transforms.

3.4.4 Derivatives of Probability Plots

A variety of statistical procedures originate from the probability plotting method, and various graphical transforms stimulated by probability plotting have been advanced. For example, the well-known Kolmogorov–Smirnov statistic may be viewed, after the appropriate probability transform of the sample, as the maximum deviation from the 45° line on a uniform P–P plot (which for the uniform distribution on (0,1) is equivalent to a Q–Q or P–Q plot). As another example, Shapiro and Wilk (1965) developed statistical testing procedures for distributional hypotheses of the normal, uniform, and exponential distributions using complete or censored samples. This approach was based on the regression

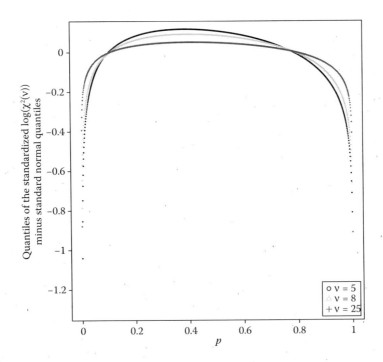

FIGURE 3.15
(See color insert.) Difference in quantiles of standardized $\log \chi^2(v)$ (v = 5, 8, 25) and the standard normal quantiles versus p.

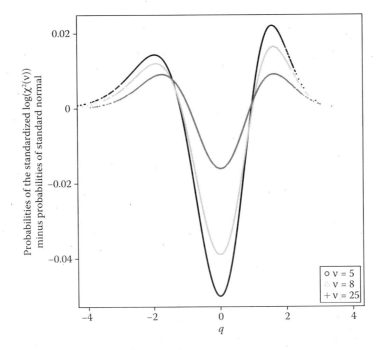

FIGURE 3.16
(See color insert.) Difference in probabilities of standardized $\log \chi^2(v)$ (v = 5, 8, 25) and the standard normal quantiles versus q.

of order statistics on expected values of standard order statistics in a Q–Q plot in order to generate test procedures for composite distributional hypotheses. The receiver operating characteristic (ROC) curve, which is a plot of sensitivities versus specificities, is a special case of a P–P plot. ROC curves are discussed in Chapter 8. Related plots are Lorenz curves and total time on test (TTT) curves.

3.5 Probability Plots as Informal Auxiliary Information to Inference

Probability plotting procedures can be usefully employed within complex objectives associated with the analysis of variance (ANOVA). The method of ANOVA was developed by Fisher (1925) and is a collection of statistical models used to model the differences between group means and their associated quantities, for example, variation among and between groups. It is typical in ANOVA modeling that many aspects and unanticipated characteristics of the same data require investigation. For instance, inference about main effects and interaction terms may be masked by the presence of outliers and violations of distributional assumptions. In practice, ANOVA is used heavily as a biomedical research tool. It provides a method for attributing components of the variance to a set of experimental conditions and random noise within each variance component as estimated through a set of mean squared error terms. It is important to provide statistical procedures for the simultaneous comparisons of the mean squares without narrowing the specification of objectives. Such procedures are termed *internal comparison* methods (e.g., see Wilk and Gnanadesikan 1961, 1964; Wilk et al. 1966). These procedures offer a statistical measure to assist in the assessment of relative magnitudes, which may be nonintuitive, particularly in large sample sizes. Furthermore, this procedure can provide perception into various inadequacies of the statistical models and is not overly influenced by some data-independent aspects, such as a necessity to pre-specify an error term (Wilk and Gnanadesikan 1968).

The principle of a probability plot, as a descriptive inference tool, is given by plotting the ordered sample values against some representative values from a presumed null distribution. For example, in a 2^k (k is the number of factors) experiment with a univariate response, a new sample of $2k - 1$ main effects and interactions can be obtained. The ordered values of these $2k - 1$–derived quantities may be plotted against representative values from a standard normal distribution. Under certain null statistical conditions, this will lead to a straight line passing through the origin. The slope of the line indicates the underlying error standard deviation. The plot allows us to distinguish the presence of real effects and the violation of distributional assumptions, or outliers, and of the heterogeneities of variance that result in distortions of the linear configuration of the plot. In addition, the plot provides a graphical summary in a simple and palatable fashion, focusing on the large effects and groupings among them.

In probability plotting, representative values involve both practical convenience and conceptual insight. Two conceptual categories may be considered: (1) The representative values are corresponding quantiles based on the reference distribution. The plots of the ordered sample values against the quantiles of the reference distribution corresponding to any of the fractions, that is, $(i-1/2)/k$, will not be very different unless very small sample sizes are involved. (2) The representative values are determined by the expected values of the standard order statistics from the reference distribution (Wilk and Gnanadesikan 1968). Note that, in general, the resulting configurations will be similar whether quantiles or expected value plotting positions are employed.

In straightforward cases, it is more convenient to employ quantiles instead of expected values, from both a computational and a conceptual standpoint. However, in more complex cases, for example, in the cases of independent unequal statistical components with different degrees of freedom or in the cases of dependent equal or unequal components that arise in ANOVA, the notion of an expected value can be well defined conceptually, while the meaning of the notion of a quantile may be unclear or even inapplicable.

This section reviews some probability plotting techniques, providing insight into the assessment of relative magnitudes, the adequacy of the statistical models, and so forth.

3.5.1 Specific Internal Comparison Probability Plotting Techniques

Various probability plotting techniques are available based on different orthogonal analyses of variance situations. The classification of orthogonal analysis of variance situations distinguishes univariate response scenarios from multivariate response scenarios, and for each of these gives three categories of decomposition of the treatment structure: all single degrees of freedom, all multiple but equal degrees of freedom, and the general mixed degrees of freedom case.

Full-normal and half-normal probability plotting methods are proposed for a univariate response with the decomposition of the treatment structure, each with single degrees of freedom. To illustrate, we consider data of the injection molding with 20 observations in a 2^8 fractional factorial design from Box et al. (1978). Figure 3.17 shows the full-normal Q–Q plot (left) and the half-normal Q–Q plot (right) for the injection molding data, produced as follows:

```
> # install.packages("FrF2")
> library(FrF2)
> data(BM93.e3.data, package="BsMD") # Injection Molding data.
> iMdat <- BM93.e3.data[1:16,2:10] # only original experiment
> # make data more user-friendly
> colnames(iMdat) <- c("MoldTemp","Moisture","HoldPress","CavityThick",
  "Boost Press",
+                      "CycleTime","GateSize","ScrewSpeed", "y")
> # a linear model with all main effects and 2-factor interactions
> iM.lm <- lm(y ~ (.)^2, data=iMdat)
>
> par(mar=c(3.2,3.2,2,2),mfrow=c(1,2))
> DanielPlot(iM.lm,code=TRUE,main="Normal Q-Q plot")
> DanielPlot(iM.lm,half=TRUE,code=TRUE,main="Half-normal Q-Q plot")
```

In particular, the full-normal plot gives the ordered effects plotted against the $(i–1/2)/k$ quantiles of the standard normal, while the half-normal plot shows the ordered absolute effects plotted against the $(i–1/2)/k$ quantiles of the half-normal distribution.

The normal Q–Q plot and the half-normal Q–Q plot, shown in Figure 3.17, suggest that the main effects of holding pressure (C) and booster pressure (E), as well as the interaction effect (AE) between mold temperature and booster pressure, are comparatively large, thus giving a strong indication of real effects against a background of a stable error configuration.

The use of half-normal plotting in two-level factorial experiments was suggested by Daniel (1959). From the null hypothesis viewpoint, the sign of the contrast is irrelevant, under which case half-normal plotting can be used, providing a more stable and focused display. However, when the actual signs of the individual or groups of contrasts are of interest, the full-normal plot should be employed. In addition, the full-normal plot assists in exhibiting

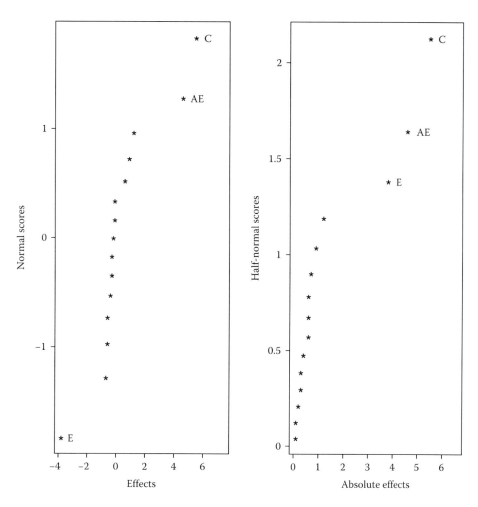

FIGURE 3.17
Full-normal plot (left) and half-normal plot (right) for the injection molding data from Box et al. (1978), where A
is the mold temperature factor, C is the holding pressure factor, and E is the booster pressure factor.

possible distributional peculiarities, when some of the contrasts reflect real experimental effects, which may be concealed when the distribution is folded. While the latter contingency may only arise rarely, it is suggested to include both full- and half-normal plots routinely in the analysis of 2^k experiments. For details, we refer the reader to Daniel (1959) and Wilk et al. (1962a, 1962b, 1963a).

For a univariate response with decomposition of the treatment structure of all v degrees of freedom, Wilk et al. (1962a, 1962b, 1963b) considered gamma plotting with the shape parameter $\eta = v/2$. Note that half-normal plotting on absolute contrasts is equivalent to gamma plotting of squared contrasts with the shape parameter $\eta = 1/2$. For a univariate response with decomposition of the treatment structure of mixed degrees of freedom, a technique of generalized probability plotting was proposed by Wilk et al. (1966), which consists of plotting the ordered ANOVA mean squares against representative values defined as expected values of appropriately conditioned order statistics of standardized mean squares.

In the multivariate single degree of freedom case, Wilk and Gnanadesikan (1961, 1964), as well as Wilk et al. (1962a, 1962b), proposed gamma plotting of generalized squared distances, that is, positive semidefinite quadratic forms in the elements of the contrast vectors, using estimated shape parameters from a collection of the smaller of these squared distances. For more details, we refer the reader to Wilk and Gnanadesikan (1968).

3.5.2 Residuals in Regression Analysis

In regression analysis, it has been traditional to base inferences on the mean squared error, that is, the sum of squares of residuals (observed-model estimates) from the fitted model divided by the degrees of freedom. The use of only this summary precludes the employment of one of the most sensitive and informative tools in regression studies, namely, plots of various kinds of individual residuals. Such plots may be used to check the adequacy of the model, the appropriateness of independent variables, the existence of outliers, the relevance of extraneous variables, and distributional peculiarities. One such plot, by no means the most important, is a probability plot of the residuals.

To illustrate, we revisit the Old Faithful geyser data described in Section 3.2. Figure 3.18 shows the full-normal Q–Q plot of standardized residuals by fitting a linear regression model of the eruption time on the waiting time. The full-normal Q–Q plot indicates that the residuals may deviate from the normal distribution. Note that there are formal tests for normality, such as the Kolmogorov–Smirnov test and the Shapiro–Wilk test, but these are not as flexible as the Q–Q plot. It should also be noted that residuals are not independent random variables, and thus subtly violate formal tests of normality. For smaller sample sizes, formal tests may lack the power to detect departures from normality, while with large sample sizes, even mild deviations from nonnormality may be detected, even though there would be little reason to abandon least squares because the effects of nonnormality are mitigated by large sample sizes.

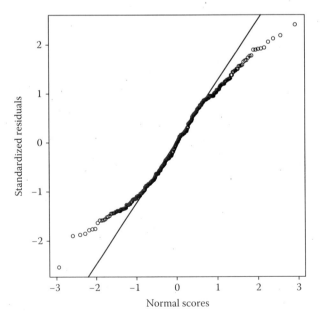

FIGURE 3.18
Full-normal plot of the standardized residuals for the Old Faithful geyser data.

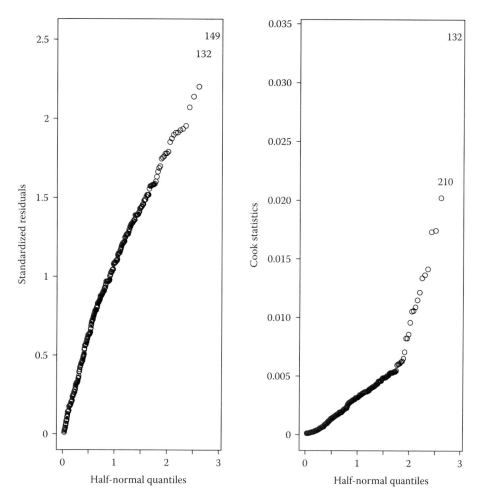

FIGURE 3.19
Half-normal plot of the standardized residuals (left) and Cook's distance (right) for the Old Faithful geyser data.

Moreover, data points with large residuals (outliers) or highly influential points that may distort the outcome and accuracy of a regression can be detected via probability plotting of related statistics such as residuals, Cook's distance, or leverage. Note that we are usually not looking for a linear relationship here since we do not necessarily expect a positive normal distribution for quantities such as Cook's distance. Instead, we are looking for outliers or highly influential points that will be apparent as points that diverge substantially from the rest of the data. Figure 3.19 shows the half-normal plot of corresponding standardized residuals of the Old Faithful geyser data in the left panel, while the right panel indicates the half-normal plot of Cook's distances. The observation 132 shows up clearly as unusual in both plots.

3.5.3 Other Applications

Other applications of probability plotting in the analysis of variance framework are the cases of collections of regression coefficients and residuals in multiway tables. Typically, these involve dealing with order statistics of correlated or singular random variables.

3.6 Heat Maps

The heat map is a graphical technique to represent data where colors and darkness are used to represent the individual values contained in a data matrix. The heat maps are often used to look for similarities between variables, for example, genes, and between samples. Heat maps can also be made from dissimilarity matrices, which are particularly useful when clustering patterns might not be easily visible in the data matrix, as with absolute correlation distance (van der Laan and Pollard 2003). Various color-coding schemes can be used to illustrate the heat map, with perceptual advantages and disadvantages for each. For example, rainbow color maps are often used, as humans can perceive more shades of color than they can of gray, and this would purportedly increase the amount of detail perceivable in the image. However, in many cases, rainbow color maps may make actual gradients less prominent and sometimes actually obscure detail rather than enhancing it, while grayscale or blackbody spectrum color maps can keep the natural perceptual ordering. In the microarray data analysis, the red–green color map is the most commonly used, ranging from pure green at the low end, through black in the middle, to pure red at the high end.

3.6.1 Visualization of Data in the Heat Map Manner

To identify patterns contained in data, rows and columns of the data are often ordered in heat maps, according to some set of values (e.g., row or column means) within the restrictions imposed by the dendrogram. A dendogram is a tree diagram (the Greek *dendro* "tree" + *gramma* "drawing"). Commonly, in the heat map context, row dendrograms display the distance (or similarity) between rows and which nodes each row belongs to as an output of the clustering calculation, whereas column dendrograms show the distance (or similarity) between the variables (the selected cell value columns). Clustering is often used to provide this ordering, by identifying groups of rows and columns of the data matrix or the dissimilarity matrix in terms of certain pre-specified dissimilarity measures and then arranging the groups so that the closest ones are adjacent. This ordering makes heat maps most effective; for example, groups of samples that have similar expression-level patterns and genes that are similar across samples can be identified.

Figure 3.20 presents a heat map of a microarray data matrix reflecting gene expression values in the control small interfering RNA (siRNA) transfection group treated with vehicle or androgens, where rows and columns are arranged according to separate hierarchical clustering of samples and genes.

We start by installing and loading the relevant package we need in R:

```
> # install.packages("gplots")   # only install it for the first time
> library(gplots)
```

The *gplots* package contains various R programming tools for plotting data. Here we show how to generate a smoothly varying set of colors, for example, *greenred* for the green-black-red color panel.

```
> cols = greenred(35)
```

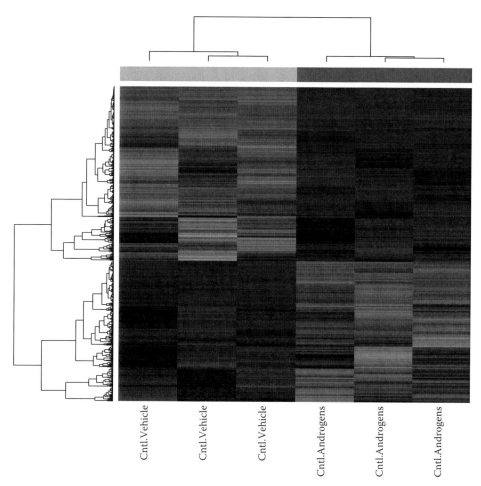

FIGURE 3.20
(See color insert.) Heat map generated from microarray data reflecting gene expression values in the control siRNA transfection group with two different treatments: vehicle or androgens.

It can be applied to colors used for the heat map, as shown in Figure 3.20. Here we used the *heatmap.2* function, which provides a number of extensions to the standard R *heatmap* function, to produce the heat map, specifying 1 – correlation as the dissimilarity measures.

```
> # specify the dissimilarity function
> dist2 <- function(x){as.dist(1-cor(t(x), method="pearson"))}
>
> # use colors to annotate data columns by the treatment group (trt.grp)
> supervised.col=as.character(factor(trt.grp,labels=c("red","green")))
>
> # produce the heat map use the pre-specified greenred colorpanel,
> # i.e. col=cols
> heatmap.2(as.matrix(dat), distfun=dist2, col=cols,
+           ColSideColors=supervised.col,
+           scale="row", symkey=FALSE,
```

```
+            key=FALSE, # the color key can be turned on setting key=TRUE
+            density.info="none", trace="none", cexRow=0.45, cexCol=0.85,
+            labRow=FALSE, margins=c(8,5))
```

The heat map shown in Figure 3.20 clearly characterizes two treatment groups of biolog-ical replicates that have been treated with vehicle or androgens, and visibly shows andro-gen downregulated genes and androgen upregulated genes by color blocks.

3.6.2 Graphical Comparisons of Statistical Tests

In addition to the use of pattern identification in data, heat maps can be used for clear visualization of power comparisons for various tests across various significance levels or based on data with different sample sizes.

To illustrate this usage, we reconsider the power comparison of seven tests for equal-ity of population means described in Chapters 5 and 6, including the two-sample t-test with unpooled variances or pooled variances, the paired two-sample t-test, the Mann–Whitney U-test, the Wilcoxon signed-rank test, the Kolmogorov–Smirnov test, and the empirical likelihood test. Details regarding these tests can be found in subsequent chapters. The empirical powers are calculated for all tests with various sample sizes $n = 10, 25, 50, 75, 100$, and 200. The powers are compared at the 0.05 significance level using the Monte Carlo (MC) technique, simulating data from the normal distribution with mean 1, standard deviation $\sqrt{5}$, and the normal distribution with mean 2, standard deviation 1, respectively.

The MC technique, a well-known approach for obtaining accurate approximations to the distribution of the test statistics, is employed to obtain the empirical powers. By simulating data from the underlying data distribution of interest, that is, $X \sim N(1,\sqrt{5})$, $Y \sim N(2,1)$ in the current considered scenario, for a relatively large number of MC repetitions, for example, MC = 10,000, the distribution of test statistics can be well approximated under the nonnull considered. Following the decision rule for the test procedures, the MC powers can be calculated as the proportion of rejections of the null hypothesis in MC repetitions. (The MC strategy to calculate critical values, p-values, and powers of statistical tests is further explained in Chapter 16.) The following codes illustrate the use of the MC method for the two-sample t-test with pooled variances (denoted as t.eq.var) and the empirical likelihood test (EL) based on data with a sample size 25 at the 0.05 significance level in the above-mentioned scenario, that is, $X \sim N(1,\sqrt{5})$, $Y \sim N(2,1)$:

```
> n<-25
> MC<-10000
> alpha<-0.05
> powers.indx<-sapply(1:MC,function(b){
+    set.seed(b)
+    x<-rnorm(n,1,sqrt(5))
+    y<-rnorm(n,2,1)
+
+    # indicator or rejection for t.test with pooled variances
+    t.reject<-t.test(x,y,var.equal=TRUE)$p.value<alpha
+
+    # indicator or rejection for EL test
+    EL.reject<-EL.means(x,y)$p.value<alpha
+    return(c(t.reject,EL.reject))
```

```
+ })
> # obtain powers as the proportion of rejections
> powers<-apply(powers.indx,1,mean)
> names(powers)<-c("t.eq.var","EL")
```

For clarification and better presentation, especially when the number of tests to be compared is large and the number of sample sizes considered is large, the heat map can be employed to compare statistical powers. Figure 3.21 presents a heat map demonstrating comparisons among the empirical powers of the tests described above, using a grayscale spectrum color map to show the natural perceptual ordering of empirical powers.

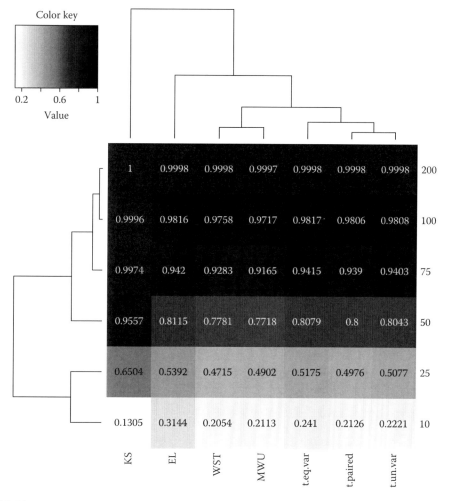

FIGURE 3.21
(See color insert.) Grayscale heat map for comparisons among the empirical powers of several tests for equality of means where $X \sim N(1,\sqrt{5})$, $Y \sim N(2,1)$ with various sample sizes ($n = 10, 25, 50, 75, 100, 200$) at the 0.05 significance level. The tests considered include the two-sample t-test with unpooled variances (t.un.var) or pooled variances (t.eq.var), the paired two-sample t-test (t.paired), the Mann–Whitney U-test (MWU), the Wilcoxon signed-rank test (WST), the Kolmogorov–Smirnov test (KS) and the empirical likelihood test (EL).

This heat map manifests itself with comparisons of powers, with column names presenting test procedures considered and row names presenting sample sizes. A color key shown in the left upper corner demonstrates the one-to-one correspondence between the grayness and the numerical value, where the black color represents large values of powers and the white color characterizes smaller values of powers. It can be noted that the Kolmogorov–Smirnov test has a great power property, with powers greater than 0.95 starting from the sample size 50. The empirical likelihood test works comparatively well in the case of very small sample sizes, that is, $n = 10$. Note that the Kolmogorov–Smirnov test, which is a test for the equality of two one-dimensional (1D) continuous probability distributions and can compare distributions that do not even have a mean, is not exactly appropriate here. For example, we consider the situation where two samples are from different underlying distributions, both of them with equal means, for example, $X \sim N(1,1)$, $Y \sim \exp(1)$. This scenario depicts a situation where the Kolmogorov–Smirnov test fails in the Type I error control, while other tests for equality of means, such as the empirical likelihood test, have the corresponding to the null hypothesis, $EX = EY$, Type I error under control.

Moreover, with the addition of the dendrogram, the heat map can aid in clustering test procedures and sample sizes under investigation. As can be seen in Figure 3.21, the clustering result of test procedures is shown at the top side of the heat map; a dendrogram on the left side of the heat map clusters the sample sizes considered. It can easily tell how similar various tests and sample sizes considered are. As in the hierarchical clustering method, different numbers of clusters or different height cutoff values specified will lead to different clustering results. For example, we consider two clusters for sample sizes and test procedures. Considering all seven tests in general, sample sizes 10 and 25 corresponding to comparatively low powers are well separated from the other sample sizes. Considering all sample sizes in general, the seven tests can be divided into two groups: one containing the Kolmogorov–Smirnov test, which leads to comparatively high powers, and the remaining six tests fall in the other group. Note that instead of considering a variety of sample sizes at a pre-specified significance level, the performance of difference tests at various significance levels can be considered and compared visually using the heat map method with a fixed sample size, as the case studied in Figure 3.14.

In general, heat maps are very useful in visualization of data, with great application to compare powers when a large number of methods and sample sizes or significance levels are of interest.

3.7 Concluding Remarks

The graphical methods presented in this chapter are informal tools for the statistical analysis of data and may be used for summarization and examination of the underlying data structure. While using statistical assumptions and models to generate the graphical display or for the analysis of the given data using empirical plots, the methods do not guarantee the interpretation independent of a judgment of the assumption adequacy. Thus, these techniques have many of the desirable characteristics of data-analyzing methodology as discussed by Tukey and Wilk (1966). Note that most of the approaches discussed in the earlier sections of this chapter can be implemented routinely in data analysis.

3.8 Supplement

1. Gnanadesikan and Lee (1970) proposed probability plotting methods for two summary statistics derived from equal degree of freedom sums of product matrices. This approach is useful for graphical internal comparisons of the magnitudes of the sums of product matrices. There are various possible applications with multiresponse data, including the simultaneous assessment of all the main effects, or of all the interactions of the same order, in a factorial experiment with $m \geq 3$ levels for each factor, and the comparison of several observed covariance matrices. For example, consider within-group covariance matrices in a multiresponse analysis of variance or discriminant analysis, each based on the same number of replicate observations. The authors illustrated the applications of the method to three sets of data. The first set simulates the results of a 30-cell experiment with four replications per cell based on computer-generated trivariate normal data. The second set of data originates from an experiment focused on identifying persons according to speech spectrograms of their utterances of specific words. The third example, Monte Carlo data, employs independent sets of three random observations, each generated from a nonspherical quadrivariate normal distribution, where 20 sums of product matrices were obtained, that is, $p = 4$, $v = 3$, and $k = 20$.

2. Anscombe (1973) discussed the importance of the use of ordinary scatterplots and "triple" scatterplots in regression analysis. The author illustrated the use of graphical displays by four fictitious data sets, each consisting of 11 (x, y) pairs.

3. Graphical methods have been widely applied to assess the validity of a probability model and for estimating location and scale parameters. Consider data of independent observations $Y_1, \ldots, Y_n$ for a continuous random variable Y with a distribution function that is believed to have some particular form $F((y - \mu)/\sigma)$. Typically, the ordered sample values, $Y_{(1)} \leq Y_{(2)} \leq \ldots \leq Y_{(n)}$, are plotted against quantities $F^{-1}(\xi_i)$, where $\xi_i = F((y_{(i)} - \mu)/\sigma)$, to display a fit between the theoretical distribution and the empirical distribution of Y. However, the preferred choices of plotting positions ξ_i should vary with the form of the probability model and reflect the predominant aim of interest, the model validation, or the parameter estimation. Barnett (1975) investigated probability plotting estimators in terms of the estimation problem with known properties of estimates of expected values of order statistics. The author also presented some general observations on biased estimates of the expected value of order statistics using the minimum mean squared error.

4. Doksum and Sievers (1976) considered simple graphical statistical methods that can assist in making conclusions regarding how two populations, say X and Y, are different in the context of their distributional properties. The problem was analyzed using a response function $\Delta(X)$ with its property that $X + \Delta(X)$ has the same distribution as Y. The authors considered both general and parametric models for the response function computed by employing independent samples from two populations. Doksum and Sievers (1976) proposed the method based on the simultaneous confidence band. In statistical terms, evaluating a function $f(x)$ using

its point estimator $\hat{f}(x)$, we can define a simultaneous confidence band $\hat{f}(x) \pm \omega(x)$ with coverage probability $1 - \alpha$ that satisfies the following condition:

$$\Pr\left\{\hat{f}(x) - \omega(x) \leq f(x) \leq \hat{f}(x) + \omega(x) \text{ for all } x\right\} = 1 - \alpha$$

The authors illustrated the method with the data from an experiment designed to study undesirable effects of ozone, one of the components of California smog. One group of 22 seventy-day-old rats were kept in an ozone environment for 7 days and their weight gains Y_i noted. Another group of 23 similar rats of the same age were kept in an ozone-free environment for 7 days and their weight gains x noted.

5. Fienberg (1979) outlined some of the highlights in the historical development of statistical graphics and some recent advances in the use of graphical methods for statistical analysis. The author introduced a simple taxonomy that can be used to characterize the current use of graphical methods, which can be used to describe the evolution of the use of graphics in some major statistical and related scientific journals.

6. To summarize and objectively evaluate the information contained in probability plots, the use of the correlation coefficient is suggested in Looney and Gulledge (1985). The authors examined the use of the Pearson product–moment correlation coefficient as a technique for constructing a test statistic based on a normal probability plot. Using empirical sampling methods, the authors generated the null distribution for the normal distribution for several commonly used plotting positions, and concluded that use of the plotting position (a list of the fractions of values at or below each quantity given a set of ordered quantities) $p_i = (i - 0.375)/(n + 0.25)$, $i = 1, ..., n$, yields a competitive regression-type test of fit for normality.

7. Wainer (1990) reviewed and examined the importance and different aspects of fundamental graphical tools, as well as areas of current and future graphical concerns. The authors focused on the following aspects: (1) how fundamental graphic tools have become integral tools for the scientist, (2) three instances where modern views of graphics have remained unchanged since Playfair's time, and (3) one area where there has been new innovations.

8. Sawitzki (1994) presented a survey of some well-known and recent proposals to present a distribution drawn on the line, based on sample data. The authors claimed that a diagnostic plot is only as good as the hard statistical theory that is supporting it. Similarly, Cook and Weisberg (1999) argued in detail that useful graphs must have a context induced by associated theory, and that a graph without the well-understood statistical context is hardly worth drawing.

9. Kernel smoothing provides a simple way to display data structures without parametric assumptions on data distributions. It can be applied to many important curve testing problems, such as the evaluation of probability density functions, spectral densities, and hazard rate functions. For example, the R command *density* computes kernel density estimates for univariate observations. For details regarding kernel smoothing, we refer the reader to Wand and Jones (1994). Kernel methods also may be a way to smooth more jagged empirical approaches, such as the histogram and EDF plots.

10. In a dynamite plot, the height of a bar shows the mean, and the vertical line on top of it denotes the standard deviation (or standard error). It is sometimes used to present data. However, there is a lot of criticism regarding its utility in data presentation, and more intelligible ways are suggested, such as a boxplot. For example, dynamite plots hide the raw data and typically only show one-sided confidence intervals; the confidence interval is usually assumed to be symmetric, and it masks the actual range of the data. For more details, we refer the reader to Drummond and Vowler (2011).

11. Chen et al. (2007) noted that visualization of the data is an essential step in the data analysis. The authors reviewed modern data visualization methods from both theoretical and practical aspects, for example, mosaic plots, parallel coordinate plots, and linked views. Various graphical methods for particular areas of statistics, for example, Bayesian analysis, genomic data, and cluster analysis, are also presented.

12. Klemelä (2009) noted that it is important to incorporate visualization tools, for example, smoothing, into the density estimation. The author depicted a new look at some classical visualization tools and at cluster analysis.

13. Fu and Wang (2012) provided and demonstrated applications of various statistical graphical tools for analyzing water quality data.

14. To recognize patterns in temporal point data, a TT-plot can be used. A TT-plot transforms the 3D data consisting of two spatial and one temporal axis to a 2D representation and reduces the spatial component to an interevent distance matrix, introducing a second time axis by creating a matrix of spatial distances for every time point to all other time points.

4

A Brief Ode to Parametric Likelihood

J. Bertrand said it this way: "Give me four parameters and I shall describe an elephant; with five, it will wave its trunk."

Le Cam (1990)

4.1 Introduction

One of the traditional instruments used in medical experiments and drug development is the testing of statistical hypotheses based on the *t*-test statistic or its different modifications. Despite the fact that these tests are straightforward with respect to their applications in clinical trials, it should be noted that there has been much literature on the criticism of *t*-test-type statistical tools. One major issue that has been widely recognized is the significant loss of efficiency of these procedures under nonnormal distributional assumptions. The legitimacy of *t*-test-type procedures also comes into question in the context of inflated Type I errors seen when data distributions differ from normal and the number of observations is fixed. This can pose serious problems when data based on biomarker measurements are available for statistical testing. The recent biostatistical literature has well addressed the arguments that show the values of biomarker measurements tend to follow skewed distributions, for example, a lognormal distribution (Limpert et al. 2001). Hence, the use of *t*-test-type techniques in this setting is suboptimal, and is accompanied by significant difficulties in controlling the corresponding Type I error.

Consider the following example, based on data from a study evaluating biomarkers related to atherosclerotic coronary heart disease (Schisterman et al. 2001): A cross-sectional population-based sample of randomly selected residents (ages 35–79) of Erie and Niagara Counties of the State of New York was the focus of this experiment. The New York State Department of Motor Vehicles driver's license rolls were employed as the sampling frame for adults between the ages of 35 and 65, whereas the elderly sample (ages >65–79) was randomly selected from the Health Care Financing Administration database. Participants provided a 12-hour fasting blood specimen for biochemical analysis at baseline, and a number of characteristics were evaluated from fresh blood samples. Samples presented 50 measurements (mg/dl) of the biomarker high-density lipoprotein (HDL) cholesterol obtained from healthy patients. These measurements were divided into two groups: *X* and *Y*. The following R code shows the input of the data and the construction of histograms of the data, as seen in Figure 4.1.

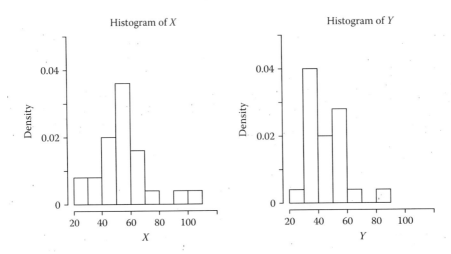

FIGURE 4.1
R data analysis output based on measurements of the HDL cholesterol levels in healthy individuals.

```
> X<-c(61.6,96.8,50.6,37.4,22.0,52.8,41.8,61.6,46.2,55.0,57.2,48.4,105.6,
  55.0,35.2,48.4,63.8,41.8,59.4,26.4,70.4,57.2,59.4,63.8,50.6)
> Y<-c(46.2,33.0,48.4,37.4,57.2,57.2,22.0,81.4,57.2,35.2,30.8,48.4,55.0,
  44.0,50.6,33.0,39.6,60.2,55.0,50.6,35.2,46.2,33.0,37.4,33.0)
> a<-min(c(X,Y))-10
> b<-max(c(X,Y))+20
> par(pty="s",mfrow=c(1,2),mar=c(1,4,0,1))
> hist(X,xlim=c(a,b),ylim=c(0,0.045),freq=FALSE)
> hist(Y,xlim=c(a,b),ylim=c(0,0.045),freq=FALSE)
```

Although one can reasonably expect the samples to be from the same population, the *t*-test result shows a significant difference of their distributions, as demonstrated below via the use of the function t.test in R.

```
> t.test(X,Y)
        Welch Two Sample t-test
data: X and Y
t = 2.0655, df = 43.859, p-value = 0.04482
alternative hypothesis: true difference in means is not equal to 0
95 percent confidence interval:
 0.2254395 18.4305605
sample estimates:
mean of x mean of y
 54.736 45.408
```

Perhaps, in order to investigate reasons for this incorrect output of the *t*-test, the following issues should be taken into account:

The histograms displayed in Figure 4.1 indicate that the distributions of the variables X and Y appear skewed. In a nonasymptotic context, when the sample sizes are relatively small, one can show that the *t*-test statistic is a product of likelihood ratio–type considerations, based on normally distributed observations (Lehmann and Romano 2006). That is, the *t*-test is a parametric test, and the normality assumption seems to be violated in this example.

Thus, in many settings, it may be reasonable to propose an approach for developing statistical tests, attending to data distributions, in order to provide procedures that are as efficient as the *t*-test based on normally distributed observations. Toward this end, the likelihood methodology can be employed.

The likelihood methodology is addressed extensively in the literature. There are a multitude of books that consider different likelihood-based methods and their applications to testing statistical hypotheses. In this chapter, we briefly introduce several principles and aspects of tests based on the likelihood ratio statistic.

4.2 Likelihood Ratio Test and Its Optimality

Let us start by first outlining the likelihood principle. When the forms of data distributions are assumed to be known, the likelihood principle is a central tenet for developing powerful statistical inference tools for use in clinical experiments. The *likelihood method*, or simply the *likelihood*, is arguably the most important concept for inference in parametric modeling when the underlying data are subject to various assumed stochastic mechanisms and restrictions related to medical and epidemiological studies; for example, in the context of the analysis of survival data, one would assume potentially right-skewed and censored data. Likelihood-based testing was first proposed and formulated in a series of foundational papers published in the period of 1928–1938 by Jerzy Neyman and Egon Pearson (1928, 1933, 1938). In 1928, the authors introduced the generalized likelihood ratio test and its association with chi-square statistics. Five years later, the Neyman–Pearson lemma was introduced, showing the optimality of the likelihood ratio test. These seminal works provided us with the familiar notions of simple and composite hypotheses and errors of the first and second kind, thus defining formal decision-making rules for testing. Without loss of generality, the principle idea of the proof of the Neyman–Pearson lemma can be shown by using the trivial inequality

$$(A - B)(I\{A \ge B\} - \delta) \ge 0, \tag{4.1}$$

for all A, B, where $\delta \in [0,1]$ and $I\{\cdot\}$ denotes the indicator function. For example, suppose we would like to classify independent identically distributed (i.i.d.) biomarker measurements $\{X_i, i = 1, \ldots, n\}$ corresponding to hypotheses of the following form: H_0: X_1 is from a density function f_0 versus H_1: X_1 is from a density function f_1. In this context, to construct the likelihood ratio test statistic, we should consider the ratio between the joint density function of $\{X_1, \ldots, X_n\}$ obtained under H_1 and the joint density function of $\{X_1, \ldots, X_n\}$ obtained under H_0, and then define $\prod_{i=1}^{n} f_1(X_i) / \prod_{i=1}^{n} f_0(X_i)$ as the likelihood ratio. In this case, the likelihood ratio test is uniformly most powerful. This proposition directly follows from the expected value under H_0 of the inequality (4.1), where we define $A = \prod_{i=1}^{n} f_1(X_i)/f_0(X_i)$, B to be a test threshold (i.e., the likelihood ratio test rejects H_0 if and only if $L \ge B$) and δ is assumed to represent any decision rule based on $\{X_i, i = 1, \ldots, n\}$. The appendix and Section 7.7.1 contain details of the proof. This simple proof technique was used to show optimal aspects of different statistical decision-making policies, based on the likelihood ratio concept applied in clinical experiments (Vexler and Wu 2009; Vexler et al. 2010b; Vexler and Gurevich 2011; Vexler and Tarima 2011).

4.3 Likelihood Ratio Based on the Likelihood Ratio Test Statistic Is the Likelihood Ratio Test Statistic

The Neyman–Pearson testing concept, given by fixing the probability of a Type I error, has come under some criticism by epidemiologists and others. One of the critical points is the importance of paying attention to Type II errors. For example, Freiman et al. (1978) pointed out the results of 71 clinical trials that reported no "significant" differences between the compared treatments. The authors found that in the great majority of these trials, the strong effects of new treatment were reasonable. It was argued that the investigators in these trials failed to reject the null hypothesis when it appeared that the alternative hypothesis was more likely the underlying truth, which probably resulted in an increase in Type II errors. In the context of likelihood ratio–based tests, we present the following result that demonstrates an association between the probabilities of Type I and II errors.

Suppose we would like to test for H_0 versus H_1, employing the likelihood ratio $L = f_{H_1}(D)/f_{H_0}(D)$ based on data D, where f_H defines a density function that corresponds to the data distribution under the hypothesis H. Say, for simplicity, we reject H_0 if $L > C$, where C is a presumed threshold. In this case, we can then show that

$$f_{H_1}^L(u) = u\, f_{H_0}^L(u),\tag{4.2}$$

where $f_H^L(u)$ is the density function of the test statistic L under the hypothesis H and $u > 0$. Details of the proof of this fact are shown in the appendix. Thus, we can obtain the probability of a Type II error in the form of

$$\Pr\left\{\text{the test does not reject } H_0 \,|\, H_1 \text{ is true}\right\} = \Pr\left\{L \le C \,|\, H_1 \text{ is true}\right\} = \int_0^C f_{H_1}^L(u)\,du = \int_0^C u f_{H_0}^L(u)\,du.$$

Now, if in order to control the Type I error the density function $f_{H_0}^L(u)$ is assumed to be known, then the probability of the Type II error can be easily computed.

The likelihood ratio property $f_{H_1}^L(u)/f_{H_0}^L(u) = u$ can be applied to solve different issues related to performing the likelihood ratio test. For example, in terms of the bias of the test, one can request to find a value of the threshold C that maximizes

$$\Pr\{\text{the test rejects } H_0 | H_1 \text{ is true}\} - \Pr\{\text{the test rejects } H_0 | H_0 \text{ is true}\},$$

where the probability $\Pr\{\text{the test rejects } H_0 | H_1 \text{ is true}\}$ depicts the power of the test. This equation can be expressed as

$$\Pr\left\{L > C \,|\, H_1 \text{ is true}\right\} - \Pr\left\{L > C \,|\, H_0 \text{ is true}\right\} = \left(1 - \int_0^C f_{H_1}^L(u)\,du\right) - \left(1 - \int_0^C f_{H_0}^L(u)\,du\right).$$

Set the derivative of the above formula equal to zero and solve the equation:

$$\frac{d}{dC}\left[\left(1 - \int_0^C f_{H_1}^L(u)\,du\right) - \left(1 - \int_0^C f_{H_0}^L(u)\,du\right)\right] = -f_{H_1}^L(C) + f_{H_0}^L(C) = 0.$$

By virtue of the property (4.2), this implies $-C f_{H_0}^L(C) + f_{H_0}^L(C) = 0$ and then $C = 1$, which provides the maximum discrimination between the power and the probability of the Type I error in the likelihood ratio test.

In other words, the interesting fact is that the likelihood ratio $f_{H_1}^L / f_{H_0}^L$ based on the likelihood ratio $L = f_{H_1}/f_{H_0}$ comes to be the likelihood ratio, that is, $f_{H_1}^L(L)/f_{H_0}^L(L) = L$. Interpretations of this statement in terms of information we leave to the reader's imagination.

4.4 Maximum Likelihood: Is It the Likelihood?

Various real-world data problems require considerations of statistical hypotheses with structures that depend on unknown parameters. In this case, the maximum likelihood method proposes to approximate the most powerful likelihood ratio test, employing a proportion of the maximum likelihoods, where the maximizations are over values of the unknown parameters belonging to distributions of observations under the corresponding null and alternative hypotheses. We shall assume the existence of essential maximum likelihood estimators. The influential Wilks' theorem provides the basic rationale as to why the maximum likelihood ratio approach has had tremendous success in statistical applications (Wilks 1938). Wilks showed that under regularity conditions (see the appendix for details), asymptotic null distributions of maximum likelihood ratio test statistics are independent of the nuisance parameters. That is, the Type I error rate in the maximum likelihood ratio tests can be controlled asymptotically, and approximations to the corresponding p-values can be computed.

Thus, if certain key assumptions are met, one can show that parametric likelihood methods are very powerful and efficient statistical tools. We should emphasize that the role of the discovery of the likelihood ratio methodology in statistical developments can be compared to the development of the assembly line technique of mass production. The likelihood ratio principle gives clear instructions and technique manuals on how to construct efficient statistical decision rules in various complex problems related to clinical experiments. For example, Vexler et al. (2011c) developed a likelihood ratio type test for comparing populations based on incomplete longitudinal data subject to instrumental limitations.

Although many statistical publications continue to contribute to the likelihood paradigm and are very important in the statistical discipline (an excellent account can be found in Lehmann and Romano 2006), several significant questions naturally arise about the maximum likelihood approach's general applicability. Conceptually, there is an issue specific to classifying maximum likelihoods in terms of likelihoods that are given by joint density (or probability) functions based on data. Integrated likelihood functions, with respect to their arguments related to data points, are equal to 1, whereas accordingly integrated maximum likelihood functions often have values that are indefinite. Thus, while likelihoods present full information regarding the data, the maximum likelihoods might lose information conditional on the observed data. Consider the below simple example.

Suppose we observe X_1, which is assumed to be from a normal distribution $N(\mu, 1)$ with mean parameter μ. In this case, the likelihood has the form $(2\pi)^{-0.5} \exp(-(X_1 - \mu)^2/2)$ and, correspondingly, $\int (2\pi)^{-0.5} \exp(-(X_1 - \mu)^2/2) dX_1 = 1$, whereas the maximum likelihood, that is, the likelihood evaluated at estimated μ, $\hat{\mu} = X_1$, is $(2\pi)^{-0.5}$, which clearly does not represent the data and is not a proper density. This demonstrates that since the Neyman–Pearson lemma is fundamentally founded on the use of the density-based constitutions of likelihood ratios, maximum likelihood ratios cannot be optimal in general. That is, the likelihood ratio principle is generally not robust when the hypothesis tests have corresponding nuisance parameters to consider, for example, testing a hypothesized mean given an unknown variance.

An additional inherent difficulty of the likelihood ratio test occurs when a clinical experiment is associated with an infinite-dimensional problem and the number of unknown parameters is relatively large. In this case, Wilks' theorem should be reevaluated, and nonparametric approaches should be considered in the contexts of reasonable alternatives to the parametric likelihood methodology (Fan et al. 2001).

The ideas of likelihood and maximum likelihood ratio testing may not be fiducial and applicable in general nonparametric function estimation/testing settings. It is also well known that when key assumptions are not met, parametric approaches may be suboptimal or biased compared to their robust counterparts across the many features of statistical inferences. For example, in a biomedical application, Ghosh (1995) proved that the maximum likelihood estimators for the Rasch model are inconsistent, as the number of nuisance parameters increases to infinity (Rasch models are often employed in clinical trials that deal with psychological measurements, e.g., abilities, attitudes, and personality traits). Due to the structure of likelihood functions based on products of densities, or conditional density functions, relatively insignificant errors in classifications of data distributions can lead to vital problems related to the applications of likelihood ratio–type tests (Gurevich and Vexler 2010). Moreover, one can note that given the wide variety and complex nature of biomedical data (e.g., incomplete data subject to instrumental limitations or complex correlation structures), parametric assumptions are rarely satisfied. The respective formal tests are complicated or oftentimes not readily available.

Example 4.1

Assume that a sample of i.i.d. measurements $X_1, X_2, ..., X_n$ follow an exponential distribution with the rate parameter λ, that is, $X_1, ..., X_n \sim f(x) = \lambda \exp(-\lambda x)$. We then describe the maximum likelihood ratio test statistic for the composite hypothesis $H_0: \lambda = 1$ versus $H_1: \lambda \neq 1$. The log-likelihood function is

$$l(\lambda) = l(\lambda; X_1, X_2, ..., X_n) = \sum_{i=1}^{n} \log f(X_i) = n\log\lambda - \lambda \sum_{i=1}^{n} X_i.$$

To calculate the maximum likelihood estimation, we solve the equation $\dfrac{dl(\lambda)}{d\lambda} = \dfrac{n}{\lambda} - \sum_{i=1}^{n} X_i = 0$. The maximum likelihood estimator of λ is $\hat{\lambda} = n \Big/ \sum_{i=1}^{n} X_i = \bar{X}^{-1}$.

Therefore, the likelihood ratio test statistic is

$$\Lambda = 2[l(\hat{\lambda}) - l(1)] = 2n[-\log(\bar{X}) - 1 + \bar{X}].$$

The distribution of Λ under H_0 is approximately χ_1^2 and the 95% critical value is $\chi_{1,0.95}^2 = 3.84$. We reject H_0 if $\Lambda > 3.84$ at the 0.05 significance level.

4.4.1 Reconsideration of Data Example

Let's revisit the HDL data shown in Section 4.1 and Figure 4.1; we would like to test $H_0: \mu_1 = \mu_2$ versus $H_1: \mu_1 \neq \mu_2$. Note that oftentimes measurements related to biological processes follow a lognormal distribution (see Section 1.5 of Chapter 1). Based on the Shapiro–Wilk test for normality, the X deviates from the normal distribution, while the hypotheses that the logarithm-transformed X and Y follow normal distributions are not rejected. Therefore, we conduct the maximum likelihood ratio test based on $X_i^* = \log(X_i)$, $i = 1, ..., n$, and $Y_j^* = \log(Y_j)$, $j = 1, ..., m$.

Under the null hypothesis, the log-likelihood function is

$$\log L_0(\mu, \sigma_1^2, \sigma_2^2) = -\frac{n+m}{2}\log(2\pi) - \frac{n}{2}\log(\sigma_1^2) - \frac{m}{2}\log(\sigma_2^2) - \frac{\sum_{i=1}^{n}(X_i^* - \mu)^2}{2\sigma_1^2} - \frac{\sum_{j=1}^{m}(Y_j^* - \mu)^2}{2\sigma_2^2}.$$

Then under the null hypothesis, the maximum likelihood estimators of μ, σ_1^2 and σ_2^2 can be easily found to maximize $\log L_0$. Therefore, the maximum log-likelihood under H_0 is $\max_{\mu, \sigma_1^2, \sigma_2^2} L_0\left(\mu, \sigma_1^2, \sigma_2^2\right)$.

Under the alternative hypothesis, the maximum log-likelihood function is

$$\log L_1(\hat{\sigma}_1^2, \hat{\sigma}_2^2) = -\frac{n+m}{2}\log(2\pi) - \frac{n}{2}\log(\hat{\sigma}_1^2) - \frac{m}{2}\log(\hat{\sigma}_2^2) - \frac{n+m}{2}.$$

The distribution of the maximum log-likelihood ratio statistic, which has the form of $2\log L_1(\hat{\sigma}_1^2, \hat{\sigma}_2^2) - 2\log \log L_0(\mu, \sigma_1^2, \sigma_2^2)$, under H_0 is approximately χ_1^2 and $\chi_{1,0.95}^2 = 3.84$. In this case, the maximum likelihood ratio statistic has the value of 3.086, that is less than the critical value 3.84, and therefore we fail to reject H_0 at the 0.05 significance level.

The R code for implementation is presented below.

```
> shapiro.test(X)
        Shapiro-Wilk normality test

data: X
W = 0.9091, p-value = 0.02916
> shapiro.test(Y)
        Shapiro-Wilk normality test

data: Y
W = 0.9471, p-value = 0.2158

>
> shapiro.test(log(X))
        Shapiro-Wilk normality test

data: log(X)
W = 0.9427, p-value = 0.1711
> shapiro.test(log(Y))
        Shapiro-Wilk normality test

data: log(Y)
W = 0.972, p-value = 0.6954

> # logarithm of the normal density function
> log.pdf<-function(xx,mu,sigma2) -log(sqrt(2*pi))-(xx-mu)^2/(2*sigma2)
>
> get.MLR<-function(x,y){
+    # likelihood ratio under H1
+    logL.H1<-sum(log.pdf(x,mean(x),mean((x-mean(x))^2)))+sum(log.
        pdf(y,mean(y),mean((y-mean(y))^2)))
```

```
+
+    # likelihood ratio under H0
+    get.L0<-function(par,x,y){
+      mu<-par[1]
+      sigma2.x<-par[2]
+      sigma2.y<-par[3]
+      -(sum(log.pdf(x,mu,sigma2.x))+sum(log.pdf(y,mu,sigma2.y)))
+    }
+    obj.H0<-optim(c(100,50,50),get.L0,x=x,y=y)
+
+    # maximum likelihood ratio statistic
+    Lambda<-2*logL.H1/(-obj.H0$value)
+    cat(paste0("The maximum likelihood ratio statistic is",
+      round(Lambda,3),"\n"))
+    cat(paste0("The decision rule is that we ",ifelse(Lambda>qchisq(0.95,
+      df=1),"reject H_0","fail to reject H_0")),"\n")
+    return(Lambda)
+ }
>
>
> get.MLR(x=log(X),y=log(Y))
The maximum likelihood ratio statistic is 3.086
The decision rule is that we fail to reject H_0
[1] 3.086216
```

4.5 Supplement

The theoretical and applied literature has extensively addressed various statistical like-lihood ratio–type procedures. We outline several publications in which health-related researchers may be interested.

1. Barlow (1968) considered likelihood ratio tests for some geometrically restricted families of distributions. For example, define

$$\mathbf{F}_0 = \{F \,|\, F(0) = 0 \text{ and } -\log[1 - F(x)]x^{-1} \text{ nondecreasing in } x \geq 0\}.$$

Then $\mathbf{F}_0$ is known as the increasing failure rate average (IFRA) family of distribu-tions. These distributions are very important in the theoretical parts of reliability. Nonetheless, the family is nonparametric and there is no sigma-finite measure relative to which all $F \in \mathbf{F}_0$ are absolutely continuous. Thus, the maximum likeli-hood estimate concept does not suffice. Let $F_1, F_2 \in \mathbf{F}$ and let $f(\cdot\,; F_1, F_2)$ denote the Radon–Nikodym derivative of F_1 with respect to the measure induced by $F_1 + F_2$. In the problem of testing $H_0: F \in \mathbf{F}_0$ against the alternative $H_1: F \in \mathbf{F} - \mathbf{F}_0$, where $\mathbf{F}_0 \subset \mathbf{F}$, based on a random sample $\mathbf{X}$, the author defined the likelihood ratio statis-tic $\Lambda_n(\mathbf{X})$ and investigated the properties of the likelihood ratio statistic $\Lambda_n(\mathbf{X})$ for various restricted families of distribution $\mathbf{F}_0 \subset \mathbf{F}$. Two unbiased tests for testing for constant versus increasing (or decreasing) failure rate were proposed based on likelihood ratio statistics.

2. By means of simple diagrams, Buse (1982) presented an intuitive discussion of the concept of the likelihood ratio, the Lagrange multiplier, as well as Wald test procedures. The elementary logic of the likelihood ratio (LR) test is to take the ratio of likelihoods with and without the restrictions of the null hypothesis enforced. Suppose that the vector θ of interest consists of only one component, such that $\bar{\theta} = \theta_0$, where θ_0 is the value of θ specified in a simple null hypothesis and the alternative hypothesis $\theta \neq \theta_0$. Then the asymptotic distribution of the LR test statistic is $LR = 2(\log L(\hat{\theta}) - \log L(\bar{\theta})) \sim \chi_g^2$, where $\hat{\theta}$ is the unrestricted estimate of the population vector, $\bar{\theta}$ is the restricted estimate, and g is the number of restrictions specified in the null hypothesis. The three test statistics were shown to be numerically identical and have χ^2-distributions for all sample sizes under the null hypothesis if the log-likelihood function is quadratic.

3. The typical asymptotic chi-square distribution for the likelihood ratio test statistic assumes that the parameter is taken under the null hypothesis and that the data follow the parametric model under consideration. Kent (1982) examined the distribution of the likelihood ratio statistic when the "nearest" member of the parametric family still satisfies the null hypothesis, instead of the case where the data follow the assumed parametric model. In this scenario, the likelihood ratio statistic no longer follows an asymptotic chi-square distribution. For parametric models for which the likelihood ratio test is nonrobust, the author proposed an alternative statistic based on the union-intersection approach, which was shown to follow an asymptotic χ_p^2-distribution for all reasonable underlying distributions.

4. Let f_λ be a kernel estimate (with window width λ) of the density f. Its performance can be assessed by the Kullback–Leibler information distance $I(f, f_\lambda) = \int f \log f - \int f \log f_\lambda$. Note that only the second term, $R_\lambda = \int f \log f_\lambda = \int f \log f_\lambda \, dF$, is relevant for comparing different values of λ. Focusing on the term R_λ, Wong (1983) provided conditions for the asymptotic equivalence and the common limiting value of the cross-validation estimate, as well as the jackknife estimate. The cross-validation estimate has the form of $\hat{R}_\lambda^{(CV)} = \frac{1}{n} \sum_{i=1}^{n} \log f_\lambda(X_i, X_{(i)})$, where $X_{(i)} = X \backslash \{X_i\}$ and the jackknife estimate corrects for the bias by subtracting from $\bar{R}_\lambda = \int \log f_\lambda d\hat{F} = \frac{1}{n} \sum_{i=1}^{n} \log f_\lambda(X_i; X)$ the jackknife estimate of bias $E^{(Jack)}(\bar{R}_\lambda - R_\lambda)$, which is an approximation to the bootstrap expected amount of overestimation $E^{(boot)}(\bar{R}_\lambda - R_\lambda) = E_* \left[\sum_{i=1}^{n} (P_i^* - \frac{1}{n}) \log f_\lambda(X_i, X^*) \right]$. It provided a useful "modified likelihood" criterion for choosing λ (Duin 1976; Habbema et al. 1974).

5. Davison (1986) provided a predictive likelihood, which expands posterior likelihood and approximates both Bayes and maximum likelihood predictive inference. The approximations were derived from a posterior predictive density and may be viewed as Bayesian approaches with available prior information. The approximation is different from exact Bayes posterior predictive density by $O_p(n^{-2})$, and from exact predictive likelihood by $O_p(n^{-1})$, but does not depend on the availability of prior information. When exact predictive likelihood cannot be found, it is also applicable. Using the generalized extreme-value distribution, the results were applied to the prediction of extremes.

6. Suppose that we draw independent observations such that k have a known density $g(x)$ and $n-k$ have a known density $f(x)$. McLeish and Small (1986) considered the discrimination issue of assigning observations to their parent densities based on the rule of minimizing the expected number of misclassifications as a function of k and estimators of k. Based on the order statistics, properties of the likelihood function of k were studied. It was concluded that a mixture model analysis performs well independent of the mechanism, stochastic or deterministic, that produced k and the correct allocation.

7. Berger et al. (1988) addressed the following issues regarding the likelihood principle (LP): (a) LP depends on the assumptions of exact knowledge of the model or data distribution, which may lead to hasty rejection of the LP, and (b) LP only provides a way that any method of analysis should follow, but does not specify the way to perform a statistical analysis. Based on examples and appeals to practical use and common sense, the author argued that the LP is sensible and introduced a generalized version of the LP, which removes the restriction of an exactly known likelihood function. The implementation of the LP was presented, and it was argued that Bayesian analysis (see Chapter 7) is the most realistic and sensible method of implementation.

8. Le Cam (1990) presented some examples where maximum likelihood estimates may misbehave. The author provided a list of principles leading to the construction of good estimates, and the main principle noted that one should study each problem for its own purpose and aim to simply believe in principles.

9. For maximum likelihood estimators, Pal and Berry (1992) considered the property of invariance to non-one-to-one parameter transformations and discussed three approaches to maximum likelihood estimation. It was shown that the invariance depends on the approach adopted where sufficient conditions for invariance to hold under all three approaches were presented.

10. When fitting models jointly for the mean and dispersion of a response, there is some controversy about estimating the dispersion parameters. Nelder and Lee (1992) investigated finite sampling properties of several dispersion estimators based on simulation for the maximum extended quasi-likelihood estimator, the maximum pseudolikelihood estimator, and the maximum likelihood estimator, if it exists. Among these estimators, the maximum extended quasi-likelihood estimator was shown to be superior in minimizing the mean squared error.

11. Newton and Raftery (1994) studied the extent to which a new bootstrap procedure, the weighted likelihood bootstrap (WLB), can be used by applied Bayesian statisticians as a way to simulate approximately based on a posterior distribution. WLB, a Monte Carlo method, is easy to implement in models where maximum likelihood estimation is feasible, for example, regression models, iteratively reweighted least-squares models, and generalized linear models. In the generic weighting scheme, under general conditions, the WLB is first-order correct. The second-order properties of the WLB were shown by asymptotic expansions, which is a generalization of Rubin's Bayesian bootstrap. Using the WLB as a source of samples in the sampling importance resampling (SIR) algorithm that allows incorporation of particular prior information, inaccuracies can be removed. The SIR-adjusted WLB can be viewed as a competitive integration method. The authors also considered the calculation of approximate Bayes factors for model comparison. It can be noted that for a sample simulated from the posterior distribution, the marginal likelihood may be simulation consistently

estimated by the harmonic mean of the associated likelihood values. It can also be noted that a modification of this estimator avoids instability. For a wide class of models, these methods provided simple approaches to calculating approximate Bayes factors and posterior model probabilities.

12. The method of estimating functions (Godambe 1991) is commonly used to make inference about parameters of interest with an unknown full distribution of the observation. Nevertheless, the use of this approach may be limited due to multiple roots for the estimating function, a poorly behaved Wald test, or lack of a goodness-of-fit test. Under the case where either one of these three problems occurs, Hanfelt and Liang (1995) presented approximate likelihood ratios that can be used together with estimating functions. The authors showed that the approximate likelihood ratio offers correct large sample inference under very general circumstances, for example, based on clustered data or misspecified weights in the estimating function. Two methods of constructing the approximate likelihood ratio were compared and shown to be closely related. One was based on the quasi-likelihood approach, and the other was based on the linear projection approach. It was demonstrated that quasi-likelihood is the limit of the projection approach.

13. Martingale methods are a useful and powerful tool for making inference of dependent variables. Estimators have distributions that are approximated in first order by the distribution of a martingale, and martingales have asymptotic properties that hold under weak conditions. Nevertheless, a major weakness of martingale methods is that for small samples, the quality of the approximation in the martingale central limit theorems (CLTs) can be quite poor. In order to correct this problem, Mykland (1995) introduced the concept of dual likelihood as a method of improving accuracy in inference situations, depending on martingale estimating equations. Asymptotic results were given for the dual likelihood ratio statistic, and the structure of the family of alternatives was investigated. The dual likelihood ratio (LR) is a reasonably natural construction, and its statistic gives rise to tests and confidence intervals with good accuracy properties. Note that in the case of independent data, the dual LR statistic coincides with Owen's empirical LR statistic (see Chapter 6 for details). There are similar connections to point process likelihoods in survival analysis. In both cases, this connection reduces nonparametric LR statistics to parametric statistics. The authors also presented applications to survival analysis and to time series, likelihood inference, and independent observations.

14. Meeker and Escobar (1995) outlined their approach to construct confidence regions or intervals based on maximum likelihood (ML) estimation and described how to present the ideas to students, focusing on a wide range of practical applications.

15. Choi et al. (1996) studied tests of hypotheses about finite-dimensional parameters in a semiparametric model from Pitman's moving alternative or local approach, based on Le Cam's (1986) local asymptotic normality concept. When a real parameter was tested, asymptotically uniformly most powerful (AUMP) tests were characterized for one-sided hypotheses and AUMP unbiased tests for two-sided ones. For multidimensional hypotheses, an asymptotic invariance principle was introduced, and AUMP invariant tests were presented. Assume that we observe a normally distributed random variable with mean vector Bu and known variance matrix B, where the normal variable is the score vector, B the information, and u the shift in the parameter under local alternatives. Results based on Choi et al.'s methods were shown to

be parallel to those for testing hypotheses about part of a vector u in large samples. When the test is one-sided about a real component $u = (u_1, u_2)$ one way to derive a uniformly most powerful (UMP) test is based on a maximal invariant statistic, as well as on a sufficient and complete statistic under a group of nonsingular linear transformations for the whole vector (Lehmann 1986). However, this theory can be avoided—thereby avoiding a need for dealing with asymptotic sufficiency and completeness. An alternative derivation, a UMP unbiased test, was to fix a null value of the nuisance parameter u_2 by confining attention to a restricted alternative of a hyperplane, that is, focusing on level α tests of $u = (0, u_2^0)$ versus u in the hyperplane $\{u : u_1 \in \Re, u_2 = u_2^0 - B_{22}^{-1} B_{21} u_1\}$, which considers only effective observations—and requiring invariance only for effective observations. These provided the optimality property, when constructions are feasible, for Wald, Rao (score), Neyman–Rao (effective score), and likelihood ratio tests in parametric models, and for Neyman–Rao tests in semiparametric models. Note that inversions may result in asymptotically uniformly most accurate confidence sets. The authors illustrated examples for one-, two-, and k-sample problems, a linear regression model with unknown error distribution, and a proportional hazards regression model with arbitrary baseline hazards.

16. Reid (1996) summarized the recent developments in higher-order asymptotic theory for statistical inference, for example, using the likelihood function to approximate cumulative distribution functions. The author presented the versatility of the likelihood approach by providing examples of problems solved and solvable by this approach. The author considered generalizations and extensions with suggestions for further development and briefly outlined the re-expression of the saddlepoint approximation for the density and distribution function of the sample mean using the likelihood function.

17. For a real parameter in the presence of an infinite-dimensional nuisance parameter, Murphy and Van der Vaart (1997) investigated likelihood ratio tests and related confidence intervals and demonstrated that the estimator of the real parameter has an asymptotic normal distribution in all cases. Nevertheless, the estimator of the nuisance parameter may not follow Gaussian asymptotically or may converge to the true parameter value at a slower rate than the square root of the sample size. The likelihood ratio statistic was shown to possess an asymptotic chi-square distribution. The examples considered were tests concerning survival probabilities based on doubly censored data, a test for the presence of heterogeneity in the gamma frailty model, a test for significance of the regression coefficient in Cox's regression model for current status data, and a test for a ratio of hazards rates in an exponential mixture model. In the last examples, the rate of convergence of the estimator of the nuisance parameter was shown to be less than the square root of the sample size.

18. Mykland (1999) studied the connection between large- and small-deviation results for the likelihood ratio statistic R^2 and its signed square root R, both for likelihoods and for likelihood-like criterion functions. It was noted that they both depend on cumulants (cum), where the cumulants have different orders in the two types of expansion. The author presented that $\mathrm{cum}_q(R) = O(n^{-q/2})$ for $3 \le q < p$, whereas $\mathrm{cum}_q(R) = k_p n^{-(p-2)/2} + O(n^{-p/2})$, provided that (a) $p - 1$ Bartlett identities are satisfied to the first order, and (b) the pth identity is violated to this order. It was demonstrated that the large-deviation behavior of R is determined by the values of p and k_p, which was also valid for more general statistics. Affine (additive or multiplicative) correction to R and R^2 was shown to be a special case corresponding

to $p = 3$ or 4. The cumulant behavior of R offers a way of measuring the extent to which R-statistics based on criterion functions other than log-likelihoods can be expected to behave like ones derived from true log-likelihoods, by looking at the number of Bartlett identities that are satisfied. Based on the "dual criterion functions," empirical and nonparametric survival analysis–type likelihoods were analyzed.

19. In order to test whether the contamination of a known density f_0 by another density of the same parametric family reduces to f_0, Lemdani and Pons (1999) studied the asymptotic distribution of the likelihood ratio statistic. Noticing that the classical asymptotic theory for the likelihood ratio statistic fails, the authors proposed a reparameterization that guarantees regularity properties and demonstrated locally asymptotic normality in $n^{-1/2}$ neighborhoods of the true parameter values. The likelihood ratio statistic converges to the supremum of a squared truncated Gaussian process under the null hypothesis. The result was extended to the case of the contamination of a mixture of p known densities by q other densities of the same family. Examples were presented for Gaussian densities and binomial densities.

20. The Wald statistic may fail in some cases (Fears et al. 1996). Consider a simple normal random effects model based on a balanced data set, $y_{ij} = u + a_i + e_{ij}$, where u is the grand mean, the person effect a_i is i.i.d. $N(0, \sigma_a^2)$, the residual effect e_{ij} is i.i.d. $N(0, \sigma^2)$, and the a_i's and e_{ij}'s are independent. The analysis of variance table and the standard F test for $H_0 : \sigma_a^2 = 0$ can be constructed, and the fallibility of the Wald statistic may manifest in this case. Note that one tends to rely on the Wald test in complicated or nonnormal models where there are no exact tests to serve as a gold standard in practice. Pawitan (2000) explained the failure of the Wald test based on the profile likelihood functions, which appear to be nonnormal graphically.

21. Reid (2000) provided general introductions to the concept of the likelihood function and its informal use in inference. The author presented an illustration of the likelihood function using the data obtained from a study conducted at the University of Toronto and concluded that the risk of a traffic accident increased fourfold when the driver was using a cellular telephone (Redelmeier and Tibshirani 1997).

22. Hoff (2000) discussed a new technique for calculating maximum likelihood estimators (MLEs) of probability measures in the case where the measures are assumed to constrain to a compact, convex set. In such sets, measures can be characterized as mixtures of simple measures, and so the problem of maximizing the likelihood in the constrained measures becomes an issue of maximizing in an unconstrained mixing measure. Such convex constraints arise in many modeling situations, such as empirical likelihood and estimation under stochastic ordering constraints. The author described the mixture representation technique for these two situations and presented a data analysis of an experiment in cancer genetics, assuming a partial stochastic ordering and incomplete data.

23. Pawitan (2001) concentrated on the likelihood and Fisherian methods of taking into account uncertainty when studying a statistical problem, considering the concept of the likelihood as the best method for combining statistical modeling and theory of inference. The likelihood principle was emphasized as an important tool for modeling. The method was illustrated with realistic examples, including a simple comparison of two accident rates and complex studies requiring generalized linear or semiparametric modeling.

24. Fan et al. (2001) presented that maximum likelihood ratio test statistics may not exist in general in nonparametric function estimation settings, and even if they exist, they are hard to find and cannot be optimal. The authors introduced the generalized likelihood statistics to deal with the weaknesses of nonparametric maximum likelihood ratio statistics. The authors demonstrated that a family of the generalized likelihood statistics based on certain suitable nonparametric estimators are asymptotically distribution-free and follow χ^2-distributions under null hypotheses for a number of useful hypotheses and a variety of useful models, including Gaussian white noise models, nonparametric regression models, varying coefficient models, and generalized varying coefficient models. Generalized likelihood ratio statistics were shown to be asymptotically optimal in terms of rates of convergence. The generalized likelihood ratio statistics based on function estimation were demonstrated to be general and powerful for nonparametric testing problems.

25. Hall et al. (2001) advised locally parametric methods for estimating curves in various spatial problems, for example, boundaries of density supports or fault lines in response surfaces. Based on spatial approximations to the local likelihood that the curve passes through a given point in the plane, the local likelihood methods may be a regular likelihood computed locally with kernel weights (e.g., in the case of support boundary estimation) or a local version of a likelihood ratio statistic (e.g., in fault line estimation). The local likelihood surface represents a function that is relatively large near the target curve, and relatively small elsewhere in either case. Consequently, the curve can be estimated as a ridge line of the surface, requiring only a numerical algorithm for tracking the projection of a ridge into the plane. This approach has the following advantages: (a) we can plot the local likelihood surface, and assess the degree of "ridginess" graphically to emphasize the ridge and the curve adequately based on the variation of the level of local smoothing in different spatial locations; (b) we do not need to compute the local likelihood surface in anything like its entirety, where we can track it following the ridge line once we have a reasonable approximation to a point on the curve; and (c) the method is appropriate without change for many different types of spatial explanatory variables. The authors studied three examples, including (a) fault lines in response surfaces and in intensity or density surfaces, (b) the estimation of support boundaries of point process intensities or probability densities, and (c) temporary curve approximation problems involving estimation from spatial data.

26. Banerjee and Wellner (2001) studied the problem of testing for equality at a fixed point in the setting of nonparametric estimation of a monotone function. The likelihood ratio test for this hypothesis was presented in the particular case of interval censoring (or current status data) and obtained the limiting distribution, which is that of the integral of the difference of the squared slope processes corresponding to the problem involving Brownian motion and greatest convex minorants thereof. Pointwise confidence intervals for the unknown distribution function were derived based on inversion of the family of test yields. The authors investigated the statistic under local and fixed alternatives. The following examples were presented: (a) monotone density function; (b) interval censoring, current status data; (c) panel count data; (d) monotone hazard function with right-censored data; and (e) monotone regression function.

27. The pth cumulant of the signed square root of the likelihood ratio, the R-statistic, is typically of the form $n^{-p/2}k_p + O(n^{-(p+2)/2})$, where $R = \text{sgn}(\hat{\theta} - \theta)(l(\hat{\theta}) - l(\theta))^{1/2}$, l is the log-likelihood, $\hat{\theta}$ is the maximum likelihood estimator, and n is the number

of observations. Mykland (2001) presented the computation k_p without invoking the Bartlett identities and showed how the family of alternatives influences the coverage accuracy of R.

28. Schweder and Hjort (2002) presented a new version of the Neyman–Pearson lemma, demonstrating that the confidence distribution based on the natural statistic in exponential models for continuous data has less dispersion than all other confidence distributions, independent of the way to measure dispersion. Note that approximations are necessary for both discrete data and in many models with nuisance parameters, and in such cases, approximate pivots may be useful, where likelihood in the parameter of interest, along with a confidence distribution, is determined by a pivot based on a scalar statistic. This proper likelihood was reduced of all nuisance parameters, and was suitable for meta-analysis and updating of information. The reduced likelihood was shown to be different from the confidence density generally.

29. Based on interval-censored data, Vandal et al. (2005) proposed a reduction technique, versions of the expectation–maximization (EM) algorithm, and the vertex exchange method to conduct constrained nonparametric maximum likelihood estimation of the cumulative distribution function. The constrained vertex exchange method can be employed to construct likelihood intervals for the cumulative distribution function in practice. The method was illustrated with the following data: (a) breast cosmesis data, which consist of interval-censored and right-censored times to cosmetic deterioration in women with breast cancer assigned to two treatment arms, radiotherapy alone and radiotherapy with adjuvant chemotherapy (RTC), and (b) data obtained from a historical cohort of subjects who underwent fasciotomy after trauma-induced acute compartment syndrome (Vaillancourt et al. 2004).

30. Vexler et al. (2011c) developed a likelihood function by implementing the autoregressive process of outcomes. Considering both the limit of detection problem and the dropout process, the method incorporated the characteristics of the longitudinal data in biomedical research. The method provided powerful tests to detect a difference between study populations in terms of the growth rate and dropout rate. With the formal notation of the likelihood function, one may easily adapt the proposed method for a variety of different scenarios in terms of the number of groups and a variety of growth trend patterns. The inferential properties for the proposed method benefit from many well-developed theorems regarding the likelihood approach, for example, asymptotic results and good power properties. The method was illustrated with three data sets obtained from mouse tumor experiments: (a) a gene (Thoc1) deficiency study, (b) an animal tumor immunotherapy experiment (Koziol et al. 1981), and (c) a tumor xenograft model (Tan et al. 2002).

31. Probability ratio $P(h|e)/P(h)$, which has been said to measure the degree of inductive support or confirmation that evidence e provides to hypothesis h, and likelihood ratio measures of inductive support and related notions have appeared as theoretical tools for probabilistic approaches. For the purpose of conceptual clarification, axiomatic foundations for the two families of measures were created and have been criticized for their dependence on unduly demanding or poor assumptions. Crupi et al. (2012) denoted $P(e|h)/P(e|-h)$ as the likelihood ratio and demonstrated that probability ratio and likelihood ratio measures can be axiomatized in a way that overcomes these difficulties.

4.5.1 One-Sided Likelihood

1. A sufficient condition for the validity of the one-sided tests is that the underlying density $p(x, w)$ is a "monotone likelihood ratio," where x is the observed variable and w is the unknown parameter. Note that only monotone functions of the observed variable x should be used as potential estimating functions of w. Karlin and Rubin (1956) investigated the case where the test statistic has the property of sufficiency, indicating that one can control the risk of error in the test by the appropriate use of the single test statistic as if we used the detailed data of the individual observations. This restriction enables one to consider the case where we are dealing only with a single observation. The authors focused on distributions that obey inequality $p(x_1, w_1) p(x_2, w_2) - p(x_1, w_2) p(x_2, w_1) \geq 0$. The most important class of such distributions includes the exponential family of distributions, that is, distributions whose density can be represented as $p(x|w) = \beta(w) e^{xw} f(x)$. For these densities, we have $p(x_1 | w_1) p(x_2 | w_2) - p(x_1 | w_2) p(x_2 | w_1) = \beta(w_1) \beta(w_2) [e^{(x_1 - x_2)(w_1 - w_2)} - 1] f(x_1) f(x_2)$ $e^{x_1 w_2 + x_2 w_1}$, which is positive if $x_1 > x_2$ and $w_1 > w_2$. A simple criterion often useful in determining whether a density $p(x, w)$ has a monotone likelihood ratio is that $\dfrac{\partial^2}{\partial w \, \partial x} \log p(x, w)$ should be nonnegative.

2. When the population is univariate normal, the ordinary one-sided test using either the normal or the t-distribution functions can be employed to determine whether the means are slipped to the right given a multivariate normal population with known variance matrix; that is, the problem is to test the hypothesis $H : \theta_1 = \theta_2 = 0$ against the bivariate one-sided alternative $K : (\theta_1, \theta_2) \in \Theta$, where $\Theta = \{(\theta_1, \theta_2); \theta_1 \geq 0, \theta_2 \geq 0, \max(\theta_1, \theta_2) > 0\}$. Kudo (1963) developed a multivariate analogue of the one-sided test of significance and defined a $\bar{\chi}^2$-statistic based on the likelihood ratio criterion. The authors discussed its existence and geometric nature. The computation and the distribution function of the $\bar{\chi}^2$-statistic were presented, assuming that either the variance–covariance matrix of the population is known or an estimate is available with enough accuracy to be taken as the population value. Two further extensions of the results were given; one was to make the null hypothesis more general and the other was to replace the assumptions about the variance–covariance matrix with somewhat less restrictive ones. Noticing that Kudo's $\bar{\chi}^2$ is not optimal in general, and hence it is meaningful to propose test statistics derived from other principles, Shirahata (1978) proposed a new test procedure for a one-sided alternative concerning the mean vector in a bivariate normal population with a known covariance matrix from a new principle. In addition, extensions to the two-sided case and multivariate case were presented. Shirahata's procedure was shown to be more powerful when the population correlation is negative based on Monte Carlo studies.

3. Consider the problem to test the null hypothesis $H_0 : u_1 = \ldots = u_k$ against the simple ordered alternative hypothesis $H_A : u_1 \leq \ldots \leq u_k$ with at least one strict inequality, in the usual balanced one-way fixed-effects analysis of variance (ANOVA) model $X_{ij} = u_i + \varepsilon_{ij} (1 \leq j \leq n; 1 \leq i \leq k)$, where the ε_{ij} are independent $N(0, \sigma^2)$ random variables and u_i is the mean of the ith treatment $(1 \leq i \leq k)$. The likelihood ratio test (LRT) of Bartholomew (1961) can be used; it is sensitive to specifications of the treatment means satisfying the order restriction, but suffers from the disadvantage of not having a convenient inversion to a set of simultaneous confidence intervals for useful contrasts of the treatment means. Hayter (1990) considered

a simple multiple-contrast test procedure, which may be viewed as a one-sided studentized range test (OSRT). The OSRT rejects the null hypothesis H_0 if and only if the statistic $\max_{1 \le i < j \le k}(\bar{X}_j - \bar{X}_i)/(S/\sqrt{n})$ exceeds a suitable critical value, where $\bar{X}_i$ is the sample mean of the ith treatment ($1 \le i \le k$), and S^2 is an unbiased estimate of σ^2, which is distributed independently of the $\bar{X}_i$ as a $\sigma^2 \chi_v^2 / v$ random variable. By employing this test procedure, we can simply construct exact simultaneous one-sided confidence intervals of the form (d_{ij}, ∞) for all of the ordered pairwise differences of the treatment means $u_j - u_i$ ($1 \le i < j \le k$). These confidence intervals yield the shortest possible ones of this kind and can be extended to produce exact simultaneous confidence intervals for all nonnegative contrasts of the treatment means $\sum_{i=1}^{k} c_i u_i$ where $\sum_{i=1}^{k} c_i = 0$ and $\sum_{i=1}^{j} c_i \le 0$ ($1 \le j \le k-1$). The critical points of the two-sided studentized range test (SRT) were obtained by solving a two-dimensional integral equation, independent of the number of treatments k. It was shown that for $3 \le k \le 9$, the critical points may be obtained by solving no more than a three-dimensional integral equation. Modifications of the OSRT for an unbalanced ANOVA model were provided. The natural modification that provides a conservative test procedure when applied to the SRT was shown to give a possibly liberal test if applied to the OSRT.

4. Let **H** and **G** be independently distributed according to the Wishart distributions $W_m(M, \Phi)$ and $W_m(M, \psi)$, respectively. Kuriki (1993) derived the limiting null distributions of the likelihood ratio criteria for testing $H_0 : \Phi = \Psi$ against $H_1 - H_0$ with $H_1 : \Phi \ge \Psi$, and for testing $H_0^{(R)} : \Phi \ge \Psi$, rank($\Phi - \Psi$) $\le$ R (for given R) against $H_1 - H_0^{(R)}$, which are special cases of the chi-bar-square distributions.

5. Silvapulle (1997) presented a simple but interesting example that involves the maximum likelihood estimator and the likelihood ratio test. Let $X \sim N(u, \Omega)$, where $X = (X_1, X_2)$, $u = (u_1 - u_2)$, $\Omega_{11} = \Omega_{22} = 1$, and $\Omega_{12} = \Omega_{21} = 0.90$. For a random sample from $N(u, \Omega)$, suppose that the sample mean $\bar{X} = (-3, -2)$; thus, every observed value of X_1 and X_2 can be negative. Then, for a suitable hypothesis testing problem with $u_1 = 0$ being the null hypothesis and $\bar{X}_1$ being the test statistic, one would accept that $u_1 < 0$, and similarly, one would accept that $u_2 < 0$. However, the likelihood ratio test of $H_0 : u = 0$ against $H_1 : u > 0$ and $u \ne 0$, would reject H_0 and accept H_1. The author pointed out that the hypothesis $H_1 : u \ge 0$ and $u \ne 0$ does not allow negative values for u_1 or u_2. This phenomenon has subdivisions for testing against restricted multiparameter hypotheses in more general situations.

6. Let $Y_i = (X_{1i}, ..., X_{pi})^T$, $i = 1, ..., n$, denote independent p–dimensional random variables distributed as multivariate $u = (u_{1i}, ..., u_p)^T$ and covariance matrix Σ. Consider testing the hypothesis $H_0 : u_i = 0$ versus $H_1 : u_i \ge 0$ ($i = 1, ..., p$), with strict inequality for some i, assuming Σ is unknown. Perlman (1969) derived the likelihood ratio test (LRT) statistic $U(\Theta)$ and the sharp upper and lower bounds on its null distribution, where Θ is the positive orthant. The author also showed that the LRT is biased. Tang (1994) proposed a class of half-space tests that are uniformly more powerful than the LRT. Nonetheless, the critical values for these tests are independent of the parameter space, thus limiting the advantage of these tests. Wang and McDermott (1998) derived the conditional likelihood ratio test, given $V = \sum_{i=1}^{n} Y_i Y_i^T$, for significance of a multivariate mean having nonnegative components. Under the null hypothesis, V is the complete and sufficient statistic for the nuisance parameter Σ,

and consequently, the conditional distribution of $\overline{Y}$ given V does not depend on Σ. The test used the information about the alternative parameter space more effectively and was shown to be uniformly more powerful than the LRT and the half-space tests proposed by Tang and Hotelling's T^2-test. The consistency, invariance, and unbiasedness of the new test were presented. The test was illustrated with data from a randomized, double-blind crossover trial of an inhaled active drug versus placebo, where 17 patients with asthma or chronic obstructive airway disease participated in the trial, which had a secondary objective of investigating the effect of the drug on three measures of respiratory function: peak expiratory flow rate (PEFR), forced expiratory volume (FEV1), and forced vital capacity (FVC).

7. Jensen (1995) provided a detailed review of a wide range of methods on improving the accuracy of the standard normal approximation to the distribution of the signed root of the likelihood ratio statistic R, based mainly on saddlepoint approximations, which improve the accuracy in the asymptotic normal approximation to the distribution of R from first to second, or even to third, order. DiCiccio et al. (2001) proposed two methods based on the signed root of the likelihood ratio statistic R for one-sided testing of a simple null hypothesis about a scalar parameter in the presence of nuisance parameters. The first method employs a standard normal approximation to the distribution of a mean- and variance-corrected version of R. The second method is based on tail probabilities of the distribution of R itself, obtained under a choice of parameter value equal to the null hypothesis constrained maximum likelihood estimator. The required tail probability was estimated through Monte Carlo simulation. The second method can be viewed as a null hypothesis parametric bootstrap procedure, which corresponds to simulation using a parameter value equal to the maximum likelihood estimate. If such an approach is employed, then the resulting inferences are generally only second-order accurate. In order to achieve third-order accuracy, the application of Monte Carlo simulation must be employed as in the second method. Both methods have the following properties: (a) are third-order accurate, (b) use simulation to avoid the need for onerous analytical calculations characteristic of competing saddlepoint procedures, (c) do not require specification of ancillary statistics, and (d) respect the conditioning associated with similar tests up to an error of third order, and conditioning on ancillary statistics to an error of second order.

8. Bloch et al. (2001) introduced an intersection-union test (IUT) for multiple-endpoint problems with multivariate one-sided alternative hypotheses. The test incorporates the essential univariate and multivariate features of the treatment effects to be compared. This formulation provides a new test statistic that is powerful for the alternative hypothesis. To avoid the analytic complexity of the test statistic, the authors presented a bootstrap test and its large sample theory. The method was compared with existing methods in a simulation study and applied to data on rheumatoid arthritis patients receiving one of two treatments. However, IUT does not utilize the appropriate multivariate one-sided test. Toward this end, Perlman and Wu (2004) modified and obtained an alternative IUT that does utilize the appropriate one-sided test. Empirical and graphical evidence showed that the proposed test is more appropriate.

9. Hinkley (1977) derived two tests for testing the mean of a normal distribution with known a coefficient of variation (CV) for right alternatives. They are the locally most powerful (LMP) and the conditional tests based on the ancillary

statistic for u. Bhat and Rao (2007) derived the likelihood ratio (LR) and Wald tests for the one- and two-sided alternatives, as well as the two-sided version of the LMP test. The performances of these tests were compared with those of the classical t-, sign, and Wilcoxon signed-rank tests, where the following points can be addressed: (a) the latter three tests do not use the information on CV; (b) normal approximation was used to approximate the null distribution of the test statistics except for the t-test; (c) based on simulation results, all the tests were shown to maintain the Type I error rates; that is, the attained level is close to the nominal level of significance of the tests; (d) based on simulation results, the power functions of the tests indicated that for one-sided alternatives, the LMP test is the best test, whereas for the two-sided alternatives, the LR or Wald test is the best test; (e) the t-, sign, and Wilcoxon signed-rank tests have lower power than the LMP, LR, and Wald tests at various alternative values of u; (f) based on simulation results, the t-, sign, and Wilcoxon signed-rank tests were shown to have considerably lower power even for the alternatives that are far away from the null hypothesis when the CV is large; and (g) Bhat and Rao's tests were shown to maintain the Type I error rates for moderate values of CV.

10. The statement that likelihood ratio, score, and Wald tests statistics are asymptotically equivalent is widely known to hold true under standard conditions. In the situation when the parameter space is constrained and the null hypothesis lies on the boundary of the parameter space, such as, for example, in variance component testing, knowledge is scattered across the literature and considerably less well-known among practitioners. Motivated from simple but generic examples, Molenberghs and Verbeke (2007) showed there is quite a market for asymptotic one-sided hypothesis tests, in the scalar as well as in the vector case. The three standard tests can be used here as well and are asymptotically equivalent, but a somewhat more elaborate version of the score and Wald test statistics is needed. Null distributions were proven to have the form of mixtures of χ^2-distributions. Statistical and numerical considerations lead one to formulate pragmatic guidelines as to when to prefer which of the three tests. The following examples were considered: (a) the rat data resulted from a randomized longitudinal experiment, in which 50 male Wistar rats were randomized to either a control group or one of the two treatment groups, where treatment consisted of a low or high dose of the testosterone inhibitor Decapeptyl; (b) the toenail data obtained from a randomized, double-blind, parallel-group, multicenter study for the comparison of two oral treatments for toenail dermatophyte onychomycosis; and (c) the NTP data where the dose–response relationship was investigated in mice of the potentially hazardous chemical compound ethylene glycol.

11. The two one-sided tests (TOST) procedure, like classical point null hypothesis testing, is subject to multiplicity issues when more comparisons are made. Lauzon and Caffo (2009) provided a condition that bounds the family-wise error rate (FWER) (see Chapter 14) using TOST and presented a simple solution for controlling the FWER. The authors demonstrated that if all pairwise comparisons of k independent groups are evaluated for equivalence, then simply scaling the nominal Type I error rate down by $(k-1)$ is sufficient to maintain the FWER at the desired value or less. The resulting rule was shown to be much less conservative than the equally simple Bonferroni correction. The method was applied to an example of equivalence testing in a non–drug development setting.

12. An integrated likelihood depends only on the parameter of interest and the data, so it can be used as a standard likelihood function for likelihood-based inference. Consider a model with a scalar parameter of interest ψ, a d-dimensional nuisance parameter λ taking values in a set Λ, and the likelihood function $L(\psi, \lambda)$. Likelihood inference about ψ is often based on a pseudolikelihood function, a function of ψ, and the data with properties similar to those of a genuine likelihood. Severini (2010) focused on a particular type of pseudolikelihood, integrated likelihood, which is of the form $\int_\Lambda L(\psi, \lambda) \pi(\lambda \mid \psi) d\lambda$, where π is a nonnegative weight function on Λ. The author presented the higher-order asymptotic properties of the signed integrated likelihood ratio statistic for a scalar parameter of interest. These results were used to construct a modified integrated likelihood ratio statistic and to suggest a class of prior densities to use in forming the integrated likelihood. The properties of the integrated likelihood ratio statistic were compared to those of the standard likelihood ratio statistic. Examples showed that the integrated likelihood ratio statistic can be a useful alternative to the standard likelihood ratio statistic.

13. Ledwina and Wyłupek (2012) proposed, implemented, and investigated a new nonparametric two-sample test for detecting stochastic dominance. Motivated by drawbacks of standard procedures that may result in serious errors in inference, the authors posed the question of detecting the stochastic dominance in a novel way. This procedure matched testing and model selection. The authors reparameterized the testing problem in terms of Fourier coefficients of well-known comparison densities, and the estimated Fourier coefficients were used to form a kind of signed–smooth rank statistic. Therefore, the number of Fourier coefficients incorporated into the statistic is a smoothing parameter, which is determined via certain flexible selection rules and established the asymptotic properties of the new test under null and alternative hypotheses. The finite sample performance of the new solution was confirmed by Monte Carlo studies. The method was illustrated with an application to a set of survival times in days of the guinea pigs analyzed in Doksum (1974).

14. Lehmann (2012) discussed a large class of situations in which likelihood ratio tests perform very poorly, and analyzed just how intuition misleads us; he also presented an alternative approach that in these situations is optimal.

4.6 Appendix

4.6.1 The Most Powerful Test

The most powerful statistical decision rule is to reject H_0 if and only if $\prod_{i=1}^{n} f_1(X_i)/f_0(X_i) \geq B$, for a fixed test threshold B. The term *most powerful* induces us to formally define how to compare statistical tests. Since the ability to control the Type I error (TIE) rate of statistical tests has an essential role in statistical decision making, without loss of generality, we compare tests with equivalent probabilities of the TIE, $\Pr_{H_0}\{\text{test rejects } H_0\} = \alpha$, where the subscript H_0 indicates that we consider the probability, given that the null hypothesis is correct. The level of significance α is the probability of making a TIE. In practice, the researcher should choose a value of α, for example, $\alpha = 0.05$, before performing the test. Thus, we should compare the likelihood ratio test with δ, any decision rule based on $\{X_i, i = 1, \ldots, n\}$ setting up $\text{Pr}_{H_0}\{\delta \text{ rejects } H_0\} = \alpha$ and $\text{Pr}_{H_0}\left\{\prod_{i=1}^{n} f_1(X_i)/f_0(X_i) \geq B\right\} = \alpha$. This comparison is with respect to the power $\text{Pr}_{H_1}\{\text{test rejects } H_0\}$. Notice that to derive the mathematical expectation, in the context of a problem related to testing statistical hypotheses, one must define whether the expectation should be conducted under the H_0 or H_1 regime. For example,

$$E_{H_1}\varphi(X_1, X_2, \ldots, X_n) = \int \varphi(x_1, x_2, \ldots, x_n)f_1(x_1, x_2, \ldots, x_n)dx_1 dx_2 \ldots dx_n$$

$$= \int \varphi(x_1, x_2, \ldots, x_n)\prod_{i=1}^{n} f_1(x_i)\prod_{i=1}^{n} dx_i,$$

where the expectation is considered under the alternative hypothesis. The indicator $I\{C\}$ of the event C can be considered as a random variable with values 0 and 1. By virtue of the definition, the expected value of $I\{C\}$ is

$$EI\{C\} = 0 \times \text{Pr}\{I\{C\} = 0\} + 1 \times \text{Pr}\{I\{C\} = 1\} = \text{Pr}\{I\{C\} = 1\} = \text{Pr}\{C\}.$$

Taking into account the comments mentioned above, we derive the expectation under H_0 of the inequality $(A - B)(I\{A \geq B\} - \delta) \geq 0$, where $A = \prod_{i=1}^{n} f_1(X_i)/f_0(X_i)$, B is a test threshold, and δ represents any decision rule based on $\{X_i, i = 1, \ldots, n\}$. One can assume that $\delta = 0, 1$ and when $\delta = 1$, we reject H_0. Thus, we obtain

$$E_{H_0}\left(\left(\prod_{i=1}^{n} \frac{f_1(X_i)}{f_0(X_i)} - B\right)I\left\{\prod_{i=1}^{n} \frac{f_1(X_i)}{f_0(X_i)} \geq B\right\}\right) \geq E_{H_0}\left(\left(\prod_{i=1}^{n} \frac{f_1(X_i)}{f_0(X_i)} - B\right)\delta\right).$$

And hence,

$$E_{H_0}\left(\prod_{i=1}^{n} \frac{f_1(X_i)}{f_0(X_i)} I\left\{\prod_{i=1}^{n} \frac{f_1(X_i)}{f_0(X_i)} \geq B\right\}\right) - BE_{H_0}\left(\prod_{i=1}^{n} I\left\{\frac{f_1(X_i)}{f_0(X_i)} \geq B\right\}\right)$$

$$\geq E_{H_0}\left(\prod_{i=1}^{n} \frac{f_1(X_i)}{f_0(X_i)}\delta\right) - BE_{H_0}(\delta),$$

where $E_{H_0}(\delta) = E_{H_0}(I\{\delta = 1\}) = \text{Pr}_{H_0}\{\delta = 1\} = \text{Pr}_{H_0}\{\delta \text{ rejects } H_0\}$. Since we compare the tests with the fixed level of significance

$$E_{H_0}\left(I\left\{\prod_{i=1}^{n} \frac{f_1(X_i)}{f_0(X_i)} \geq B\right\}\right) = \text{Pr}_{H_0}\left\{\prod_{i=1}^{n} \frac{f_1(X_i)}{f_0(X_i)} \geq B\right\} = \text{Pr}_{H_0}\{\delta \text{ rejects } H_0\} = \alpha,$$

we have

$$E_{H_0}\left(\prod_{i=1}^{n} \frac{f_1(X_i)}{f_0(X_i)} I\left\{\prod_{i=1}^{n} \frac{f_1(X_i)}{f_0(X_i)} \geq B\right\}\right) \geq E_{H_0}\left(\prod_{i=1}^{n} \frac{f_1(X_i)}{f_0(X_i)}\delta\right). \tag{4.3}$$

Consider

$$
E_{H_0}\left(\prod_{i=1}^{n}\frac{f_1(X_i)}{f_0(X_i)}\delta\right) = E_{H_0}\left(\prod_{i=1}^{n}\frac{f_1(X_i)}{f_0(X_i)}\delta(X_1,\ldots,X_n)\right)
$$

$$
= \int\prod_{i=1}^{n}\frac{f_1(x_i)}{f_0(x_i)}\delta(x_1,\ldots,x_n)f_0(x_1,\ldots,x_n)dx_1\ldots dx_n
$$

$$
= \int\frac{\prod_{i=1}^{n}f_1(x_i)}{\prod_{i=1}^{n}f_0(x_i)}\delta(x_1,\ldots,x_n)\prod_{i=1}^{n}f_0(x_i)dx_1\ldots dx_n \qquad (4.4)
$$

$$
= \int\delta(x_1,\ldots,x_n)\prod_{i=1}^{n}f_1(x_i)\,dx_1\ldots dx_n
$$

$$
= E_{H_1}\delta = \mathrm{Pr}_{H_1}\left\{\delta \text{ rejects } H_0\right\}.
$$

Since δ represents any decision rule based on $\{X_i, i = 1, \ldots, n\}$ including the likelihood ratio–based test, Equation 4.4 implies

$$
E_{H_0}\left(\prod_{i=1}^{n}\frac{f_1(X_i)}{f_0(X_i)}I\left\{\prod_{i=1}^{n}\frac{f_1(X_i)}{f_0(X_i)}\geq B\right\}\right) = \mathrm{Pr}_{H_1}\left\{\prod_{i=1}^{n}\frac{f_1(X_i)}{f_0(X_i)}\geq B\right\}.
$$

Applying this equation and (4.4) to (4.3), we complete the proof that the likelihood ratio test is a most powerful statistical decision rule.

4.6.2 The Likelihood Ratio Property $f_{H_1}^{L}(u) = f_{H_0}^{L}(u)u$

In order to obtain this property, we consider

$$
\mathrm{Pr}_{H_1}\{u-s\leq L\leq u\} = E_{H_1}I\{u-s\leq L\leq u\} = \int I\{u-s\leq L\leq u\}f_{H_1}
$$

$$
= \int I\{u-s\leq L\leq u\}\frac{f_{H_1}}{f_{H_0}}f_{H_0} = \int I\{u-s\leq L\leq u\}Lf_{H_0}.
$$

This implies the inequalities

$$
\mathrm{Pr}_{H_1}\{u-s\leq L\leq u\} \leq \int I\{u-s\leq L\leq u\}uf_{H_0} = u\mathrm{Pr}_{H_0}\{u-s\leq L\leq u\}
$$

and

$$
\mathrm{Pr}_{H_1}\{u-s\leq L\leq u\} \geq \int I\{u-s\leq L\leq u\}(u-s)f_{H_0} = (u-s)\mathrm{Pr}_{H_0}\{u-s\leq L\leq u\}.
$$

Dividing these inequalities by s and employing $s \to 0$, we obtain $f_{H_1}^L(u) = f_{H_0}^L(u)u$, where $f_{H_0}^L(u)$ and $f_{H_1}^L(u)$ are the density functions of the statistic $L = f_{H_1}/f_{H_0}$ under H_0 and H_1, respectively.

4.6.3 Wilks' Theorem

Suppose $\mathbf{x} = \{X_1, \ldots, X_n\}$, where $X_1, \ldots, X_n$ are i.i.d. observations, each with the density function $f(x|\boldsymbol{\theta})$, where $\boldsymbol{\theta}$ is a real-valued vector of parameters. We are interested in testing whether the vector $\boldsymbol{\theta}$ is in a specified subset Ω_0 of the parametric space Ω, that is, $H_0: \boldsymbol{\theta} \in \Omega_0$ versus $H_1: \in \Omega_0^c$, where Ω_0^c is a complement to Ω_0 in Ω. Let $L(\boldsymbol{\theta}|\mathbf{x}) = \prod_{i=1}^n f(X_i|\boldsymbol{\theta})$ be the likelihood function. The *likelihood ratio* test statistic is $\Lambda(\mathbf{x}) = \sup_{\theta \in \Omega^c} L(\boldsymbol{\theta}|\mathbf{x})/\sup_{\theta \in \Omega_0} L(\boldsymbol{\theta}|\mathbf{x})$.

Then under the null hypothesis, the distribution of $2\log \Lambda(\mathbf{x})$ follows a χ_d^2-distribution as $n \to \infty$, where the degrees of freedom d equal to the difference in dimensionality of Ω^c and Ω_0. This proposition requires that the regularity conditions hold. For simplicity and clarity of exposition, we present the regularity conditions in the one-dimension case:

1. The parameter space Ω is an open interval (not necessarily finite).
2. The distribution P_θ of X_i have common support, so that the set $A = \{x : f(x|\theta) > 0\}$ is independent of θ.
3. For every $x \in A$, the log of density function $f(x|\theta)$ is third differentiable with respect to θ, and the third derivative is continuous in θ.
4. The integral $\int f(x|\theta)d\mu(x)$ can be third differentiated under the integral sign, where μ is a sigma-finite measure for the density function $f(x|\theta)$.
5. The Fisher information $I(\theta) = E(-\partial^2\log f(x|\theta)/\partial\theta^2) = E(\partial\log f(x|\theta)/\partial\theta)^2$ satisfies $0 < I(\theta) < \infty$.
6. For any given $\theta_0 \in \Omega$, there exist a positive number c and a function $M(x)$ (both of which may depend on θ_0) such that $|\partial^3 \log f(x|\theta)/\partial\theta^3| \le M(x)$ for all $x \in A$, $\theta_0 - c < \theta < \theta_0 + c$, and $E_{\theta_0}[M(X_1)] < \infty$.
7. The maximum likelihood estimator $\hat{\theta}$ of θ satisfies $\hat{\theta} \xrightarrow{p} \theta$, as $n \to \infty$.

Consider the case where θ is a one-dimension parameter where $d = 1$; that is, we are interested in testing $H_0 : \theta = \theta_0$ versus $H_0 : \theta \ne \theta_0$. Let $l(\theta|x) = \log L(\theta|x)$ and $\hat{\theta}$ be the maximum likelihood estimator (MLE) of θ under H_1, that is, $\hat{\theta} = \arg\max_\theta L(\theta)$, provided that $\hat{\theta}$ exists. Expand $l(\theta_0|\mathbf{x})$ in a Taylor series around $\hat{\theta}$, that is,

$$l(\theta_0 | \mathbf{x}) = l(\hat{\theta} | \mathbf{x}) + (\theta_0 - \hat{\theta})l'(\hat{\theta} | \mathbf{x}) + (\theta_0 - \hat{\theta})^2 \frac{l''(\hat{\theta} | \mathbf{x})}{2} + R,$$

where the remainder term $R = (\theta_0 - \hat{\theta})^3 \dfrac{l'''(\tilde{\theta} | \mathbf{x})}{6}$, for some real number $\tilde{\theta}$ between $\hat{\theta}$ and θ. Based on the regularity condition that $|\partial^3 \log f(x|\theta)/\partial\theta^3| \le M(x)$ for all $x \in A$, $\theta_0 - c < \theta < \theta_0 + c$ with $E_{\theta_0}[M(X)] < \infty$, and the fact that $|\theta_0 - \hat{\theta}| = O_p(n^{-1/2})$ (Lehmann and Casella 1998), we can obtain $R = O_p(n^{-3/2}n) = O_p(n^{-1/2}) = o_p(1)$. Noting that $l'(\hat{\theta} | \mathbf{x}) = 0$, we have

$$l(\theta_0 | \mathbf{x}) = l(\hat{\theta} | \mathbf{x}) + (\theta_0 - \hat{\theta})^2 \frac{l''(\hat{\theta} | \mathbf{x})}{2} + o_p(1).$$

By substituting $l(\theta_0|x)$ with its corresponding Taylor expansion, we conclude that

$$2\log \Lambda(x) = 2l(\hat{\theta}\,|\,x) - 2l(\theta_0\,|\,x) = -(\theta_0 - \hat{\theta})^2 l''(\hat{\theta}\,|\,x) + o_p(1)$$

$$= \left\{\sqrt{n}(\theta_0 - \hat{\theta})\right\}^2 (-n^{-1}l''(\hat{\theta}\,|\,x)) + o_p(1) = \left\{\sqrt{n}(\theta_0 - \hat{\theta})\sqrt{(-n^{-1}l''(\hat{\theta}\,|\,x))}\right\}^2 + o_p(1).$$

Under the regularity conditions, we have $\sqrt{n}(\theta_0 - \hat{\theta}) \to N(0, 1/I(\theta_0))$ in distribution (Lehmann and Casella 1998) and $-n^{-1}l''(\hat{\theta}\,|\,x) \to I(\theta_0)$ in probability. As a result of Slutsky's theorem (Grimmett and Stirzaker 1992), $\sqrt{n}(\theta_0 - \hat{\theta})\sqrt{(-n^{-1}l''(\hat{\theta}\,|\,x))}$ converges to $N(0,1)$ in distribution, and therefore $2\log \Lambda(x)$ converges to χ_1^2 in distribution.

5

Tests on Means of Continuous Data

5.1 Introduction

Two data characteristics, the mean and the standard deviation, are the primary descriptors of continuous data in practice. Therefore, tests for means have very important roles in health-related experiments. It is frequently of interest to compare two independent groups with respect to their mean scores of a continuous measure. Does a sample mean equal to a pre-specified population mean, or, instead, do two or more samples have the same population mean? These inquiries can be answered by hypothesis testing about a single mean in the univariate setting or testing the equality means in the k-group setting. In this chapter, we also present an exact likelihood ratio test for the joint equality of means and variances of two populations.

5.2 Univariate and p-Dimensional Likelihood Ratio Tests of Location Given Normally Distributed Data

Given a random sample of independent and identically distributed (i.i.d.) observations $X_1, \ldots, X_n$ from a normal distribution with mean μ and variance σ^2, suppose we would like to test the simple hypothesis

$$H_0 : \mu = \mu_0 \text{ versus } H_1 : \mu = \mu_1.$$

In this circumstance, the likelihood function is

$$\left(\sigma\sqrt{2\pi}\right)^{-n} \exp\left\{-\sum_{i=1}^{n}(X_i - \mu)^2 \Big/ \left(2\sigma^2\right)\right\}.$$

Thus, the likelihood ratio has the form

$$L = \left(\sigma_1/\sigma_0\right)^{-n} \exp\left\{-\sum_{i=1}^{n}(X_i - \mu_1)^2 \Big/ \left(2\sigma_1^2\right) + \sum_{i=1}^{n}(X_i - \mu_0)^2 \Big/ \left(2\sigma_0^2\right)\right\},$$

where σ_0 and σ_1 are the standard deviation of observations under H_0 and H_1, respectively. In the case where $\sigma_0 = \sigma_1 = \sigma$, we have

$$\log L \propto \sum_{i=1}^{n}(X_i - \mu_0)^2 - \sum_{i=1}^{n}(X_i - \mu_1)^2 = 2(\mu_1 - \mu_0)\sum_{i=1}^{n}X_i - n(\mu_1^2 - \mu_0^2).$$

We reject H_0 if $L > C_\alpha$, where the test threshold C_α is selected for a specified value for the significance level α, the Type I error rate. Thus, when $\sigma_0 = \sigma_1 = \sigma$ and the values of μ_0 and μ_1 are known, we can use this most powerful likelihood ratio test.

5.3 *t*-Type Tests

As a case in point of the maximum likelihood methodology, we present *t*-test-type decision rules, which are widely used in practice. Toward this end, we assume the following constraints: (1) the data is a simple random sample from the population and each sample observation is independent from the others, and (2) the sample observations were drawn from a normal distribution, so *t*-tests can be easily conducted to test means of continuous data. The one-sample *t*-test can be applied to test for the equality of the sample mean to a presumed value when the population variance is unknown. To determine if two independent sets of data are significantly different from each other, the two-sample *t*-test can be applied. In the case of multivariate hypothesis testing, the multivariate *t*-test (Hotelling's *T*-squared-test), as a generalization of Student's *t*-statistic, can be used.

5.3.1 One-Sample *t*-Test

In testing the null hypothesis that the population mean is equal to a specified value μ_0, that is, $H_0 : \mu = \mu_0$ versus $H_1 : \mu \neq \mu_0$, based on the observed data $X_1, \ldots, X_n$, one uses the statistic

$$t = \frac{\bar{X} - \mu_0}{s/\sqrt{n}},$$

where n is the sample size, $\bar{X} = n^{-1}\sum_{i=1}^{n}X_i$ is the sample mean, and $s^2 = (n-1)^{-1} \times \sum_{i=1}^{n}(X_i - \bar{X})^2$ is the sample standard deviation. At the α significance level, the null hypothesis can be rejected if $|t| \geq t_{\alpha/2, n-1}$, where $t_{\alpha/2, n-1}$ is the $(1 - \alpha/2)$th quantile of *t*-distribution with $n - 1$ degrees of freedom. We express the pth quantile for a random variable as the value x, so that the probability that the random variable will be less than x is at most p, and the likelihood that the random variable will be more than x is at least $1 - p$. Note that the population does not need to be normally distributed for a large sample size (greater than 30, as a rule of thumb). By the central limit theorem, the distribution of the population of sample means, $\bar{X}$, will be approximately normal for a sufficiently large sample size (Box et al. 1978).

5.3.2 Two-Sample *t*-Test

The two-sample *t*-test is used to determine if two independent population means are equal, that is, $H_0 : \mu_1 = \mu_2$ versus $H_1 : \mu_1 \neq \mu_2$. Given two samples of i.i.d. observations $X_{i1}, \ldots, X_{in_i}, i = 1, 2,$ we denote the sample size, the sample mean, and the unbiased estimator of the variance of the two samples as n_i, $\bar{X}_i = n_i^{-1} \sum_{j=1}^{n_i} X_{ij}$ and $s_i^2 = (n_i - 1)^{-1} \sum_{j=1}^{n_i} (X_{ij} - \bar{X}_i)^2, i = 1, 2,$ respectively. The *t*-statistic to test whether the means are equal can be calculated as follows:

$$t = \frac{\bar{X}_1 - \bar{X}_2}{s_d} .$$

Based on the equivalence of the population variance in two groups, the equal variances case and the unequal variances case are considered separately, and the estimator s_d can be calculated accordingly.

5.3.2.1 Equal Variances

When the two distributions are assumed to have the same variance, the estimator is $s_d = s_p \sqrt{n_1^{-1} + n_2^{-1}}$, where the pooled sample deviation

$$s_p = \sqrt{\left((n_1 - 1)s_1^2 + (n_2 - 1)s_2^2\right) / (n_1 + n_2 - 2)}$$

is an estimator of the common standard deviation of the two samples. At the α significance level, the null hypothesis of equal means can be rejected if $|t| \geq t_{\alpha/2, n_1 + n_2 - 2}$, where $t_{\alpha/2, n_1 + n_2 - 2}$ is the $(1 - \alpha/2)$th quantile of the *t*-distribution with $n_1 + n_2 - 2$ degrees of freedom. Note that s_p^2 is an unbiased estimator of the common variance whether or not the population means are the same.

5.3.2.2 Unequal Variances (Welch's t-Test)

When the two population variances are not assumed to be equal, the estimator is $s_d = \sqrt{s_1^2/n_1 + s_2^2/n_2}$. Note that in this case, s_d^2 is not a pooled variance. At the α significance level, the null hypothesis of equal means can be rejected if $|t| \geq t_{\alpha/2, df}$, where $t_{\alpha/2, df}$ is the $(1 - \alpha/2)$th quantile of the *t*-distribution with

$$df = \frac{\left(s_1^2/n_1 + s_2^2/n_2\right)^2}{\left(s_1^2/n_1\right)^2 / (n_1 - 1) + \left(s_2^2/n_2\right)^2 / (n_2 - 1)}$$

degrees of freedom.

5.3.3 Paired *t*-Test

In clinical trials, the generalized treatment effect can be used to compare treatments or interventions based on the difference in mean outcomes between pre- and post-treatment measurements. In the case of one paired sample, paired *t*-tests can be conducted to test for a paired difference. Given a paired sample $X_{k1}, \ldots, X_{kn}$ of pre-treatment ($k = 1$) and post-treatment ($k = 1$) measurements, to test whether the difference μ_D in means between post- and pre-treatment measurements is μ_0, the t-statistic is

$$t = \frac{\bar{X}_D - \mu_0}{s_D/\sqrt{n}},$$

where n is the number of pairs, $X_{Di} = X_{2i} - X_{1i}$,

$$\bar{X}_D = n^{-1} \sum_{i=1}^{n} X_{Di},$$

and

$$s_D^2 = (n-1)^{-1} \sum_{i=1}^{n} \left(X_{Di} - \bar{X}_D \right)^2.$$

is the sample mean and sample variance of differences between all pairs, respectively. At the α significance level, the null hypothesis can be rejected if $|t| \geq t_{\alpha/2,\, n-1}$, where $t_{\alpha/2,\, n-1}$ is the $(1 - \alpha/2)$th quantile of the t-distribution with $n - 1$ degrees of freedom.

We exemplify the use of the paired t-test with a real-life example of the effect of asthma education on pediatric patients' acute care visits (Riffenburgh 2012).

Example 5.1: One Sample t-Test Using R

Let the study sample consist of 32 patients who satisfy inclusion criteria and present over a period of time. The number of acute care visits during a year is recorded. After a standardized course of asthma training, the number of acute care visits for the following year is recorded again. The changes per patient, that is, the before-and-after difference in the number of visits, were 1, 1, 2, 4, 0, 5, –3, 0, 4, 2, 8, 1, 1, 0, –1, 3, 6, 3, 1, 2, 0, –1, 0, 3, 2, 1, 3, –1, –1, 1, 1, and 5. It is of interest to test if the training affects the number of visits (Riffenburgh 2012).

The following R code can be used to carry out the two-tailed test $H_0 : \mu_D = 0$ against $H_1 : \mu_D \neq 0$:

```
> # input the data: difference (before-after)
> D <-c(1,1,2,4,0,5,-3,0,4,2,8,1,1,0,-1,3,6,3,1,2,0,-1,0,3,2,1,3,-1,
-1,1,1,5)
> alpha <- 0.05 # pre-specified significance level
> # check the normality by the histogram
> hist(D,xlab="Difference",main="Histogram of the Differences")
>
> # calculate the test statistic
> n <- length(D) # the sample size, i.e., the number of pairs
> t.stat <- (mean(D)-0)/(sd(D)/sqrt(n))
> t.stat
[1] 4.034031
>
> # obtain the critical value and the p-value
> crit <- qt(1-alpha/2,df=n-1)
> crit
[1] 2.039513
> pval <- 2*(1-pt(t.stat,df=n-1)) # a two-sided test
> pval
[1] 0.0003323025
```

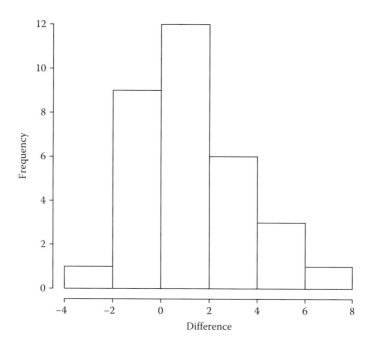

FIGURE 5.1

Histogram of the differences in the number of acute care visits pre- and post-asthma training.

Alternatively, one may use the built-in function *t.test* setting *paired=TRUE* and *alternative="two.sided"* in R to conduct the two-sided paired *t*-test. It yields the following output:

```
> t.test(D,rep(0,n),paired=TRUE,alternative="two.sided")
        Paired t-test
data: D and rep(0, n)
t = 4.034, df = 31, p-value = 0.0003323
alternative hypothesis: true difference in means is not equal to 0
95 percent confidence interval:
 0.818888 2.493612
sample estimates:
mean of the differences
          1.65625
```

The form of the histogram of the differences, shown in Figure 5.1, suggests an approximately normal shape; thus, we may assume that the data points are distributed satisfying the normal distribution assumption. The test statistic is $t = 4.034$, which is greater than the critical value $t_{\alpha/2,\,df=31} = 2.04$ at the $\alpha = 0.05$ significance level. We can state that we are 95% sure that the asthma training was efficacious.

5.3.4 Multivariate *t*-Test

Hypothesis testing of the equality of means can be constructed in the multivariate case, say p-dimensional. Assuming that the samples are independently drawn from two independent multivariate normal distributions with the same covariance, that is, for the ith sample, $\mathbf{X}_{ij} \sim N_p(\boldsymbol{\mu}_i, \Sigma)$, $i = 1, 2$, $j = 1,\ldots, n_i$, the hypothesis is H_0: $\boldsymbol{\mu}_1 = \boldsymbol{\mu}_2$ versus H_a: $\boldsymbol{\mu}_1 \neq \boldsymbol{\mu}_2$. Define $\overline{\mathbf{X}}_i = n_i^{-1}\sum_{j=1}^{n_i} \mathbf{X}_{ij}$, $i = 1, 2$, as the sample means, and

$\mathbf{W} = \left(n_1 + n_2 - 2\right)^{-1} \sum_{i=1}^{2} \sum_{j=1}^{n_i} \left(\mathbf{X}_{ij} - \overline{\mathbf{X}}_i\right)\left(\mathbf{X}_{ij} \quad \overline{\mathbf{X}}_i\right)^{T}$ as the unbiased pooled sample covariance matrix estimate; then, Hotelling's two-sample T^2-statistic is

$$t^2 = \frac{n_1 n_2}{n_1 + n_2}\left(\overline{\mathbf{X}}_1 - \overline{\mathbf{X}}_2\right)^{T} \mathbf{W}^{-1}\left(\overline{\mathbf{X}}_1 - \overline{\mathbf{X}}_2\right).$$

Note that Hotelling's two-sample T^2-statistic follows Hotelling's T^2-distribution with parameters p and $n_1 + n_2 - 2$, that is, $t^2 \sim T^2\ (p, n_1 + n_2 - 2)$. The null hypothesis is rejected if $t^2 > T^2\ (\alpha;\ p, n_1 + n_2 - 2)$ at the α significance level. (Here the matrix transpose operation ^{T} means $\begin{bmatrix} a \\ b \end{bmatrix}^{T} = \begin{bmatrix} a & b \end{bmatrix}$ and $\begin{bmatrix} a & b \end{bmatrix}^{T} = \begin{bmatrix} a \\ b \end{bmatrix}$.)

In the following example, we will demonstrate how to simulate multivariate normal data in R using the function *mvrnorm* introduced in Chapter 2 and conduct Hotelling's two-sample T^2-test.

Example 5.2: Hotelling's Two-Sample T^2-Test

We consider an example in which age and measurements of weight (in kg) are recorded for each patient in two independent groups. Assume that for the first group, $n_1 = 50$ patients' measurements are randomly sampled from the population $N_2\left(\begin{pmatrix} 25 \\ 65 \end{pmatrix}, \begin{pmatrix} 5 & 1 \\ 1 & 9 \end{pmatrix}\right)$, while for the second group, $n_2 = 70$ patients' measurements are randomly sampled from the population $N_2\left(\begin{pmatrix} 25 \\ 70 \end{pmatrix}, \begin{pmatrix} 5 & 1 \\ 1 & 9 \end{pmatrix}\right)$. We simulate the data and test if the means are equal.

For each group, we assume a bivariate normal data distribution with a common population covariance matrix. The following R code simulates bivariate normal data and conducts Hotelling's two-sample T^2-test for the equality of means:

```
> # Check if packages are aleady installed.
> check.pkg <- c("ICSNP", "MASS") %in% rownames(installed.packages())
> if(any(!check.pkg)) install.packages(c("ICSNP", "MASS")[!check.pkg])
> # load packages
> library(ICSNP)
> library(MASS)
> # simulate data
> set.seed(123)
> n1 <- 50
> n2 <- 70
> Sigma <- matrix(c(5,1, 1,9), byrow=TRUE, ncol=2) # common covariance
> # matrix
> X1 <- mvrnorm (n1, mu=c(25, 65), Sigma=Sigma)
> X2 <- mvrnorm (n2, mu=c(25, 70), Sigma=Sigma)
> X <- rbind(X1, X2)
> Group <- factor(rep(1:2, c(n1,n2)))
> HotellingsT2(X ~ Group)
```

It yields the following output:

```
        Hotelling's two sample T2-test
data: X by Group
T.2 = 35.3461, df1 = 2, df2 = 117, p-value = 9.823e-13
alternative hypothesis: true location difference is not equal to c(0,0)
```

With the obtained p-value far less than 0.001, we reject the null hypothesis at the 0.05 significance level. We can conclude that there is a statistically significant difference in the bivariate means from our example data.

5.4 Exact Likelihood Ratio Test for Equality of Two Normal Populations

In this section, we introduce an exact likelihood ratio test that compares the means and variances of two populations simultaneously. Let $\{X_1, ..., X_n\}$ and $\{Y_1, ..., Y_m\}$ be two independent random samples from normal populations $N(\mu_1, \sigma_1^2)$ and $N(\mu_2, \sigma_2^2)$, respectively. Suppose it is of interest to test

$$H_0 : \mu_1 = \mu_2 \text{ and } \sigma_1^2 = \sigma_2^2 \text{ versus } H_1 : \mu_1 \neq \mu_2 \text{ or } \sigma_1^2 \neq \sigma_2^2 .$$

Pearson and Neyman (1930) considered the likelihood ratio test

$$\lambda_{n,m} = \frac{\left[\sum_{i=1}^{n} (X_i - \bar{X})^2 / n \right]^{n/2} \left[\sum_{j=1}^{m} (Y_j - \bar{Y})^2 / m \right]^{m/2}}{\left\{ \left[\sum_{i=1}^{n} (X_i - u)^2 + \sum_{j=1}^{m} (Y_j - u)^2 \right] / (n+m) \right\}^{(n+m)/2}},$$

where $\bar{X}$, $\bar{Y}$, and u are the sample means of the X sample, the Y sample, and the combined sample, respectively. For $\lambda \in (0, 1)$, Zhang et al. (2012) derived the exact distribution of $\lambda_{n,m}$ as

$$\Pr\left(\lambda_{n,m} \leq \lambda\right) = 1 - C \int\int_D w_1^{(n-1)/2-1} w_2^{(m-1)/2-1} / \sqrt{1 - w_1 - w_2} \, dw_1 dw_2$$

$$= 1 - C \int_{r_1}^{r_2} w_1^{(n-3)/2} \int_{z/w_1^{n/m}}^{1-w_1} w_2^{(m-3)/2} / \sqrt{1 - w_1 - w_2} \, dw_2 \, dw_1,$$

where

$$z = \frac{\lambda^{2/m} n^{n/m} m}{(n+m)^{(n+m)/m}}, \quad C = \frac{\Gamma\left((n+m-1)/2\right)}{\Gamma\left((n-1)/2\right)\Gamma\left((m-1)/2\right)\Gamma\left(1/2\right)},$$

$$D = \left\{(w_1, w_2) : w_1 > 0, w_2 > 0, w_1 + w_2 < 1, w_1^{n/2} w_2^{m/2} (n+m)^{(n+m)/2} / (n^{n/2} m^{m/2}) > \lambda \right\},$$

$\Gamma(\cdot)$ is the gamma function and $r_1 < r_2$ are the two roots (for the variable w_1) of

$$1 - w_1 - z/w_1^{n/m} = 0.$$

Note that the double integral can be computed using the Gaussian quadrature, implemented with the R function *plrt*.

5.5 Supplement

The issue of testing for equality between means is well addressed in the literature. In this section, we outline a limited number of publications in which health-related researches may be interested.

1. In order to assess the mean of asymmetrical distributions, Johnson (1978) proposed some modified t-tests, which can be applied to a wide range of parent distributions from the normal distribution to an asymmetric distribution, such as an exponential distribution for sample sizes as small as 13. In many practical scenarios, due to the cost of the sampling procedures, the skewness of the parent distribution can be greater than those studied by Johnson and the sample sizes can be quite small, possibly as small as 10, under which cases Johnson's test can be quite inaccurate. To deal with this issue, Sutton (1993) suggested a composite test to improve Johnson's upper-tailed t-test and Chen (1995) proposed a test procedure for the upper-tailed test for the mean of positively skewed distributions. Based on a Monte Carlo study, Chen's test was shown to be more accurate and more powerful than both Johnson's modified t-test and Sutton's composite test for a variety of positively skewed distributions with a small sample.

2. Fagerland and Sandvik (2009a) investigated the appropriateness of the practice of interpreting the results of tests for comparing the locations of two independent populations as evidence for or against equality of means or medians. The authors investigated the performance of five frequently used tests: the two-sample T-test, the Welch U-test, the Yuen–Welch test, the Wilcoxon–Mann–Whitney test, and the Brunner–Munzel test. These tests are associated with different null hypotheses. Under violations of both normality and variance homogeneity, the true significance level and power of the tests depend on a complex interplay of several factors. Based on simulation studies, the authors investigated a variety of scenarios differing in skewness, skewness heterogeneity, variance heterogeneity, sample size, and sample size ratio. It was shown that small differences in distribution properties can affect test performance dramatically, therefore confounding the effort to present simple test recommendations. The Welch U-test is suggested for use most frequently, but it cannot be considered an omnibus test.

3. In order to assess a monotonic dose–response relationship between exposure and disease in epidemiological and clinical studies, the Mantel-extension chi-square test for overall trend and an asymptotically equivalent test based on logistic regression can be used. Nonetheless, these tests have two disadvantages: (a) a parametric model of linear form on the logit scale is assumed, and (b) an a priori choice of scores to code for the exposure categories is imposed. Note that if made incorrectly, the linear assumption can lead to an invalid result, and the choice of scores is arbitrary. Leuraud and Benichou (2001) compared several tests, including the test based on isotonic regression, the t-test based on contrasts, a test based on adjacent contrasts (Dosemeci–Benichou test), and the Mantel-extension test for overall trend. The authors investigated their statistical properties, including Type I error and power. By generating cohort and case-control data, the authors considered one- and two-sided versions of the tests, and studied the tests under the null hypothesis of no relationship between exposure and disease and under various alternative patterns of monotonic or nonmonotonic dose–response relationships.

It was confirmed that the commonly used trend tests can lead to the erroneous conclusion of a monotonic dose–response relationship. The test based on isotonic regression does not stand for a favorable alternative, as it tends to be too powerful in the case of nonmonotonic dose–response relationship patterns. The tests based on contrasts may have better performance, for example, Type I error close to the nominal level, high power for monotonic alternatives, and low power for nonmonotonic alternatives. These results were illustrated with case-control data on occupational risks of bladder cancer.

4. Due to the inability to provide a measure for the magnitude of the mean effect, the p-value from the two-sample t-test has sometimes been criticized. However, with the knowledge of the p-value and the sample size, a relationship was shown with Cohen's effect size (Cohen 1969) and exact confidence limits on the effect size. Browne (2010) considered using confidence limits to create graphs of the normal density consonants with the data. Additionally, for treatments X and Y, the author derived exact confidence limits for $\Pr(X > Y)$ and the odds of X being greater than Y, where t-test results can be denoted based on differences between individuals randomly chosen from the two populations instead of differences in population means. The author described the limitations of $p < 0.05$ and $p < 0.0001$ that are widely considered in practice.

5. Robust statistics is an extension of classical parametric statistics taking into account the fact that the assumed parametric models are only approximate. Farcomeni and Ventura (2012) reviewed and outlined the robustness of inferential procedures that may be applied in the biomedical research. The authors presented numerical illustrations for the t-test, regression models, logistic regression, survival analysis, and receiver operating characteristic (ROC) curves, showing that robust methods are more appropriate than standard procedures.

6

Empirical Likelihood

> I suppose it is tempting, if the only tool you have is a hammer, to treat everything as if it were a nail.
>
> **Abraham Maslow***

6.1 Introduction

As mentioned in Chapter 1, when using robust statistical testing methods, which minimize the assumptions regarding the underlying distributions, it is important to still maintain a high level of efficiency compared to their parametric counterparts. Toward this end, the recent biostatistical literature has shifted focus toward robust and efficient nonparametric and semiparametric developments of various "artificial" or "approximate" likelihood techniques. These methods have a wide variety of applications related to clinical experiments. Many nonparametric and semiparametric approximations to powerful parametric likelihood procedures have been used routinely in both statistical theory and practice. Well-known examples include the quasi-likelihood method, which is approximations of parametric likelihoods via orthogonal functions, techniques based on quadratic artificial likelihood functions, and the local maximum likelihood methodology (Claeskens and Hjort 2004; Fan et al. 1998; Wang 2006; Wedderburn 1974). Various studies have shown that artificial or approximate likelihood-based techniques efficiently incorporate information expressed through the data, and have many of the same asymptotic properties as those derived from the corresponding parametric likelihoods. The empirical likelihood (EL) method is one of a growing array of artificial or approximate likelihood-based methods currently in use in statistical practice (Owen 2001). Interest and the resulting impact in EL methods continue to grow rapidly. Perhaps more importantly, EL methods now have various vital applications in expanding numbers of areas of clinical studies.

In this chapter, we focus on the performance of EL constructions relative to ordinary parametric likelihood ratio–based procedures in the context of clinical experiments. Our desire to incorporate several recent developments and applications in these areas in an easy-to-use manner provides one of the main impetuses for this chapter. The EL method for testing has been dealt with extensively in the literature within a variety of settings (Lazar and Mykland 1998; Owen 1990; Qin and Lawless 1994; Vexler et al. 2009a, 2014d; Yu et al. 2010).

---

* Toward a Psychology of Being.

6.2 Classical Empirical Likelihood Methods

As background for the development of EL-type techniques, we first outline the classical EL approach. The classical EL takes the form $\prod_{i=1}^{n}(F(X_i) - F(X_i-))$, which is a functional of the cumulative distribution function F and independent and identically distributed (i.i.d.) observations X_i, $i = 1, ..., n$. This EL technique is "distribution function based" (Owen 2001). In the distribution-free setting, an empirical estimator of the likelihood takes the form of $L_p = \prod_{i=1}^{n} p_i$, where the components p_i, $i = 1, ..., n$, estimators of the probability weights, should maximize the likelihood L_p, provided that $\sum_{i=1}^{n} p_i = 1$ and empirical constraints based on $X_1, ..., X_n$ hold. For example, suppose we would like to test the hypothesis

$$H_0: Eg(X_1, \theta) = 0 \text{ versus } H_1: Eg(X_1, \theta) \neq 0, \tag{6.1}$$

where $g(.,.)$ is a given function and θ is a parameter, then, in a nonparametric fashion, we define the EL function of the form $EL(\theta) = L(X_1, ..., X_n \mid \theta) = \prod_{i=1}^{n} p_i$, where $\sum_{i=1}^{n} p_i = 1$. Under the null hypothesis, the maximum likelihood approach requires one to find the value of the p_i, $i = 1, ..., n$, that maximize the EL given the empirical constraints $\sum_{i=1}^{n} p_i = 1$ and $\sum_{i=1}^{n} p_i g(X_i, \theta) = 0$ that present an empirical version of the condition under H_0 that $Eg(X_1, \theta) = 0$ (the null hypothesis is assumed to be rejected when there are no $0 < p_1, ..., p_n < 1$ to satisfy the empirical constraints). In this case, using Lagrange multipliers, one can show that

$$EL(\theta) = \sup_{0 < p_1, p_2, ..., p_n < 1, \sum p_i = 1, \sum p_i g(X_i, \theta) = 0} \prod_{i=1}^{n} p_i = \prod_{i=1}^{n}(n + \lambda g(X_i, \theta))^{-1}, \tag{6.2}$$

where λ is a root of $\sum g(X_i, \theta)(n + \lambda g(X_i, \theta))^{-1} = 0$. Since under H_1 the only constraint under consideration is $\sum p_i = 1$, we have

$$EL = \sup_{0 < p_1, p_2, ..., p_n < 1, \sum p_i = 1} \prod_{i=1}^{n} p_i = \prod_{i=1}^{n} n^{-1} = (n)^{-n}. \tag{6.3}$$

Combining Equations 6.2 and 6.3, we obtain the empirical likelihood ratio (ELR) test statistic $ELR(\theta) = EL/EL(\theta)$ for the hypothesis test of H_0 versus H_1. For example, when the function $g(u, \theta) = u - \theta$, the null hypothesis corresponds to the expectation $EX_1 = \theta$.

Owen (1988) showed that the nonparametric test statistic $2 \log ELR(\theta)$ has an asymptotic chi-square distribution under the null hypothesis. This result illustrates that Wilks' theorem–type results continue to hold in the context of this infinite-dimensional problem. Consequently, there are techniques for correcting forms of ELRs to improve the convergence rate of the null distributions of ELR test statistics to chi-square distributions. These techniques are similar to those applied in the field of parametric maximum likelihood ratio procedures (Vexler et al. 2009a). The statement of the hypothesis testing above can easily be inverted with respect to providing nonparametric confidence interval estimators.

In terms of the accessibility of this method, it should be noted that the number of EL software packages continues to expand, particularly the R-based software packages.

For example, see the *library(emplik)* and *library(EL)* of R packages that include the R functions *el.test()* and *EL.test()*. These simple R functions can be very useful for the EL analysis of data from clinical studies.

For an illustrative example, we revisit the high-density lipoprotein (HDL) cholesterol data shown in Figure 4.1 in Chapter 4. Now, we use the empirical likelihood ratio test for means. The following R output shows the result of the empirical likelihood comparison between the means of the groups X and Y:

```
> library(EL)
> EL.means(X,Y)

Empirical likelihood mean difference test

data: X and Y
-2 * LogLikelihood = 3.547, p-value = 0.05965
95 percent confidence interval:
 -0.4900842 19.0138090
sample estimates:
Mean difference
       10.17393
```

Perhaps, in this example, the ELR test outperforms the *t*-test that claims to reject the hypothesis $E(X) = E(Y)$, when X and Y are the measurements related to the same group of patients.

Example 6.1: EL Test of the Mean

Assume that we have a sample of i.i.d. measurements $X_1, ..., X_{25}$ simulated from the following distributions: (1) normal distribution $N(0,1)$ and (2) $F(x) = (1 - \lambda exp(- \lambda(x + 1)))$ $I \{x + 1 > 0\}$, where λ is the rate parameter. We would like to test H_0: $EX = 0$ versus H_1: $EX \neq 0$ at the $\alpha = 0.05$ significance level. For both scenarios, we fail to reject H_0 based on either the EL methodology or the *t*-test. However, in the case (2), the result of the *t*-test application is not valid since the distributional assumption is not satisfied. The following code implements the procedures:

```
> library(emplik)
> n<-25
>
> ## (1) N(0,1)
> X<-rnorm(n,0,1)
> el.obj<-el.test(X,mu=0)
> el.obj$Pval
[1] 0.1673519
> t.test(X,mu=0)$p.value
[1] 0.2019836
>
> ## (2) exp(1)-1
> X<-rexp(n,rate=1)-1
> el.obj<-el.test(X,mu=0)
> el.obj$Pval
[1] 0.2043935
> t.test(X,mu=0)$p.value
[1] 0.1463612
```

The classical EL methodology has been shown to have properties that make it attractive for testing hypotheses regarding parameters (e.g., moments) of distributions (Owen 1988;

Qin and Lawless 1994). However, statisticians working on clinical experiments, for example, case-control studies, commonly face a variety of distribution-free comparisons or evaluations over all distribution functions of complete and incomplete data subject to different types of measurement errors. In this framework, the *density-based* empirical likelihood methodology shown in Section 6.4 figures prominently.

6.3 Techniques for Analyzing Empirical Likelihoods

In this section, we consider the hypothesis described in (6.1) and the simple form of the ELR test statistic defined above via Equations 6.2 and 6.3. The analysis is relatively clear and has the basic ingredients for more general cases. We posit that the following results can be associated with deriving different properties of EL-type procedures, including the power and Type I error analysis of ELR type tests.

Properties of many statistical quantities based on parametric likelihoods can be studied by using the fact that parametric likelihood functions are often highly peaked about their maximum values (e.g., DasGupta 2008). The modern statistical literature considers a variety of semi- and nonparametric procedures created by proposing to use EL functions in efficient parametric schemes instead of parametric likelihoods. For example, in this context, the results of Qin and Lawless (1994) have a remarkable utility with respect to operations with ELs in a manner similar to those related to parametric maximum likelihoods. The following lemma illustrates a strong similarity between behaviors of empirical and parametric likelihood functions. Suppose the function $g(x, \theta)$ appearing in Equations 6.1 and 6.2 is differentiable with respect to the second argument θ; then, we have

Lemma 6.1. Let θ_M be a root of the equation $n^{-1} \sum_{i=1}^{n} g(X_i, \theta_M) = 0$, where $\partial g(X_i, \theta)/\partial \theta < 0$ (or $\partial g(X_i, \theta)/\partial \theta > 0$) for all $i = 1, 2, \ldots, n$. Then the argument θ_M is a global maximum of the function

$$EL(\theta) = \max\left\{ \prod_{i=1}^{n} p_i : 0 < p_i < 1, \sum_{i=1}^{n} p_i = 1, \sum_{i=1}^{n} p_i g(X_i, \theta) = 0 \right\}$$

which follows from the fact that it increases and decreases monotonically for $\theta < \theta_M$ and $\theta > \theta_M$, respectively.

The proof scheme of Lemma 6.1 is presented in Vexler et al. (2013a, 2014d).

For example, when $g(u, \theta) = u - \theta$, we obtain $\theta_M = \bar{X} = n^{-1} \sum_{i=1}^{n} X_i$; if, for a given function $z(u)$, $g(u, \theta) = z(u) - \theta^2$, $\theta > 0$, then $\theta_M^2 = n^{-1} \sum_{i=1}^{n} z(X_i)$.

Turning to the task of developing asymptotic methods based on ELs, we provide the proposition below. Without loss of generality and for simplicity of notation, we set $g(u, \theta) = u - \theta$ in the definition of the function $ELR(\theta)$ via Equations 6.2 and 6.3. Thus, $EL(\theta) = \prod_{i=1}^{n} p_i$, $\log ELR(\theta) = \sum_{i=1}^{n} \log\{1 + \lambda(X_i - \theta)/n\}$, with $p_i = \{n + \lambda(X_i - \theta)\}^{-1}$, where $\lambda = \lambda(\theta)$ is a root of

$$\sum_{i=1}^{n} (X_i - \theta)(n + \lambda(X_i - \theta))^{-1} = 0. \tag{6.4}$$

Then, defining $\lambda' = d\lambda(\theta)/d\theta$, $\lambda'' = d^2\lambda(\theta)/d\theta^2$, $\lambda^{(k)} = d^k\lambda(\theta)/d\theta^k$, $k = 3, 4$, and using (6.4), one can show the following proposition:

Proposition 6.1. We have the following equations:

$$d\log ELR(\theta)/d\theta = -\lambda(\theta), \quad \lambda' = -n\sum_{i=1}^{n} p_i^2 \Big/ \sum_{i=1}^{n} (X_i - \theta)^2 p$$

$$\lambda'' = -\left\{ 2\lambda'^2 \sum_{i=1}^{n} (X_i - \theta)^3 p_i^3 + 4n\lambda' \sum_{i=1}^{n} (X_i - \theta) p_i^3 - 2n\lambda \sum_{i=1}^{n} p_i^3 \right\} \Big/ \sum_{i=1}^{n} (X_i - \theta)^2 p_i^2$$

$$\lambda^{(3)} = \left\{ 6\lambda'\lambda'' \sum_{i=1}^{n} (X_i - \theta)^3 p_i^3 + 6n\lambda'' \sum_{i=1}^{n} (X_i - \theta) p_i^3 - 6\lambda'^3 \sum_{i=1}^{n} (X_i - \theta)^4 p_i^4 \right.$$

$$\left. -18n\lambda'^2 \sum_{i=1}^{n} (X_i - \theta)^2 p_i^4 + 12n\lambda' \sum_{i=1}^{n} p_i^3 - \left(18n^2\lambda' + 6n\lambda^2\right) \sum_{i=1}^{n} p_i^4 \right\} \Big/ \sum_{i=1}^{n} (X_i - \theta)^2 p_i^2$$

$$\lambda^{(4)} = \left\{ \left(8\lambda'\lambda^{(3)} + 6\lambda''^2\right) \sum_{i=1}^{n} (X_i - \theta)^3 p_i^3 + 8n\lambda^{(3)} \sum_{i=1}^{n} (X_i - \theta) p_i^3 - 36\lambda'^2\lambda'' \sum_{i=1}^{n} (X_i - \theta)^4 p_i^4 \right.$$

$$- 72n\lambda'\lambda'' \sum_{i=1}^{n} (X_i - \theta)^2 p_i^4 - \left(36n^2\lambda'' - 18n\lambda\lambda'\right) \sum_{i=1}^{n} p_i^4 + 24n\lambda'' \sum_{i=1}^{n} p_i^3$$

$$+ 24\lambda'^4 \sum_{i=1}^{n} (X_i - \theta)^5 p_i^5 + 96n\lambda'^3 \sum_{i=1}^{n} (X_i - \theta)^3 p_i^5 - 72n\lambda' \sum_{i=1}^{n} (X_i - \theta) p_i^4$$

$$+ \left(144n^2\lambda'^2 + 24n\lambda^2\lambda'\right) \sum_{i=1}^{n} (X_i - \theta) p_i^5 - \left(72n^2\lambda\lambda' + 24n\lambda^3\right) \sum_{i=1}^{n} p_i^5 \right\} \Big/ \sum_{i=1}^{n} (X_i - \theta)^2 p_i^2.$$

This proposition can support a variety of evaluations of $ELR(\theta)$-type procedures. To show the relevant examples, we should note that $\log ELR(\theta_M) = 0$, since, in this case, $p_i = 1/n$, for all i, and $EL(\theta_M) = EL$. It is also clear that when $\theta = \theta_M$, $\lambda(\theta) = 0$, since $p_i = 1/n$, $i = 1, \ldots, n$ maximize $EL \geq EL(\theta)$ for all θ and satisfy automatically the constraint $\sum p_i g(X_i, \theta) = 0$ when $\theta = \theta_M$, by virtue of the definition of θ_M. Thus, one can use Proposition 6.1 to obtain the Taylor expansion for the function $\log ELR(\theta)$ at argument $\theta_M = \bar{X}$, in the form of

$$\log ELR(\theta) \approx \log ELR(\bar{X}) + (\theta - \bar{X}) \frac{d\log ELR(\bar{X})}{d\theta}\bigg|_{\theta = \bar{X}}$$

$$+ \frac{(\theta - \bar{X})^2}{2!} \frac{d^2 \log ELR(\bar{X})}{d\theta^2}\bigg|_{\theta = \bar{X}} + \frac{(\theta - \bar{X})^3}{3!} \frac{d^3 \log ELR(\bar{X})}{d\theta^3}\bigg|_{\theta = \bar{X}}$$

$$= \frac{1}{2}\left(n^{0.5}(\theta - \bar{X})\right)^2 \Big/ \left[\frac{1}{n}\sum_{i=1}^{n}(X_i - \bar{X})^2\right] + \frac{1}{3}n(\theta - \bar{X})^3 \Big/ \left[\frac{1}{n}\sum_{i=1}^{n}(X_i - \bar{X})^2\right]^3.$$

This approximation depicts Wilks' theorem when $\theta = EX_1$ and $E|X_1|^3 < \infty$. (In the case of $\theta = EX_1$ and $n \to \infty$, $n^{0.5}(\theta - \bar{X})$ has a normal distribution, $n(\theta - \bar{X})^3 \overset{p}{\to} 0$, and

$\sum_{i=1}^{n} (X_i - \bar{X})^2 / n \rightarrow \text{var}(X_1)$.) Using Proposition 6.1 to figure more terms in the Taylor expansion one can provide high-order approximations to the null distribution of the ELR test, for example, to obtain the Bartlett correction of the ELR structure (e.g., Vexler et al. 2009a). Under the alternative hypothesis $\theta \neq EX_1$, the approximation above shows the power of the ELR test. Lazar and Mykland (1998) considered a general form of ELRs and the case where $|\theta - EX_1| \sim O(n^{-0.5})$. The authors compared the local power of EL to that of an ordinary parametric likelihood. Their notable research shows that there is no loss of efficiency in using the EL model up to a second-order approximation.

In a similar manner to Proposition 6.1, more complicated ELR structures can be analyzed. For example, one can consider the null hypothesis $H_0 : E(X_1) = \theta_1$ and $E(X_1^2) = \theta_2$. In this case, under the null hypothesis, the EL function is given as

$$EL(\theta_1, \theta_2) = \max \left\{ \prod_{i=1}^{n} p_i : \sum_{i=1}^{n} p_i = 1, \sum_{i=1}^{n} p_i X_i = \theta_1, \sum_{i=1}^{n} p_i X_i^2 = \theta_2 \right\}.$$

Then using the Lagrangian

$$\Lambda = \sum_{i=1}^{n} \log p_i + \lambda \left(1 - \sum_{i=1}^{n} p_i \right) + \lambda_1 \left(\theta_1 - \sum_{i=1}^{n} p_i X_i \right) + \lambda_2 \left(\theta_2 - \sum_{i=1}^{n} p_i X_i^2 \right),$$

we obtain $p_i = \{n + \lambda_1 (X_i - \theta_1) + \lambda_2 (X_i^2 - \theta_2)\}^{-1}$, where λ_1 and λ_2 are roots of $\sum (X_i - \theta_1) p_i = 0$ and $\sum (X_i^2 - \theta_2) p_i = 0$. In this case, the appendix presents several results that are similar to those related to the evaluations of $ELR(\theta)$ mentioned above.

Example 6.2: Comparison of LR versus ELR Function Forms

Let $x = \{X_1, \ldots, X_n\}$ denote a random sample from the following distributions: (1) normal distribution $N(\theta,1)$ and (2) exponential(θ), where $\theta = 1$ is the rate parameter. We would like to test $H_0 : EX_1 = 1$ versus $H_1 : EX_1 \neq 1$ at the $\alpha = 0.05$ significance level. Define $\bar{X} = n^{-1} \sum_{i=1}^{n} X_i$. In the normal case, the log-likelihood ratio test statistic is $\log LR(\theta) = -n\bar{X}^2 + 2n\theta\bar{X} - n\theta^2$ and the log-empirical likelihood ratio is $\log ELR(\theta) = \sum_{i=1}^{n} \log\{1 + \lambda(X_i - \theta)/n\}$, where λ is a root of $\sum_{i=1}^{n} (X_i - \theta)(n + \lambda(X_i - \theta))^{-1} = 0$. In the case of the exponential distribution, the log-likelihood ratio test statistic is $\log LR(\theta) = n \log \theta - n\theta\bar{X} + n \log \bar{X} + n$ and the log-empirical likelihood ratio is $\log ELR(\theta) = \sum_{i=1}^{n} \log\{1 + \lambda(X_i - 1/\theta)/n\}$, where λ satisfies $\sum_{i=1}^{n} (X_i - 1/\theta)(n + \lambda(X_i - 1/\theta))^{-1} = 0$.

Figure 6.1 presents the plot of the log-likelihood ratio and the log-empirical likelihood ratio versus the parameter θ based on samples of sizes $n = 25, 50, 150$, where the black solid line and the red dashed line represent the log-empirical likelihood ratio and the log-likelihood ratio when the underlying distribution is normal, respectively, while the green dotted line and the blue dot-dash line represent the log-empirical likelihood ratio and the log-likelihood ratio when the underlying distribution is exponential, respectively. Figure 6.1 illustrates Lemma 6.1. The figure shows that the empirical likelihood ratio behaves in a manner similar to that of the parametric likelihood ratio and

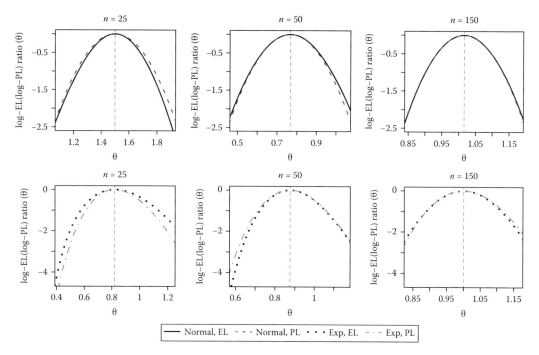

FIGURE 6.1

(See color insert.) The log-empirical likelihood ratios and the log-likelihood ratios based on samples of sizes $n = 25, 50, 150$, where the black solid line and the red dashed line represent the log-empirical likelihood ratios and the log-likelihood ratios when the underlying distribution is normal, respectively, while the green dotted line and the blue dot-dash line represent the log-empirical likelihood ratio and the log-likelihood ratio when the underlying distribution is exponential, respectively.

approaches the parametric likelihood ratio asymptotically. Furthermore, as the sample size n increases, the log-empirical likelihood ratio approximates the log-likelihood ratio well in the neighborhood of the maximum likelihood estimator (MLE) of θ. The log-empirical likelihood (ratio) increases monotonically up to the maximum likelihood estimator and then decreases monotonically.

The R code for implementation of the procedure is shown below:

```
> library(emplik)
> theta0<-1
> n.seq<-c(25, 50, 150)
>
> # normal
> plot.norm<-function(X){
+ get.elr<-function(theta) sapply(theta,function(pp)
  el.test(X,mu=pp)$'-2LLR'/(-2)) # log EL
+ get.plr<-function(theta) sapply(theta,function(pp)
  sum(-(X-pp)^2/2)-sum(-(X-mean(X))^2/2)) # log(PL)
+ rg<-6/sqrt(length(X))
+ curve(get.elr,xlim=c(max(0,mean(X)-rg),mean(X)+rg),type="l",lty=1,
  lwd=2,add=TRUE,col=1)
+ curve(get.plr,xlim=c(max(0,mean(X)-rg),mean(X)+rg),type="l",lty=2,
  lwd=2,add=TRUE,col=2)
+ }
>
> # exponential
> plot.exp<-function(X){
```

```
+ get.elr.exp<-function(theta) sapply(theta,function(pp)
  el.test(X,mu=1/pp)$'-2LLR'/(-2)) # log EL
+ get.l.exp<-function(theta) sum(log(dexp(X,rate=theta)))
+ get.plr.exp<-function(theta) sapply(theta,function(pp)
  get.l.exp(pp)-get.l.exp(1/mean(X))) # log(PL)
+ rg<-6/sqrt(length(X))
+ curve(get.elr.exp,xlim=c(max(0.1,1/mean(X)-rg),1/mean(X)+rg),type="l",
  lty=3,lwd=2,add=TRUE,col=3)
+ curve(get.plr.exp,xlim=c(max(0.1,1/mean(X)-rg),1/mean(X)+rg),type="l",
  lty=4,lwd=2,add=TRUE,col=4)
+ }
>
> # add legend for the plot
> add_legend <- function(...) {
+ opar <- par(fig=c(0, 1, 0, 1), oma=c(0, 0, 0, 0),
+ mar=c(0, 0, 0, 0), new=TRUE)
+ on.exit(par(opar))
+ plot(0, 0, type='n', bty='n', xaxt='n', yaxt='n')
+ legend(...)
+ }
> par(mar=c(5.5, 4, 3.5, 1.5),mfrow=c(2,3),mgp=c(2,1,0))
>
> # normal
> for (n in n.seq){
+ rg<-2/sqrt(n) +
+ X<-rnorm(n,theta0,1)
+ plot(theta0,1,xlim=c(max(0,mean(X)-rg),mean(X)+rg),xlab=expression
  (theta), ylim=c(-2.5,0.005),ylab=expression(paste("log-EL(log-PL)
  ratio (",theta,")")),.main=paste0("n=",n),cex.axis=1.2)
+ plot.norm(X)
+ abline(v=mean(X),lty=2,col="grey")
+ }
> # exponential
> for (n in n.seq){
+ rg<-2/sqrt(n)
+ X<-rexp(n,rate=theta0)
+ plot(theta0,1,xlim=c(max(0,1/mean(X)-rg),1/mean(X)+rg),xlab=expression
  (theta), ylim=c(-4.5,0.005),ylab=expression(paste("log-EL(log-PL)
  ratio (",theta,")")), main=paste0("n=",n),cex.axis=1.2)
+ plot.exp(X)
+ abline(v=1/mean(X),lty=2,col="grey")
+ }
>
> add_legend("bottom", legend=c("Normal, EL","Normal, PL","Exp,
  EL","Exp, PL"), lwd=2,
+ lty=1:4, col=1:4, horiz=TRUE, bty='n', cex=1.1)
```

6.4 Density-Based Empirical Likelihood Methods

According to the Neyman–Pearson lemma, density-based likelihood ratios can provide uniformly most powerful tests. Using this as a starting point, Vexler and Gurevich (2010b) proposed an alternative to the distribution function–based EL methodology. The authors employed the approximate density-based likelihood, which has the following form:

$$L_f = \prod_{i=1}^{n} f(X_i) = \prod_{i=1}^{n} f_i, \; f_i = f(X_{(i)}),$$

where $X_{(1)} \leq X_{(2)} \leq \ldots \leq X_{(n)}$ are the order statistics based on $X_1, \ldots, X_n$, and $f_1, \ldots, f_n$ take on the values that maximize L_f given the empirical constraint corresponding to $\int f(u)\,du = 1$. This density-based EL approach was used successfully in order to construct efficient entropy-based goodness-of-fit test procedures. The density-based EL methodology has been satisfactorily applied to develop a test for symmetry based on paired data (Vexler et al. 2013b). This test significantly outperforms classical procedures. Gurevich and Vexler (2011) extended the density-based EL approach to a two-sample nonparametric likelihood ratio test. Vexler and Yu (2011) used the density-based EL concept to present two-group comparison principles based on bivariate data with a missing pattern as a consequence of data collection procedures. Further, the density-based EL methods were used to efficiently address nonparametric problems of complex composite hypothesis testing in children, in social and behavioral studies based on randomized prospective experiments (Vexler et al. 2012a). In many practical settings, the density-based ELRs can provide simple and exact tests. Some distinctive characteristics of the density-based EL method test statistic compared to the typical EL approach are summarized in Table 6.1.

We note that Table 6.1 cannot reflect all relevant EL techniques. For example, Hall and Owen (1993) developed large sample methods for constructing distribution function–based EL confidence bands in problems of nonparametric density estimation. Einmahl and McKeague (2003) proposed localizing the distribution function–based EL approach using one or more time variables implicit in the given null hypothesis. Integrating the log-likelihood ratio over those variables, the authors constructed exact-test procedures for detecting a change in distribution, testing for symmetry about zero, testing for exponentiality, and testing for independence.

It is a common practice to conduct medical trials in order to compare a new therapy with a standard of care based on paired data consisting of pre- and post-treatment measurements. In such cases, there is often great interest in identifying treatment effects within each therapy group, as well as detecting a between-group difference. Nonparametric comparisons between distributions of new therapy and control groups, as well as detecting treatment effects within each group, may be based on multiple-hypothesis tests. Toward this end, one can create relevant tests combining, for example, the Kolmogorov–Smirnov

TABLE 6.1

Comparison of the Classical EL and Density-Based EL Approaches

Characteristics	Classical EL Methods	Density-Based EL Methods
Construction of the likelihood function	Distribution based	Density based
Usage of Lagrange multipliers method	Yes	Yes
Usage of constraints for maximization	Yes	Yes
Common focus of the test	Parameters (e.g., moments)	Overall distributions
Critical value	Asymptotic	Exact
Form of the test statistic	Numeric approach is required for calculating values of Lagrange multipliers	No numeric approach

test and the Wilcoxon signed-rank test. The use of the classical procedures commonly requires complex considerations about combining the known nonparametric tests, preserving the Type I error control, and maintaining reasonable power of the resulting test. Alternatively, the density-based ELR technique provides a direct distribution-free approach for efficiently analyzing a variety of tasks occurring in clinical trials. The density-based EL method can easily be applied, to test nonparametrically for different composite hypotheses. In this case, the density-based EL approach implies a standard scheme to develop highly efficient procedures, approximating nonparametrically the most powerful Neyman–Pearson test rules, given aims of clinical studies. For example, Vexler et al. (2012a) developed a density-based ELR methodology that was efficiently used to compare two therapy strategies for treating children's attention-deficit/hyperactivity disorder (ADHD) and severe mood dysregulation (SMD). It was demonstrated that various composite hypotheses in a paired data setting (e.g., before vs. after treatment) can be tested with the density-based ELR tests, which give more emphasis to the overall distributional difference rather than to certain location parameter differences.

The R software can be employed in order to implement a computer program that realizes a density-based EL strategy. For example, programs of this type are presented in the *Statistics in Medicine* journal's web domain: http://onlinelibrary.wiley.com/doi/10.1002/sim.4467/suppinfo.

Miecznikowski et al. (2013) developed the R package *dbEmpLikeGOF* for nonparametric density-based likelihood ratio tests for goodness-of-fit and two-sample comparisons. See also http://cran.r-project.org/web/packages/dbEmpLikeNorm/ for the R package "*dbEmpLikeNorm*: Test for Joint Assessment of Normality," as well as Section 6.9.2. Vexler et al. (2014c) presented a package entitled "Novel and Efficient Density Based Empirical Likelihood Procedures for Symmetry and K-Sample Comparisons" in STATA, a general-purpose statistical software language. It is available over the web at http://sphhp.buffalo.edu/biostatistics/research-and-facilities/software/stata.html.

In order to exemplify the density-based empirical likelihood method, we employ the data of measurements of HDL cholesterol levels from the clinical study that is mentioned in Chapter 4. This study was designed as a case-control study of biomarkers for coronary heart disease. In accordance with the biomedical literature, the HDL biomarker has been suggested as having strong discriminatory ability for myocardial infarction (MI). To define cases, we consider the sample Y that consists of 25 measurements of the HDL biomarker in individuals who recently survived an MI. In order to represent controls, 25 HDL biomarker measurements on healthy subjects are denoted as $X_1, \ldots, X_{25}$. The following R code inputs the data and constructs the histograms of the data, as shown in Figure 6.2:

```
> X<-c(96.8,57.2,37.4,44.0,55.0,41.8,46.2,41.8,41.8,59.4,44.0,52.8,
    33.0,52.8,41.8,44.0,52.8,59.4,37.4,77.0,39.6,57.2,57.2,41.8,39.6)
> Y<-c(26.4,33.0,30.8,35.2,44.0,48.4,61.6,41.8,26.4,28.6,55.0,61.6,
    63.8,24.2,37.4,48.4,52.8,46.2,57.2,68.2,46.2,37.4,46.2,52.8,35.2)
> a<-min(c(X,Y))-20
> b<-max(c(X,Y))+20
> par(pty="s",mfrow=c(1,2),oma=c(0,0,0,0),mar=c(0,4,0,0))
> hist(X,xlim=c(a,b),ylim=c(0,0.05),freq=FALSE)
> hist(Y,xlim=c(a,b),ylim=c(0,0.05),freq=FALSE)
```

The classical empirical likelihood ratio test can be conducted via the R function EL.means. With the p-value of 0.101 as shown below, we fail to reject that $E(X) = E(Y)$ at the 0.05 significance level.

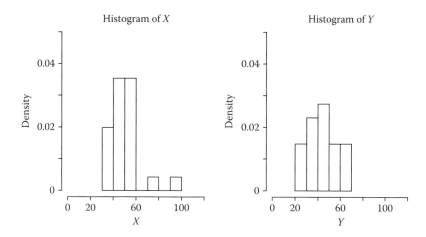

FIGURE 6.2
R data analysis output based on measurements of the HDL cholesterol levels, X and Y, related to individuals with and without the disease, respectively.

```
> EL.means(X,Y)
        Empirical likelihood mean difference test
data: X and Y
-2 * LogLikelihood = 2.6898, p-value = 0.101
95 percent confidence interval:
  -1.066513 13.850197
sample estimates:
Mean difference
        5.720065
```

Thus, in this example, the classical ELR test cannot be used efficiently to demonstrate the discriminatory ability of the HDL biomarker with respect to the MI disease. In this case, the two-sample density-based empirical likelihood ratio test proposed by Gurevich and Vexler (2011) shows p-value < 0.043, supporting rejection of the hypothesis regarding equivalency of distributions of X and Y. For the sake of completeness, we present in the appendix an example of R procedures for executing the two-sample density-based ELR test. In addition, note that Vexler et al. (2014e) proposed a simple, but very efficient, density-based empirical likelihood ratio test for independence and provided the R code to run the procedure.

6.5 Combining Likelihoods to Construct Composite Tests and Incorporate the Maximum Data-Driven Information

Strictly speaking, "distribution function/density-based" EL techniques and parametric likelihood methods are closely related concepts. This provides the impetus for an impressive expansion in the number of EL developments, based on combinations of likelihoods of different types (Qin and Zhang 2005).

Consider a simple example where we observe independent couples given as (X, Y). In this case, the likelihood function can be denoted as $L(X, Y)$. Suppose values of X's are observed completely, whereas a proportion of the observed data for the Y's is incomplete. Assume a model of Y given X, $Y|X$, is well defined, for example, $Y_i = \beta X_i + \varepsilon_i$, where β denotes the model parameter and ε_i is a normally distributed error term, for $i = 1, \ldots, n$. Then, we refer to Bayes's theorem to represent $L(X, Y) = L(Y|X) L(X)$, where $L(X)$ can be substituted by the EL to avoid parametric assumptions regarding distributions of X's.

In this context, Qin (2000) shows an inference on incomplete bivariate data, using a method that combines the parametric model and ELs. This method also incorporates auxiliary information from variables in the form of constraints, which can be obtained from reliable resources such as census reports. This approach makes it possible to use all available bivariate data, whether completely or incompletely observed. In the context of a group comparison, constraints can be formed based on null and alternative hypotheses, and these constraints are incorporated into the EL. This result was extended and applied to the following practical issues.

Malaria remains a major epidemiological problem in many developing countries. In endemic areas, an individual may have symptoms attributable either to malaria or to other causes. From a clinical viewpoint, it is important to attend to the next tasks: (1) to correctly diagnose an individual who has developed symptoms, so that the appropriate treatments can be given, and (2) to determine the proportion of malaria-affected cases in individuals who have symptoms, so that policies on an intervention program can be developed. Once symptoms have developed in an individual, the diagnosis of malaria can be based on the analysis of the parasite levels in blood samples. However, even a blood test is not conclusive, as in endemic areas, many healthy individuals can have parasites in their blood slides. Therefore, data from this type of study can be viewed as coming from a mixture distribution, with the components corresponding to malaria and nonmalaria cases. Qin and Leung (2005) constructed new EL procedures to estimate the proportion of clinical malaria using parasite-level data from a group of individuals with symptoms attributable to malaria. Yu et al. (2010) and Vexler et al. (2010c) proposed two-sample EL techniques based on incomplete data to analyze a pneumonia risk study in an intensive care unit (ICU) setting. In the context of this study, the initial detection of ventilator-associated pneumonia (VAP) for inpatients at an ICU requires composite symptom evaluation, using clinical criteria such as the clinical pulmonary infection score (CPIS). When the CPIS is above a threshold value, bronchoalveolar lavage (BAL) is performed, to confirm the diagnosis by counting actual bacterial pathogens. Thus, CPIS and BAL results are closely related, and both are important indicators of pneumonia, whereas BAL data are incomplete. Yu et al. (2010) and Vexler et al. (2010c) derived EL methods to compare the pneumonia risks among treatment groups for such incomplete data. In semi- and nonparametric contexts, including EL settings, Qin and Zhang (2005) showed that the full likelihood can be decomposed into the product of a conditional likelihood and a marginal likelihood, in a manner similar to that of the parametric likelihood considerations. These techniques augment the study's power by enabling researchers to use any observed data and relevant information.

6.6 Bayesians and Empirical Likelihood: Are They Mutually Exclusive?

The statistical literature has shown that Bayesian methods (see Chapter 7 for details) can be applied for various tasks of clinical experimentations, for example, when data are subject to complex missing data problems (e.g., parts of data are not manifested as numerical scores) (Daniels and Hogan 2008). Commonly, the application of a Bayesian approach requires the assumption of functional forms corresponding to the distribution of the underlying data and parameters of interest. However, in cases with data subject to complex missing data problems, parametric estimation is complicated and formal tests for the relevant goodness of fit are often not available. The statistical literature has shown that tests derived from empirical likelihood methodology possess many of the same asymptotic properties as those based on parametric likelihoods. This leads naturally to the idea of using empirical likelihood instead of parametric likelihood as the basis for Bayesian inference.

Lazar (2003) demonstrated the potential for constructing nonparametric Bayesian inference based on ELs. The key idea is to substitute the parametric likelihood (PL) with the EL in the Bayesian likelihood construction relative to the component of the likelihood used to model the observed data. It is demonstrated that the EL function is a proper likelihood function and can serve as the basis for robust and accurate Bayesian inference. This Bayesian empirical likelihood method provides a robust nonparametric data-driven alternative to the more classical Bayesian procedures (Vexler et al. 2016). Furthermore, Vexler et al. (2013a) recommended applying EL functions to create Bayes factor (BF) type nonparametric procedures (we refer the reader to Chapter 7 for details). The EL concept was shown to be very efficient when it is employed for modifying BF-type procedures to the nonparametric setting.

Vexler et al. (2014d) developed the nonparametric Bayesian posterior expectation fashion by incorporating the EL methodology into the posterior likelihood construction. The asymptotic forms of the EL-based Bayesian posterior expectation are shown to be similar to those derived in the well-known parametric Bayesian and frequentist statistical literature. In the case when the prior distribution function depends on unknown hyperparameters, a nonparametric version of the empirical Bayesian method, which yields double empirical Bayesian estimators, can be obtained. This approach yields a nonparametric analogue of the well-known James–Stein estimation that has been well addressed in the literature dealing with multivariate normal observations. Note that when the data are normally distributed, the estimator is comparable to the MLE. When informative priors are used and the data are generated from either a normal or lognormal distribution, the estimator provides significantly smaller variances than the classical estimator $\bar{X}$ and the MLE. This in turn yields much narrower confidence intervals. The asymptotic approximations to the EL-based posterior expectations are shown to be quite accurate.

The EL Bayesian procedures can serve as a powerful approach to incorporating external information into the inference process about given data, in a distribution-free manner. In the following sections, we briefly present the works of Lazar (2003) and Vexler et al. (2014d).

6.6.1 Bayesian Empirical Likelihood

Let $X_1, \ldots, X_n$ be independent identically distributed observations from some unknown distribution F, which has a d-dimensional mean vector μ and a nonsingular $d \times d$ covariance matrix Σ. We are interested in inference concerning some functional of F, say $\theta(F)$. For simplicity, we assume that $d = 1$. To proceed with the Bayesian analysis, the profile empirical likelihood function may serve as the likelihood part of Bayes's theorem. Lazar (2003) considered putting a prior on θ, the functional of interest, focusing on the specific case of the mean, μ.

Consider an alternative likelihood, L_a, to the data likelihood, built for a functional θ of the underlying unspecified distribution. A definition of validity of an alternative likelihood

L_a with which to perform Bayesian inference is suggested based on the coverage properties of posterior sets, along with a numerical technique that may be used to invalidate certain likelihoods (Monahan and Boos 1992). A posterior density based on L_a is valid by coverage for the model $f(y|t)$ if and only if $\Pr\{\theta \in S_\alpha(y)\} = \alpha$ for every $S_\alpha(y)$, a posterior coverage set function of level α under the measure $p(t)\,f(y|t)$, where $p(t)$ is the prior. The likelihood L_a is proper in terms of coverage if and only if the posterior $p_a(t|y)$ is valid by coverage for every absolutely continuous prior. To verify properness, one can calculate, in the one-dimensional case,

$$H = \int_{-\infty}^{\theta} p_a(t\,|\,y)\,dt.$$

This corresponds to posterior coverage set functions of the form $(-\infty, t_a^\alpha)$, where t_a^α is the ath percentile point of the posterior density $p_a(t|y)$. If $p_a(t|y)$ is valid by coverage, then H is distributed as $Uniform(0,1)$. Moreover, if there exists a prior for which the distribution of H is not uniform, then $L_a(y|t)$ is not a proper likelihood for Bayesian inference.

When $\theta(F)$ can be determined by an estimating equation $Eg(x_i,\theta) = 0$, following Section 6.2, the empirical likelihood function is defined as $EL(\theta) = \prod_{i=1}^{n} \left(n + \lambda g\left(X_i, \theta\right) \right)^{-1}$, where λ is a root of $\sum_{i=1}^{n} g\left(X_i,\theta\right)\left(n + \lambda g(X_i,\theta)\right)^{-1}$. Then by setting $L_a = EL(\theta)$, one can calculate the statistic H. It is demonstrated that even for the most diffuse of the priors, the distribution of H calculated from empirical likelihood lies very close to the quantiles of the uniform distribution, confirming that empirical likelihood gives valid posterior intervals. Furthermore, empirical likelihood is robust to the choice of prior to a certain extent and is reasonable to use within the Bayesian paradigm.

6.6.2 Empirical Likelihood–Based Empirical Bayesian Posterior

Suppose we have independent identically distributed observations $X_1, \ldots, X_n$ from a density function $f(x|\theta)$, where θ is the parameter to be evaluated.

6.6.2.1 Nonparametric Posterior Expectations of Simple Functionals

For convenience of exposition and without loss of generality, we assume the parameter θ is one-dimensional and consider nonparametric posterior expectations of simple functionals here; for the case of general functionals, we refer the reader to Vexler et al. (2014d).

When the form of the density function f is assumed to be known, the Bayesian point estimator of θ can be defined as the posterior expectation

$$\hat{\theta} = \frac{\int \theta \prod_{i=1}^{n} f(X_i\,|\,\theta)\pi(\theta)d\theta}{\int \prod_{i=1}^{n} f(X_i\,|\,\theta)\pi(\theta)d\theta},$$

where $\pi(\theta)$ is the prior distribution.

In the case where the density function f is unknown, instead of the parametric likelihoods, one can use the EL function. Following Section 6.2, the simple EL function with respect to the mean of $X_1, \ldots, X_n$ can be defined as $EL(\theta) = \prod_{i=1}^{n} (n + \lambda(X_i - \theta))^{-1}$ and the EL ratio has the form of $ELR(\theta) = EL(\theta)n^n$, where λ is a root of $\sum_{i=1}^{n} (X_i - \theta)(n + \lambda(X_i - \theta))^{-1}$. Thus, the nonparametric posterior expectation is

$$\hat{\theta} = \frac{\int_{X_{(1)}}^{X_{(n)}} \theta e^{\log EL(\theta)} \pi(\theta) d\theta}{\int_{X_{(1)}}^{X_{(n)}} e^{\log EL(\theta)} \pi(\theta) d\theta} = \frac{\int_{X_{(1)}}^{X_{(n)}} \theta e^{\log ELR(\theta)} \pi(\theta) d\theta}{\int_{X_{(1)}}^{X_{(n)}} e^{\log ELR(\theta)} \pi(\theta) d\theta}, \tag{6.5}$$

where $X_{(1)}, \ldots X_{(n)}$ are the order statistics based on the sample $X_1, \ldots, X_n$.

Proposition 6.2. Assume $E|X_1|^4 < \infty$, $\int |\theta| \pi(\theta) d\theta < \infty$, and $\pi(\theta)$ is twice continuously differentiable in a neighborhood of $\bar{X} = n^{-1} \sum_{i=1}^{n} X_i$; then the estimator defined in (6.5) satisfies

$$\hat{\theta} = \frac{\int \theta \exp\left[-\frac{n(\bar{X} - \theta)^2}{2\sigma_n^2}\right] \pi(\theta) d\theta}{\int \exp\left[-\frac{n(\bar{X} - \theta)^2}{2\sigma_n^2}\right] \pi(\theta) d\theta} + \frac{M_n^3}{\sigma_n^2 n} + g_n,$$

where $\sigma_n^2 = n^{-1} \sum_{i=1}^{n} (X_i - \bar{X})^2$, $M_n^3 = n^{-1} \sum_{i=1}^{n} (X_i - \bar{X})^3$, and $g_n = O_p(n^{-3/2+\epsilon})$ for all $\epsilon > 0$, as $n \to \infty$.

Corollary 6.1. Let $\pi(\theta) = (2\pi\sigma_\pi^2)^{-1/2} \exp\left[-(\theta - \mu_\pi)^2/2\sigma_\pi^2\right]$, where μ_π and σ_π^2 are known hyperparameters, and the conditions of Proposition 6.2 hold. Then, the posterior expectation (6.5) can be approximated as

$$\hat{\theta} = \tilde{\theta} + \frac{M_n^3}{\sigma_n^2 n} + O_p(n^{-3/2+\epsilon}), \quad \tilde{\theta} = \frac{(\mu_\pi \sigma_n^2 + \bar{X}\sigma_\pi^2 n)}{(n\sigma_\pi^2 + \sigma_n^2)} = \frac{(\sigma_\pi^2)^{-1} \mu_\pi}{(\sigma_\pi^2)^{-1} + n(\sigma_n^2)^{-1}} + \frac{n(\sigma_n^2)^{-1} \bar{X}}{(\sigma_\pi^2)^{-1} + n(\sigma_n^2)^{-1}}.$$

The estimator $\tilde{\theta}$ is equivalent to the form of the parametric posterior expectation derived under the normal–normal model (e.g., Carlin and Louis, 2011).

The integral mentioned in Proposition 6.2 can sometimes be obtained analytically, depending on the form of $\pi(\theta)$. Following the process of the asymptotic evaluation of the parametric posterior expectations, one can easily show Corollary 6.2.

Corollary 6.2. Under the conditions of Proposition 6.2, let $\pi(\theta)$ be a prior function with $|d^3 \log(\pi(\theta))/d\theta^3| < \infty$ for all θ. Then we have

$$\hat{\theta} = \frac{n\bar{X} + \sigma_n^2 \{\log \pi(\bar{X})\}' - \sigma_n^2 \{\log \pi(\bar{X})\}'' \bar{X}}{n - \sigma_n^2 \{\log \pi(\bar{X})\}''} + \frac{M_n^3}{\sigma_n^2 n} + O_p(n^{-3/2+\epsilon}), \epsilon > 0, \text{ as } n \to \infty.$$

Now, we consider the normal prior, $\pi(\theta)$, when μ_π and σ_π^2 are unknown. Following the empirical Bayes concepts (e.g., Carlin and Louis 2011), the unknown hyperparameters can be estimated by, for example, maximizing the respective marginal distributions.

This method can be applied to the nonparametric posterior expectation yielding double empirical posterior estimation. In this case, we define

$$\hat{\theta}_E = \frac{\int \theta \exp[\log EL(\theta)] \exp[-(\theta - \hat{\mu}_\pi)^2 / 2\hat{\sigma}_\pi^2] d\theta}{\int \exp\left[\log EL(\theta)\right] \exp[-(\theta - \hat{\mu}_\pi)^2 / 2\hat{\sigma}_\pi^2] d\theta}, \tag{6.6}$$

where $\left(\hat{\mu}_\pi, \hat{\sigma}_\pi^2\right) = \arg\max_{\mu,\sigma} [(2\pi\sigma^2)^{-1/2} \int_{-\infty}^{\infty} \exp\{\log EL(\theta)\} \exp\{-(\theta - \mu)^2 / 2\sigma^2\} d\theta]$. The next result implies a simple asymptotic form of $\hat{\theta}_E$.

Corollary 6.3. Assume $E|X_1|^4 < \infty$; then the posterior expectation $\hat{\theta}_E$ satisfies

$$\hat{\theta}_E = \frac{\hat{\mu}_\pi \sigma^2 + \bar{X}\hat{\sigma}_\pi^2 n}{n\hat{\sigma}_\pi^2 + \sigma_n^2} + \frac{M_n^3}{\sigma_n^2 n} + O_p\left(n^{-3/2 + \varepsilon}\right),$$

where $\hat{\mu}_\pi - \bar{X} \to 0$, $\hat{\sigma}_\pi^2 - \max\{0, \sigma_n^2 - \sigma^2\} \to 0$, $\sigma^2 = \text{var}(X_1)$, and $\varepsilon > 0$ as $n \to \infty$.

Note that the approximations of nonparametric posterior expectation are similar to those related to parametric Bayesian point estimators. The following remark presents the asymptotic distribution of the nonparametric posterior expectations.

Vexler et al. (2014d) demonstrated that the estimators of the posterior expectation based on ELs are more efficient than the classic nonparametric procedures, even when incorrect priors are employed. When forms of the nonparametric posterior estimators use informative priors, the nonparametric estimation based on ELs generally outperforms the relevant maximum likelihood estimation.

6.6.2.2 Nonparametric Analogue of James–Stein Estimation

Let us begin by outlining the classic James–Stein estimation process assuming the observations $X_1, X_2, \ldots, X_n$, are independent and identically distributed as multivariate normal with corresponding mean vector $\theta = (\theta_1, \theta_2, \ldots, \theta_k)$ and covariance matrix Σ, that is, $X_i = (X_{i1}, X_{i2}, \ldots, X_{ik})^T \sim N((\theta_1, \theta_2, \ldots, \theta_k)^T, \Sigma)$ $i = 1, 2, \ldots, n$. In this case, Stein (1956) proved that for $K \geq 3$, the MLE of θ is inadmissible; that is, there exists another estimator with frequentist risk (MSE) that is less than or equal to that of the MLE. Through the analysis of the quadratic loss function, one such dominating estimator was derived by James and Stein (1961). Efron and Morris (1972) showed that the James–Stein estimator belongs to a class of the parametric empirical Bayes (PEB) point estimators related to the Gaussian–Gaussian model.

When $K = 1$ and the prior function is a normal density function, it has been shown above that the proposed nonparametric posterior expectation is asymptotically equivalent to the parametric posterior expectation derived under assumptions of the Gaussian–Gaussian model. In this section, we assume $X_1, X_2, \ldots, X_n$ are independent random vectors, $X_i = (X_{i1}, X_{i2}, \ldots, X_{ik})^T$, with an unknown distribution, and $E|X_{ij}|^4 < \infty, j = 1, \ldots, K, i = 1, 2, \ldots, n$. Under these sets of assumptions, we propose a nonparametric estimate of the mean $(\theta_1, \theta_2, \ldots \theta_k)^T$ using the double empirical posterior estimation, in the form of

$$\hat{\theta}_{Ej} = \frac{\int \theta \exp\{\log EL_{4j}(\theta)\} \exp(-\theta^2 / 2\tilde{\sigma}_\pi^2) d\theta}{\int \exp\{\log EL_{4j}(\theta)\} \exp(-\theta^2 / 2\tilde{\sigma}_\pi^2) d\theta} \tag{6.7}$$

with

$$\tilde{\sigma}_\pi^2 = \arg\max_{\sigma^2} \sum_{j=1}^{K} \log\left[\left(2\pi\sigma^2\right)^{-1/2} \int \exp\{\log EL_{4j}(\theta)\} \exp(-\theta^2/2\sigma^2)d\theta\right],$$

where $EL_{4j}(\theta_j) = \max\left\{\prod_{i=1}^{n} p_{ij} : 0 < p_{ij} < 1, \sum_{i=1}^{n} p_{ij} = 1, \sum_{i=1}^{n} p_{ij} X_{ij} = \theta_j\right\}$, $j = 1, 2, \ldots, K$. In Proposition 6.3, we show the proposed distribution-free estimation is asymptotically equivalent to the parametric version of the James–Stein estimator.

Proposition 6.3. For all $\varepsilon > 0$ and as $n \to \infty$, the double empirical posterior estimator (6.7) has the following asymptotic form

$$\hat{\theta}_{Ej} = \left\{1 - \frac{(K-2)/n}{\bar{X}^T S^{-1} \bar{X}}\right\}\bar{X}_j + \frac{1}{n}\sum_{r=1}^{K} \frac{\sum_{i=1}^{n}\left(X_{ir} - \bar{X}_r\right)^3}{\sum_{i=1}^{n}\left(X_{ir} - \bar{X}_r\right)^2} + O_p\left(n^{-3/2+\varepsilon}\right) \quad \text{for } j = 1,\ldots,K,$$

where $\bar{X} = \left(\bar{X}_1, \ldots, \bar{X}_K\right)^T \bar{X}_j = n^{-1}\sum_{i=1}^{n} X_{ij}$ and S is the sample estimator of Σ.

In the multivariate setting, with prior functions defined to be normal distributions with unknown hyperparameters, the double empirical Bayesian estimation yields a nonparametric version of the well-known James–Stein estimator.

6.7 Three Key Arguments That Support the Empirical Likelihood Methodology as a Practical Statistical Analysis Tool

One of the important advantages of EL techniques is their general applicability and an assessment of their performance under conditions that are commonly unrestricted by parametric assumptions. When one is in doubt about the best strategy for constructing statistical decision rules, the following arguments can be accepted in favor of EL methods:

Argument 6.1. The EL methodology employs the likelihood concept in a simple nonparametric fashion in order to approximate optimal parametric procedures. The benefit of using this approach is that the EL techniques are often robust as well as highly efficient. In this context, we also may apply EL functions to replace parametric likelihood functions in known and well-developed constructions. Consider the following example. The statistical literature widely suggests applying Bayesian methods for various tasks of clinical experiments, for example, when data are subject to complex missing data problems (e.g., parts of data are not manifested as numerical scores) (Daniels and Hogan 2008). Commonly, to apply a Bayesian approach, one needs to assume functional forms corresponding to the distribution of the underlying data and parameters of interest. Lazar (2003) demonstrated potentials of constructing nonparametric Bayesian inference based on ELs that take the role of model-based likelihoods. This research demonstrated that the EL is a valid function for Bayesian inference. Vexler et al. (2013a) recommended applying EL functions to create Bayes factor (BF)–type nonparametric procedures. The BF, a practical tool of applied biostatistics, has been dealt with extensively in the literature in the context of hypothesis testing (e.g., Carlin and Louis 1997, 2011). The EL concept was shown to be very efficient when it was employed for modifying BF-type procedures to the nonparametric setting.

Argument 6.2. Similar to the parametric likelihood concept, the EL methodology gives relatively simple systematic directions for constructing efficient statistical tests that can be applied in various complex clinical experiments.

Argument 6.3. Perhaps the extreme generality of EL methods and their wide scope of usefulness partly follow abilities to easily set up EL-type statistics as components of composite parametric/semi- and nonparametric likelihood-based systems, efficiently attending to any observed data and relevant information. Parametric, semiparametric, and empirical likelihood methods play roles complementary to one another, providing powerful statistical procedures for complicated practical problems.

   In conclusion, we note that EL-based methods are employed in much of modern statistical practice, and we cannot describe all relevant theory and examples. The reader interested in EL methods will find more details and many pertinent articles across the statistical literature.

6.8 Supplement

1. DiCiccio et al. (1989) presented a detailed study of differences between parametric and empirical likelihood functions or surfaces and derived the exact order of difference between the nonparametric and parametric log-likelihood functions. The differences between parametric and empirical log-likelihood functions are exactly of order $n^{-1/2}$ when evaluated at the true parameter value. In general, empirical likelihood and parametric likelihood intervals based on Stein's least favorable family approximation to the profile likelihood share the same orders of accuracy. The errors in coverage of one-sided and two-sided intervals are typically of orders $n^{-1/2}$ and n^{-1}, respectively. However, empirical likelihood intervals are Bartlett adjustable such that the order of coverage error in two-sided intervals is n^{-2}. In situations where the functional of interest is a smooth function of vector means, first- and second-order expansions for log-likelihood functions were developed. For some exponential family models, it was demonstrated that empirical and parametric log-likelihood ratios are maximized at exactly the same point. They agree to first order as functions but differ to second order. In general, the surfaces do not require agreeing to first order. However, the surfaces can be quite close in a distributional sense in certain exponential family models. Furthermore, empirical likelihood can be viewed as an approximation to a true parametric likelihood based on a parametric least favorable family.

2. Let $\mathbf{x} = \{X_1, ..., X_n\}$ denote a r - variate random sample that depends in some way on an unknown s - vector quantity $\theta = \theta_0$ and $\hat{\theta}$ be its estimator. Likelihood-based confidence regions are constructed as follows. Let $\hat{Q}$ be an estimate of the asymptotic variance matrix Q of $n^{1/2}\hat{\theta}$, and f be the density of $\hat{\eta}_0 = \hat{Q}^{-1/2}\left(\hat{\theta} - \theta_0\right)$. Hall (1990) showed that empirical likelihood confidence regions are approximately the same

as pseudolikelihood regions, but are based on $\hat{\xi}_0 \equiv \left(Q^{1/2} \hat{Q}^{-1} Q^{1/2} \right)^{1/2} Q^{-1/2} \left(\hat{\theta} - \theta_0 \right)$ instead of $\hat{\eta}_0$. Hall demonstrated that empirical likelihood does draw contours that approximate those of a pseudolikelihood (the qualifier *pseudo* is used since f is the density of a certain function of the data but not the likelihood of the entire data set) function and are second-order correct except for a location term. Nevertheless, this pseudolikelihood is not used commonly to construct a likelihood-based confidence region except in the one-dimension scenario. Hall showed that empirical likelihood regions can be adjusted for location to be second-order correct. The location-adjusted empirical likelihood regions are Bartlett correctable. When applying a simple empirical scale correction to location-adjusted empirical likelihood, it reduces coverage error by an order of magnitude. Nevertheless, the form of the Bartlett correction is altered by the location adjustment. Although both empirical likelihood regions and bootstrap likelihood regions are based on statistics whose centered distributions agree to second order, they differ to second order.

3. Hall and La Scala (1990) examined the main features of empirical likelihood and discussed some developments, including Bartlett correction and location adjustment. The authors presented algorithms for implementing empirical likelihood in several important cases, for example, to means, variances, and correlation coefficients. It was shown that empirical likelihood is a strong competitor to all bootstrap methods such as percentile-t and accelerated bias correction, as well as to classical methods such as normal approximation. Empirical likelihood has the following advantages: (a) It does not impose prior constraints on region shape. (b) It does not require construction of a pivotal statistic. (c) The shapes of empirical likelihood regions, such as the degree of asymmetry in the case of a confidence interval, are determined "automatically" by the sample rather than in a pre-determined way. (d) Empirical likelihood regions do not require estimation of scale or skewness. (e) Empirical likelihood regions are range preserving and transformation respecting. (f) Empirical likelihood regions are Bartlett correctable and allow very low coverage error. For example, in some cases, an empirical correction for scale reduces the order of magnitude of coverage error from n^{-1} to n^{-2}, where n denotes sample size.

4. The empirical likelihood method for constructing confidence regions for parameters, expressed as functionals $\theta(F)$ of an unknown distribution function F, introduced by Owen (1988, 1990) has sampling properties similar to those of the bootstrap. While the bootstrap uses resampling, the empirical likelihood method computes the profile likelihood of a general multinomial distribution based on data points. In a two-sample problem where one sample comes from a distribution specified up to a parameter and the other sample comes from an unspecified distribution, Qin (1991) generalized Owen's empirical likelihood and provided a likelihood ratio–based confidence interval for the difference of two sample means. Qin (1993) introduced empirical likelihood in the biased sampling problem. Wilks' theorem leading to an empirical likelihood ratio confidence interval for the mean, as well as some extensions, discussion, and simulations, was presented.

5. When constructing confidence intervals for a population quantile (in particular, for the median), empirical likelihood intervals are identical to the sign-test intervals or binomial-method intervals. They both have relative large coverage

errors of size $n^{-1/2}$, even though they are two-sided intervals. Chen and Hall (1993) showed that the coverage accuracy may be improved from order $n^{-1/2}$ to order n^{-1} by appropriately smoothing the empirical likelihood method. The improvement is available for a wide range of choices of the smoothing parameter so that accurate choice of an "optimal" value of the parameter is not necessary. A very general version of Wilks' theorem was presented in the context of empirical likelihood for quantiles with necessary and sufficient conditions on the smoothing parameter for the error in the chi-square approximation to be $O(n^{-1})$. Furthermore, the authors showed that smoothed empirical likelihood is Bartlett correctable and an empirical correction for scale can reduce the size of coverage error from order n^{-1} to order n^{-2}.

6. The property that the the empirical likelihood is nonparametric in nature reflects emphasis on the observed data and hence has considerable potential for the construction of nonparametric confidence bands in curve estimation. Hall and Owen (1993) presented the construction of an empirical likelihood functional, rather than a function, and contoured it to produce confidence bands. In an infinite parameter setting, analogues of Wilks' theorem were established based on kernel estimates. Note that the kernel function introduces bias into the problem, leading to confidence bands for the expected value of the function estimator instead of for the function itself. The issue can be dealt with by a bias correction or by undersmoothing so that bias is negligible. The authors also suggested a bootstrap calibration approach to selecting the appropriate contour. The bands were shown to have asymptotically correct coverage based on the developed large sample theory.

7. Chen (1994) compared the powers of empirical likelihood and bootstrap tests for a mean parameter against a series of local alternative hypotheses, that is, to test H_0: $\mu = \mu_0$ versus H_1: $\mu = \mu_0 + n^{-1/2}\Sigma^{1/2}\tau$, where both μ_0 and τ are constant p-dimensional vectors. The comparison was conducted by developing Edgeworth expansions. For univariate and bivariate cases, practical rules were proposed for choosing the more powerful test. In the univariate case, the empirical likelihood test is more powerful than the bootstrap test when $\tau\alpha_3 > 0$ and vice versa when $\tau\alpha_3 < 0$, where α_3 is the population skewness parameter. Similar rules hold for higher-dimensional cases.

8. For the problems in which one may have more estimating equations than parameters in constructing confidence regions for functionals $\theta(F)$ of an unknown distribution function F, Qin and Lawless (1994) proposed the empirical likelihood method. By assuming that information about F and θ is available in the form of unbiased estimating functions, the authors proposed linking estimating functions or equations and empirical likelihood, as well as developed methods of combining information about parameters. It was shown that the maximized empirical likelihood estimates for both parameters and distribution function are asymptotically efficient. Efficiency results for estimates of both θ and F were obtained. The authors also demonstrate that empirical likelihood ratio statistics for parameters have asymptotic χ^2-distributions. Many theorems based on empirical likelihood and parametric likelihood were shown to share analogous versions. It was demonstrated that the method proposed by Qin and Lawless combines information in the form of estimating functions in an optimal way.

9. Let (X, Y) be a pair of positive random variables with cumulative distribution function F_0 and G_0. We say that X is left truncated by Y (and thus Y is right truncated by X)

if the pair (X, Y) is observable only when $X > Y$. Given a randomly left-truncated data set consisting of n i.i.d. draws $(X_1, Y_1), \ldots, (X_n, Y_n)$ from $L((X, Y)|X > Y)$, where X and Y are independent, one important goal is to draw inferences on the proportion of individuals in the population whose lifetimes would not exceed a specified $a > 0$, that is, $F_0(a) = P(X \leq a)$. The commonly used method of interval estimation of probabilities for randomly truncated data is based on the normal approximation of the product-limit estimator. However, the drawbacks include (a) that it may produce intervals containing impossible values outside the range [0, 1] and (b) its unsatisfactory small sample performance. Alternatively, Li (1995) proposed an exact nonparametric analogue of the classical parametric likelihood ratio theory, to derive inference procedures for F_0 directly based on a conditional nonparametric likelihood ratio. The resulting confidence intervals were shown to be range preserving and have a better small sample performance based on Monte Carlo simulation studies. The author generalized this approach to obtain confidence intervals for the ratio of two probabilities, make joint inferences on any finite number of probabilities, and test goodness of fit of a given distribution function. The method was illustrated using the Centers for Disease Control's transfusion-related acquired immune deficiency syndrome data (Kalbfleisch and Lawless 1989), which consist of 295 cases. In this study, the dates of infection were ascertained retrospectively for patients who were diagnosed with AIDS and were thought to be infected by blood transfusion, where the incubation time (in months) is right-truncated by the time (in months) from the HIV infection to the end of the study, and the individual's age at the time of transfusion.

10. Since the percentile-t method only uses the "derived sample" in the variance estimation, undersmoothing produces erratic variance estimates. A conflict between the prescribed undersmoothing and the explicit variance estimate required by the percentile-t method leads to the coverage discrepancy that confidence intervals produced by the kernel-based percentile-t bootstrap do not have the coverage claimed by the theory. To deal with this issue, Chen (1996) suggested using empirical likelihood in conjunction with the kernel method to construct confidence intervals for the value of a probability density f at a point x. By studentizing internally, empirical likelihood avoids the problem faced by the bootstrap, and produces better confidence intervals. The author showed that the empirical likelihood produces confidence intervals consistent with theoretical coverage accuracy of the same order of magnitude as the bootstrap, and which are also empirically more accurate. The method was illustrated and was shown to be robust for analyzing a data set from a line transect aerial survey of southern bluefin tuna (Buckland et al. 2005). The kernel method has been shown to be robust for analyzing line transect data.

11. In some scenarios, it may not be reasonable to assume a statistical model in a parametric form completely, but we still are interested in inference for the mean of the distribution. For example, one might assume that a random variable has a distribution that is roughly normal for a specific range of the data, for example, in the center of the distribution, while outside that range, for example, with tails, it is left arbitrary. To tackle the problems, Qin and Wong (1996) proposed using methods that are insensitive to the shape of the tails based on the semiparametric likelihood function. The semiparametric likelihood function consists of the parametric likelihood function for data in the center or one tail of the distribution and the empirical

likelihood function for the rest of the data. The authors showed that Wilks' theorem still holds for the semiparametric model; that is, the semiparametric likelihood ratio statistic has asymptotically a chi-square distribution. Consequently, confidence intervals and observed levels of significance for the mean can be obtained from the semiparametric likelihood ratio statistic. The method was applied to a study of the times between successive failures of air conditioning equipment in a Boeing 720 airplane (Cox and Snell 1981; Lawless 2011).

12. Li et al. (1996) derived confidence bands for quantile functions using a nonparametric likelihood ratio approach. The method has the following properties: (a) It is easy to implement. (b) It is general and can be applied to both right-censored and other important missing data schemes, including random truncation, for example, left-truncated data. (c) The nonparametric likelihood ratio confidence bands are valid under much weaker conditions, involving neither density estimation nor the requirement of the existence of a density. In contrast, the methods based on bootstrap were derived under the strong condition that F_0 has a bounded second derivative, where F_0 is the distribution functions of survival time. The performance of the proposed method was confirmed by a Monte Carlo study. The author presented the application of the method to a real data set consisting of survival times following treatment for malignant melanoma (Gill et al. 1997), where the analysis was restricted to the 87 males under study, of whom 31 were observed to die from the disease and the remaining were censored observations.

13. Exponential empirical likelihood, an alternative nonparametric likelihood, may be constructed using Efron's (1981, 1982) method of nonparametric tilting. Let $X_1, \ldots, X_n$ be a sample of independent and identically distributed random variables and $p_1, \ldots, p_n$ be a probability vector that assigns probability mass p_i to observation i. By restricting the p_i to be of the form $p_i(\tilde{t}) = \exp(\tilde{t}X_i) / \sum_{j=1}^{n} \exp(\tilde{t}X_j)$, the exponential empirical log-likelihood ratio is then given by $\tilde{W}_u = 2\sum_{i=1}^{n} \log\{np_i(\tilde{t})\}$, where $\tilde{t}$ satisfies $\sum_{i=1}^{n} p_i(\tilde{t})(X_i - u) = 0$. Jing and Wood (1996) showed that exponential empirical likelihood is not Bartlett correctable, by comparing the relevant expansions for empirical likelihood and exponential empirical likelihood.

14. When developing or extending a median test for censored cases, one may face two questions. One is the way to handle the ambiguous observations, that is, the censored observations that are less than the pooled-sample median. The other is the definition of the pooled median. The empirical likelihood approach may answer these questions naturally. Naik-Nimbalkar and Rajarshi (1997) adopted the empirical likelihood approach for testing the equality of k medians based on censored data. This test does not require the assumption of the underlying k survival functions being identical under the null hypothesis, which is common in most of the existing tests. The author supplemented some details to the proof of Thomas and Grunkemeier (1975) and proved that the asymptotic distribution of the test statistic is chi-square with $k - 1$ degrees of freedom, when the null hypothesis of equality of k median holds.

15. Lazar and Mykland (1998) compared local power and conditional properties (concentrating specifically on the search for approximate ancillaries) of empirical

and dual likelihood. Focusing on tests of a scalar parameter or functional of interest, empirical likelihood was compared with ordinary parametric likelihoods based on the local power, while also compared with quasi-likelihood based on conditional properties. The authors showed that there is no loss of efficiency in using a dual or empirical likelihood model, to the second order. Either the artificial likelihood or the true likelihood test could be more efficient to the third order; this is determined by the Fisher information, the distance between the null and the alternative hypotheses, and the statistical curvature of the models. Without the presence of overdispersion or, more generally, an unknown amount of dispersion, it was shown that there is little difference in the ancillaries for conditional inference based on empirical likelihood or on other possible likelihoods, such as a quasi-likelihood. However, when the quantity of dispersion is assumed to be known, it was shown to be correct to base inference on the quasi-likelihood.

16. Baggerly (1998) suggested that the empirical likelihood method can be considered one of the allocating probabilities to an n-cell contingency table such that a goodness-of-fit criterion is minimized. When considering the empirical likelihood for the mean, one has the goodness-of-fit criterion $-2\sum \log(np_i)$ and the constraint $\sum p_i X_i = u_0$. Define the Cressie–Read power-divergence statistic as

$$CR(\lambda) = \frac{2}{\lambda(\lambda+1)} \sum_{i=1}^{k} o_i \left\{ \left(\frac{o_i}{e_i} \right)^{\lambda} - 1 \right\} \quad (-\infty < \lambda < \infty),$$ where k is the number of distinct

cells in the table, o_i and e_i are the observed and expected cell counts, respectively, and λ is a user-specified parameter. It was shown that when the Cressie–Read power-divergence statistic is used as the criterion, confidence regions enjoying the same convergence rates as those found for empirical likelihood can be obtained for the entire range of values of the Cressie–Read parameter λ, including –1, maximum entropy, 0, empirical likelihood, and 1, Pearson's χ^2. In the power-divergence family, empirical likelihood was shown to be the only member that is Bartlett correctable. However, simulation results suggest that, for the mean, using a scaled F-distribution yields more accurate coverage levels for moderate sample sizes.

17. Lee and Young (1999) showed that higher-order correction to the confidence interval can be obtained by a variety of techniques, including asymptotic adjustment to the chi-square percentiles, bootstrapping the nonparametric likelihood ratio, and direct substitution of truncated asymptotic expansions for the confidence interval endpoints. In a smooth-function model setting, the authors proposed the construction of two-sided nonparametric confidence intervals based on Stein's least favorable family. The approach shares the same asymptotic properties and the advantages of empirical likelihood, such as having a data-driven shape. In addition, the method does not require nested levels of bootstrap sampling, and thus is computationally less intensive. Based on the method, one may propose and analyze asymptotic and bootstrapping techniques as a way of reducing coverage error to levels. Based on a simulation study, the coverage error was shown to be substantially reduced by simple analytic adjustment of the nonparametric likelihood interval. Moreover, it was suggested that bootstrapping the distribution of the nonparametric likelihood ratio results in very desirable coverage accuracy.

18. Consider the problem of estimating a mixture proportion based on data from two different distributions, as well as from a mixture of them. Qin (1999) developed an empirical likelihood ratio–based statistic for constructing confidence intervals for the mixture proportion, assuming that the log-likelihood ratio of the two densities is linear in the observations. Under some regularity conditions, this statistic was shown to converge to a chi-square random variable. The performance of this statistic was shown to be satisfactory based on simulation studies. The author also presented estimators for the two distribution functions, as well as the connections between case-control studies and discrimination analysis.

19. When nuisance parameters are present, Lazar and Mykland (1999) investigated the higher-order asymptotic behavior of the empirical likelihood ratio statistic from the aspect of dual likelihood for the simplest case of two parameters, one parameter of interest and one nuisance parameter. It was demonstrated that, as introduced via a system of estimating equations, the asymptotic expansion for the signed square root of the empirical likelihood ratio statistic has a nonstandard form. Specifically, the mean- and variance-adjusted version of the empirical likelihood ratio statistic was shown to be nonstandard normal to the high level of accuracy achieved in the function of means case for empirical likelihood and in general for ordinary parametric likelihood. It implies that the empirical likelihood ratio statistic itself does not admit a Bartlett correction.

20. In survey sampling, measurement errors may persist. Consider the case where several different imperfect instruments and one perfect instrument are used independently to measure some characteristic of a population. Zhong et al. (2000) investigated the problem of combining this information to make statistical inference on parameters of interest, specifically the population mean and cumulative distribution function. The authors developed maximum empirical likelihood estimators and examined their asymptotic properties. The finite sample efficiency of these estimators was shown by simulation results.

21. Under the commonly used constrained estimation model and the selection bias model, Chen and Chen (2000) examined Bahadur representations of the empirical likelihood quantiles. Under the selection bias model, it is assumed that in addition to the random sample from F, there is a second independent random sample from the weighted F population G defined by $G(y) = W^{-1} \int_{-\infty}^{y} w(x)dF(x)$, where $W = \int_{-\infty}^{\infty} w(x)dF(x)$, and $w(x)$ is a known, nonnegative continuous real function that satisfies $0 < W < \infty$. It was shown that the additional model information improves the quantile estimation in large samples.

22. Qin (2000) demonstrated that empirical likelihood can effectively incorporate auxiliary information if it can be summarized as unbiased estimating equations. The auxiliary information can be summarized as $E\{\psi(X, \theta)\} = 0$, where $\psi(\cdot)$ is a $q \times 1$ known vector-valued function of X and θ. The author showed that the combined empirical and parametric likelihoods can produce valid inferences for the underlying parameters. A Wilks-type theorem was proved for the combined likelihood ratio statistic. The performance of the combined likelihood ratio confidence interval was shown to be better than that based on a normal approximation based on simulation.

23. Kitamura (2001) examined the asymptotic size and power, that is, the asymptotic efficiency, of moment restrictions tests, based on large deviations. Let α_n and β_n denote the Type I and Type II error probabilities of a test. Consider (competing) tests that satisfy $\limsup\limits_{n\to\infty} n^{-1}\log\alpha_n \leq -\eta$ for a given $\eta > 0$. The generalized Neyman–Pearson criterion states that among such tests, a test is optimal if it minimizes $\limsup\limits_{n\to\infty} n^{-1}\log\beta_n$ uniformly over all multinomial distributions with the same support. Kitamura demonstrated that for the empirical likelihood ratio test for moment restrictions with a possibly continuous distribution, the generalized Neyman–Pearson optimality result holds.

24. Owen (2001) presented one of the first books published on empirical likelihood. The author showed how to apply empirical likelihood to various problems, from simple problems, such as the construction of a confidence region for a univariate mean under random sampling, to problems defined through smooth functions of means, regression models, generalized linear models, estimating equations, or kernel smoothing, and to sampling with nonidentically distributed data. The concepts and techniques were reinforced with a large number of figures and examples from a wide range of disciplines. Detailed descriptions of algorithms were presented as well.

25. Wang and Rao (2002a) pointed out that the imputed data by the kernel regression imputation are not i.i.d., and thus it is invalid to make empirical likelihood–based inference based on the complete imputed data assuming they were i.i.d. To this end, the authors developed an adjusted empirical likelihood approach to inference for the mean of the response variable under kernel regression imputation for missing response data. The authors proposed a nonparametric version of Wilks' theorem for the adjusted empirical log-likelihood ratio, that is, with an asymptotic standard chi-square limiting distribution. In order to compare the adjusted empirical likelihood and the normal approximation methods, a simulation study was conducted to examine the coverage accuracies and average lengths of confidence intervals. The empirical likelihood–based estimator and other related estimators were also compared in terms of bias and standard error. It depicted that the adjusted empirical likelihood method performs competitively. It was confirmed that auxiliary information helps provide improved inferences.

26. Let $\tilde{X}$ be the surrogate variables and X be the true variables. Assuming that independent validation data $\left\{\left(X_i, \tilde{X}_i\right)_{i=N+1}^{N+n}\right\}$ are available in addition to the primary data $\left\{\left(Y_i, \tilde{X}_i\right)_{i=1}^{N}\right\}$, Wang and Rao (2002b) developed empirical likelihood methods in the presence of errors in covariates by considering linear errors-in-covariate models. The authors proved that their asymptotic distribution is a weighted sum of independent standard χ_1^2 random variables with unknown weights. The authors constructed an estimated empirical likelihood confidence region for the regression parameter vector by consistently estimating the unknown weights. An adjusted empirical log-likelihood was suggested whose asymptotic distribution is a standard χ^2. A partially smoothed bootstrap empirical log-likelihood for constructing a confidence region was proposed in order to avoid estimating the unknown weights or the adjustment factor, which has asymptotically correct coverage probability. Based on a simulation study, the proposed methods were

shown to be better than a method based on a normal approximation in terms of coverage accuracy and average length of the confidence interval.

27. Zou et al. (2002) considered a partial profile empirical likelihood for a semiparametric mixture model based on observations from K mixtures with common component densities f and g satisfying the exponential tilt model (Andersen 1970), $g(x) = \exp(\beta_0 + x\beta_1) f(x)$. The partial likelihood is the conditional likelihood with replacing the nuisance parameters by their estimators from the full likelihood. Note that the conditional likelihood implies alternative estimators. Zou and Fine (2002) demonstrated that the partial likelihood estimator is more efficient than an estimator with known nuisance parameters. The practical implications of this counterintuitive result are discussed.

28. Bravo (2003) investigated the asymptotic efficiency of empirical goodness-of-fit test statistics using the conventional Pitman approach based on the comparison of local power. Focusing on the second-order local power properties of a broad class of nonparametric likelihood tests recently introduced by Baggerly (1998), the authors showed that in the multiparameter setting, the well-known result that first-order efficiency implies second-order efficiency (Bickel et al. 1981) does not hold in general unless one considers the average power criterion. Therefore, none of the members of the empirical goodness-of-fit class of tests is uniformly superior in terms of its second-order local power. Note that a test has the property of local maximinity if it has maximum power, when compared to other tests in the same class based on the minimum power that can be achieved by alternatives within a given distance from the null hypothesis. In terms of local maximinity, a test based on the empirical likelihood ratio was shown to enjoy an optimality property.

29. Einmahl and McKeague (2003) constructed omnibus tests for various nonparametric hypotheses based on the empirical likelihood method. The authors specifically studied four nonparametric problems: tests for symmetry about zero, changes in distribution, independence, and exponentiality. The method localizes the empirical likelihood using one or more suitable time variables implicit in the null hypothesis, with the localized empirical likelihood ratio $R(x) = \sup\{L(\tilde{F}) : \tilde{F}(x) = F_0(x)\}/\sup\{L(\tilde{F})\}$, where $L(\tilde{F}) = \prod_{i=1}^{n} (\tilde{F}(X_i) - \tilde{F}(X_i -))$. Then the test statistics are constructed by integrating the log-likelihood ratio statistic over those variables. The authors established the asymptotic null distributions of these statistics and showed that the proposed statistics are more efficient with greater power than corresponding Cramer–von Mises-type statistics based on simulation studies.

30. Consider a k-variate data set $X = \{X_1, \ldots, X_n\}$ drawn from a two-term mixture distribution, each having independent components $F(x) = \pi \prod_{j=1}^{k} F_{j1}(x_j) + (1-\pi) \prod_{j=1}^{k} F_{j2}(x_j)$, where π denotes the mixture proportion, F_{jr} is the univariate distribution function of the jth marginal in the rth population π_r, and $x = (x_1, \ldots, x_k)$. Hall and Zhou (2003) considered nonparametric methods for estimating r and F_{jr} for $1 < j < k$ and $r = 1, 2$, using only the data X. When $k = 1$, neither π nor F_{jr} is nonparametrically identifiable. When $k = 2$, the authors showed that the problem is almost identifiable where the set of all possible representations can be expressed, in terms of any one of those representations, as a two-parameter family. When $k > 3$ and under mild regularity

conditions, the problem is identifiable from the nonparametric aspect. The authors introduced root $-n$ consistent nonparametric estimators of the $2k$ univariate marginal distributions and the mixing proportion and described finite sample and asymptotic properties of the estimators.

31. Li and Wang (2003) developed an adjusted empirical likelihood for the vector of regression coefficients using a synthetic data approach in the linear regression analysis of right-censored data. Noticing that it may not be hard to profile the nuisance parameters involved in constrained optimization in high-dimensional situations, one may replace the nuisance parameters by their least-squares estimates and adjust empirical likelihood with an appropriate adjustment factor. The adjusted empirical likelihood was shown to have a central chi-square limiting distribution. Furthermore, an adjusted empirical likelihood method for linear combinations of the regression coefficients was also developed. The way to incorporate auxiliary information was discussed. The empirical likelihood confidence intervals were shown to have more accurate coverage probabilities than the normal-based intervals in a simulation study. The method was illustrated with the Stanford heart transplant data (Miller 1976), which include the lengths of survival (in days) after transplantation, ages at time of transplant, and T5 mismatch scores for 69 patients who received heart transplants.

32. When a population consists of many zero values and the sample size is not very large, parametric models, for example, commonly used based on normal, Poisson, or gamma distribution, may have poor coverage probabilities and have to be modified. When an appropriate mixture model can be found, the problem can be reduced by constructing parametric likelihood ratio intervals. Nevertheless, usually minimal assumptions about the population of interest are preferred in the context of survey sampling. Toward this end, Chen et al. (2003a) investigated the coverage properties of nonparametric empirical likelihood confidence intervals for the population mean. Under a variety of hypothetical populations, the authors showed that empirical likelihood intervals often outperformed parametric likelihood intervals by having more balanced coverage rates and larger lower bounds. The method was illustrated with a data set from the Canadian Labour Force Survey for the year 2000.

33. Noticing that the empirical likelihood ratio test has size distortion in a small sample, Tanizaki (2004) compared empirical likelihood ratio tests of population means with different size corrections in the case of small sample size. Considering the Bartlett correction and the bootstrap method, the author compared the t-test and the empirical likelihood ratio tests with respect to the sample power, as well as the empirical size based on Monte Carlo experiments.

34. Suppose a random variable Y that can be partitioned as $Y = (Y_1, Y_2)$, possibly after a transformation, has a density $f_y(y, \phi)$ depending on a vector parameter $\phi = (\theta, \eta)$; then the full parametric likelihood can be decomposed into the product of a conditional likelihood and a marginal likelihood, that is, $f_y(y, \phi) = f_{Y_1}(y_1, \phi) f_{Y_2|Y_1}(y_2|y_1, \phi)$. Qin and Zhang (2005) showed that this property can be extended from parametric likelihood to the empirical likelihood method. The authors discussed applications in case-control studies, genetic linkage analysis, genetic quantitative trait analysis, tuberculosis infection data, and unordered-pair data, all of which can be treated as

semiparametric finite mixture models. The authors considered the estimation problem in detail in the simplest case of unordered-pair data, where one can only observe the minimum and maximum values of two random variables; the identities of the minimum and maximum values are lost. The profile empirical likelihood approach was used for maximum semiparametric likelihood estimation. Some large sample results and a simulation study were presented.

35. Let X and Y be some characteristic of the new treatment and the control treatment, respectively. One may compare the average treatment effects based on $\Delta = E(X) - E(Y)$, the probability of one treatment being better than the other based on $\Delta = \Pr(X < Y)$ or $\Delta = \Pr(X > Y)$, or the probability of death before a given time in survival analysis based on $\Delta = \Pr(X < t_0) - \Pr(Y < t_0)$. Standard statistical approaches such as maximum likelihood can be used under parametric data distribution assumptions. For the treatment effect in the two-sample problem with censoring, Zhou and Liang (2005) proposed a unified method of semiparametric inference when the model for one sample is parametric and that for the other is nonparametric. The semiparametric confidence interval based on the empirical likelihood principle was shown to improve its counterpart constructed from the common estimating equation. The empirical likelihood ratio was shown to be asymptotically chi-square. The method based on the empirical likelihood was shown to outperform the method based on the estimating equation via simulation studies. The method was illustrated with a litter-matched study of the tumorigenesis of a drug (Mantel et al. 1977), where one rat was randomly selected from each of 50 litters and given the drug, while two rats from each litter were selected as controls and given a placebo.

36. Wu (2005) developed computational algorithms and R codes for the pseudoempirical likelihood method in survey sampling. In addition, algorithms for obtaining the maximum pseudoempirical likelihood estimators under nonstratified sampling and the pseudoempirical likelihood ratio confidence intervals were developed. The functions and codes were shown to perform very well and can directly be used for survey applications and simulation experiments.

37. For time series instrumental variable models specified by nonlinear moment restrictions when identification may be weak, Guggenberger and Smith (2005) examined the performance of generalized empirical likelihood (GEL) methods. The authors demonstrated that under weak identification, all GEL estimators are first-order equivalent, and each is inconsistent and has a nonstandard asymptotic distribution. New GEL test statistics were proposed and shown to have asymptotic chi-square distributions under the null hypothesis, regardless of the strength or weakness of identification. When the parameters not under test were strongly identified, modified versions of the statistics were presented for tests of hypotheses on parameter subvectors. Tests based on these statistics were shown to have competitive power properties and good size properties even when conditional heteroscedasticity is present, based on Monte Carlo simulation for the linear instrumental variable regression model with a wide range of error distributions. The tests were shown to work well especially for thick-tailed or asymmetric error distributions.

38. Based on a local empirical likelihood approach, Cao and Van Keilegom (2006) investigated the problem of testing whether two populations have the same law by comparing kernel estimators of the two density functions. The authors derived

the asymptotic distribution of the test statistic and proposed a bootstrap approximation to calibrate the test. Note that the method can be extended to multiple samples and multivariate distributions. The proposed method was compared with two competitors based on a simulation study. A method to select the bandwidth parameter was studied. The method was applied to a data set obtained from a study to determine the effect of a calcium supplement on the total body bone mineral content (Akritas and Van Keilegom, 2001).

39. In order to accommodate the within-group correlation in longitudinal partially linear regression models, You et al. (2006) proposed a block empirical likelihood procedure using working independence. As a result, in this case, the within-subject correlation structure can be ignored. A nonparametric version of Wilks' theorem was established. Compared with normal approximations, the method does not require a consistent estimator for the asymptotic covariance matrix. Therefore, it is easier to conduct inference on the parametric component of the model. The method was illustrated with data from a longitudinal hormone study (Zhang et al. 1998).

40. In the context of partial linear models, Xue and Zhu (2007) proposed a block empirical likelihood method by centering longitudinal data. Asymptotic normality of the maximum empirical likelihood estimator of the regression coefficients and a nonparametric version of Wilks' theorem were proposed. However, their method does not take the within-subject correlation structure of the longitudinal data into account.

41. In the usual case where measurement error is present, assuming that all the imperfect instruments are unbiased, Wu and Zhang (2007) considered the problem of combining information of measurement errors based on the pooled samples to make statistical tests for parameters more relevant. The empirical likelihood ratio functions were defined and their asymptotic distributions were obtained in the presence of measurement error.

42. Fan and Jiang (2007) selectively overviewed nonparametric inferences and proposed testing various null hypotheses versus nonparametric alternatives based on generalized likelihood ratio (GLR) statistics. The authors emphasized the trade-off between the flexibility of alternative models and the power of the statistical tests. Noticing a great potential for developing the GLR tests, the authors discussed Wilks' phenomena for a variety of semi- and nonparametric models.

43. Yang and Zhao (2007) developed a new χ^2-test of treatment effect by combining the weighted log-rank statistics and using the empirical likelihood (EL) method. For a variety of combinations of the short-term and long-term treatment effects, the performance of the test was shown to be good compared with other related ones based on extensive simulation studies.

44. Consider partially linear models of the form $Y = X^T\beta + v(Z) + \varepsilon$, where the covariate X is measured with error, the response variable Y is sometimes missing with missingness probability π depending on (X, Z), and $v(Z)$ is an unspecified smooth function. The missingness scheme here is missing not at random, instead of the usual missing at random. In this case, Liang et al. (2007) proposed a family of semiparametric estimators for β and the population mean $E(Y)$. It was shown that the resulting estimators are consistent and

asymptotically normal under general assumptions. The authors proposed an empirical likelihood–based statistic, which was shown to be chi-square distributed asymptotically, in order to construct a confidence region for β. The methods were illustrated with an AIDS clinical trial data set of the pediatric AIDS clinical trial group PACTG 338 study, where one of the purposes was to investigate the effectiveness of antiretroviral medicines and the effect of CD4 cell counts on the amount of HIV in the blood, the HIV viral load (Liang et al. 2004).

45. In a missing response problem, Qin and Zhang (2007) proposed an empirical likelihood (EL) estimator for improving the inverse probability weighting estimation. The empirical likelihood estimator is defined as $\hat{\mu}_{EL} = \sum_{i=1}^{n} r_i p_i^{EL} y_i$, where weights p_i^{EL} are defined for complete case observations (i.e., when $r_i = 1$). The empirical log-likelihood function $l = \sum_{i=1}^{n} r_i \log p_i^{EL}$ is maximized subject to constraints $p_i^{EL} \geq 0$, $\sum_{i=1}^{n} r_i p_i^{EL} = 1$, $\sum_{i=1}^{n} r_i p_i^{EL} \pi\left(x_i; \hat{\beta}\right) = \hat{\theta}$, and $\sum_{i=1}^{n} r_i p_i^{EL} a\left(x_i; \hat{\beta}\right) = \hat{a}$, where $a = (a_1, ..., a_p)$ is a fixed vector function of $p < n$ dimensions, $\hat{\theta} = n^{-1} \sum_{i=1}^{n} \pi(x_i; \hat{\beta})$ and $\hat{a} = n^{-1} \sum_{i=1}^{n} a(x_i)$. Based on simulation studies, it was shown that the finite sample performance of the EL estimator is better than certain existing estimators with large sample results for the estimator. Note that this EL estimator is computed in a two-step manner, which would be much easier to implement, unlike the single-step estimator discussed in Qin and Lawless (1994). Furthermore, for estimation from an overidentified system of estimating equations and optimally combining estimating equations, the EL estimator of Qin and Zhang (2007) is also different from the general empirical likelihood methodologies of Qin and Lawless (1994).

46. For the regression model of mean quality-adjusted lifetime with right censoring, Zhao and Wang (2008) proposed an empirical likelihood method of testing for the vector of the regression parameters. It was demonstrated that the empirical log-likelihood ratio is asymptotically a weighted sum of independent chi-square random variables. The authors adjusted this empirical log-likelihood ratio such that the limiting distribution is a standard chi-square. Empirical likelihood methods were shown to outperform the normal approximation methods in terms of coverage probability based on simulation studies. The methods were illustrated with a data example from a randomized clinical trial that examined two treatments for the node-positive breast cancer: short-duration chemotherapy and long-duration chemotherapy (Cole et al. 1993).

47. Based on an empirical likelihood methodology, Qin and Zhang (2008) investigated the uncertainty of structural differences, for example, mean and distribution function differences between populations, in terms of a confidence interval (CI). The authors presented a method for estimating CIs for differences between characteristics of populations with missing values, where a simple random hot-deck imputation method was employed. The power of this CI estimation was illustrated by using the method as a new machine learning technique for distinguishing spam from nonspam emails in a spam base data set.

48. In order to address noncompliance problems in randomized trials, causal approaches based on the potential outcome framework can be used as a useful tool.

Considering randomized clinical trials with noncompliance, Cheng et al. (2009) proposed a new estimator of causal treatment effects by using the empirical likelihood approach to construct a profile random sieve likelihood and considering the mixture structure in outcome distributions. The estimator is robust to parametric distribution assumptions and provides substantial finite sample efficiency gains over the standard instrumental variable estimator. The estimator was shown to be asymptotically equivalent to the standard instrumental variable estimator and can be applied to outcome variables with a continuous, ordinal, or binary scale. The method was illustrated with a randomized trial of an intervention to improve the treatment of depression among depressed elderly patients in primary care practices (Bruce et al. 2004).

49. In a sequential clinical trial whose stopping rule depends on the primary endpoint, in order to address the problem of substantial bias that may result from ignoring the possibility of early stopping based on the primary endpoint, a commonly used approach is to develop bias correction by estimating the bias in the case of bivariate normal outcomes. Lai et al. (2009) proposed a new approach based on resampling and a novel ordering scheme in the sample space of sequential statistics observed up to a stopping time. It was shown that this approach provides accurate inference in complex clinical trials, including time-sequential trials with survival endpoints and covariates.

50. Consider a random sample of d-dimensional random vectors $X_1, \ldots, X_n$. Let $\mu \in R^p$ be a parameter of interest and $v \in R^q$ be some nuisance parameter, where the unknown, true parameters (μ_0, v_0) are uniquely determined by the system of equations $E\{g(X, \mu_0, v_0)\} = 0$, where $g = (g_1, \ldots, g_{p+q})$ is a vector of $p + q$ functions. Molanes Lopez et al. (2009) developed an empirical likelihood (EL) method to make inference for the parameter μ_0, which is valid under very mild conditions on the vector of criterion functions g, for example, in the case where $g_1, \ldots, g_{p+q}$ are unsmooth in μ or v. The asymptotic limit of the empirical log-likelihood ratio was presented and small sample performance was evaluated via a small simulation study.

51. Chan et al. (2009) proposed empirical likelihood methods based on characteristic functions with application to Lévy processes, which are widely applied for pricing the dynamics of financial securities due to the ability to capture jumps. This method is based on the integrated distance of characteristic functions and can be applied in (a) the estimation of parameters, (b) testing the belonging of a characteristic function to a particular parametric class, and (c) testing the symmetry of the underlying distribution around an unknown mean. The effectiveness of the method was confirmed by simulation studies.

52. In small samples or high dimensions, the empirical likelihood method is very poorly calibrated, leading to test results with a higher Type I error than the nominal level, and it suffers from a limiting convex hull constraint. One of the methods to address this problem is to supplement the observed data set with an artificial data point. Emerson and Owen (2009) investigated the consequences of this approach and described a limitation of the method in settings when the sample size is relatively small compared with the dimension. The authors proposed a modification to the extra data approach that involves two additional points and changing the location of the extra points. This modification results in better calibration, especially in difficult cases, as well as a small sample connection between the modified empirical likelihood method and Hotelling's T^2 test. It was shown that a continuum of

tests can be established by varying the location of the added data points that range from the unmodified empirical likelihood statistic to Hotelling's T^2 statistic.

53. Vexler et al. (2009a) investigated the performance of the asymptotic evaluation of the Type I error of empirical likelihood (EL) ratio–type tests based on a nonparametric version of Wilks' theorem when the EL is based on finite samples obtained from various distributions. The authors demonstrated that the classical EL procedure and Student's t-test share a similar Type I error control asymptotically. Note that the efficiency of the EL method can be affected by data with skewed distributions. In order to improve the EL ratio test, modifications of t-type tests can be undertaken. The authors also modified the t-test proposed by Chen (1995) to the EL ratio test and showed that Chen's approach leads to a location change of observed data, while the classical Bartlett method is known to be a scale correction of the data distribution. The EL ratio test was modified via both the Chen and Bartlett corrections. Monte Carlo simulations and a real data example from a study that evaluates biomarkers related to atherosclerotic coronary heart disease were used to study the performance of the test.

54. Consider a continuous response variable longitudinal regression model: $y_{ij} = X_{ij}^T \beta + \varepsilon_{ij}$, $i = 1, \ldots n$, $j = 1, \ldots, m_i$, where n is the total number of subjects, m_i is the number of repeated measurements for the ith subject, y_{ij} is the jth measurement on the ith subject, X_{ij} and β are a q-vector of covariate values and unknown regression coefficients, respectively, and ε_{ij} is a zero-mean random variable with variance σ_{ij}^2. Based on this model, Wang et al. (2010) proposed two generalized empirical likelihood–based methods that incorporate the within-subject correlation structure of the repeated measurements. A nonparametric version of Wilks' theorem for the empirical likelihood ratios, as well as inference for linear combinations of the regression parameters for both proposed methods, was addressed. One of the proposed methods was shown to be locally efficient among a class of within-subject variance–covariance matrices. Based on a simulation study, the proposed methods were shown to be more efficient than existing methods that ignore the correlation structure, for example, the block empirical likelihood method by You et al. (2006), and to be better in terms of coverage than the normal approximation with correctly specified within-subject correlation. The methods were illustrated with the well-known ongoing longitudinal Framingham Heart Study, which has produced 50 years of data collected from residents of Framingham and identified major risk factors associated with heart disease, strokes, and other diseases.

55. When individuals have concentrations at or below the laboratory limits of detection and many zero values, it is necessary to employ estimation procedures that allow for data with many zero values in order to compare mean concentrations between individuals with and without disease. Kang et al. (2010) examined parametric methods and proposed nonparametric likelihood methods based on empirical likelihood methodology for comparing data sets with many zero observations. The empirical likelihood interval for the mean and mean difference of two independent populations with mass at zero was derived, and the coverage probability of the intervals was examined. The authors illustrated and compared the parametric likelihood interval estimation and the empirical likelihood interval estimation based on the data from the organochlorine pesticides exposure and risk of endometriosis study.

56. Aiming to compare the pneumonia risks among treatment groups for incomplete data, Yu et al. (2010) derived a method that combines nonparametric empirical likelihood ratio techniques with classical testing for parametric models. This method increases the study power by enabling one to use any observed data. The asymptotic property of the proposed method was investigated theoretically. Both asymptotic results and excellent power properties of the method were confirmed by Monte Carlo simulations. The method was applied to the data obtained in clinical practice settings and compares the ventilator-associated pneumonia risks among treatment groups.

57. In the analysis of randomized clinical trials and observational studies, covariate adjustment, when properly used, can be used to increase efficiency and power and reduce possible bias (Armitage, 1981). Wu and Ying (2011) proposed a nonparametric approach to covariate adjustment based on the empirical likelihood method. This approach automatically employs covariate information in an optimal way without fitting nonparametric regression. This empirical likelihood ratio–based test was shown to have a nonparametric Wilks-type result of convergence to a χ^2-distribution, and the corresponding maximum empirical likelihood estimator was shown to have an asymptotic normal distribution. It was demonstrated that the resulting test is asymptotically most powerful and that the estimator for the treatment effect achieves the semiparametric efficiency bound. The authors applied the new method to the Global Use of Strategies to Open Occluded Coronary Arteries (GUSTO) I trial. In this study, the primary endpoint was 30-day death, where 6.29% of 10,366 patients were randomly assigned to tissue plasminogen activator (TPA), 7.32% of 10,354 patients were randomly assigned to streptokinase (SK) with IV heparin, 6.99% of 10,303 patients were randomly assigned to a combination of SK and TPA, and 7.24% of 9773 patients were randomly assigned to SK with SQ heparin.

58. Yu, Vexler, Kim, and Hutson (2011) proposed a series of two-sample median-specific empirical likelihood–based tests. The way of incorporating the relevant constraints into the empirical likelihood function for in-depth median testing was presented. Based on an extensive Monte Carlo study, the resulting tests were shown to have excellent operating characteristics even under unfavorable situations, for example, nonexchangeability under the null hypothesis. The proposed methods were illustrated with biomarker data from Western blot analysis to compare normal cells with bronchial epithelial cells from a case-control study that consists of 48 subjects, including 18 normal and 30 abnormal observations.

59. Vexler and Yu (2011) proposed and examined the method for comparing two treatment groups based on the incomplete bivariate data in the context of the ventilator-associated pneumonia study. A semiparametric methodology employing the density-based empirical likelihood approach was proposed in order to compare two treatments with bivariate observed data exhibiting this pattern of missingness. The method provides a nonparametric analogue to Neyman–Pearson-type test statistics. The empirical likelihood approach has both parametric and nonparametric components. The nonparametric component is based on the observations for the nonmissing cases, while the parametric component tackles the case where observations are missing with respect to the invasive variable. The method was illustrated with the actual data obtained from an institutional randomized clinical trial studying oral health and ventilator-associated pneumonia to determine the effect of chlorhexidine gluconate application (once or twice per day)

against the control group on the reduction of oral colonization by pathogens in subjects in an ICU (Scannapieco et al. 2009).

60. Note that when only a small part of parameters is of interest, using a profile empirical likelihood method to construct confidence regions could be computationally costly. In order to overcome this computational burden, Li et al. (2011) proposed a jackknife empirical likelihood method. This method is easy to implement and works well in practice.

61. Qin et al. (2011) defined a profile empirical likelihood ratio for the sensitivity of a continuous-scale diagnostic test and demonstrated that its limiting distribution is a scaled chi-square distribution. Two empirical likelihood–based confidence intervals for the sensitivity of the test at a fixed level of specificity were proposed by using the scaled chi-square distribution. The finite sample performance of the empirical likelihood–based intervals was compared with that of the existing intervals for sensitivity in terms of coverage probability based on simulation studies. The authors illustrated the application of the proposed methods to assess the diagnostic accuracy of carbohydrate antigenic determinant CA19-9 in the detection of pancreatic cancer.

62. Vexler et al. (2012b) investigated both parametric and nonparametric techniques to analyze repeated measures data or pooled data subject to measurement error (ME) problems. It was concluded that the likelihood methods based on a mixture of both pooled and unpooled data (a hybrid pooled–unpooled design) are very efficient and powerful in the presence of ME. Furthermore, novel EL ratio test statistics that can aid in constructing the confidence interval estimation based on pooled–unpooled data and repeated measures data were developed. The performance of empirical likelihood–based methods was confirmed by an extensive Monte Carlo study. The efficiency of the methods was demonstrated via a data set from a study on coronary heart disease investigating the discriminatory ability of a cholesterol biomarker for myocardial infarction.

63. For composite hypotheses related to treatment effects, Vexler et al. (2012a) proposed exact nonparametric tests to provide efficient tools that compare study groups based on paired data. When data distributions are correctly specified, parametric likelihood ratios are optimal to detect a difference in distributions of two samples based on paired data. The authors adapted density-based empirical likelihood methods to deal with various testing scenarios involved in the two-sample comparisons based on paired data. It was shown that the procedures outperform classical approaches and can be easily applied to a variety of testing problems in practice. The authors applied the density-based empirical likelihood technique to compare two therapies of attention-deficit/hyperactivity disorder and severe mood dysregulation.

64. When the current sample size is too small due to cost and time constraints, in order to accurately and efficiently estimate parameters of interest, Wang et al. (2012) proposed a robust semiparametric empirical likelihood method to integrate all available information from multiple samples with a common center of measurements. Two different sets of estimating equations were used to improve the classical likelihood inference on the measurement center. The methods do not require knowledge of the functional forms of the probability density functions of related populations. The performance of the method in terms of the mean squared errors, coverage probabilities, and average lengths of confidence intervals was shown to

be better than that of the classical likelihood method. More informative and efficient inference can be offered based on Wang's method than on the conventional maximum likelihood estimator if a certain structural relationship exists among the parameters of relevant samples.

65. Noticing that the empirical likelihood estimator proposed by Qin and Zhang (2007) does not have a uniformly smaller asymptotic variance than other existing estimators in general, Chan (2012) considered several modifications to the empirical likelihood estimator. Under missing at random, it was shown that Chan's estimator dominates the empirical likelihood estimator and several other existing estimators in terms of asymptotic efficiencies. The estimator was shown to attain the minimum asymptotic variance among estimators having influence functions in a certain class and to have certain double-robustness properties.

66. In order to implement empirical likelihood for inference about a multivariate mean, Yang and Small (2013) developed an R package termed *el.convex*. Targeting the same goal, five functions employing various optimization algorithms are included in the package. These functions are based on the theory of convex optimization, including Newton, Davidon–Fletcher–Powell (DFP), Broyden–Fletcher–Goldfarb–Shanno (BFGS), conjugate gradient method (FRPR), and damped Newton. Note that among these methods, damped Newton and DFP are ensured to succeed theoretically. Newton runs fastest, but it is the least stable. Using FRPR should be avoided. Furthermore, these functions were compared with the function `el.test` in the existing R package *emplik*. No theoretical result can guarantee that the `el.test` function converges to the global minimum. Even if it does converge eventually, it may be very slow. In general, DFP, BFGS, and damped Newton need more iterations but are more stable than `el.test`. Consequently, to conduct the empirical likelihood method, one may consider using `el.test` first and checking whether the weights sum up to 1. If they do not, the authors suggested using package *el.convex*, and the `el.test.damped` function is probably the best choice.

67. In order to test for the equality of marginal distributions given that sampling is from a continuous bivariate population, Vexler et al. (2013b) developed an empirical likelihood (EL) ratio approach. In various shift alternative scenarios, the proposed exact test was demonstrated to be superior to the classic nonparametric procedures. Note that classic nonparametric procedures may break down completely or are frequently inferior to the density-based EL ratio test, which is specifically true for the skewed data distribution or in the case where a nonconstant shift exists under the alternative. The proposed test was shown to have excellent operating characteristics based on an extensive Monte Carlo study. The density-based EL ratio test was applied to the following medical studies: (a) a data set consisting of measurements of 56 assay pairs of cyclosporine (Hawkins 2002) and (b) a study examining the feasibility and efficacy of a group-based therapy program for children with ADHD and SMD.

68. In many biomedical studies, differences in upper quantiles represent the upper range of biomarkers or may be used as the cutoff value for a disease classification. Based on the empirical likelihood methodology, Yu et al. (2014) investigated two-group comparisons of an upper quantile. The classical empirical likelihood and "plug-in" empirical likelihood were employed to construct the test statistics. Though the plug-in method was developed in the frame of the empirical likelihood, the test statistic is not obtained by maximizing the empirical likelihood. It is simplified in its construction by using an indicator function.

Based on extensive simulation results, the plug-in empirical likelihood approach was shown to perform better than upper quantiles across various underlying distributions and sample sizes. The authors applied the methods to test the differences in upper quantiles in two different studies: (a) the oral colonization of pneumonia pathogens for intensive care unit patients treated by two different oral treatments and (b) the biomarker expressions of normal and abnormal bronchial epithelial cells.

6.9 Appendix

6.9.1 Several Results That Are Similar to Those Related to the Evaluations of *ELR* (θ)

One can show that the logarithm of the ELR test statistic for the null hypothesis $H_0: E(X_1) = \theta_1$ and $E(X_1^2) = \theta_2$ has the form of $\log ELR(\theta_1, \theta_2) = \sum_{i=1}^{n} \log\{1 + \lambda_1(X_i - \theta_1)/n + \lambda_2(X_i^2 - \theta_2)/n\}$. In this case, $\partial \log ELR/\partial\theta_1 = -\lambda_1$ and $\partial \log ELR/\partial\theta_2 = -\lambda_2$. At point $\left(\theta_1 = \bar{X} = \sum_{i=1}^{n} X_i/n, \theta_2 = \bar{X}^2 = \sum_{i=1}^{n} X_i^2/n\right)$, we have $\log ELR(\theta_1, \theta_2) = \lambda_1 = \lambda_2 = 0, p_i = 1/n$ and the following derivative values:

$$\frac{\partial \lambda_1}{\partial \theta_1} = \frac{n^2 \sum_{i=1}^{n}\left(X_i^2 - \bar{X}^2\right)^2}{\Delta}, \frac{\partial \lambda_2}{\partial \theta_2} = \frac{n^2 \sum_{i=1}^{n}\left(X_i - \bar{X}\right)^2}{\Delta}, \frac{\partial \lambda_1}{\partial \theta_2} = \frac{\partial \lambda_2}{\partial \theta_1} = \frac{n^2 \sum_{i=1}^{n}\left(X_i - \bar{X}\right)\left(X_i^2 - \bar{X}^2\right)}{\Delta},$$

$$\frac{\partial^2 \lambda_1}{\partial \theta_1^2} = \frac{1}{n\Delta}\left[2\sum_{i=1}^{n}\left(X_i^2 - \bar{X}^2\right)\left\{\frac{\partial \lambda_1}{\partial \theta_1}\left(X_i - \bar{X}\right) + \frac{\partial \lambda_2}{\partial \theta_1}\left(X_i^2 - \bar{X}^2\right)\right\}^2 \sum_{i=1}^{n}\left(X_i - \bar{X}\right)\left(X_i^2 - \bar{X}^2\right)\right.$$
$$\left. -2\sum_{i=1}^{n}\left(X_i - \bar{X}\right)\left\{\frac{\partial \lambda_1}{\partial \theta_1}\left(X_i - \bar{X}\right) + \frac{\partial \lambda_2}{\partial \theta_1}\left(X_i^2 - \bar{X}^2\right)\right\}^2 \sum_{i=1}^{n}\left(X_i^2 - \bar{X}^2\right)^2\right],$$

$$\frac{\partial^2 \lambda_2}{\partial \theta_1^2} = \frac{1}{n\Delta}\left[2\sum_{i=1}^{n}\left(X_i - \bar{X}\right)\left\{\frac{\partial \lambda_1}{\partial \theta_1}\left(X_i - \bar{X}\right) + \frac{\partial \lambda_2}{\partial \theta_1}\left(X_i^2 - \bar{X}^2\right)\right\}^2 \sum_{i=1}^{n}\left(X_i - \bar{X}\right)\left(X_i^2 - \bar{X}^2\right)\right.$$
$$\left. -2\sum_{i=1}^{n}\left(X_i^{\,2} - \bar{X}^2\right)\left\{\frac{\partial \lambda_1}{\partial \theta_1}\left(X_i - \bar{X}\right) + \frac{\partial \lambda_2}{\partial \theta_1}\left(X_i^2 - \bar{X}^2\right)\right\}^2 \sum_{i=1}^{n}\left(X_i - \bar{X}\right)^2\right],$$

$$\frac{\partial^2 \lambda_1}{\partial \theta_2^2} = \frac{\partial^2 \lambda_2}{\partial \theta_1 \partial \theta_2} = \frac{1}{n\Delta}\left[2\sum_{i=1}^{n}\left(X_i^2 - \bar{X}^2\right)\left\{\frac{\partial \lambda_1}{\partial \theta_2}\left(X_i - \bar{X}\right) + \frac{\partial \lambda_2}{\partial \theta_2}\left(X_i^2 - \bar{X}^2\right)\right\}^2 \sum_{i=1}^{n}\left(X_i - \bar{X}\right)\left(X_i^2 - \bar{X}^2\right)\right.$$
$$\left. -2\sum_{i=1}^{n}\left(X_i - \bar{X}\right)\left\{\frac{\partial \lambda_1}{\partial \theta_1}\left(X_i - \bar{X}\right) + \frac{\partial \lambda_2}{\partial \theta_1}\left(X_i^2 - \bar{X}^2\right)\right\}^2 \sum_{i=1}^{n}\left(X_i^2 - \bar{X}^2\right)^2\right],$$

$$\frac{\partial^2 \lambda_2}{\partial \theta_1^2} = \frac{\partial^2 \lambda_1}{\partial \theta_1 \partial \theta_2} = \frac{1}{n\Delta} \left[2 \sum_{i=1}^{n} \left(X_i - \bar{X} \right) \left\{ \frac{\partial \lambda_1}{\partial \theta_1} \left(X_i - \bar{X} \right) + \frac{\partial \lambda_2}{\partial \theta_1} \left(X_i^2 - \bar{X}^2 \right) \right\}^2 \sum_{i=1}^{n} \left(X_i - \bar{X} \right) \left(X_i^2 - \bar{X}^2 \right) \right.$$

$$\left. -2 \sum_{i=1}^{n} \left(X_i^2 - \bar{X}^2 \right) \left\{ \frac{\partial \lambda_1}{\partial \theta_1} \left(X_i - \bar{X} \right) + \frac{\partial \lambda_2}{\partial \theta_1} \left(X_i^2 - \bar{X}^2 \right) \right\}^2 \sum_{i=1}^{n} \left(X_i - \bar{X} \right)^2 \right]$$

where $\Delta = \left\{ \sum_{i=1}^{n} \left(X_i - \bar{X} \right) \left(X_i^2 - \bar{X}^2 \right) \right\}^2 - \sum_{i=1}^{n} \left(X_i - \bar{X} \right)^2 \sum_{i=1}^{n} \left(X_i^2 - \bar{X}^2 \right)^2$.

6.9.2 R Procedures for Executing the Two-Sample Density-Based ELR Test

```
###########sample data with the sample sizes n1=n2=25###########
n1=25
n2=25

x<-sample(control,n1)
y<-sample(case,n2)

delta<-0.1
z<-c(x,y)
sx<-sort(x)
sy<-sort(y)
sz<-sort(z)


##################################################
#######obtaining the ELR based on the sample X###
##################################################

m<-c(round(n1^(delta+0.5))):min(c(round((n1)^(1-delta)),round(n1/2))))
###generate a vector of "m"
a<-replicate(n1,m) ###store repeated values of the vector "m"
rm<-as.vector(t(a)) ###transpose the previous length(m)*n1 matrix and
  #make it to be a vector
rm<-rep(m, each = n1) ###repeat the vector of "m" n1 times
L<-c(1:n1)- rm ###order from (1-m) to (n1-m)
LL<-replace(L, L <= 0, 1 ) ###replace values that are <=0 with 1 when
  #(1-m) <=0
U<-c(1:n1)+ rm ###order from (1+m) to (n1+m)
UU<-replace(U, U > n1, n1) ###replace values that are n1 with n1 when
  #(n1+m) >n1

xL<-sx[LL] ###obtain x(i-m)
xU<-sx[UU] ###obtain x(i+m)
F<-ecdf(z)(xU)-ecdf(z)(xL) ### the empirical distribution function
F[F==0]<-1/(n1+n2)
I<-2*rm/(n1*F) ### a (n1*length(m)) vector of (2*m)/(n1*empirical
  #distribution function)
ux<-array(I, c(n1,length(m))) ### make the previous vector as a
  #n1*length(m) matrix
tstat1<-log(min(apply(ux,2,prod))) ###get the part of the test statistic
  #based on the sample X
```

```
##################################################
#######obtaining the ELR based on the sample Y###
##################################################

m<-c(round(n2^(delta+0.5))):min(c(round((n2)^(1-delta)),round(n2/2))))
   ###generate a vector of "m"
a<-replicate(n2,m) ###store repeated values of the vector "m"
rm<-as.vector(t(a)) ###transpose the previous length(m)*n2 matrix and
   #make it to be a vector
rm<-rep(m, each = n2) ###repeat the vector of "m" n2 times

L<-c(1:n2)-rm ###order from (1-m) to (n2-m)
LL<-replace(L, L <= 0, 1) ###replace values that are <=0 with 1 when
   #(1-m) <=0
U<-c(1:n2)+ rm ###order from (1+m) to (n2+m)
UU<-replace(U, U > n2, n2) ###replace values that are>n2 with n2 when
   #(n2+m)>n2
yL<-sy[LL] ###obtain y(i-m)
yU<-sy[UU] ###obtain y(i+m)

F<-ecdf(z)(yU)-ecdf(z)(yL) ###the empirical distribution function
F[F==0]<-1/(n1+n2)

I<-2*rm/(n2*F) ### the (n2*length(m)) vector of (2*m)/(n2*empirical
   #distribution fuction)
uy<-array(I, c(n2,length(m))) ### make the previous vector as a
   #n2*length(m) matrix
tstat2<-log(min(apply(uy,2, prod))) ###get ELR_Y
finalts<-tstat1+tstat2 ### the final test statistic log(V)
```

7

Bayes Factor–Based Test Statistics

"Essay towards Solving a Problem in Doctrine of Chance"

Thomas Bayes*

7.1 Introduction

Statistical science has over the years developed two schools of thought as it applies to statistical inference. One school is termed frequentist methodology, and the other school of thought is termed Bayesian methodology. There has been a decades-long debate between both schools of thought on the optimality and appropriateness of the other's approach. The fundamental difference between the two schools of thought is philosophical in nature regarding the definition of probability, which ultimately one could argue is axiomatic in nature. The frequentist approach denotes probability in terms of long-run averages, for example, the probability of getting heads when flipping a coin infinitely many times would be half, given a fair coin. Inference within the frequentist context is based on the assumption that a given experiment is one realization of an experiment that could be repeated infinitely many times; for example, the notion of the Type I error discussed earlier (Chapter 1) is that if we were to repeat the same experiment infinitely many times, we would falsely reject the null hypothesis a fixed percentage of the time.

The Bayesian approach defines probability as a measure of an individual's objective view of scientific truth based on his or her current state of knowledge. The state of knowledge, given as a probability measure, is then updated through new observations. We take the approach that both the Bayesian and frequentist methods are useful, and that in general there should not be much disagreement between the approaches in the practical setting. Our ultimate goal is to provide a road map for tools that are efficient in a given setting. In general, Bayesian approaches are more computationally intensive than frequentist approaches; hence, their use has been limited historically. However, due to advances in computing power, Bayesian methods have emerged as an increasingly effective and practical alternative to the corresponding frequentist methods. In fact, there have been many attempts to reconcile the two approaches that go beyond the scope of this textbook. This chapter provides a basic introduction to the Bayesian view of statistical testing strategies with a focus on Bayes factor–type principles.

As an introduction to the Bayesian approach as it contrasts to frequentist methods, first consider the simple hypothesis test H_0: $\theta = \theta_0$ versus H_1: $\theta = \theta_1$, where the parameters θ_0 and θ_1 are known. Given an observed random sample $X = \{x_1, \ldots, x_n\}$, we can then construct the likelihood ratio test statistic $L = f(X|\theta_1)/f(X|\theta_0)$ for the purpose of determining which hypothesis is more probable, when f denotes a density function of X. The decision-making

---

* *Philosophical Transactions of the Royal Society (London),* 53, 376–398, 1763.

143

procedure is to reject H_0 for large values of L. In this case, the decision-making rule based on the likelihood ratio test is uniformly most powerful. See the appendix and Section 4.2 for details. Although this classical hypothesis testing approach has a long and celebrated history in the statistical literature and continues to be a favorite of practitioners, it can be applied in a straightforward manner only in the case of a simple hypothesis; that is, the parameter under the alternative hypothesis, θ_1, is known.

Various practical hypothesis testing problems involve the consideration of the scenarios where the parameter under the alternative, θ_1, is unknown, for example, testing the composite hypothesis $H_0: \theta = \theta_0$ versus $H_1: \theta \neq \theta_0$. In general, when the alternative parameter is unknown, the parametric likelihood ratio test is not applicable since it is not well defined. When a hypothesis is composite, Neyman and Pearson suggested replacing the density at a single parameter value with the maximum of the density over all parameters in that hypothesis. As a result of this groundbreaking theory, the maximum likelihood ratio test became a key method in statistical inference (see details in Chapter 4).

It should be noted, however, that several criticisms pertaining to the maximum likelihood ratio test may be made. First, in a decision-making process, we do not generally need to estimate the unknown parameters under H_0 or H_1. We just need to make a binary decision regarding whether to reject the null hypothesis. Another criticism is that in practice, we rely on the function $f(X|\hat{\theta})$ in place of $f(X|\theta)$, which technically does not yield a likelihood function; that is, it is not a proper density function. Therefore, the maximum likelihood ratio test may lose efficiency compared to the likelihood ratio test of interest.

Alternatively, one can provide testing procedures substituting the unknown alternative parameter with variables that do not depend on the observed data. Such approaches can be extended to provide test procedures within a Bayes factor–type framework. We can integrate test statistics through variables that represent the unknown parameters with respect to a function commonly called a *prior* distribution. This approach can be generalized to be applied to more complicated hypotheses and models.

In the following sections, we describe and explore topics regarding the use of representative values instead of unknown parameters, as well as Bayes factor principles. Under Bayes factor type of statistical decision-making mechanisms, external information is incorporated into the evaluation of evidence about a hypothesis, and functions that represent possible parameter values under the alternative hypothesis are considered. These functions can be interpreted in the light of our current state of knowledge, such as belief where we would like to be most powerful regarding the external, or prior information on the parameter of interest under the alternative hypothesis; for example, a physician may expect the median survival rate for a new compound to behave in a certain way with a given degree of probability. Without loss of generality, we focus on basic scenarios of testing that could be easily extended to more complicated situations of statistical decision-making procedures.

7.2 Representative Values

Without loss of generality, we consider a straightforward example that introduces the basic ingredients for further explanations in this chapter.

Assume that we observe independent and identically distributed (i.i.d.) data points $X_1, \ldots, X_n$ and are interested in testing the hypothesis $H_0: X \sim f_0(x)$ versus $H_1: X \sim f_0(x) \cdot \exp(\theta_1 x + \theta_2)$, where f_0 is a density function (known or unknown), and quantities

θ_1, θ_2 are unknown when $f_0(x) \cdot \exp(\theta_1 x + \theta_2)$ is a density function with argument x; θ_2 can depend on n and θ_1. Let the sign of θ_1 be known, for example, $\theta_1 > 0$. Under this statement of hypothesis testing, the statistic $\exp\left(a \sum_{i=1}^{n} X_i + b \right)$ is the most powerful test statistic, where a and b can be chosen arbitrarily and a is of the same sign of θ_1; that is, $a > 0$ in this example. The proof is deferred to the appendix. Note that if θ_1 and θ_2 are assumed to be known, then the most powerful test is the likelihood ratio test. Since θ_1 and θ_2 are unknown, one can propose estimating θ_1 and θ_2 by using the maximum likelihood method in order to approximate the likelihood test statistics. In this case, the efficiency of the test may be lost completely. The optimal method based on the test statistic $\exp\left(a \sum_{i=1}^{n} X_i + b \right)$ can be referred to as a simple representative method, since we employ arbitrarily chosen numbers to represent the unknown parameters θ_1 and θ_2.

The statement of the problem above is quite general. For example, when $X \sim N(\mu, 1)$ the considered hypothesis could have the form of H_0: $\mu = 0$ versus H_0: $\mu \neq 0$. In this case, we have $f_0(x) = \exp(-x^2/2)/\sqrt{2\pi}$ and $f_1(x) = f_0(x) \exp(\theta_1 x + \theta_2)$, with $\theta_1 = \mu/2$ and $\theta_2 = \mu^2/2$, respectively.

7.3 Integrated Most Powerful Tests

In the previous section, we studied the simple representative method, which can be easily extended by integrating test statistics through variables that represent unknown parameters with respect to a function that can display corresponding weights to the variables. This approach can be referred to as Bayes factor–type decision-making mechanisms, which will be described formally below.

Assume for quality of explanation that we have a sample $\mathbf{x} = \{X_1, \ldots, X_n\}$ and are interested in the composite hypothesis H_0: $\theta = \theta_0$ versus H_1: $\theta \neq \theta_0$. Classical statistics are operationalized solely by the use of sample information (the data obtained from the statistical investigation) in terms of making inferences about θ, in general, without utilizing prior knowledge of the parameter space (i.e., the set of all possible values of the unknown parameter). However, in the decision-making process, attempts are made to combine the sample information with other relevant facets of the problem in order to make an optimal decision.

Typically, two kinds of external information are relevant. The first source of information is a set of rules regarding the possible cost of any given decision. Usually this information, referred to as the loss function, can be quantified by determining the incurred loss for each possible decision across all values of θ. The second source of information can be termed prior information, that is, prior belief (weights) on the possible values of θ being true under the alternative hypothesis across the parameter space. This is information about the parameter of interest θ obtained from sources other than the statistical investigation; for example, information comes from past experience about similar situations involving similar parameters of interest θ (see Berger [1980] for more details). In the clinical trial setting, one may, for example, gain insight into the behavior of the process in early-stage clinical investigations and can then apply this information to the later stages of investigation.

More formally, let $\pi(\theta)$ represent our level of belief (probability-based weights) of the possible consequences of the decisions or the possible values of θ under the alternative hypothesis. One can extend the technique of the previous section in general hypothesis testing to propose the test statistic of the form

$$B_n(X_1, ..., X_n) = \frac{\int f_{H_1}(X_1, ..., X_n \mid \theta) \pi(\theta) \, d\theta}{f_{H_0}(X_1, ..., X_n \mid \theta_0)}.$$

The decision rule is to reject the null hypothesis for large values of the test statistic. One can show that this decision rule provides the integrated most powerful test with respect to the function $\pi(\theta)$. The proof is deferred to the appendix. Note that the definition of the test statistic $B_n(X_1, ..., X_n)$ corresponding to the point null hypothesis $\theta = \theta_0$ is widely addressed in the Bayesian statistical literature (e.g., Berger 1985, pp. 148–150, eq. (4.15); Bernardo and Smith 1994, pp. 391–392; Kass 1993).

Following this result, we can reconsider $\pi(\theta)$ with respect to the area under which it would yield the most powerful decision-making rule. For example, if $\pi(\theta) = I\{\theta \in [G_1, G_2]\}$, where $I\{\cdot\}$ is the indicator function, then $B_n(X_1, ..., X_n)$ will provide the integrated most powerful test with respect to the interval $[G_1, G_2]$. The values of G_1 and G_2 can be set up based on the practical meaning of the parameter θ under the alternative hypothesis.

Remark 7.1

The function $\pi(\theta)$ can be chosen in a conservative fashion, oftentimes known as a flat prior, or in an anticonservative fashion, such that we put a lot of weight on a narrow range of values for θ, or it can be chosen anywhere between. The benefit of the anticonservative approach is that if our prior belief about the location of θ is corroborated by the observed data values, we have a very powerful decision rule. In general, the following principles can be considered: (1) the function $\pi(\theta)$ depicts our belief of how good values of θ represent the unknown parameter, weighting θ's values; (2) $\pi(\theta)$ displays a function form of the prior information; and (3) the function $\pi(\theta)$ can be chosen depending on the area under which we would like to obtain the most powerful decision rule by virtue of the result regarding the integrated most powerful property of the Bayes factor–based test statistics shown above. We also refer the reader to Section 7.4.2 for more details regarding the choice of $\pi(\theta)$.

7.4 Bayes Factor

The Bayesian approach to hypothesis testing was developed by Jeffreys (1935, 1961) as a major part of his program for scientific theory. A large statistical literature has been devoted to the development of Bayesian methods on various testing problems. The Bayes factor, as the centerpiece in Bayesian evaluation of evidence, closely presents human considerations of decision-making mechanisms based on formal statistical tests. In a probabilistic manner, the Bayes factor efficiently combines the information on a parameter based on data (or likelihood) and prior knowledge of the parameter.

A formal Bayesian analysis for analyzing the collected data x involves the specification of a prior distribution for all parameters of interest, say θ, denoted by $\pi(\theta)$, and a sampling distribution for $\mathbf{x}$, denoted by $\Pr(\mathbf{x}|\theta)$. Then the posterior distribution of θ given the data $\mathbf{x}$ is

$$\Pr(\theta|\,\mathbf{x}) = \frac{\Pr(\mathbf{x}|\theta)\pi(\theta)}{\displaystyle\int \Pr(\mathbf{x}|\theta)\pi(\theta)\,d\theta},$$

which provides a basis for performing formal Bayesian analysis.

Assume that the data $\mathbf{x}$ have arisen from one of the two hypotheses H_0 and H_1 according to a probability density $\Pr(\mathbf{x}|H_0)$ or $\Pr(\mathbf{x}|H_1)$. Given a priori (prior) probabilities $\Pr(H_0)$ and $\Pr(H_1) = 1 - \Pr(H_0)$, the data produce a posteriori (posterior) probabilities $\Pr(H_0|\mathbf{x})$ and $\Pr(H_1|\mathbf{x}) = 1 - \Pr(H_0|\mathbf{x})$. Based on Bayes's theorem, we then have

$$\frac{\Pr(H_1|\,\mathbf{x})}{\Pr(H_0|\,\mathbf{x})} = \frac{\Pr(\mathbf{x}|\,H_1)}{\Pr(\mathbf{x}|\,H_0)}\frac{\Pr(H_1)}{\Pr(H_0)}.$$

The transformation from the prior probability to the posterior probability is simply multiplication by

$$B_{10} = \frac{\Pr(\mathbf{x}|\,H_1)}{\Pr(\mathbf{x}|\,H_0)}, \tag{7.1}$$

which is named the *Bayes factor*. Therefore, posterior odds (odds = probability/[1 − probability]) is the product of the Bayes factor and the prior odds. In other words, the Bayes factor is the ratio of the posterior odds of H_1 to its prior odds, regardless of the value of the prior odds. When there are unknown parameters under either or both of the hypotheses, the densities $\Pr(\mathbf{x}|H_k)$ ($k = 0, 1$) can be obtained by integrating (not maximizing) over the parameter space, that is,

$$\Pr(\mathbf{x}|H_k) = \int \Pr(\mathbf{x}|\theta_k, II_k)\pi(\theta_k|H_k)\,d\theta_k, \quad k = 0, 1,$$

where θ_k is the parameter under H_k, $\pi(\theta_k|H_k)$ is its prior density, and $\Pr(\mathbf{x}|\theta_k, H_k)$ is the probability density of $\mathbf{x}$ given the value of θ_k or the likelihood function of θ_k. Here θ_k may be a vector, and in what follows we will denote its dimension by d_k. When multiple hypotheses are involved, we denote B_{jk} as the Bayes factor for H_k versus H_j. In this case, as a common practice, one of the hypotheses is considered the null and is denoted by H_0. Kass and Raftery's (1995) outstanding paper provided helpful details related to the Bayes factor mechanism.

7.4.1 Computation of Bayes Factors

Bayes factors involve computation of integrals usually solved via numerical integration. Many integration techniques have been adapted to problems of Bayesian inference, including the computation of Bayes factors.

Define the density (integral) in the numerator or the denominator of the Bayes factor described in Equation 7.1 as

$$I = \Pr(\mathbf{x}|H) = \int \Pr(\mathbf{x}|\theta, H)\pi(\theta|H)\,d\theta.$$

For simplicity and for ease of exposition, the subscript k ($k = 0$, 1) as the hypothesis indicator is eliminated in the notation H here.

In some cases, the density (integral) I may be evaluated analytically. For example, an exact analytic evaluation of the integral I is possible for exponential family distributions with conjugate priors, including normal linear models (DeGroot 2005; Zellner 1996). Exact analytic evaluation is best in the sense of accuracy and computational efficiency, but it is feasible only for a narrow class of models.

More often, numerical integration, also called quadrature, is required when the analytic evaluation of the integral I is intractable. Generally, most relevant software is inefficient and of little use for the computation of these integrals. One reason is that when sample sizes are moderate or large, the integrand becomes *highly peaked* around its maximum, which may be found more efficiently by other techniques. In this instance, general-purpose quadrature methods that do not incorporate knowledge of the likely maximum are likely to have difficulty finding the region where the integrand mass is accumulating. In order to demonstrate this intuitively, we first show that an important approximation of the log-likelihood function is based on a quadratic function of the parameter, for example, θ. We do not attempt a general proof, but provide a brief outline in the unidimensional case. Suppose the log-likelihood function $l(\theta)$ is twice differentiable. Informally, consider a Taylor approximation to the log-likelihood function $l(\theta)$ of second order around the maximum likelihood estimator (MLE) $\hat{\theta}$, that is,

$$l(\theta) \approx l\left(\hat{\theta}\right) + (\theta - \hat{\theta})l'\left(\hat{\theta}\right) + \frac{(\theta - \hat{\theta})^2}{2!}l''\left(\hat{\theta}\right).$$

Note that at the MLE, $\hat{\theta}$, the first derivative of the log-likelihood function $l'(\hat{\theta}) = 0$. Thus, in the neighborhood of $\hat{\theta}$, the log-likelihood function $l(\theta)$ can be expressed in the form

$$l(\theta) \approx l\left(\hat{\theta}\right) + \frac{(\theta - \hat{\theta})^2}{2!}l''\left(\hat{\theta}\right).$$

(See Section 7.4.1.1 for more details.)

The following example provides some intuition about the quadratic approximation of the log-likelihood function.

Example 7.1: Examination of the log-likelihood in the frequentist and Bayesian context

Let $\mathbf{x} = \{x_1, \ldots, x_n\}$ denote a random sample from a gamma distribution with unknown shape parameter θ and known scale parameter κ_0. The density function of the gamma distribution is $f(x; \theta, \kappa_0) = x^{\theta-1}\exp(-x/\kappa_0)/(\Gamma(\theta)\kappa_0^\theta)$, where the gamma function $\Gamma(\theta) = \int_0^\infty t^{\theta-1}\exp(-t)\,dt$. The likelihood function of θ is

$$l(\theta) = (\theta - 1)\sum_{i=1}^n \log(x_i) - n\log(\Gamma(\theta)) - n\theta\log(\kappa_0) - \sum_{i=1}^n x_i/\kappa_0.$$

The first and second derivatives of the log-likelihood function are

$$l'(\theta) = -n\Gamma'(\theta)/\Gamma(\theta) + \sum_{i=1}^n \log(x_i) - n\log(\kappa_0),$$

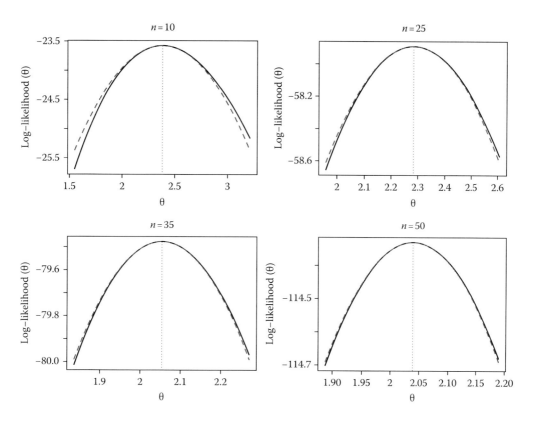

FIGURE 7.1
(See color insert.) Plot of log-likelihood (black solid line) and its quadratic approximation (red dashed line) versus the shape parameter θ based on samples of sizes $n = 10, 25, 35, 50$ from a gamma distribution with a true shape parameter of $\theta_0 = 2$ and a known scale parameter of 2.

$$l''(\theta) = -n\frac{d^2}{d\theta^2}\log(\Gamma(\theta)) = n\int_0^1 \frac{t^{\theta-1}\log(t)}{1-t}\,dt < 0,$$

respectively. In this case, there is no closed-form solution of the MLE of the shape parameter $\hat{\theta}$, which can be found by solving $l'(\hat{\theta}) = 0$ numerically. Correspondingly, the value of the second derivative of the log-likelihood function at the MLE, $l''(\hat{\theta})$, can be computed. Figure 7.1 presents the plot of log-likelihood (black solid line) and its quadratic approximation (red dashed line) versus the shape parameter θ based on samples of size $n = 10, 25, 35, 50$ from a gamma distribution with a true shape parameter of $\theta_0 = 2$ and a known scale parameter of $\kappa_0 = 2$. It is obvious from Figure 7.1 that as the sample size n increases, the quadratic approximation to the log-likelihood function $l(\theta)$ performs better in the neighborhood of the MLE of θ.

Implementation of Figure 7.1 is shown in the following R code:

```
> n.seq<-c(10,25,35,50)
> N<-max(n.seq)
> shape0<-2
> scale0<-2
> X<-rgamma(N,shape=shape0,scale = scale0)
```

```
>
> # Quadratic approximation to the log-likelihood function
> par(mar=c(3.5, 4, 3.5, 1),mfrow=c(2,2),mgp=c(2,1,0)) > for (n in
  n.seq).{
+   x<-X[sample(1:N,n,replace=FALSE)]
+   # log-likelihood as a function of the shape parameter theta
+   loglike<-function(theta) (theta-1)*sum(log(x))-n*log(gamma(theta))-
    n*theta*log(scale0)-sum(x)/scale0
+   neg.loglike<-function(theta)-loglike(theta)
+
+   # the first derivative from the log-likelihood
+   loglike.D<-function(theta) sum(log(x)) - n*digamma(theta)-
    n* log(scale0)
+   # the second derivative of log-likelihood
+   loglike.DD<-function(theta) -n*trigamma(theta)
+
+   # one-dimensional optimization that maximize log-likelihood with
+   # respect to the shape parameter
+   init<-mean(x)^2/var(x) # set initial value
+   theta.mle<-optim(init,neg.loglike,method="L-BFGS-B", lower=init-6*
    (-loglike.DD(init)^(-1/2))/sqrt(n), upper=init+6*(-loglike.DD
    (init)^(-1/2))/sqrt(n))$par
+
+   loglike.DD.mle <- loglike.DD(theta.mle) # second derivative at MLE
+
+   # approximation of log-likelihood
+   loglike.est<-function(theta) loglike(theta.mle)+loglike.DD.
    mle*((theta-theta.mle)^2)/2
+
+   # plot: the plotting limit of x-axis
+   tc<-theta.mle
+   rg<-6*((-loglike.DD.mle)^(-1/2) )/sqrt(n) # half range
+
+   # plot the true log-likehood
+   plot(Vectorize(loglike),c(tc-rg,tc+rg),xlim=c(tc-rg,tc+rg),type="l",
    lty=1,lwd=2,cex.lab=1.2,xlab=expression(theta),ylab=expression(paste
    ("Log-likelihood( ",theta,")")), main=paste0("n=",n))
+   # plot the approximation to the log-likehood
+   curve(loglike.est,from=tc-rg,to=tc+rg,type="l",lty=2,lwd=2,add=TRUE,
    col=2)
+   lines(c(theta.mle,theta.mle), c(-1e+5,loglike(theta.mle)),lty=3)
+   }
>
```

Thus, it can be easily shown that the likelihood function $\Pr(\mathbf{x}|\theta)$ is highly peaked near the MLE $\hat{\theta}$, for example, in the cases of large samples. In such cases, the posterior density function $\Pr(\theta|\mathbf{x})$ is highly peaked about its maximum $\tilde{\theta}$, that is, the posterior mode (generalized MLE), at which the log-posterior is maximized and has slope zero. Assume that $\tilde{\theta}$ exists and the prior $\pi(\theta)$ (positive), as well as the log-likelihood function $l(\theta)$, is twice differentiable near the posterior mode $\tilde{\theta}$. Then the posterior density $\Pr(\theta|\mathbf{x})$ for a large sample size n can be approximated by a normal distribution with mean $\tilde{\theta}$ and covariance matrix $\tilde{\Sigma} = (\mathbf{I}\tilde{l}(\tilde{\theta}))^{-1}$, where the generalized observed Fisher information matrix $\mathbf{I}\tilde{l}(\tilde{\theta}) = -\mathbf{H}\tilde{l}(\tilde{\theta})$, that is, minus the Hessian matrix (second derivative matrix) of the log-posterior evaluated at $\tilde{\theta}$. More specifically, component-wise, $\mathbf{I}\tilde{l}(\tilde{\theta})_{ij} = -\left[\dfrac{\partial^2 \tilde{l}(\theta)}{\partial\theta_i\,\partial\theta_j}\right]_{\theta=\tilde{\theta}}$. Consequently, in such cases, for large sample size n, the Bayes factor is approximately equivalent to the maximum likelihood ratio.

In addition, the asymptotic distribution of the posterior mode depends on the Fisher information and not on the prior (Le Cam 1986). Intuitively, consistent with the Bayes factor methodology, when we have quite enough information from data, that is, n is relatively large, the impact of the prior information vanishes up to 0.

For ease of exposition, we outline the proof of the normal approximation informally in a unidimensional case. Denote the nonnormalized posterior $h(\theta) = \Pr(\mathbf{x}|\theta, H)\,\pi(\theta|H)$ and $\tilde{l}(\theta) = \log(h(\theta))$. Similar to the way of obtaining the approximation to the log-likelihood function, applying a second order Taylor expansion of $\tilde{l}(\theta)$ at the posterior mode $\tilde{\theta}$, intuitively, we have

$$\Pr(\mathbf{x}|\theta) \propto \Pr(\mathbf{x}|\theta, H)\pi(\theta|H) = \exp\left(\tilde{l}(\theta)\right) \approx \exp\left\{\tilde{l}(\tilde{\theta}) + \tilde{l}''(\tilde{\theta})(\theta - \tilde{\theta})^2/2\right\} \propto N\left(\tilde{\theta}, \left(-\tilde{l}''(\tilde{\theta})\right)^{-1}\right),$$

where $\propto$ represents proportionality. Note that the posterior mode always lies between the peak of the prior and that of the likelihood, because it combines information from the prior density and the likelihood. This posterior density approximation technique is often referred to as the modal approximation because θ is estimated by the posterior mode. It is also called the first-order approximation, where the relative error is of order $O(n^{-1})$.

For relatively large samples, the choice of the prior density is generally not that relevant, and in fact, the prior $\pi(\theta)$ might be ignored in the above derivation. In such cases, the posterior mode $\tilde{\theta}$ is replaced by the MLE $\hat{\theta}$, and the generalized observed Fisher information is replaced by the observed Fisher information $-l''(\hat{\theta})$. This may also be considered a case where frequentist and Bayesian methods align in some regards. To illustrate this idea, we consider the example of the gamma-distributed sample displayed above and a uniform prior where $\theta \sim Uniform$ [0.5, 3.5]. Figure 7.2 presents the plot of posterior function (black solid line) and its normal approximation (red dashed line) versus the shape parameter θ based on a uniform prior and samples of sizes $n = 10, 25, 50, 250$ from a gamma distribution with a true shape parameter of $\theta_0 = 2$ and a known scale parameter of 2. It can be noted that the normal approximations to the posterior density perform well even in comparatively small sample sizes, and the posterior density is highly peaked about its maximum for large samples.

The R code to create Figure 7.2 is

```
> n.seq<-c(10,25,50,250)
> N<-max(n.seq)
> shape0<-2
> scale0<-2
> X<-rgamma(N, shape=shape0, scale = scale0)
>
> par(mar=c(3.5, 4, 3.5, 1),mfrow=c(2,2),mgp=c(2,1,0))
> for (n in n.seq){
+    x<-X[sample(1:N,n,replace=FALSE)]
+
+    # Derive the MLE of shape parameter theta
+    loglike<-function(theta) (theta-1)*sum(log(x))-n*log(gamma(theta))-
     n*theta*log(scale0)-sum(x)/scale0
+    neg.loglike<-function(theta) -loglike(theta) # negative log-likelihood
+    loglike.DD<-function(theta) -n*trigamma(theta) #second derivative
+    init<-mean(x)^2/var(x) # set initial value
```

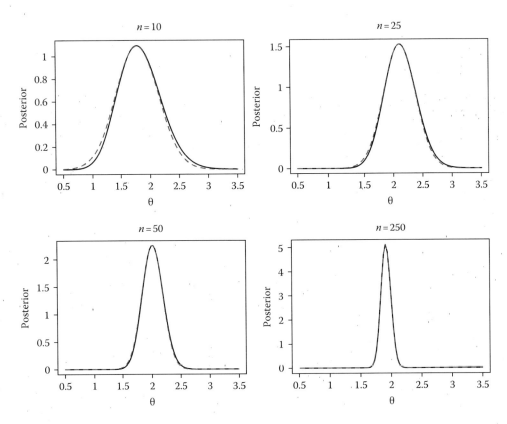

FIGURE 7.2
(See color insert.) Plot of the posterior function (black solid line) and its normal approximation (red dashed line) versus the shape parameter θ. The prior is based on a uniform distribution function. The samples are from a gamma distribution with a true shape parameter of $\theta_0 = 2$ and a known scale parameter of 2. $n = 10, 25, 50, 250$.

```
+    theta.mle<-optim(init,neg.loglike,method="L-BFGS-B", lower=init-6*
     (-loglike.DD(init)^(-1/2))/sqrt(n), upper=init+6*(-loglike.DD
     (init)^(-1/2))/sqrt(n))$par
+    loglike.DD.mle <- loglike.DD(theta.mle) # value at MLE
+
+    like <-function(theta) exp(loglike(theta))
+    prior <- function(theta) (1/(2*rg))*(theta<=3.5)*(theta>=0.5) # Uniform
+    post.raw <- function(theta) like(theta)*prior(theta)
+    norm.constant<- integrate(Vectorize(post.raw),0.5,3.5)$value
+    post <- function(theta) post.raw(theta)/norm.constant
+    var<-(-loglike.DD.mle)^(-1)
+    #post.est <- function(theta) sqrt(2*pi*var)*exp(loglike(theta.mle))*
     dnorm(theta,theta.mle,sqrt(var))
+
+    # plot posterior function
+    plot(Vectorize(post),c(0.5,3.5),xlim=c(0.5,3.5), type="l",lty=1,
     lwd=2,ce x.lab=1.2,xlab=expression(theta),ylab="posterior",main=
     paste0("n=",n))
+    curve(dnorm(x,theta.mle,sqrt(var)), add=TRUE,lty=2,lwd=2, col="red")
+    }
```

In general, in order to estimate the posterior moments and quantiles, the corresponding features of the approximating normal density can be employed. However, when the true posterior differs significantly from normal, the estimates of the posterior moments and quantiles based on this approximation may be poor.

The fact that some problems are of high dimension may also lead to intractable analytic evaluation of integrals. In this case, Monte Carlo methods may be used, but these too need to be adapted to the statistical context. Bleistein and Handelsman (1975), as well as Evans and Swartz (1995), reviewed various numerical integration strategies for evaluating the integral *I*. In this section, we simply introduce several techniques available to evaluate the Bayes factor, including the asymptotic approximation method, the simple Monte Carlo, importance sampling, and Gaussian quadrature strategies, as well as approaches based on simulating from the posterior distributions. For general discussion and references, see, for example, Kass and Raftery (1995), Han and Carlin (2001), and Sinharay and Stern (2001).

7.4.1.1 Asymptotic Approximations

7.4.1.1.1 Laplace's Method

The Laplace approximation (De Bruijn 1970; Tierney and Kadane 1986) to the marginal density *I* of the data is obtained by approximating the posterior with a normal distribution. It is assumed that the posterior density, which is proportional to the nonnormalized posterior $h(\theta) = \Pr(\mathbf{x}|\theta, H)\,\pi(\theta|H)$, is highly peaked about its maximum $\tilde{\theta}$, that is, the posterior mode. The assumption will usually be satisfied if the likelihood function $\Pr(\mathbf{x}|\theta, H)$ is highly peaked near its maximum $\hat{\theta}$, for example, the case for large samples. Denote $\tilde{l}(\theta) = \log(h(\theta))$. Expanding $\tilde{l}(\theta)$ as a quadratic about $\tilde{\theta}$ and then exponentiating it yields an approximation to $h(\theta)$ that has the form of a normal density with mean $\tilde{\theta}$ and covariance matrix $\tilde{\Sigma} = \left(-\mathbf{H}\tilde{l}(\tilde{\theta})\right)^{-1}$, where $\mathbf{H}\tilde{l}(\tilde{\theta})$ is the Hessian matrix of second derivatives of the log-posterior evaluated at $\tilde{\theta}$. More specifically, component-wise, $\mathbf{H}\tilde{l}(\tilde{\theta})_{ij} = \left[\dfrac{\partial^2 \tilde{l}(\theta)}{\partial \theta_i \, \partial \theta_j}\right]_{\theta=\tilde{\theta}}$. Integrating the approximation to $h(\theta)$ with respect to θ yields

$$\hat{I}_L = (2\pi)^{d/2}\,|\tilde{\Sigma}|^{1/2}\,\Pr\!\left(\mathbf{x}\,|\,\tilde{\theta}, H\right)\pi\!\left(\tilde{\theta}\,|\,H\right),$$

where *d* is the dimension of θ. Under conditions specified by Kass et al. (1990), it can be derived that $I = \hat{I}_L(1 + O(n^{-1}))$ as $n \to \infty$; that is, the relative error of Laplace's approximation to *I* is $O(n^{-1})$. Therefore, when Laplace's method is applied to both the numerator and denominator of B_{10} in Equation 7.1, the resulting approximation leads to a relative error of order $O(n^{-1})$.

Laplace's method yields accurate approximations and is often computationally efficient. By employing Laplace's method, one can show that the asymptotic properties of Bayes factor–type procedures based on data are close to those based on maximum likelihood methods.

7.4.1.1.2 Variants on Laplace's Method

Laplace's method may be applied in alternative forms by omitting part of the integrand from the exponent when performing the expansion. (For general formulation, see Kass and Vaidyanathan [1992], which followed Tierney et al. [1989] and Mosteller and Wallace [1964]). An important variant on the approximation $\hat{I}$ is

$$\hat{I}_{\mathrm{MLE}} = (2\pi)^{d/2} \, | \, \hat{\Sigma} \, |^{1/2} \, \Pr(\mathbf{x} \, | \, \hat{\theta}, H) \pi(\hat{\theta} \, | \, H),$$

where $\hat{\Sigma}^{-1}$ is the observed information matrix, that is, the negative Hessian matrix of the log-likelihood evaluated at the maximum likelihood estimator $\hat{\theta}$. This approximation again has a relative error of order $O(n^{-1})$.

Consider nested hypotheses, where there must be some parameterization under H_1 of the form $\theta = (\beta, \psi)^T$ such that H_0 is obtained from H_1 when $\psi = \psi_0$ for some ψ_0, with parameter (β, ψ) having prior $\pi(\beta, \psi)$ under H_1 and then H_0: $\psi = \psi_0$ with prior $\pi(\beta|H_0)$. For instance, it is desired to check whether the collected data, denoted by $\mathbf{x}$, could be described as a random sample from some normal distribution with mean μ_0, assuming that they may be described as a random sample from some normal distribution with unknown mean μ and unknown variance σ^2. In this case, notation-wise, $\psi_0 = \mu_0$, $\psi = \mu$, and $\beta = \sigma^2$. Applying the approximation $\hat{I}_{\mathrm{MLE}}$, one can show that

$$2 \log B_{10} \approx \Lambda + \log \pi(\hat{\beta}, \hat{\psi} \, | \, H_1) - \log \pi(\hat{\beta}^*, H_0) + (d_1 - d_0) \log(2\pi) + \log | \hat{\Sigma}_1 | - \log | \hat{\Sigma}_0 |,$$

where $\Lambda = 2(\log \Pr(\mathbf{x} \, | \, (\hat{\beta}, \hat{\psi}), H_1) - \log \Pr(\mathbf{x}| \, \hat{\beta}, H_0)$ is the log-likelihood ratio statistic having approximately a chi-square distribution with degrees of freedom $(d_1 - d_0)$ and $\hat{\beta}^*$ denotes the MLE under H_0. Here the covariance matrices $\hat{\Sigma}_k$ could be either observed or expected information, under which case the approximation of $2 \log B_{10}$ has a relative error of order $O(n^{-1})$ or $O(n^{-1/2})$, respectively. For more information, we refer the reader to Kass and Raftery (1995).

Alternatively, we may consider the following MLE-based approach. We do not attempt a general proof, but instead provide an informal outline for the unidimensional case. Recall that the log-likelihood function $l(\theta)$ attains its maximum at the MLE $\hat{\theta}$, and $l(\theta)$ increases up to MLE $\hat{\theta}$ and decreases afterwards. Define $\phi_n = c/n^{1/2-\gamma}$, where c is a constant and $\gamma < 1/2$. Then the marginal can be divided into three components:

$$I = \int_{-\infty}^{\infty} \exp(l(\theta))\pi(\theta) \, d\theta = I_1 + I_2 + \int_{\hat{\theta}-\phi_n}^{\hat{\theta}+\phi_n} \exp(l(\theta))\pi(\theta) \, d\theta,$$

where $I_1 = \int_{-\infty}^{\hat{\theta}-\phi_n} \exp(l(\theta))\pi(\theta) \, d\theta$ and $I_2 = \int_{\hat{\theta}+\phi_n}^{\infty} \exp(l(\theta))\pi(\theta) \, d\theta$. We first consider the component I_1. Based on the fact that the log-likelihood function $l(\theta)$ is a nondecreasing function of θ for $\theta \in (-\infty, \hat{\theta} - \phi_n)$ and that $l(\hat{\theta} - \phi_n) \to -\infty$ as $n \to \infty$, it can be derived that

$$I_1 \le \exp(l(\hat{\theta} - \phi_n)) \int_{-\infty}^{\infty} \pi(\theta) \, d\theta = \exp(l(\hat{\theta} - \phi_n)) \to 0 \, , \text{ as } n \to \infty.$$

Similarly for the component I_2—since the log-likelihood function $l(\theta)$ is a nonincreasing function of θ for $\theta \in (\hat{\theta} + \phi_n, \infty)$ and $l(\hat{\theta} + \phi_n) \to -\infty$ as $n \to \infty$, we have

$$I_2 \le \exp(l(\hat{\theta} + \phi_n)) \int_{-\infty}^{\infty} \pi(\theta) \, d\theta = \exp(l(\hat{\theta} + \phi_n)) \to 0 \text{ as } n \to \infty.$$

Therefore, we have $I \approx \int_{\hat{\theta}-\phi_n}^{\hat{\theta}+\phi_n} \exp(l(\theta))\pi(\theta)\,d\theta$ as $n \to \infty$. In a more formal manner, Vexler et al. (2014d) showed the asymptotic approach for constructing nonparametric Bayesian point estimators, where the empirical likelihood method (see Chapter 6) was used instead of the parametric likelihood in a Bayesian posterior expectation calculation.

7.4.1.1.3 *Schwarz Criterion*

It is possible to avoid the introduction of the prior densities $\pi_k \,(\theta_k|H_k)$ in Equation 7.1 by using

$$S = \log \Pr\left(\mathbf{x} \,|\, \hat{\theta}_1, H_1\right) - \log \Pr\left(\mathbf{x} \,|\, \hat{\theta}_0, H_0\right) - \frac{1}{2}(d_1 - d_0)\log(n),$$

where $\hat{\theta}_k$ is the MLE under H_k, d_k is the dimension of θ_k, $k = 0, 1$, and n is the sample size. The second term in S acts as a penalty term that corrects for differences in dimension between H_k, $k = 0, 1$. The quantity S is often called the Schwarz criterion. The Bayesian information criterion (BIC) can be defined as minus twice the Schwarz criterion; sometimes an arbitrary constant is added. Schwarz (1978) showed that

$$\frac{S - \log B_{10}}{\log B_{10}} \to 0 \text{ as } n \to \infty.$$

Thus, the quantity $\exp(S)$ provides a rough approximation to the Bayes factor that is independent of the priors on the θ_k. Kass and Raftery (1995) provided excellent discussion regarding the method mentioned above.

The benefits of asymptotic approximations in this context include the following: (1) numerical integration is replaced with numerical differentiation, which is computationally more stable; (2) asymptotic approximations do not involve random numbers, and consequently, two different analysts can produce a common answer based on the same data set, model, and prior distribution; and (3) in order to investigate the sensitivity of the result to modest changes in the prior or the likelihood function, the computational complexity is greatly reduced; for more detail, we refer the reader to Carlin and Louis (2011). Among the asymptotic approximations described above, the Schwarz criterion is the easiest approximation to compute and requires no specification of prior distributions. In addition, as long as the number of degrees of freedom involved in the comparison is reasonably small relative to sample size, the analysis based on the Schwarz criterion will not mislead in a qualitative sense.

However, asymptotic approximations also have the following limitations: (1) in order to obtain a valid approximation, the posterior distribution must be unimodal, or at least nearly unimodal; (2) the size of the data set must be fairly large, but it is hard to judge how large is large enough; (3) the accuracy of asymptotic approximations cannot be improved without collecting additional data; (4) the correct parameterization, on which the accuracy of the approximation depends, for example, θ versus $\log(\theta)$, may be difficult to ascertain; (5) when the dimension of θ is moderate or high, say, greater than 10, Laplace's method becomes unstable and numerical computation of the associated Hessian matrices will be prohibitively difficult; and (6) when the number of degrees of freedom involved in the comparison is large and the prior is very different from that for which the approximation is best, the asymptotic approximation based on the Schwarz criterion can be very poor; for example, McCulloch and Rossi (1991) illustrated the poor approximation by the Schwarz criterion with an example of 115 degrees of freedom. For more details, we refer the reader to, for example, Kass and Raftery (1995) and Carlin and Louis (2011). Therefore, in such cases, practitioners may turn to alternative methods, for example, Monte Carlo sampling, importance sampling, and Gaussian quadrature. These methods typically require longer run times, but can be programmed easily and can be applied in more general scenarios, which are the subject of the following section in this chapter.

7.4.1.2 Simple Monte Carlo Evaluations, Importance Sampling, and Gaussian Quadrature

Dropping the notational dependence on the hypothesis indicator H_k, the integral I becomes $I = \Pr(\mathbf{x}) = \int \Pr(\mathbf{x}\,|\,\theta)\pi(\theta)\,d\theta$. The simplest Monte Carlo integration estimate of I is

$$\hat{\Pr}_1(D) = \frac{1}{m}\sum_{i=1}^{m}\Pr\left(\mathbf{x}\,|\,\theta^{(i)}\right),$$

where $\{\theta^{(i)}: i = 1, \ldots, m\}$ is a sample from the prior distribution; this is the average of the likelihoods of the sampled parameter values (e.g., Hammersley and Handscomb 1964).

The precision of simple Monte Carlo integration can be improved by importance sampling. It involves generating a sample $\{\theta^{(i)}: i = 1, \ldots, m\}$ from a density $\pi^*(\theta)$. Under general conditions, a simulation-consistent estimate of I is

$$\hat{I}_{MC} = \frac{\sum_{i=1}^{m} w_i\,\Pr\left(\mathbf{x}\,|\,\theta^{(i)}\right)}{\sum_{i=1}^{m} w_i},$$

where $w_i = \pi\,(\theta^{(i)})/\pi^*(\theta^{(i)})$; the function $\pi^*(\theta)$ is known as the importance sampling function. Then the approximation of the Bayes factor can be computed accordingly; for general discussion, see Geweke (1989). Although the Monte Carlo integration and importance sampling methods are less precise and more computationally demanding, they may be the only applicable methods in complex models.

Genz and Kass (1997) demonstrated the evaluation of integrals that are peaked around a dominant mode and provided an adaptive Gaussian quadrature method. This method is efficient, especially when the dimensionality of the parameter space is modest.

7.4.1.3 Simulating from the Posterior

Several methods can be applied to simulate from posterior distributions, including direct simulation and rejection sampling for the simplest cases. In more complex cases, Markov chain Monte Carlo (MCMC) methods (e.g., Smith and Roberts 1993), particularly the Metropolis–Hastings algorithm and the Gibbs sampler, as well as the weighted likelihood bootstrap (Smith and Roberts 1993), provide general schemes.

These methods provide a sample approximately drawn from the posterior density $\Pr(\theta\,|\,\mathbf{x}) = \Pr(\mathbf{x}\,|\,\theta)\,\pi(\theta)/\Pr(\mathbf{x})$. Substituting into $\hat{I}_{MC}$ defined in Section 7.4.1.2 yields as an estimate for $\Pr(\mathbf{x})$

$$\hat{\Pr}(\mathbf{x}) = \left\{\frac{1}{m}\sum_{i=1}^{m}\Pr(\mathbf{x}\,|\,\theta^{(i)})^{-1}\right\}^{-1},$$

the harmonic mean of the likelihood values (Newton and Raftery 1994). This converges almost surely to the correct value, Pr(**x**), as $m \to \infty$, but it does not generally satisfy a Gaussian central limit theorem. See Kass and Raftery (1995) for additional modifications and discussion. Note that the MCMC methods have not yet been applied in many demanding problems and may require large numbers of likelihood function evaluations, resulting in difficulty in some cases.

7.4.1.4 Combining Simulation and Asymptotic Approximations

When it is possible to simulate observations from the posterior distributions by employing Markov chain Monte Carlo or other techniques, DiCiccio et al. (1997) provided a simulated version of Laplace's method. Follow the notations of $\tilde{\theta}$ and $\tilde{\Sigma}$ described in Section 7.4.1.1.1; that is, let $\tilde{\theta}$ be the posterior mode and let covariance matrix $\tilde{\Sigma}$ be minus the inverse of the Hessian of the log-posterior evaluated at $\tilde{\theta}$. If no analytical form can be obtained, then $\tilde{\theta}$ and $\tilde{\Sigma}$ can be estimated via simulation. The normal approximation to the posterior is $\phi(\cdot) = \phi(\cdot; \tilde{\theta}, \tilde{\Sigma})$, where $\phi(\cdot; \mu, \Sigma)$ denote a normal density with mean vector μ and covariance matrix Σ. Let $B = \left\{ \theta \in \Theta; \| (\theta - \tilde{\theta})' \tilde{\Sigma}^{-1} (\theta - \tilde{\theta}) \|^2 < \delta^2 \right\}$, which has volume

$$\upsilon = \delta^p \pi^{p/2} \,|\, \tilde{\Sigma}^{1/2} \,|\, / \Gamma(p/2 + 1). \text{ Let } \Pr(B) = \int_B \Pr(\theta \,|\, \mathbf{x}) d\theta \text{ and } \Phi(B) \equiv \int_B \Phi(\theta; \tilde{\theta}, \tilde{\Sigma}) d\theta = \alpha.$$

A modification of Laplace's method can be obtained that simply estimates the (unknown) value of the posterior probability density at the mode using the (simulated) probability assigned to a small region around the mode divided by its area. Observing that

$$I = \frac{\Pr(D \,|\, \tilde{\theta}) \pi(\tilde{\theta})}{\Pr(\tilde{\theta} \,|\, \mathbf{x})} = \frac{\Pr(\mathbf{x} \,|\, \tilde{\theta}) \pi(\tilde{\theta})}{\phi(\tilde{\theta})} \frac{\phi(\tilde{\theta})}{\Pr(\tilde{\theta} \,|\, \mathbf{x})} \approx \frac{\Pr(\mathbf{x} \,|\, \tilde{\theta}) \pi(\tilde{\theta})}{\phi(\tilde{\theta})} \frac{\alpha}{\Pr(B)},$$

the volume-corrected estimator has the form

$$\hat{I}_L^* = \frac{\Pr(\mathbf{x} \,|\, \tilde{\theta}) \pi(\tilde{\theta})}{\phi(\tilde{\theta})} \frac{\alpha}{\hat{P}},$$

where $\hat{P}$ is the Monte Carlo estimate of $\Pr(B)$, that is, a proportion of the sampled values inside B. DiCiccio et al. (1997) demonstrated that the simulated version of Laplace's method with local volume correction approximates the Bayes factor accurately, which is especially useful in the case of costly likelihood function evaluations.

The importance sampling techniques can be modified by restricting them to small regions about the mode. To improve the accuracy of approximations, Laplace's method can be combined with the simple bridge sampling technique proposed by Meng and Wong (1996). For detailed information, we refer the reader to DiCiccio et al. (1997).

7.4.2 Choice of Prior Probability Distributions

Implementation of Bayes factor approaches requires the specification of priors, as is the case in all Bayesian analysis. In principle, priors formally represent available external information, providing a way to combine other information about the values of the target parameter with the data.

Typically, prior distributions are specified based on information accumulated from past studies or from the opinions of subject area experts. The *elicited prior* is a means of drawing information from subject area experts, who have a great deal of information about the substantive question but are not involved in the model construction process, with the goal of constructing a probability structure that quantifies their specific knowledge and experiential intuition about the studied effects.

In order to simplify the subsequent computational burden, for example, make computation of the posterior distribution easier, experimenters often limit the choice of priors by restricting $\pi(\theta)$ to some familiar distributional family. In choosing a prior belonging to a specific distributional family, some choices may have more computational advantages than others. In particular, if the prior probability distribution $\pi(\theta)$ is in the same distributional family as the resulting posterior distribution $\Pr(\theta|\mathbf{x})$, then the prior and posterior are called conjugate distributions, and the prior is called a *conjugate prior* for the likelihood function. For example, the Gaussian family is conjugate to itself (or self-conjugate) with respect to a Gaussian likelihood function. That is, if the likelihood function is Gaussian, choosing a Gaussian prior over the mean will guarantee the Gaussian posterior distribution.

Often in practice, there is no reliable prior information regarding θ that exists, or it is desired to make an inference based solely on the data. In such cases, the *noninformative prior* plays a major role in Bayesian analyses. Oftentimes, using noninformative priors aligns to their frequentist likelihood-based counterparts in the sense of being a more data-driven approach, for example, being a similar maximum likelihood estimation. A noninformative prior can be constructed by some formal rule that contains "no information" with respect to θ in the sense that no one θ value is favored over another, provided all values are logically possible. The simplest and oldest rule to determine a noninformative prior is the principle of indifference, which assigns equal probabilities to all possibilities. Noninformative priors can express objective information such as "the variable is within a certain range." For example, if we have a bounded continuous parameter space, say, $\Theta = [a, b]$, $-\infty < a < b < \infty$, then the uniform distribution $\pi(\theta) = 1/(b - a)$ $I\{a \le \theta \le b\}$, where $I\{\cdot\}$ is the indicator function, is arguably noninformative for θ. If the parameter space is unbounded, that is, $\Theta = (-\infty, \infty)$, then the appropriate uniform prior may be $\pi(\theta) = c$, $c > 0$. It is worth emphasizing that even if this distribution is *improper* in that $\int \pi(\theta)d\theta = \infty$, Bayesian inference is still possible provided that $\int \Pr(\mathbf{x}|\theta)d\theta = K$, $K < \infty$. Then

$$\Pr(\theta|\mathbf{x}) = \frac{\Pr(\mathbf{x}|\theta)c}{\int \Pr(\mathbf{x}|\theta)c\,d\theta} = \frac{\Pr(\mathbf{x}|\theta)}{K}.$$

Since $\int \Pr(\theta|\mathbf{x})d\theta = 1$, the posterior density is indeed proper, and hence Bayesian inference may proceed as usual. Note that when employing improper priors, proper posteriors will not always result and extra care must be taken.

Krieger et al. (2003) have proposed several forms of a prior $\pi(\theta)$ and the corresponding distribution $H(\theta) = \int^{\theta} \pi(\theta)d\theta$ in the context of sequential change-point detection. This method of choices of a prior can be adapted for the problem stated in this chapter. For example, if we suspect that the observations under the alternative hypothesis have a distribution that differs greatly from the distribution of the observations under the null (Φ is the standard normal distribution function), the distribution of the prior could be chosen as

$$H(\theta) = \Phi^{-1}\left(\frac{\mu}{\sigma}\right)\left(\Phi\left(\frac{\theta-\mu}{\sigma}\right) - \Phi\left(-\frac{\mu}{\sigma}\right)\right)^{+}, \tag{7.2}$$

where $a^{+} = aI\{a > 0\}$.

And a somewhat broader prior is

$$H(\theta) = \frac{1}{2}\left(\Phi\left(\frac{\theta-\mu}{\sigma}\right) + \Phi\left(\frac{\theta+\mu}{\sigma}\right)\right). \tag{7.3}$$

Note that the parameters μ and $\sigma > 0$ of the distributions $H(\theta)$ can be chosen arbitrarily. Krieger et al. (2003) recommended the specification of $\mu = 0$, and $\sigma = 1$ so that the two forms of $H(\theta)$ specified above are simplified. In accordance with the rules shown in Marden (2000), where the author reviewed the Bayesian approach applied to hypothesis testing, the function H can be defined, for example, for a fixed $\sigma > 0$, in the form

$$H \in \Theta = \left\{\frac{1}{2}\left(\Phi\left(\frac{\theta-\mu}{\sigma}\right) + \Phi\left(\frac{\theta+\mu}{\sigma}\right)\right), \mu \in (\mu_{lower}, \mu_{upper})\right\}. \tag{7.4}$$

Here Θ is a set of distribution functions. For more details, we refer the reader to Vexler and Wu (2009). The following R code shows the way to plot the distribution functions of priors specified in Equations 7.2 through 7.4, as shown in Figure 7.3.

```
> # The distribution function defined by Equation (4.5.1).
> H1<-function(theta,mu,sigma) {
+    tmp<-pnorm((theta-mu)/sigma)-pnorm(-mu/sigma)
+    H<-ifelse(tmp>0,tmp,0)/pnorm(mu/sigma)
+    return(H)
+ }
>
> # The distribution function defined by Equations (4.5.2) and (4.5.3).
> H2<-function(theta,mu,sigma) {
+    H<-(pnorm((theta-mu)/sigma)+pnorm((theta+mu)/sigma))/2
+    return(H)
+ }
> par(mfrow=c(1,2),mar=c(4,4,2,2))
> theta.seq<-seq(0,4,.1)
> H1.dist<-sapply(theta.seq,H1,mu=0,sigma=1)
> plot(theta.seq,H1.dist,type="l",xlim=c(-4,4),lty=1,lwd=2,xlab="theta",
  ylab="Probability")
>
> theta.seq2<-seq(-4,4,.1)
> H2.dist<-sapply(theta.seq2,H2,mu=0,sigma=1)
> lines(theta.seq2,H2.dist,lty=2,lwd=2)
>
> # fix sigma=1
> mu.seq<-seq(-5,5,1)
```

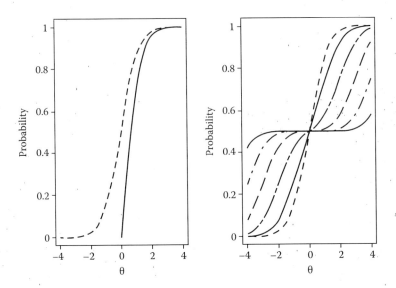

FIGURE 7.3
Cumulative distribution functions that correspond to the priors (7.2) through (7.4). The solid line and the
dashed line in the left panel present $H(\theta)$ defined by Equations 7.2 and 7.3, with $\mu = 0$ and $\sigma = 1$, respectively.
The right panel presents $H(\theta)$ defined by Equation 7.4, where $\mu = -5, ..., 5$.

```
> H2.dist<-sapply(theta.seq2,H2,mu=mu.seq[1],sigma=1)
> plot(theta.seq2,H2.dist,lty=3,lwd=2,type="l",xlim=c(-4,4),ylim=c(0,1),x
  lab="theta",ylab="Probability")
> for (i in 2:length(mu.seq)){
+    H2.dist<-sapply(theta.seq2,H2,mu=mu.seq[i],sigma=1)
+    lines(theta.seq2,H2.dist,lty=i+2,lwd=2)
+ }
```

In Figure 7.3, the solid line and the dashed line in the left panel present $H(\theta)$ defined by
Equations 7.2 and 7.3, with $\mu = 0$ and $\sigma = 1$, respectively, and the right panel presents $H(\theta)$
defined by Equation 7.4 for μ changing from –5 to 5.

Example 7.2

As a specific example of the choice of the prior function, Gönen et al. (2005) provided a
case study. Assuming the data Y_{ir} ($i = 1, 2, r = 1, ..., n_i$) are independent and normally distributed with means μ_i and a common variance σ^2, the goal is to test the H_0: $\delta = \mu_1 - \mu_2 = 0$
against H_1: $\delta \neq 0$. In order to obtain the usual two-sample t-statistic, prior knowledge is
modeled for δ/σ instead of δ, which can be specified as $\delta/\sigma\,|\,\{\mu,\sigma^2,\delta/\sigma \neq 0\} \sim N\left(\lambda,\sigma_\delta^2\right)$.
For sample size calculations, prior information to suggest the expected effect size λ is rou-
tinely used. The large sample size calculation formula for two-sample tests is given by

$$n = \frac{2\left(z_{1-\alpha/2} + z_{1-\beta}\right)^2}{\left(\delta/\sigma\right)^2},$$

where $n = n_1 = n_2 = 2n_\delta$ is the sample size per group, δ/σ is the pre-specified anticipated
standardized effect size, and α, β are the Type I and II error probabilities, respectively.

Note that the value σ_δ can be expressed as a function of the prior probability that the effect is in the wrong direction. For example, in the case of $\alpha = 0.05$, $\beta = 0.2$, $\lambda = (1.96 + 0.84)n_\delta^{-1/2} = 2.80n_\delta^{-1/2}$, and one thinks $\Pr(\delta < 0 | \delta \neq 0) = 0.10$, one can obtain $\sigma_\delta = 2.19n_\delta^{-1/2}$ using normal distribution calculations. These calculations involve the choice of zero for the 10th percentile of the prior on δ/σ; other percentiles could have been selected as well. Another calibration would involve selection of σ_δ based on a prior assumed value for $\Pr(\delta/\sigma > 2\lambda | \delta \neq 0) = 0.10$. In order to ensure consistency, it would be helpful to try several such values. The remaining parameter that needs to be specified is given in terms of the probability that H_0 is true, that is, $\pi_0 = \Pr(\delta = 0)$. Observing that it is unethical to randomize patients when the outcome is certain, the quantities $\Pr(\delta \leq 0)$ and $\Pr(\delta > 0)$ should be roughly comparable. One may set $\pi_0 = 0.5$ as an "objective" value (Berger and Sellke 1987), which, in conjunction with $\Pr(\delta < 0 | \delta \neq 0) = 0.10$, yields $\Pr(\delta \leq 0) = 0.5 + 0.10 * 0.5 = 0.55$. Alternatively, the prior π_0 can be assigned to reflect prior belief in the null; one may set $\Pr(\delta \leq 0) = 0.5$, which implies $\pi_0 = 0.444$ in conjunction with $\Pr(\delta < 0 | \delta \neq 0) = 0.10$.

Note that a common criticism of Bayesian methods is that the priors must be arbitrary, or subjective in a special way. Kass (1993) discussed that the value of a Bayes factor may be sensitive to the choice of priors on parameters in the competing models. A broad range of literature has discussed the selection of priors and various techniques for constructing priors, including Jeffreys's rules and their variants; see, for example, Marden (2000), Berger (1980, 1985), Kass and Wasserman (1996), and Sinharay and Stern (2002) for additional information.

7.4.3 Decision-Making Rules Based on the Bayes Factor

The Bayes factor is a summary of the evidence provided by the data in favor of one scientific theory, represented by a statistical model, as opposed to another. Jeffreys (1961) provided a scale of interpretation for the Bayes factor in terms of evidence against the null hypothesis; see Table 7.1 for details. It is suggested to interpret B_{10} in half units on the $\log_{10}$ scale.

Probability itself provides a meaningful scale defined by betting, and so these categories are not a calibration of the Bayes factor, but rather a rough descriptive statement about standards of evidence in scientific investigation; see Kass and Raftery (1995) for a detailed review.

Asymptotic approximations to the Bayes factor are easy to compute using the output from standard packages that maximize likelihoods. Recall that we described the asymptotic behavior of the Bayes factor in Section 7.4.1.1, for example, the Schwarz criterion,

$$S = \log \Pr(\mathbf{x} | \hat{\theta}_1, H_1) - \log \Pr(\mathbf{x} | \hat{\theta}_0, H_0) - \frac{1}{2}(d_1 - d_0) \log(n),$$

TABLE 7.1

Bayes Factor as Evidence against the Null Hypothesis

$\log_{10}(B_{10})$	B_{10}	Evidence Against H_0
0 to 1/2	1 to 3.2	Weak
1/2 to 1	3.2 to 10	Substantial
1 to 2	10 to 100	Strong
>2	>100	Decisive

which provides a rough approximation to the logarithm of the Bayes factor as $n \to \infty$. Note that $\Lambda = 2(\log \Pr(x \mid \hat{\theta}_1, H_1) - \log \Pr(x \mid \hat{\theta}_0, H_0))$ is the log-likelihood ratio statistic having approximately a $\chi^2_{d_1-d_0}$ distribution; see Section 7.4.1.1 for more details. Consequently, Bayes factor–type tests can be viewed as traditional tests due to the asymptotic results, where critical values and powers can be obtained accordingly.

Example 7.3: Calculating the Bayes factor

Consider a simple but common example. Let $x = \{x_1, \ldots, x_n\}$ be a random sample from some normal distribution with mean μ and variance σ^2. It is desired to test the one-sided hypothesis $H_0: \mu \leq \mu_{X0}$ versus $H_1: \mu \leq \mu_{X0}$, where μ_{X0} is a pre-specified number of interest. Let $\bar{x}$ denote the sample mean, that is, $\bar{x} = n^{-1}\sum_{i=1}^{n} x_i$. We then consider two scenarios with known or unknown value of variance σ^2.

Scenario 1 (The variance σ^2 is assumed to be known.)
Let the prior distribution function of μ be normal, $N\left(\mu_0, \tau_0^2\right)$. Then the posterior density is

$$\Pr(\mu \mid x) \propto \pi(\mu)\Pr(x \mid \mu) \propto \exp\left(-\frac{1}{2}\left(\frac{(\mu - \mu_0)^2}{\tau_0^2} + \sum_{i=1}^{n}\frac{(x_i - \mu)^2}{\sigma^2}\right)\right),$$

which is a normal density function with the mean and the variance as

$$\mu_n = \frac{\mu_0/\tau_0^2 + n\bar{x}/\sigma^2}{1/\tau_0^2 + n/\sigma^2}, \tau_n^2 = \frac{1}{1/\tau_0^2 + n/\sigma^2},$$

respectively. Therefore, the posterior probability of H_0, denoted by q_0, is $\Pr(\mu \leq \mu_{X0} \mid x) = \Phi((\mu_{X0} - \mu_n)/\tau_n)$, where Φ is the standard normal distribution function. Denote the value of prior probability of H_0, $\Pr(\mu \leq \mu_{X0}) = \Phi((\mu_{X0} - \mu_0)/\tau_0)$, by p_0. Thus, the Bayes factor, the ratio of the posterior odds to the prior odds, has the form

$$B_{10} = \frac{\Pr(x \mid H_1)}{\Pr(x \mid H_0)} = \frac{\Pr(\mu > \mu_{X0} \mid x)}{\Pr(\mu \leq \mu_{X0} \mid x)} \Big/ \frac{\Pr(\mu > \mu_{X0})}{\Pr(\mu \leq \mu_{X0})} = \frac{(1 - q_0)p_0}{(1 - p_0)q_0}.$$

Note that the prior precision, $1/\tau_0^2$, and the data precision, n/σ^2, play equivalent roles in the posterior distribution. Thus, for large sample size n, the posterior distribution is largely determined by σ^2 and the sample mean $\bar{x}$; see Gelman et al. (2003) for detailed discussion.

Scenario 2 (The variance σ^2 is assumed to be unknown.)
Let the conditional distribution of μ given σ^2 be normal and the marginal distribution of σ^2 be a scaled-inverse χ^2-distribution, that is,

$$\mu \mid \sigma^2 \sim N\left(\mu_0, \sigma^2/\kappa_0\right), \sigma^2 \sim \text{Inverse-}\chi^2\left(\nu_0, \sigma_0^2\right),$$

where the probability density function of the scaled-inverse $\chi^2(v_0, \sigma_0^2)$-distribution is $f(y; v_0, \sigma_0^2) = \dfrac{(\sigma_0^2 v_0/2)^{v_0/2}}{\Gamma(v_0/2)} y^{-(1+v_0/2)} \exp\left(-\dfrac{v_0\sigma_0^2}{2y}\right)$, $y > 0$. Then the joint prior density, a product form of $\Pr(\mu|\sigma^2)\Pr(\sigma^2)$, is

$$\Pr\left(\mu, \sigma^2\right) \propto \sigma^{-1}\left(\sigma^2\right)^{-(v_0/2+1)} \exp\left(-\frac{v_0\sigma_0^2 + \kappa_0(\mu_0 - \mu)^2}{2\sigma^2}\right),$$

which is denoted as normal-inverse $\chi^2\left(\mu_0, \sigma^2/\kappa_0 ; v_0, \sigma_0^2\right)$.

Let s^2 denote the sample variance, that is, $s^2 = (n-1)^{-1}\sum_{i=1}^{n}(x_i - \bar{x})^2$. Correspondingly, the joint posterior density is

$$\Pr(\mu, \sigma^2 \mid \mathbf{x}) \propto \sigma^{-1}(\sigma^2)^{-(v_0/2+1)} \exp\left(-\frac{v_0\sigma_0^2 + \kappa_0(\mu_0 - \mu)^2}{2\sigma^2}\right)(\sigma^2)^{-n/2}\exp\left(-\frac{(n-1)s^2 + n(\bar{x} - \mu)^2}{2\sigma^2}\right)$$

which is normal-inverse $\chi^2(\mu_n, \sigma_n^2/\kappa_n ; v_n, \sigma_n^2)$, where

$$\mu_n = \frac{\kappa_0}{\kappa_0 + n}\mu_0 + \frac{n}{\kappa_0 + n}\bar{x}, \ \kappa_n = \kappa_0 + n, \ v_n = v_0 + n, \ v_n\sigma_n^2 = v_0\sigma_0^2 + (n-1)s^2 + \frac{\kappa_0 n}{\kappa_0 + n}(\bar{x} - \mu_0)^2.$$

To sample from the joint posterior distribution, we first draw σ^2 from its marginal posterior distribution inverse $\chi^2\left(v_n, \sigma_n^2\right)$, and then draw μ from its normal conditional posterior distribution $N(\mu_n, \sigma^2/\kappa_n)$, using the simulated value of σ^2.

The marginal posterior density of σ^2 is the scaled-inverse χ^2 distribution, that is,

$$\sigma^2 \mid \mathbf{x} \sim \text{Inv-}\chi^2\left(v_n, \sigma_n^2\right).$$

The conditional posterior density of μ, given σ^2, is proportional to the joint posterior density in scenario 1 where the value of σ^2 is assumed to be known, that is,

$$\mu \mid \sigma^2, \mathbf{x} \sim N(\mu_n, \sigma^2/\kappa_n).$$

Integration of the joint posterior density with respect to σ^2 shows that the marginal posterior density for μ follows a nonstandardized Student's t-distribution,

$$\Pr(\mu \mid \mathbf{x}) \propto \left(1 + \frac{\kappa_n(\mu_n - \mu)^2}{v_n\sigma_n^2}\right)^{-(v_n/2+1)} = t_{v_n}\left(\mu_n, \sigma_n^2/\kappa_n\right),$$

where the probability density function of the nonstandardized Student's t-distribution $t_v(\mu, \sigma)$ is

$$f(y; v, \mu, \sigma) = \frac{\Gamma((v+1)/2)}{\Gamma(v/2)\sqrt{\pi v}\sigma}\left(1 + \frac{1}{v}\left(\frac{y - \mu}{\sigma}\right)^2\right)^{-((v+1)/2)}.$$

Denote the corresponding distribution function as $T(y; v, \mu, \sigma) = \int_{-\infty}^{y} f(t; v, \mu, \sigma)dt$. In this case, the posterior probability of H_0, denoted by q_0, is $\Pr\left(\mu \leq \mu_{X0} \mid \mathbf{x}\right) = T\left(\mu_{X0}; v_n, \mu_n, \sigma_n^2/\kappa_n\right)$. The value of the prior probability of H_0, denoted by p_0, is $\Pr(\mu \leq \mu_{X0}) = \int_{-\infty}^{\mu_{X0}}\int_{0}^{\infty}\Pr(\mu, \sigma^2)d\mu d\sigma^2$, which can be computed based on previous derivation. Thus, the Bayes factor has the form of $B_{10} = \dfrac{(1 - q_0)p_0}{(1 - p_0)q_0}$.

The results based on the one-sample problem can be easily generalized to the two-sample case. A classic example would be to compare the means of two normal distributions with unknown variances. Let $\mathbf{x_1} = \{x_{11},...,x_{1n_1}\}$ and $\mathbf{x_2} = \{x_{21},...,x_{2n_2}\}$ be two independent random samples drawn from normal distributions $N(\mu_1,\sigma_1^2)$ and $N(\mu_2,\sigma_2^2)$, respectively, where μ_1, μ_2, σ_1^2, and σ_2^2 are unknown. We are interested in testing $H_0: \mu_1 = \mu_2, \sigma_1^2 = \sigma_2^2$ versus $H_1: \mu_1 \neq \mu_2, \sigma_1^2 \neq \sigma_2^2$.

Let us revisit the high-density lipoprotein (HDL) data example. Consider a subset of the study sample, which consists of 25 individuals with myocardial infarction (diseased) and 35 controls (healthy) based on published results regarding the HDL cholesterol biomarker. The histogram of measurements of HDL cholesterol levels in diseased (left panel) and healthy (right panel) individuals, as shown in Figure 7.4, suggests that the distributions may differ in the two groups.

Suppose it is of interest to test the equality of the means and variances in two groups. Based on published results regarding the HDL cholesterol biomarker, under the null hypothesis, let the conditional distribution of μ given σ^2 be normal, $\mu|\sigma^2 \sim N(49.94, \sigma^2/60)$, and the marginal distribution of σ^2 be the scaled-inverse χ^2-distribution, $\sigma^2 \sim$ inverse χ^2 (59, 138.69). Under the alternative hypothesis, for the diseased group, $\mu_1 | \sigma_1^2 \sim N(42.53, \sigma_1^2/25)$ and $\sigma_1^2 \sim$ inverse χ^2 (34, 87.37); for the healthy group, $\mu_2 | \sigma_2^2 \sim N(51.72, \sigma_1^2/35)$ and $\sigma_2^2 \sim$ inverse χ^2 (34, 134.87). In this case, the value of $\log_{10}(B_{10})$ is 2.9042, greater than 2, suggesting decisive evidence against H_0. The p-value related to a two-sample t-test is around 0.0007, also suggesting the rejection of H_0; so does the two-sample Kolmogorov–Smirnov test.

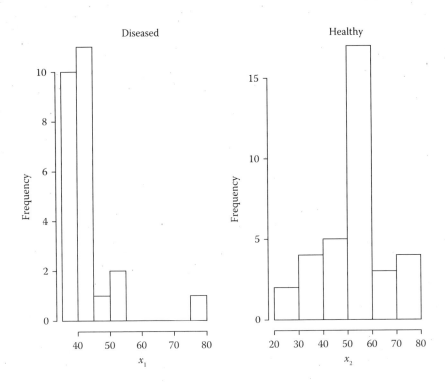

FIGURE 7.4
Histogram of measurements of HDL cholesterol levels in diseased (left) and healthy (right) individuals.

The following code shows the data and the calculation of the Bayes factor:

```
> ######## input data #####
> x1<-c(50.6,41.8,77.0,39.6,35.2,44.0,44.0,35.2,50.6,44.0,44.0,44.0,35.2,
  41.8,35.2,35.2,41.8,37.4,37.4,35.2,41.8,44.0,44.0,39.6,46.2)
> x2<-c(68.2,44.0,68.2,50.6,35.2,52.8,52.8,39.6,59.4,52.8,72.6,68.2,55.0,
  50.6,50.6,59.4,52.8,52.8,52.8,37.4,55.0,41.8,52.8,22.0,74.8,28.6,57.2,
  52.8,74.8,35.2,55.0,46.2,46.2,44.0,74.8))
>
>
> ############# prior parameters #####
> n1<-length(x1)
> n2<-length(x2)
> # prior for mu under H_0
> mu0<-49.94
> # prior for variance under H_0
> scale0<-138.69
> df0<-n1+n2-1
>
> # prior for mu1 under H_1
> mu1<-42.53
> # prior for variance of x1 under H_1
> scale1<-87.37
> df1<-n1-1
>
> # prior for mu2 under H_1
> mu2<-51.72
> # prior for variance of x2 under H_1
> scale2<-134.87
> df2<-n2-1
>
>
> # density function of the scaled inverse-chisquare distribution
> dsinvchisq<-function (x,df,scale){
+    nu<-df/2
+    ifelse(x>0,(((nu)^(nu))/gamma(nu))*(scale^nu)*(x^(-(1+nu)))*
     exp(-nu*scale/x), NA)
+ }
> ###### obtain the Pr(x|H)   ######
> Pr.x.H<-function(x,p.mu,p.K,p.scale,p.df){
+    # obtain the likelihood of the data based on N(mu,sigma2)
+    get.like<-function(x,mu,sigma2){
+      #prod(sapply(x,function(xx) dnorm(xx,mean=mu,sd=sqrt(sigma2)) ))
+      sigma2^(-1/2)*exp(-(sum(x^2)-2*mu*sum(x)+length(x)*mu^2)/
      (2*sigma2)) # proportional
+    }
+
+    # joint prior
+    get.joint.prior<-function(mu,sigma2,p.mu,p.K,p.df,p.scale){
+      #dnorm(mu,mean=p.mu,sd=sqrt(sigma2/p.K))*dsinvchisq(sigma2,p.df,
      p.scale)
```

```
+      sigma2^(-1/2-(p.df/2+1))*exp(-(p.df*p.scale+p.K*(p.mu-mu)^2)/
       (2*sigma2)) # proportional
+    }
+
+    # likelihood*joint prior
+    integrand<-function(mu,sigma2=sigma2,x=x){
+      Vectorize(get.like(x,mu,sigma2)*get.joint.prior(mu,sigma2,
       p.mu,p.K,p.df,p.scale))
+    }
+
+    # double integration with respect to mu and sigma2
+    tmp<-integrate(function(sigma2) {
+    sapply(sigma2, function(sigma2) {
+      integrate(function(mu) integrand(mu=mu,sigma2=sigma2,x=x), -Inf,
       Inf)$value
+      })
+    }, 0, Inf)$value
+    return(tmp)
+ }
>
> p0<-Pr.x.H(x=c(x1,x2),p.mu=mu0,p.K=n1+n2,p.scale=scale0,p.df=df0) # H_0
> p11<-Pr.x.H(x=x1,p.mu=mu1,p.K=n1,p.scale=scale1,p.df=df1) # x1
under H_1
> p12<-Pr.x.H(x=x2,p.mu=mu2,p.K=n2,p.scale=scale2,p.df=df2) # x2
under H_1
>
> ###### obtain the Bayes factor ######
> BF<-p11*p12/p0
> log10(BF)
[1] 2.904165
>
> t.test(x1,x2) # t-test
        Welch Two Sample t-test
data: x1 and x2
t = -3.5838, df = 57.741, p-value = 0.0006964
alternative hypothesis: true difference in means is not equal to 0
95 percent confidence interval:
 -15.420292 -4.367137
sample estimates:
mean of x mean of y
 42.59200 52.48571
> ks.test(x1, x2) # Two-sample Kolmogorov-Smirnov test
        Two-sample Kolmogorov-Smirnov test
data: x1 and x2
D = 0.5829, p-value = 9.949e-05
alternative hypothesis: two-sided
```

As mentioned above, Bayes factor–type test statistics can be used in the context of traditional tests via a control of the corresponding Type I error rate, for example, employing the asymptotic evaluations of the Bayes factor structures. We illustrate this principle in the following example.

Example 7.4

Let $\mathbf{x} = \{x_1, \ldots, x_n\}$, $n = 30$, be a random sample drawn from $Y - 1$, where $Y \sim \exp(\lambda)$, that is, $f(x; \lambda) = \lambda \exp(-\lambda (x + 1))$, $\lambda > 0$, $x > -1$, is the density function of the observations. Denote the mean of X by θ ($\theta = 1/\lambda - 1$). It is of interest to test H_0: $\theta = 0$ versus H_1: $\theta \neq 0$. Under the alternative hypothesis, the prior function for θ is assumed to be the *Uniform* [0,2]-distribution function. In this case, based on the Schwarz criterion approximation,

the relevant maximum likelihood ratio can be a well approximation to $\log B_{10} + \dfrac{1}{2}\log(n)$

as $n \to \infty$. The maximum likelihood ratio has asymptotically the χ_1^2-distribution, under the null hypothesis. Correspondingly, comparing $2\log B_{10} + \log(n)$ with the critical values related to the χ_1^2-distribution, one can provide an approach to make statistical decision rules from the traditional test perspective. Implementation of the testing procedure is presented in the following R code:

```
> n<-30
> lambda.true<-1/2
> 1/lambda.true-1 # theta.true
[1] 1
>
> set.seed(123456)
> x<-rexp(n,lambda.true)-1
> x
 [1]  0.19113728  0.01426038  1.51633983  1.11874795  1.27664726  2.94610447
  -0.86056815  4.24772281 -0.76769938
[10]  0.22111551 -0.72606026  1.06624316  0.10882527  2.32608560  3.73953110
  1.89499414  2.52307509  1.35740018
[19] -0.76989244 -0.90812499 -0.83491881  0.29580491  3.72774643 -0.01274517
  -0.57838195  2.79788529  0.74200029
[28] -0.93858993  1.18364253 -0.28730946
>
> theta0<-0 # EX under H_0
> lambda0<-(theta0+1)^(-1)
>
> neg.loglike<-function(x,theta){
+    length(x)*log(theta+1)+(sum(x)+length(x))/(theta+1)
+ }
>
> # Bayes factor
> # likelihood
> like<-function(x,theta){
+ exp(-(length(x)*log(theta+1)+(sum(x)+length(x))/(theta+1)))
+ }
>
> # prior
> ll<-0;uu<-2
> prior<-function(theta) 1/(uu-ll)*(theta<=uu)*(theta>=ll)
>
> integrand<-function(theta) like(theta,x=x) #*prior(theta)
> BF<-integrate(Vectorize(integrand), ll, uu)$value/like(theta0,x=x)
> log10(BF)
[1] 3.227941
> stat.est<-log(BF)+1/2*log(n)
> p.BF<-1-pchisq(2*stat.est,df=1)
> p.BF
[1] 1.920634e-05
> p.t<-t.test(x,mu=theta0)$p.val
> p.t
[1] 0.003940047
```

In this example, the value of $\log_{10}(B_{10})$ is 3.2279, greater than 2, suggesting decisive evidence against H_0. From the traditional test viewpoint, the approach based on the Bayes factor leads to a p-value far below 0.0001, suggesting the rejection of the null hypothesis, which is consistent with the result based on the t-test.

The following points about the Bayes factor should be emphasized: (1) Bayes factors provide a way to evaluate evidence in favor of a null hypothesis, incorporating external information; (2) Bayes factors are very general and do not require alternative models to be nested; (3) technically, Bayes factors are simpler to compute than deriving non-Bayesian significance tests, in "nonstandard" statistical models that do not satisfy common regularity conditions; (4) when estimation or prediction is of interest, Bayes factors can be converted to weights corresponding to various models so that a composite estimate or prediction may be obtained that takes account of structural or model uncertainty; and (5) it is important, and feasible, to assess the sensitivity of conclusions to the chosen prior distributions. For more details, we refer the reader to Kass and Raftery (1995) and Vexler et al. (2010b).

7.4.4 Data Example: Application of Bayes Factor

Consider a study of survival among turtles where the question of comparing two nested models is of interest. In this study, 244 turtle eggs of the same age from 31 clutches (or families) were removed from their nests in a site in Illinois on the bank of the Mississippi River and taken to the laboratory where they were incubated and hatched (Janzen et al. 2000). Several days later, the baby turtles were released from the same place where the eggs were found. The turtles that traveled successfully to the water were marked as "survived." Five days after their release, turtles not identified as survived were assumed dead. The birth weight of each turtle was collected as a covariate. The objective is to assess the effect of birth weight on survival and to determine whether there is any clutch effect on survival. Figure 7.5 shows a scatterplot of the birth weight effect on survival status, as well as the clutch effect on survival. The clutches are numbered 1 through 31 in an increasing order of average birth weight of the turtles. Figure 7.5 suggests that the heaviest turtles tend to survive and the lightest ones tend to die. It also suggests some variability in survival rates across clutches. For example, in one clutch (with average birth weight 5.41), only 2 turtles out of 12 survived, while in a second clutch (with average birth weight 7.50), 9 turtles out of 11 survived.

Let y_{ij} denote the response (survival status with 1 denoting survival) and x_{ij} the birth weight of the jth turtle in the ith clutch, $i = 1, 2, \ldots, m = 31, j = 1, 2, \ldots, n_i$. The model we fit to the data is

$$y_{ij}|p_{ij} \sim \text{bern}(p_{ij}),\ i = 1, 2, \ldots, m = 31, j = 1, 2, \ldots, n_i$$

$$p_{ij} = \phi(\alpha_0 + \alpha_1 x_{ij} + b_i),\ i = 1, 2, \ldots, m = 31, j = 1, 2, \ldots, n_i$$

$$b_i \mid \sigma^2 \overset{i.i.d.}{\sim} N(0, \sigma^2),\ i = 1, 2, \ldots, m$$

The b_i's are random effects for clutch (family). The clutch effects are assumed to be the same for all birth weights. To assess the importance of clutch effects, we compare our model (alternative model), the probit regression model with random effects, with the null model, the simple probit regression model (no random effects).

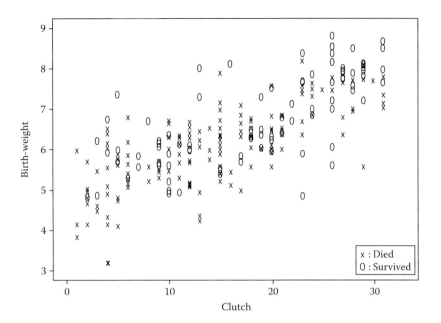

FIGURE 7.5
Snapshot from the paper by Sinharay and Stern (2002) regarding the scatterplot with the clutches sorted by average birth weight.

Suppose $p_0(\alpha)$ is the prior distribution for α under the null model, while the prior distribution for (α, θ) under the alternative model is $p(\alpha, \theta) = p(\sigma^2)\, p_1(\alpha|\sigma^2)$. Then, the Bayes factor for comparing the alternative model (M_1) against the null model (M_0) is $BF_{10} = p(y|M_1)/p(y|M_0)$, with

$$p(y\,|\,M_1) = \int p(y\,|\,\alpha, b)p(b\,|\,\sigma^2)p_1(\alpha\,|\,\sigma^2)p(\sigma^2)dbd\,\alpha d\sigma^2,$$

$$p(y\,|\,M_0) = \int p(y\,|\,\alpha, b = 0)p_0(\alpha)d\alpha.$$

For this example,

$$p(y\,|\,a, b) = \prod_{i=1}^{m}\prod_{j=1}^{n_i}\{\Phi(a_0 + a_1 x_{ij} + b_i)\}^{y_{ij}}\{1 - \Phi(a_0 + a_1 x_{ij} + b_i)\}^{1-y_{ij}},$$

$$p(y\,|\,\alpha, b = 0) = \prod_{i=1}^{m}\prod_{j=1}^{n_i}\{\Phi(a_0 + a_1 x_{ij})\}^{y_{ij}}\{1 - \Phi(a_0 + a_1 x_{ij})\}^{1-y_{ij}},$$

$$p(b\,|\,\sigma^2) \propto (\sigma^2)^{-m/2}\exp\left\{-\sum_{i=1}^{m} b_i^2/(2\sigma^2)\right\}.$$

Furthermore, we use a proper vague prior distribution on α, a bivariate normal distribution with mean 0 and variance 20.1 under both models.

The approximated value of the Bayes factor, obtained using the importance sampling method with an importance sample size of 5000 under both the models, is 0.31 with an estimated standard deviation of 0.01. The value of the Bayes factor indicates some evidence in favor of the null model.

We then investigate the sensitivity of the Bayes factor to the choice of prior distributions. The prior distributions on α under the two models do not affect the Bayes factor much because there are 244 data points in the data set. However, the prior distribution for the variance component σ^2 is influential on any posterior inference because our ability to learn about σ^2 is determined by the number of clutches rather than the number of animals. Furthermore, there is little prior information available for σ^2 because very few studies like the turtle study have been performed. To study the effect of the choice of the prior distribution for σ^2 on the Bayes factor, let BF_{10,σ^2} denote the "point mass prior Bayes factor" comparing the probit regression model with random effects, where the variance component is fixed at σ^2 against the simple probit regression model without any variance component. For a grid value of σ^2, the approximated values of the Bayes factor, $\widehat{BF}_{10,\sigma^2}$, obtained by the importance sampling method are computed. Figure 7.6 presents a plot of $\widehat{BF}_{10,\sigma^2}$ against σ^2. The figure demonstrates that $\widehat{BF}_{10,\sigma^2} = 1$ when $\sigma^2 = 0$, implying that the two models are identical at that value. The estimated Bayes factor then increases with an increase in σ^2 until it reaches its maximum value of about 4.55 at around $\sigma^2 = 0.09$. This is sensible because the restricted maximum likelihood estimate (REML) of σ^2 is 0.091. Also, when it comes to choosing between a small hypothesized value (by small here, we mean less than 0.3) of σ^2 and σ^2 equal to zero, the approximated Bayes factor favors the small positive value of σ^2. However, when it comes to choosing between a large value of σ^2 and σ^2 equal to zero, the approximated Bayes factor favors the σ^2 equal to zero; we refer the reader to Sinharay and Stern (2002) for more details.

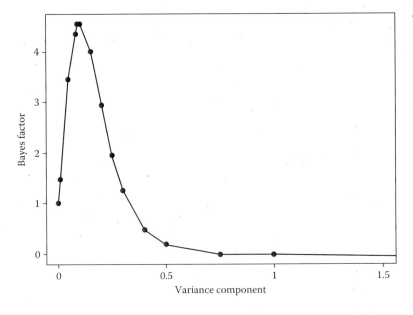

FIGURE 7.6

Snapshot from the paper by Sinharay and Stern (2002) regarding the plot of $\widehat{BF}_{10,\sigma^2}$ against σ^2.

7.5 Remarks

The Bayes factor, as the ratio of the posterior odds (not probability) of the hypothesis to its prior odds, is equal to a likelihood ratio in the simplest case (and only then); see Good (1992) for details. It can be described as a multiplicative weight of evidence. As described in Chapter 1, problems may arise when inference about the truth or believability of the null is based on the classical formulation of p-value. As alternatives to the classical formulation of p-values for testing hypotheses, Bayes factors have been suggested as a measure of the extent to which the observed data agree or disagree with a hypothesis, at the cost of requiring a prior distribution on the parameter. The use of the p-value should not be discarded all together. A small p-value does not necessarily mean that we should reject the null hypothesis and leave it at that. Rather, it is a red flag indicating that something is up; the null hypothesis may be false, possibly in a substantively uninteresting way, or maybe we got unlucky. On the other hand, a large p-value does mean that there is not much evidence against the null. For example, in many settings the Bayes factor is bounded above by the 1/p-value. Even Bayesian analyses can benefit from classical testing at the model-checking stage (see Box [1980] or the Bayesian p-values in Gelman et al. [2013]). For more details, we refer the reader to Marden (2000).

7.6 Supplement

1. Consider a situation where a test decision is based on data $\mathbf{x} = \{x_1, ..., x_n\}$ from the joint density function $f(x_1, ..., x_n)$, which is known to belong to a parametric class $\{f(x_1, ..., x_n | \mu, \eta), \mu \in \Omega_1 \subseteq \mathbf{R}^d\}$. The goal is to test the null hypothesis H_0: $(\mu, \eta) \in \Theta_0 = \{(\mu_0, \eta): \eta \in \Omega_2\}$ versus the alternative H_1: $(\mu, \eta) \in \Theta_1 = \{(\mu, \eta): \mu \neq \mu_0, \eta \in \Omega_2\} = \{\Omega_1 \times \Omega_2\} / \Theta_0$, where μ_0 is assumed to be known and fixed.

   The maximum likelihood method (or the likelihood ratio method) proposes the test statistic

$$\Lambda_n^{\mathrm{MLR}} = \frac{\sup_{(\mu,\eta)\in\Theta_1} f(\mathbf{x}|\mu,\eta)}{\sup_{\eta\in\Omega_2} f(\mathbf{x}|\mu_0,\eta)}.$$

We refer the reader to Chapter 4 for details about the maximum likelihood ratio test strategy.

   Alternatively, the method of the Bayes factor can be applied. The test statistic is the integrated likelihood ratio in the form

$$\Lambda_n^{\mathrm{ILR}} = \frac{\int f(\mathbf{x}|\mu,\eta)\,d\psi_1(\mu,\eta)}{\int f(\mathbf{x}|\mu_0,\eta)\,d\psi_0(\eta)},$$

where priors ψ_0 and ψ_1 of the parameters conditional on it are in the null or alternative, respectively (e.g., Marden 2000). Denote the Bayesian significance level of a decision rule δ in the form of

$$\bar{\alpha} = \int \delta(x_1,...,x_n) \int f(x_1,...,x_n \mid \mu_0, \eta) d\psi_0(\eta) \prod_{i=1}^{n} dx_i.$$

Vexler et al. (2010b) showed that for any δ with the fixed Bayesian significance level $\bar{\alpha}$, the statistic Λ_n^{ILR} provides the integrated most powerful test with respect to a prior ψ_A, that is,

$$\int \text{Pr}_{(\mu,\eta)}\left\{\Lambda_n^{\text{ILR}} > C_{\bar{\alpha}}\right\} d\psi_A(\mu,\eta) \geq \int \text{Pr}_{(\mu,\eta)}\left\{\delta \text{ rejects } H_0\right\} d\psi_A(\mu,\eta),$$

where the threshold $C_{\bar{\alpha}}$ is chosen by $\int \text{Pr}_{(\mu_0,\eta)}\left\{\Lambda_n^{\text{ILR}} > C_{\bar{\alpha}}\right\} d\psi_0(n) = \bar{\alpha}$.

In addition to the traditional maximum likelihood test and the Bayes factor–type test presented above, a semi-Bayes approach, a statistical test strategy between these two methods, can be considered. Consider, for example, the penalized maximum likelihood estimator of η, say

$$\hat{\eta}(\mathbf{x}) = \arg\max_a \phi(a) f(\mathbf{x} \mid \mu_0, a),$$

where ϕ is a decreasing function of a penalty. In the Bayesian framework, ϕ can be viewed as a proportion of a prior density of η (see Green 1990). Then, the estimator of the H_0-likelihood $f(\mathbf{x} \mid \mu_0, \eta)$ can be presented in the form

$$\hat{f}(\mathbf{x} \mid \mu_0, \hat{\eta}) = \phi(\hat{\eta}(\mathbf{x})) f(\mathbf{x} \mid \mu_0, \hat{\eta}(\mathbf{x})).$$

Vexler et al. (2010b) considered the semi-Bayes test statistic

$$\Lambda_n^{\text{SBLR}} = \frac{\int f(\mathbf{x} \mid \mu, \eta) d\psi_1(\mu, \eta)}{\hat{f}(\mathbf{x} \mid \mu_0, \hat{\eta})}.$$

Assume that $\mathbf{x} = \{x_1, ..., x_n\}$ are independent and identically distributed and let the function ϕ be 1 without loss of generality. O'Hagan (1995) has shown that, under standard regularity conditions (for details, see Gelfand and Dey [1994], O'Hagan [1995] and Kass and Wasserman [1995]), the numerator of the test statistic Λ_n^{SBLR} can be asymptotically expressed as

$$\psi_1\left(\hat{\mu}_{\text{MLE}}, \hat{\eta}_{\text{MLE}}\right) L_2 n^{-1} 2\pi \mid V_n \mid^{\frac{1}{2}}$$

where $L_2 = \max_{\mu,\eta} \prod_{j=1}^{n} f(x_i \mid \mu, \eta)$ is the maximized likelihood, $-nV_n^{-1}$ is the Hessian matrix of $\log f$ at the maximum likelihood estimators $\left(\hat{\mu}_{\text{MLE}}, \hat{\eta}_{\text{MLE}}\right)$, and $\psi_1(\mu,\eta)d\mu d\eta = d\psi_{1f}(\mu,\eta)$. Note that $V_n \to V$ as $n \to \infty$, where V is a constant matrix. Then

$$\Lambda = \frac{\int f(\mathbf{x} \mid \mu, \eta) d\psi_1(\mu, \eta)}{\int f\left(\mathbf{x} \mid \mu_0, \hat{\eta}_{\text{MLE},H_0}\right)} \approx \frac{L_2}{L_1} \psi_A\left(\hat{\mu}_{\text{MLE}}, \hat{\eta}_{\text{MLE}}\right) n^{-1} 2\pi \mid V \mid^{\frac{1}{2}},$$

where $L_1 = f\left(\mathbf{x} \mid \mu_0, \hat{\eta}_{\mathrm{MLE},H_0}\right)$. Under H_0,

$$2\log \Lambda \approx 2\log \frac{L_2}{L_1} + 2\log \psi_1\left(\hat{\mu}_{\mathrm{MLE}}, \hat{\eta}_{\mathrm{MLE}}\right) n^{-1} 2\pi \mid V \mid^{\frac{1}{2}},$$

which is asymptotically distributed as a χ_1^2 plus $2\log\left(\psi_A(\mu, \eta) n^{-1} 2\pi \mid V \mid^{\frac{1}{2}}\right)$.

2. The Bayesian method for hypothesis testing was developed by Jeffreys (1935) and Jeffreys (1998) for quantifying the evidence in favor of a scientific theory. The centerpiece was a number, now called the Bayes factor, which is the posterior odds of the null hypothesis when the prior probability on the null is one-half. Although there has been much discussion of Bayesian hypothesis testing in the context of criticism of p-values, less attention has been given to the Bayes factor as a practical tool of applied statistics. Kass and Raftery (1995) reviewed and discussed five scientific applications that pose problems usefully solved with the Bayes factor in the following fields: (a) genetics: to investigate if mutations leading to acetate utilization deficiency in the uvrE strain of *Escherichia coli* bacteria would occur by an unusual error-prone DNA repair mechanism, based on an experiment in molecular biology (Sklar and Strauss 1980); (b) sports: to test if erratic behavior of shooting is consistent with a stable shooting percentage rather than reflecting any real tendency for players to have good or bad streaks (Gilovich et al. 1985); (c) ecology: to examine if high levels of ozone indicate that the air is polluted (Smith 1989); (d) sociology: to study the effect of social class background, ability, and type of school attended on educational attainment (Greaney and Kellaghan 1984); and (e) psychology: to explore the interaction between human working memory failure and computer-based tasks.

3. The use of Monte Carlo integration methods was discussed for the computation of the multivariate integrals defined in the posterior moments and densities of the parameters of interest in econometric models in Chapter 3 of Van Dijk (1984). Van Dijk et al. (1987) described the computational steps of importance sampling (see Hammersley and Handscomb 1964) and presented a set of standard programs in FORTRAN that can be used for the implementation of a simple case of importance sampling.

4. Tierney and Kadane (1986) proposed easily computable second-order approximations to the posterior means and variances of positive smooth functions of a real or vector-valued parameter, as well as approximations to the marginal posterior densities of arbitrary (i.e., not necessarily positive) parameters. For asymptotic evaluation of integrals where the integrand is $f(\theta)\exp(-nh(\theta))$, and the function h is approximated by a quadratic, the authors applied Laplace's method such that the integrand is $\exp(-nh(\theta) + \log f(\theta))$, a fully exponential form. Accordingly, a second-order expansion for the ratio can be derived and the approach is feasible for any problems where maximum likelihood estimates and the observed information can be computed. The computation of more derivatives of the log-likelihood function is required in other second-order approximations (Hartigan 1965; Johnson 1970; Lindley 1980; Mosteller and Wallace 1964). Tierney and Kadane (1986) illustrated their method with data from the Stanford heart transplant program that can be described by a three-parameter model used by Turnbull et al. (1974). Tierney et al. (1989) extended the fully exponential method of Tierney and Kadane (1986) to

apply to expectations and variances of nonpositive functions. This method is formally equivalent to that of Mosteller and Wallace and that of Lindley, but does not require third derivatives of the likelihood function.

5. Efron (1986b) discussed the reason why most scientific data analysis is carried out in a non-Bayesian framework. The author argued that the Bayesian approach is difficult but Fisherian or frequentist solutions are relatively easy from a practical perspective, including a brief discussion of objectivity in statistical analyses and of the difficulties of achieving objectivity within a Bayesian framework. The author concluded with the practical advantages of Fisherian or frequentist approaches, and stated that Fisherian or frequentist approaches seem to have outweighed the philosophical superiority of Bayesianism.

6. Leonard et al. (1989) derived a Laplacian approximation to the posterior density of $\eta = g(\theta)$, which requires a conditional information matrix $\mathbf{R}_\eta$, to be positive definite for every fixed η. Nevertheless, not all $\mathbf{R}_\eta$ are positive definite in many situations, such that the computations of the approximations that cannot be normalized may fail. Instead, Hsu (1995) presented a modifiable Laplacian approximation where the corresponding conditional information matrix can be made positive definite for every fixed η, in a simpler analytical form than that proposed by Leonard et al. (1989).

7. Bayesian posterior expectations are commonly used to characterize posterior and predictive distributions and serve as Bayes analogues of frequentist point estimators based on parametric statistical models; see Tierney et al. (1989) and Carlin and Louis (1997) for details. Vexler et al. (2014d) extended the posterior expectation from parametric models to nonparametric models using empirical likelihood (see Chapter 6 for details) and developed a nonparametric analogue of the James–Stein estimation. The authors established the asymptotic approximations to the proposed posterior expectations by Laplace's method, and showed by simulation that posterior expectations are usually more efficient than the classical nonparametric procedures, particularly when the underlying data are skewed. The authors illustrated the proposed method with thiobarbituric acid reaction substances data from a case-control myocardial infarction study. See also Vexler et al. (2016).

8. The use of the posterior mean can reduce sensitivity to variations in the prior and avoid the Lindley paradox in testing point null hypotheses. Based on the use of the posterior mean of the likelihood under each model rather than the usual prior mean, Aitkin (1991) proposed a general procedure for computing Bayes factors for the comparison of arbitrary models. The author stated that the use of the posterior mean has several advantages, including reduced sensitivity to variations in the prior and the avoidance of the Lindley paradox in testing point null hypotheses.

9. In order to solve the issue of the extreme sensitivity of the Bayes factor to the priors of models under comparison, several alternative Bayes factors are proposed. In particular, some new automatic criteria are introduced to cope with the impossibility of using the Bayes factor with standard noninformative priors for model comparison, for example, the posterior Bayes factor (Aitkin 1991), the intrinsic Bayes factors (Berger and Pericchi 1996), and the partial (fractional) Bayes factor (O'Hagan 1995). Note that partial Bayes factors can be used where the training sample provides an initial informative posterior distribution of the parameters

in each model and the models are compared based on a Bayes factor calculated from the remaining data. O'Hagan (1995) discussed the properties of partial Bayes factors, whose advantages are shown in the context of weak prior information. Furthermore, the author suggested the use of the fractional Bayes factor, a variant of the partial Bayes factor, for its consistency, simplicity, robustness, and coherence. In addition to O'Hagan (1995), De Santis and Spezzaferri (1997) derived some interesting properties and uses of the fractional Bayes factor that justify its use. For example, in addition to coping with improper priors as originally introduced, the fractional Bayes factor is also useful in a robust analysis. As an example, using usual classes of priors, the authors compared several alternative Bayes factors for the problem of testing a point null hypothesis versus a two-sided alternative for the mean of the univariate normal distribution.

10. Good (1992) reviewed various aspects of the compromises occurring between Bayesian and non-Bayesian methods. An evident example of the Bayesian influence on non-Bayesian statistics is the importance of the concept of likelihood and likelihood methodology, both of which are built into Bayes's theorem even when the priors are unknown.

11. Kass and Vaidyanathan (1992) proposed asymptotic expansions to approximate Bayes factors, improving on the method used by Jeffreys (1961). Suppose that it is of interest to test the hypothesis H_0: $\psi = \psi_0$ versus H_1: $\psi \neq \psi_0$ in the presence of a nuisance parameter β and initially priors $\pi_0(\beta)$ under H_0 and $\pi(\beta, \psi)$ under H_1 are used. The authors considered the sensitivity analysis of the Bayes factor to small changes in π_0 and π. For local alternatives (which are consistent with small or moderately large values of the Bayes factor in favor of the alternative for moderate sample sizes), if β and ψ are null orthogonal parameters, then alterations in π_0 have no effect on the Bayes factor up to order $O(n^{-1})$. Under similar conditions, the authors also derived an order $O(n^{-1})$ approximation to the minimum Bayes factor over all priors π under the alternative such that the marginal prior on ψ is normal with mean ψ_0. The authors then noted that a second-order approximation due to Tierney and Kadane (1986) asymptotically provides a useful way to analyze the sensitivity to specific changes in the marginal prior on ψ.

12. In the context of comparison among two or more competing hypotheses, Bayes factors are frequently estimated by constructing a Markov chain Monte Carlo (MCMC) sampler to explore the joint space of the hypotheses. Müller and Parmigiani (1995) fitted a model to estimate a smooth function of individual points using MCMC. Gelman and Rubin (1992a, 1992b) fitted an analysis of variance (ANOVA) model to the output of multiple MCMC chains and recommended adjusting final inferences for the uncertainty from parameter estimation and computation uncertainty. Brooks and Roberts (1998) updated Gelman and Rubin's model to incorporate the time series dependence of the MCMC output. To efficiently estimate the Bayes factor in support of H_0 against the alternative H_1, Carlin and Chib (1995) recommended adjusting the prior odds in favor of H_0 such that the posterior probability is approximately 1/2, and then solving for the Bayes factor as the posterior odds divided by the prior odds. This method minimizes the standard error of estimation, while preserving the length of the MCMC chain to a computationally practical amount.

Compared to the approach that uses prior odds based on scientific input or a commonly used flat prior $\pi(H_0) = 1/2$, Carlin and Chib's method results in a more accurate Bayes factor estimate. However, it should be noted that Carlin and Chib's method suffers from the fact that several independent MCMC chains may be produced, but only one is actually used in the estimation. In general, Carlin and Chib's method applies equally well to problems where only one model is contemplated, but its proper size is not known at the outset, for example, problems involving integer-valued parameters, multiple change points (see Chapter 12), or finite mixture distributions. To illustrate, the authors applied their method on the following examples: (a) fitting two plausible straight line models to the data set of Williams and Williams (1959) and (b) analyzing a two-component normal mixture model under a noninformative prior in the context of finite mixture models (Evans et al. 1992). Suchard et al. (2005) extended the method of Carlin and Chib (1995) to incorporate the output from multiple chains. The authors proposed three statistical models that allow for the estimation of the uncertainty in the calculation of the Bayes factor and the use of several different MCMC chains even when the prior odds of the hypotheses vary from chain to chain. The first model assumes independent sampler draws and uses logistic regression to model the hypothesis indicator function for various choices of the prior odds, and the other two, more complex models relax the independence assumption by allowing for higher lag dependence within the MCMC output. The authors illustrated the use of these models to calculate Bayes factors for tests of monophyly with the following phylogenetic examples: (a) employing a Bayesian phylogenetic reconstruction model as a medical diagnostic tool on a study exploring the relationship of an unknown pathogen to a set of known pathogens, and (b) employing a Bayesian phylogenetic reconstruction model to examine the evidence in favor of intragenic recombination between different HIV-1 subtype strains.

13. In the context of model determination, within a Bayesian modeling framework, Gelfand and Dey (1994) considered the selection of models among a finite set of models based on predictive distributions. The authors presented a general predictive formulation of various Bayesian approaches and compared the asymptotic behavior of these approaches using Laplace approximations. The authors concluded that concern regarding the accuracy of these approximations for small to moderate sample sizes encourages the use of Monte Carlo techniques to carry out exact calculations. To illustrate, the authors considered a data example where the objective is to choose between nested nonlinear models.

14. For testing H_0: $\psi = \psi_0$ for the parameter of interest ψ in the presence of a nuisance parameter β, it is necessary to choose priors under the null and alternative hypotheses to compute a Bayes factor. Kass and Wasserman (1995) noted that the prior distribution on ψ under H_1 can be interpreted that "the amount of information in the prior on ψ is equal to the amount of information about ψ contained in one observation." After transforming β to be null orthogonal to ψ, it is suggested to take the marginal priors on β to be equal under the null and alternative hypotheses. Correspondingly, taking the prior on ψ to be normal, the log of the Bayes factor can be approximated with an error of order $O_p(n^{-1/2})$ instead of the usual error of order $O_p(1)$ by the Schwarz criterion (also known as the Bayes information criterion [BIC]). Therefore, the Schwarz

taken from Dawid and Skene (1979), which contain information reflecting the state of health of each patient.

24. Gönen et al. (2005) presented a Bayesian formulation of the pooled-variance two-sample *t*-statistic in the two-sided point null testing problem, which is easy to apply in practice. The authors identified a reasonable and useful prior giving a closed-form Bayes factor that can be written in terms of the distribution of the two-sample *t*-statistic under the null and alternative hypotheses, respectively. The priors are easy to use and simple to elicit, and the posterior probabilities are easily computed. The authors illustrated with a subset of the data shown by Lyle et al. (1987), which consists of blood pressure measurements on a subgroup of 21 African American subjects, 10 of whom have taken calcium supplements and 11 of whom have taken placebo.

25. Taplin (2005) proposed a new robust Bayes factor for comparing two linear models based on a pseudomodel for outliers. This Bayes factor uses a single robustness parameter to describe a priori belief in the likelihood of outliers and is more robust to outliers than the one based on the variance-inflation model for outliers. When an observation is considered an outlier for both models, the robust Bayes factor proposed by Taplin (2005) equals the Bayes factor with the outlier removed. When only one model considers an observation to be an outlier, the Bayes factor ignoring this observation should be used, but only after the application of a fixed penalty determined by the prior probability of outliers to this model for its inconsistency. For moderate outliers where the variance-inflation model is suitable, the two Bayes factors are similar. Taplin's Bayes factor employs a single robustness parameter to describe an a priori belief in the likelihood of outliers. The author illustrated the properties of the new robust Bayes factor with real and synthetic data, and highlighted the inferior properties of Bayes factors based on the variance-inflation model for outliers.

26. Emerson et al. (2005) described the evaluation of the Bayesian operating characteristics of the sequential stopping rule (see Chapter 13 for details). In particular, the authors considered a choice of probability models and a family of prior distributions that permits a concise demonstration of Bayesian properties for a specified sampling plan. The authors illustrated their approach in the context of a randomized, double-blind, placebo-controlled clinical trial of an antibody to endotoxin in the treatment of gram-negative sepsis, where a maximum of 1700 patients with proven gram-negative sepsis were to be randomly assigned in a 1:1 ratio to receive a single dose of antibody to endotoxin or placebo and the primary endpoint for this trial was the 28-day mortality rate.

27. Ashby (2006) reviewed the state of Bayesian thinking, mainly its pertinence, uses, and growth in medical analysis, in the context of major developments in Bayesian thinking and computation, referring to important books, landmark conferences, and seminal papers. Bayesian approaches have currently penetrated most of the foremost components of medical statistics, including clinical trials, epidemiology, meta-analyses and evidence synthesis, spatial modeling, longitudinal modeling, survival modeling, molecular genetics, and decision making with respect to most recent technologies.

28. The Bayes factor is very useful for evaluating sets of inequality and equality constrained models. For a constrained model with the encompassing model,

the Bayes factor reduces to the ratio of two proportions of the encompassing prior and posterior in agreement with the constraints, which enables simple estimation of the Bayes factor and the Monte Carlo error. In this context, the matter of sensitivity to model-specific prior distributions reduces to sensitivity to the prior for the encompassing model. Klugkist and Hoijtink (2007) showed that the Bayes factors for the constrained model with the unconstrained model is independent of the encompassing prior in the context of specific classes of inequality constrained models. To illustrate, the author investigated the data coming from an experiment to study the weight gain of 40 rats fed different diets, distinguished by both source and amount of proteins (Snedecor and Cochran 1967).

29. To testing the goodness of fit in multinomial models, Spezzaferri et al. (2007) proposed the application of the generalized fractional Bayes factor, a nonasymptotic method that can be used to quantify the evidence for or against a submodel. The expressions for the generalized fractional Bayes factor were presented, and the authors showed that the generalized fractional Bayes factor yields better properties than the fractional Bayes factor. To illustrate the use of the method, the author considered the following two examples: (a) the two equicorrelation models, $M_1: X|p \sim N(0, (1 - p)I + pJ)$ and $M_2: X|p, \mu \sim N(\mu 1, (1 - p)I + pJ)$, where the value of the correlation p is assumed to be known and the only unknown parameter is the mean μ in M_2, and (b) the case of model comparison with dependent data, where the generalized fractional Bayes factor appears to have more reasonable performance than that of the fractional Bayes factor.

30. In the context of receiver operating characteristic (ROC) curve (see Chapter 8 for details) estimation, Branscum et al. (2008) developed a novel Bayesian semiparametric modeling framework involving mixtures of Pólya trees for screening data with the dual purpose of diagnosing infection or disease status and assessing the accuracy of continuous diagnostic measures. In this framework, the authors derived the following results: (a) predictive probabilities of "disease" based on continuous diagnostic test outcomes in conjunction with other information, including relevant covariates and results from one or more independent binary diagnostic tests, and (b) characterization of diagnostic performance measures of continuous tests by estimating ROC curves and area under the curve, primarily when such extra information is available. To illustrate, the authors investigated the following examples: (a) the modeling of a serum enzyme-linked immunosorbent assay (ELISA) procedure for detecting antibodies to an infectious agent when used in conjunction with culture for antigen detection and (b) the data from an animal health survey for Johne's disease, where the performance of a serum ELISA was evaluated using additional information obtained from fecal culture.

31. After examining the consistency, interpretation, and application of Bayes factors constructed from standard test statistics, Johnson (2008) concluded that Bayes factors based on multinomial and normal test statistics are consistent for suitable choices of the hyperparameters (i.e., parameters of the prior distribution) used to specify alternative hypotheses, and that such constructions can be extended to obtain consistent Bayes factors based on likelihood ratio statistics. The Bayes factors based on F-statistics are closely connected to parametric Bayes factors based on normal-inverse gamma models. And similarly, Bayes factors based on chi-square statistics for multinomial data approximate accurately to Bayes factors based on multinomial or Dirichlet models. In order to illustrate how the

7.7.3 Bayes Factor Test is an Integrated Most Powerful Decision Rule

Suppose we have data points $x_1, \ldots, x_n$, then the Bayes Factor to test for H_0: $\theta = \theta_0$ vs. H_1: $\theta \neq \theta_0$, where θ is a parameter of a data density function f, can be defined as

$$B_n = \frac{\int f(x_1, \ldots, x_n \mid \theta_1)\pi(\theta_1)d\theta_1}{f(x_1, \ldots, x_n \mid \theta_0)}$$

with known θ_0 and π that is a prior density function of the unknown alternative parameter θ_1. Taking into account the inequality $(A - B)[I(A \geq B) - \delta] \geq 0$, where δ could be either 0 or 1, described in Section 7.7.1, we define $A = B_n$, $B = C$ (a test threshold: the event $\{B_n > C\}$ states to rejects H_0) and δ that represents a rejection rule of *any* test statistic based on the observations: if $\delta = 1$ we reject the null hypothesis. Then

$$E_{H_0}\left(B_n I(B_n \geq C)\right) - C E_{H_0} I(B_n \geq C) \geq E_{H_0}\left(B_n \delta - C\delta\right),$$

$$E_{H_0}\left(B_n I(B_n \geq C)\right) - C\Pr_{H_0}\{B_n \geq C\} \geq E_{H_0}\left(B_n \delta\right) - C\Pr_{H_0}\{\delta = 1\}.$$

Since we control the Type I error rate of the tests to be $\Pr\{\text{Test rejects } H_0 \mid H_1\} = \alpha$, we have

$$E_{H_0}(B_n I(B_n \geq C)) \geq E_{H_0}(B_n \delta).$$

Thus

$$\int \frac{\int f(x \mid \theta_1)\pi(\theta_1)d\theta_1}{f(x \mid \theta_0)} f(x \mid \theta_0) I(B_n \geq C)dx \geq \int \frac{\int f(x \mid \theta_1)\pi(\theta_1)d\theta_1}{f(x \mid \theta_0)} f(x \mid \theta_0)\delta(x)dx.$$

That is,

$$\int\int f(x \mid \theta_1)\pi(\theta_1)d\theta_1 I\{B_n \geq C\}dx \geq \int\int f(x \mid \theta_1)\pi(\theta_1)d\theta_1 I\{\delta(x) = 1\}dx$$

which further implies,

$$\int\int f(x \mid \theta_1)I(B_n \geq C)dx\pi(\theta_1)\theta_1 \geq \int\int f(x \mid \theta_1)\delta(x)dx\pi(\theta_1)d\theta_1.$$

This concludes that

$$\int \Pr\{B_n \text{ rejects } H_0 \mid H_1 \text{ with the alternative parameter } \theta_1\}\pi(\theta_1)\theta_1$$

$$\geq \int \Pr\{\delta \text{ rejects } H_0 \mid H_1 \text{ with the alternative parameter } \theta_1\}\pi(\theta_1)\theta_1$$

8

Fundamentals of Receiver Operating Characteristic Curve Analyses

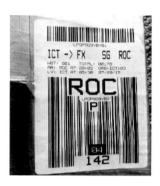

8.1 Introduction

Receiver operating characteristic (ROC) curve analysis is a popular tool for visualizing, organizing, and selecting classifiers based on their classification accuracy. The ROC curve methodology was originally developed during World War II to analyze classification accuracy in differentiating signal from noise in radar detection (Lusted 1971). Recently, the methodology has been extensively adapted to medical areas heavily dependent on screening and diagnostic tests (Lloyd 1998; Pepe 2000a, 2000b, 2003; Zhou and Mcclish 2002), in particular radiology (Eng 2005; O'Malley et al. 2001; Obuchowski 2003), bioinformatics (Lasko et al. 2005), epidemiology (Green and Swets 1966; Shapiro 1999), and laboratory testing (Campbell 1994). For example, in laboratory diagnostic tests, which are central in the practice of modern medicine, common uses of ROC-based methods include screening a specific population for evidence of disease and confirming or ruling out a tentative diagnosis in an individual patient, where the interpretation of a diagnostic test result depends on the ability of the test to distinguish between diseased and nondiseased subjects. In cardiology, diagnostic testing and ROC curve analysis play a fundamental role in clinical practice, for example, while using serum markers to predict myocardial necrosis and using cardiac imaging tests to diagnose heart disease. ROC curves are increasingly used in the machine learning field, due in part to the realization that simple classification accuracy is often a poor standard for measuring performance (Provost and Fawcett 1997). In addition to being a generally useful graphical method to visualize classification accuracy, ROC curves have properties that make them especially useful for domains with skewed discriminating distributions or unequal classification error costs. These characteristics have become increasingly important as research continues into the areas of cost-sensitive learning and learning in the presence of unbalanced classes (Fawcett 2006).

ROC analysis can also be applied generally for evaluating the accuracy of goodness of fit of a statistical model (e.g., logistic regression and linear discriminant analysis) that classifies subjects into two categories, such as diseased or nondiseased. For example, in cardiovascular research, predictive modeling to evaluate expected outcomes, such as mortality or adverse cardiac events, as functions of patient risk characteristics is common. In this setting, ROC analysis is very useful in terms of sorting out important risk factors from less important risk factors.

The ROC technique has been widely used in disease classification with low-dimensional biomarkers because (1) it does not assume a parametric form of the class probability as required, for example, in the logistic regression method; (2) it accommodates case-control designs; and (3) it allows treating false positives and false negatives in an efficient and relatively simple manner.

8.2 ROC Curve Inference

Assume, without loss of generality, that $X_1, ..., X_m$ and $Y_1, ..., Y_n$ are independent and identically distributed (i.i.d.) observations from diseased and nondiseased populations, respectively, and let F and G denote the corresponding cumulative distribution functions of X and Y. The ROC curve $R(t)$ is defined as $R(t) = 1-F(G^{-1}(1-t))$, where $t \in [0,1]$ (Pepe 1997). The ROC curve is a plot of sensitivity (the true positive rate, $1-F(t)$) against 1 minus specificity (the true negative rate, $1-G(t)$) for various values of the threshold t. Note that the ROC curve is a special case of a probability–probability plot (P–P plot). In the definition of $R(t)$, the function G^{-1} defines the inverse function of G, that is, $G^{-1}(t) : G(G^{-1}(t)) = t$. As an example, we consider three biomarkers with their corresponding ROC curves presented in Figure 8.1, where underlying distributions are $F_1 \sim N(0,1)$, $G_1 \sim N(0,1)$ for biomarker A (diagonal line); $F_2 \sim N(0,1)$, $G_2 \sim N(1,1)$ for biomarker B (dashed line); and $F_3 \sim N(0,1)$, $G_3 \sim N(10,1)$ for biomarker C (dotted line), respectively.

The following R code is used to plot the ROC curve, as shown in Figure 8.1.

```
> t<-seq(0,1,0.001)
> R1<-1-pnorm(qnorm(1-t,0,1),0,1)  # biomarker 1
> R2<-1-pnorm(qnorm(1-t,1,1),0,1)  # biomarker 2
> R3<-1-pnorm(qnorm(1-t,10,1),0,1)  # biomarker 3
> plot(R1,t,type="l",lwd=1.5,lty=1,cex.lab=1.1,ylab="Sensitivity",
  xlab="1-Specificity")
> lines(R2,t,lwd=1.5,lty=2)
> lines(R3,t,lwd=1.5,lty=3)
```

It can be seen that the farther apart the two distributions F and G are in terms of location, the more the ROC curve shifts to the top left corner. A near perfect biomarker would have a ROC curve coming close to the top left corner, and a biomarker without any discriminability would result in a ROC curve that is a diagonal line from the points (0,0) to (1,1).

There exists extensive research on estimating ROC curves from the parametric and nonparametric perspectives (Hsieh and Turnbull 1996; Pepe 1997; Wieand et al. 1989). Assuming both the diseased and nondiseased populations are normally distributed, i.e., $F \sim N(\mu_1, \sigma_1^2)$ and $G \sim N(\mu_2, \sigma_2^2)$, the corresponding ROC curve can be expressed as

$$R(t) = \Phi(a + b\Phi^{-1}(t)),$$

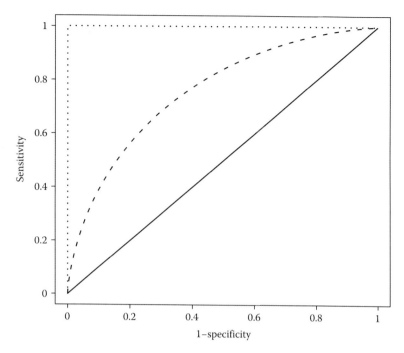

FIGURE 8.1
ROC curves related to the biomarkers. The solid diagonal line corresponds to the ROC curve of biomarker A, where $F_1 \sim N(0,1)$ and $G_1 \sim N(0,1)$. The dashed line displays the ROC curve of biomarker B, where $F_2 \sim N(0,1)$ and $G_2 \sim N(1,1)$. The dotted line close to the upper left corner plots the ROC curve for biomarker C, where $F_3 \sim N(0,1)$ and $G_3 \sim N(10,1)$.

where $a = (\mu_1 - \mu_2)/\sigma_1$, $b = \sigma_2/\sigma_1$, and Φ is the standard normal cumulative distribution function. This is oftentimes referred to as the binormal ROC curve. In this case the estimated ROC curve is obtained by substituting the maximum likelihood estimators (MLEs) of the normal parameters μ_1, μ_2, σ_1, and σ_2 into the formula above. The nonparametric estimation of the ROC curve incorporates empirical distribution functions (Hsieh and Turnbull 1996; Wieand et al. 1989) in place of their parametric counterparts. Toward this end, define the empirical distribution function of F as

$$\hat{F}_m(t) = \frac{1}{m} \sum_{i=1}^{m} I\{X_i \le t\},$$

where $I\{\cdot\}$ denotes the indicator function. The empirical distribution function $\hat{G}_n$ of G can be defined similarly. Estimating F and G by their corresponding empirical estimates $\hat{F}_m$ and $\hat{G}_n$, respectively, gives the empirical estimator of the ROC curve as

$$\hat{R}(t) = 1 - \hat{F}_m\left(\hat{G}_n^{-1}(1-t)\right),$$

which can be shown theoretically to converge to $R(t)$ for large sample sizes n and m (Hsieh and Turnbull 1996).

Figure 8.2 presents the nonparametric estimators of the ROC curves based on data related to generated values ($n = m = 1000$) of the three biomarkers described with respect to Figure 8.1, that is, $F_1 \sim N(0,1)$, $G_1 \sim N(0,1)$ for biomarker A (diagonal line); $F_2 \sim N(0,1)$, $G_2 \sim N(1,1)$ for biomarker B (dashed line); and $F_3 \sim N(0,1)$, $G_3 \sim N(10,1)$ for biomarker C (dotted line), respectively, using the following R code:

```
> if(!("pROC" %in% rownames(installed.packages()))) install.
  packages("pROC")
> library(pROC)
> n<-1000
> set.seed(123) # set the seed
> # Simulate data from the normal distribution
> X1<-rnorm(n,0,1)
> Y1<-rnorm(n,1,1)
> group<-cbind(rep(1,n),rep(0,n))
> measures<-c(X1,Y1)
> roc1<-roc(group, measures)
> plot(1-roc1$specificities,roc1$sensitivities,type="l",ylab="Sensitivity",xl
  ab="1-Specificity")
> abline(a=0,b=1,col="grey") # add the diagonal line for reference
```

It should be noted that for large sample sizes, the ROC curves are well approximated by the nonparametric estimators.

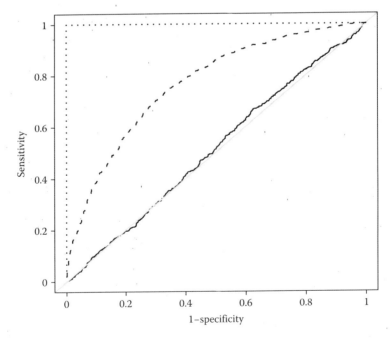

FIGURE 8.2
Nonparametric estimators of the ROC curves related to three different biomarkers based on 1000 data points. The solid diagonal line corresponds to the nonparametric estimator of the ROC curve of biomarker A, where $F_1 \sim N(0,1)$ and $G_1 \sim N(0,1)$. The dashed line displays the nonparametric estimator of the ROC curve of biomarker B, where $F_2 \sim N(0,1)$ and $G_2 \sim N(1,1)$. The dotted line close to the upper left corner plots the nonparametric estimator of the ROC curve for biomarker C, where $F_3 \sim N(0,1)$ and $G_3 \sim N(10,1)$.

In health-related studies, the ROC curve methodology is commonly related to case-control studies. As a type of observational study, case-control studies differentiate and compare two existing groups differing in outcome on the basis of some supposed causal attributes. For example, based on factors that may contribute to a medical condition, subjects can be grouped as cases (subjects with a condition or disease) and controls (subjects without the condition or disease); for example, cases could be subjects with breast cancer and controls may be healthy subjects. For independent populations, for example, cases and controls, various parametric and nonparametric approaches have been proposed to evaluate the performance of biomarkers (Bamber 1975; Hsieh and Turnbull 1996; McIntosh and Pepe 2002; Metz et al. 1998; Pepe 1997; Pepe and Thompson 2000; Wieand et al. 1989).

8.3 Area under the ROC Curve

A rough idea of the performance of a set of biomarkers, in terms of their diagnostic accuracy, can be obtained through visual examination of the ROC curve. However, judgments based solely on visual inspection of the ROC curve are far from enough to precisely describe the diagnostic accuracy of biomarkers. The area under the ROC curve (AUC) is a common summary index of the diagnostic accuracy of a binary biomarker. The AUC measures the ability of the marker to discriminate between the case and control groups (Pepe McIntosh and Pepe 2002; Pepe and Thompson 2000). Bamber (1975) noted that the area under this curve is equal to $\Pr(X > Y)$. A proof of this result is contained in the appendix. Values of the AUC can range from 0.5, in the case of no differentiation between the case and control distributions, to 1, where the case and control distributions are perfectly separated. For more details, see Kotz et al. (2003) for wide discussions regarding evaluations of the AUC-type objectives.

8.3.1 Parametric Approach

Under binormal assumptions, where for the diseased population $X \sim N\left(\mu_1, \sigma_1^2\right)$ and for the nondiseased population $Y \sim N\left(\mu_2, \sigma_2^2\right)$, a closed form of the AUC is presented as

$$A = \Phi\left(\frac{\mu_1 - \mu_2}{\sqrt{\sigma_1^2 + \sigma_2^2}}\right)$$

(Metz et al. 1998; Wieand et al. 1989). The index $A \geq 0.5$ when $\mu_1 \geq \mu_2$. We provide the proof of the AUC formula in the appendix. By substituting maximum likelihood estimators for μ_i and σ_i^2, $i = 1,2$, into the above formula, the maximum likelihood estimator of the AUC can be obtained directly. Given the estimator of the AUC under binormal distributional assumptions, one can easily construct large sample confidence interval-based tests for the AUC using the delta method; see Kotz et al. (2003) for details. For nonnormal data, a transformation of observations to normality may first be applied, for example, the Box–Cox transformation (Box and Cox 1964), prior to the parametric ROC approach being applied. In general, when data distributions are assumed to have parametric forms different than the normal distribution function for F and G, the AUC can be expressed as $\Pr(X > Y) = \int G(x)dF(x)$ and evaluated, in a similar manner to the technique above (e.g., Kotz et al. 2003).

Example 8.1: Bi-Normal ROC Curve Estimation

Assume that biomarker levels were measured from diseased and healthy populations, with i.i.d. observations $X_1 = 0.39$, $X_2 = 1.97$, $X_3 = 1.03$, and $X_4 = 0.16$, which are assumed to be from a normal distribution $N(\mu_1, \sigma_1^2)$, and i.i.d. observations $Y_1 = 0.42$, $Y_2 = 0.29$, $Y_3 = 0.56$, $Y_4 = -0.68$, and $Y_5 = -0.54$, which are assumed to be from a normal distribution $N(\mu_2, \sigma_2^2)$, respectively. In this case, the maximum likelihood estimators of the normal parameters are $\hat{\mu}_1 = 0.8875$, $\hat{\mu}_2 = 0.01$, $\hat{\sigma}_1^2 = 0.4922$, and $\hat{\sigma}_2^2 = 0.2655$. Based on the definition described in Section 8.2, $\hat{a} = (\hat{\mu}_1 - \hat{\mu}_2)/\hat{\sigma}_1 = 1.251$, $\hat{b} = \hat{\sigma}_2/\hat{\sigma}_1 = 0.734$, and therefore the ROC curve can be estimated as $\hat{R}(t) = \Phi(\hat{a} + \hat{b}\Phi^{-1}(t)) = \Phi(1.251 + 0.734\Phi^{-1}(t))$. The AUC can be estimated as $\hat{A} = \Phi((\hat{\mu}_1 - \hat{\mu}_2)/\sqrt{\hat{\sigma}_1^2 + \hat{\sigma}_2^2}) = 0.8433$, which summarizes the discriminating ability of the biomarker with respect to the disease. The interpretation of the AUC is that this particular marker accurately predicts a case to be a case and a control to be control 84% of the time, and that 16% of the time the marker will misclassify the groupings.

8.3.2 Nonparametric Approach

Conversely, a nonparametric estimator of the AUC based on continual biomarker values can be obtained as

$$\hat{A} = \frac{1}{mn} \sum_{i=1}^{m} \sum_{j=1}^{n} I(X_i > Y_j),$$

where X_i, $i = 1, ..., m$ and Y_j, $j = 1, ..., n$ are the observations for diseased and nondiseased populations, respectively (Zhou et al. 2011). It is equivalent to the well-known Mann–Whitney statistic, and the variance of this empirical estimator can be obtained using U-statistic theory (Serfling 2009). The empirical likelihood method to construct the confidence interval estimation of the AUC was introduced by Qin and Zhou (2006). Replacing the indicator function by a kernel function, one can obtain a smoothed ROC curve (Zou et al. 1997).

Example 8.2: Nonparametric ROC Curve Estimation

Biomarker levels were measured from diseased and healthy populations, providing i.i.d. observations $X_1 = 0.39$, $X_2 = 1.97$, $X_3 = 1.03$, and $X_4 = 0.16$, which are assumed to be from a continuous distribution, and i.i.d. observations $Y_1 = 0.42$, $Y_2 = 0.29$, $Y_3 = 0.56$, $Y_4 = -0.68$, and $Y_5 = -0.54$, which are also assumed to be from a continuous distribution, respectively. In this case, the empirical estimates of the distribution functions F and G have the forms $\hat{F}_4(t) = \frac{1}{4}\sum_{i=1}^{4} I(X_i < t)$ and $\hat{G}_5(t) = \frac{1}{5}\sum_{j=1}^{5} I(Y_j < t)$, respectively, and the empirical estimate of the ROC curve is $\hat{R}(t) = 1 - \hat{F}_4(\hat{G}_5^{-1}(1-t))$. The AUC can be estimated as $\hat{A} = \frac{1}{4 \times 5}\sum_{i=1}^{4}\sum_{j=1}^{5} I(X_i > Y_j) = 0.75$, suggesting a moderate discriminating ability of the biomarker with respect to discriminating the disease population from the healthy population. Note that in this case, the nonparametric estimator of the AUC is smaller than the estimator of the AUC under the normal assumption. For such a small data set used in our examples, the difference in AUC estimates is likely due more to the discreteness of the nonparametric method than any real difference between the approaches.

8.3.3 Nonparametric Comparison of Two ROC Curves

It is oftentimes of great importance for researchers to compare the discriminating ability of two biomarkers or even different diagnostic tests. If we use both diagnostic markers on the same m controls and n cases, we can represent the bivariate outcomes as (X_{1j}, X_{2j}) $(j = 1, ..., m)$ and (Y_{1k}, Y_{2k}) $(k = 1, ..., n)$, respectively. We denote the respective bivariate distributions as $F(x_1, x_2)$ and $G(y_1, y_2)$, and the marginal distributions as $F_i(x_i)$ and $G_i(y_i)$, $i = 1,2$, respectively, and we assume that the $m + n$ bivariate vectors are mutually independent. Denote the sensitivity value on the ROC curve at specificity p by $S_i(p)$, $i = 1,2$, and define

$$\Delta = \int \left(S_1(p) - S_2(p) \right) dW(p), \; S_i(p) = 1 - G_i\left(F_i^{-1}(p) \right),$$

where W is a probability measure on the open unit interval. The parameter Δ allows one to compare sensitivities on a pre-defined range of specificities of clinical interest by adjusting the weight function W accordingly. When $W(p)$ is the uniform distribution on $(0,1)$, the parameter Δ equals the difference of AUCs between two biomarkers.

Wieand et al. (1989) considered a nonparametric estimate of Δ in the form of

$$\hat{\Delta} = \int \left(\hat{S}_1(p) - \hat{S}_2(p) \right) dW(p),$$

where $\hat{S}_i(p) = 1 - \hat{G}_i\left(\hat{\xi}_{ip} \right)$, $\hat{G}_i$ is the empirical distribution of G_i and the sample quantile $\hat{\xi}_{ip}$ is the $[mp]$th order statistic among the m values of X_i, where $[mp]$ is the smallest integer that equals or exceeds mp. Assume that W is a probability measure in $(0,1)$ and that there exists $\varepsilon > 0$ such that W has a bounded derivative in $(0, \varepsilon)$ and $(1- \varepsilon, 1)$. Suppose further that $G_i(\xi_{ip})$, for $i = 1,2, ...,$ has continuous derivatives in $(0,1)$, which are monotone in $(0, \varepsilon)$ and $(1- \varepsilon, 1)$. Define $s_i(p) = S_i'(p) = -G_i'(\xi_{ip})/F_i'(\xi_{ip})$. Then, as $N = n + m$ tends to ∞ with $m/N \to \lambda$, for $0 < \lambda < 1$, $N^{1/2}(\hat{\Delta} - \Delta)$ tends to a normal distribution with variance $\sigma^2 = \sigma_{11} - 2\sigma_{12} + \sigma_{22}$, where

$$\sigma_{ii} = \int_0^1 \int_0^1 \left\{ (1-\lambda)^{-1} S_i\left(\max(p, q) \right) \left(1 - S_i\left(\min(p, q) \right) \right) \right.$$

$$\left. + \lambda^{-1} s_i(p) s_i(q) \left(\min(p, q) - pq \right) \right\} dW(p) dW(q),$$

and

$$\sigma_{12} = \int \int \left[G\left(\xi_{1p}, \xi_{2q} \right) - \left\{ 1 - S_1(p) \right\} \left\{ 1 - S_2(q) \right\} \right] dW(p) \, dW(q) / (1 - \lambda)$$

$$+ \int \int \left\{ F\left(\xi_{1p}, \xi_{2q} \right) - pq \right\} s_1(p) s_2(q) \, dW(p) \, dW(q) / \lambda.$$

Based on this asymptotic distribution of $\hat{\Delta}$, one can employ a nonparametric procedure for testing $H_0 : \Delta = 0$ versus $H_1 : \Delta > 0$. Note that the test proposed by Wieand et al. (1989) requires the estimation of densities, and selection of a satisfactory smoothing parameter may be problematic.

8.4 ROC Analysis and Logistic Regression: Comparison and Overestimation

In general, the discriminant ability of a continuous covariate, for example, a biomarker, can be considered based on logistic regression or the ROC curve methodology (Pepe and Thompson 2000). Logistic regression has been proposed for modeling the probability of disease given several test results (Richards et al. 1996). It is often used to find a linear combination of covariates that discriminates between two groups or populations, for example, diseased and nondiseased populations. Suppose we have a data set consisting of a binary outcome, $q \in \{0,1\}$, which indicates the membership of the individual, and m components in covariate vector z, including the intercept term $z_1 = 1$. Table 8.1 illustrates the connection between the ROC curve and logistic regression with a case-control study. Let X and Y represent the measurements of the biomarker in the case and control groups, respectively. Individuals in the case group ($q = 1$) have values of z given $q = 1$, that is, $X = z|q = 1$, while individuals in the control group ($q = 0$) have values of z given $q = 0$, that is, $Y = z|q = 0$.

The logistic regression models

$$\Pr\left(q = 1 \mid z\right) = \frac{e^{\beta^T z}}{1 + e^{\beta^T z}},$$

where the vector β consists of parameters of the regression.

Logistic regression relies only on an assumption about the form of the conditional probability for disease given the covariate vector z and does not require specification of the much more complex joint distribution of the covariate vector z.

It can be emphasized that logistic regression focuses on $\Pr(q = 1|z)$ and the covariant z is assumed to be fixed, whereas the ROC curve methodology attends to $\Pr(z|q)$ and z is assumed to be a random variable. Logistic regression can be used in the ROC modeling context as a dimension reduction tool.

In this section, we present the fact that using the same data to fit both the discriminant score and its estimate to its ROC curve leads to an overly optimistic estimate of the

TABLE 8.1

Outcome Levels and Biomarker Values z, where X and Y Represent Values of Measurements of the Biomarker in the Case and Control Groups, respectively

Class	z (Biomarker Values)
Case ($q - 1$)	$X - z \mid q - 1$ (values of z given $q = 1$)
Control ($q = 0$)	$Y = z \mid q = 0$ (values of z given $q = 0$)

accuracy of the test compared to how the model would perform on samples of future cases (Copas and Corbett 2002). In general, for large studies data are split into *training* samples and *validation* samples. The training sample is used to fit the model, and the validation sample is used to assess the performance of the model fit relative to how it would function on a future set of patients. This is discussed further below.

The ROC curve is a standard way of illustrating and evaluating the performance of a discriminant score or screening marker. Let s be such a score, for example, $s = \beta^T z$, where z is the covariate vector. And we have two groups or populations indexed by the binary outcome $q \in \{0,1\}$, which represents the membership of the diseased or nondiseased populations. Then threshold u gives the false positive rate

$$F_0(u) = \Pr(s \geq u \mid q = 0)$$

and the true positive rate

$$F_1(u) = \Pr(s \geq u \mid q = 1)$$

The ROC curve, R, is the graph of $F_1(u)$ against $F_0(u)$ as u ranges over all possible values,

$$R = \{(F_1(u), F_0(u)), -\infty < u < +\infty\}.$$

It is important to recognize that an empirical ROC curve, such as that shown in Figure 8.2, is a retrospective calculation, using the same data to estimate the score and assess its performance. What we really want to know is how well this particular score would perform if it were to be adopted in practice. This would involve a prospective assessment of how well the score discriminates between future and independent cases with $q = 1$ and $q = 0$. Thus, we distinguish between the retrospective (training set) ROC, $\hat{R}(\hat{\beta})$, the curve with $s = \hat{\beta}^T z$ and with F_0 and F_1 taken as the empirical distributions of s in the sample, and the prospective (validation set) ROC, $R(\hat{\beta})$, the curve with the same score $s = \hat{\beta}^T z$ but with F_0 and F_1 taken as the true population distributions of s. The term *overestimation* in the title of this section refers to the difference

$$\hat{R}(\hat{\beta}) - R(\hat{\beta}),$$

where the difference between two curves denotes the curve of differences in vertical coordinates graphed against common values for the horizontal coordinate. In other words, this is the difference in true positive rates having chosen the thresholds to match the false positive rates. Typically, the term *overestimation* is positive; that is, the retrospective ROC gives an inflated assessment of the true performance of the score.

Consider the classifier $\hat{q} = 1$ if $\hat{\beta}^T z \geq u$ and $\hat{q} = 0$ if $\hat{\beta}^T z < u$. Then it is well known that the retrospective error rate, namely, the proportion of cases in the sample for which $\hat{q} \neq q$, is a downward biased estimate of the true prospective error rate, which would be obtained if the classifier $\hat{q}$ were to be applied to the whole population. Efron (1986a) derives an asymptotic approximation of the expected bias. Efron's formula is consistent with the approximation based on the ROC curve methodology, which we present in the following subsection.

8.4.1 Retrospective and Prospective ROC

Suppose we have a total sample size of n individuals with data (z_i, q_i), where q denotes the group membership as before and there are m components in covariate vector z, including the intercept term $z_1 = 1$. We assume throughout that the data fit well to the logistic regression model

$$\Pr(q = 1 \mid z) = \frac{e^{\beta^T z}}{1 + e^{\beta^T z}}.$$

Let $\hat{\beta}$ be the maximum likelihood estimator of β. Then, if we apply the scores $\hat{u} = \hat{\beta}^T z_i$ to the data against a threshold u, the observed proportions of false and true positives are

$$\hat{F}_0(u) = \frac{1}{n(1-\bar{q})} \sum_i H(\hat{u}_i - u)(1 - q_i), \quad \hat{F}_1(u) = \frac{1}{n\bar{q}} \sum_i H(\hat{u}_i - u)q_i,$$

respectively, where $\bar{q} = \sum q_i / n$ and H is the Heaviside function: $H(z) = 1$ if $z \geq 0$ and $H(z) = 0$ if $z < 0$. The sums in these and subsequent expressions run from 1 to n. The ROC curve $\hat{R} = \hat{R}(\hat{\beta})$ is then the graph of $\hat{F}_1(u)$ against $\hat{F}_0(u)$.

For the prospective ROC fit, suppose the random q's in these data are replicated a large number of times. Then, at each x_i, we expect a proportion p_i of replicated cases to have $q = 1$, where

$$p_i = \frac{e^{u_i}}{1 + e^{u_i}}, \; u_i = \beta^T z_i$$

If the scores $\hat{u}_i$ are applied to the replicated data against a threshold v, the future proportions of false and true positives are

$$F_0(v) = \frac{1}{n(1-\bar{p})} \sum_i H(\hat{u}_i - v)(1 - p_i), \quad F_1(v) = \frac{1}{n\bar{p}} \sum_i H(\hat{u}_i - v)p_i,$$

where $\bar{p} = \sum p_i / n$. Then $R = R(\hat{\beta})$ is the graph of $F_1(v)$ and $F_0(v)$.

8.4.2 Expected Bias of the ROC Curve and Overestimation of the AUC

To simplify the notation, let $\varepsilon_i = q_i - p_i$, $H_i = H(\hat{u}_i - u)$, and $H_i^* = H(\hat{u}_i - v)$. Then we can obtain

$$\bar{q} = \bar{p} + \bar{\varepsilon},$$

and

$$n\{\hat{F}_0(u) - F_0(v)\} = \sum_i H_i \left(\frac{1 - p_i - \varepsilon_i}{1 - \bar{p} - \bar{\varepsilon}} - \frac{1 - p_i}{1 - \bar{p}} \right) - \frac{1}{1 - \bar{p}} \sum_i (H_i^* - H_i)(1 - p_i).$$

For large n, values of p_i will be close to p_u, the true value of $\Pr(y = 1|\beta^T z = u)$. Hence,

$$n\{\hat{F}_0(u) - F_0(v)\} \approx \sum_i H_i \left(\frac{1 - p_i - \varepsilon_i}{1 - \bar{p} - \bar{\varepsilon}} - \frac{1 - p_i}{1 - \bar{p}} \right) - \frac{1 - p_u}{1 - \bar{p}} \sum_i (H_i^* - H_i).$$

Similarly, we can obtain

$$n\{\hat{F}_1(u) - F_1(v)\} \approx \sum_i H_i \left(\frac{p_i + \varepsilon_i}{\bar{p} + \bar{\varepsilon}} - \frac{p_i}{\bar{p}} \right) - \frac{p_u}{\bar{p}} \sum_i (H_i^* - H_i).$$

Define v_u to be the value of v such that $n\{\hat{F}_0(u) - F_0(v)\} = 0$. We have

$$\hat{F}_1(u) - F_1(v_u) \approx n^{-1} \sum_i H_i A(i, u),$$

where

$$A(i, u) = \left(\frac{p_i + \varepsilon_i}{\bar{p} + \bar{\varepsilon}} - \frac{p_i}{\bar{p}} \right) - \frac{(1 - \bar{p}) p_u}{\bar{p}(1 - p_u)} \left(\frac{1 - p_i - \varepsilon_i}{1 - \bar{p} - \bar{\varepsilon}} - \frac{1 - p_i}{1 - \bar{p}} \right).$$

Note that $\bar{\varepsilon} = O_p(n^{-1/2})$. Let $\Omega = n^{-1} \sum_i p_i(1 - p_i) z_i z_i^T$ and $d_i^2 = z_i^T \Omega^{-1} z_i$; then we can obtain

$$S(u) = E\{\hat{F}_1(u) - F_1(v_u)\} = \frac{p_u}{n^{3/2} \bar{p}} \sum_i \left\{ d_i - \frac{1}{\bar{p}(1 - \bar{p}) d_i} \right\} \phi \left\{ \frac{n^{1/2}(u_i - u)}{d_i} \right\}.$$

The terms p_u and u_i on the right-hand side are functions of the true parameter vector β, and the terms d_i and $\bar{p}$ depend on p_i and hence are also functions of β. Estimating these in the obvious way using $\hat{\beta}$ gives the corresponding estimator $\hat{S}(u)$. The corrected ROC curve

$$R^* = \{\hat{F}_1(u) - \hat{S}(u), \hat{F}_0(u)\}$$

is an estimator of the ROC curve that would be obtained if the fitted score $\hat{\beta}^T z$ were to be validated on a large replicated sample. As expected, this indicates that this score discriminates between the two populations noticeably less well than the retrospective analysis seems to suggest.

The estimated AUC is

$$\int \hat{F}_1(u) d\hat{F}_0(u) = \frac{1}{n(1 - \bar{q})} \sum_j (1 - q_j) \hat{F}_1(\hat{u}_j).$$

Similar to the overestimation in the ROC curve described above, the overestimation in the AUC is

$$\int \{\hat{F}_1(u) - F_1(u_v)\} d\hat{F}_0(u) = \frac{1}{n(1 - \bar{q})} \sum_j (1 - q_j) \{\hat{F}_1(\hat{u}_j) - F_1(v_{\hat{u}_j})\}$$

$$= \frac{1}{n^2(1 - \bar{q})} \sum_{i,j} H(\hat{u}_i - \hat{u}_j)(1 - y_i) A(i, \hat{u}_j) \approx \frac{1}{2n^{5/2} \bar{p}(1 - \bar{p})} \sum_{i \neq j} p_i (1 - p_i) b_{ij} \phi \left\{ \frac{n^{1/2}(u_j - u_i)}{b_{ij}} \right\},$$

where $a_{ij} = (z_j - z_i)^T \Omega^{-1} z_i$, $b_{ij}^2 = a_{ij} + a_{ji} = (z_i - z_j)^T \Omega^{-1}(z_i - z_j)$. Therefore, the overestimation in the AUC is approximately

$$\frac{1}{n\bar{p}(1-\bar{p})} \bar{E}\Big[p_v (1 - p_v) f(u) \text{tr}\big\{ \Omega^{-1} \bar{\text{var}}(Z|U) \big\} \Big],$$

where $U = \beta^T Z$, and $\bar{E}(\cdot)$ denotes the empirical expectation over the empirical distribution of the sample covariate vectors $z_1, ..., z_n$. Note that the overestimation is again of the order $O(n^{-1})$. For more details see Copas and Corbett (2002).

Example 8.3: Study of TBARS and HDL

Consider a subset of the study sample, which consists of 25 individuals with myocardial infarction (diseased) and 35 controls (healthy). We would like to examine the discriminant ability of the biomarkers based on the AUC, that is, testing for H_0: AUC = 1/2 versus H_1: AUC ≠ 1/2, as well as based on the logistic regression, that is, testing for the coefficient, β, $H_0 : \beta = 0$ versus $H_1 : \beta \neq 0$.

Figures 8.3 and 8.4 present the histograms of measurements of thiobarbituric acid reactive substances (TBARS) and high-density lipoprotein (HDL) cholesterol levels in diseased (left panel) and healthy (right panel) individuals, respectively. The histograms demonstrate deviations from the normal distribution for both TBARS and HDL cholesterol measurements, and we will proceed to test for the AUC with the nonparametric method. As described in Section 8.3.2, a nonparametric estimator of the AUC is equivalent to the well-known Mann–Whitney statistic, which follows an asymptotic normal distribution, and the variance of this empirical estimator can be obtained using the U-statistic theory (Serfling 2009). Let $X_1, ..., X_m$ and $Y_1, ..., Y_n$ denote measurements from the nondiseased and diseased populations, respectively. Then the nonparametric estimator is $\hat{A} = \frac{1}{mn} \sum_{i=1}^{m} \sum_{j=1}^{n} I(X_i < Y_j)$. Let R_i be the rank of X_i's

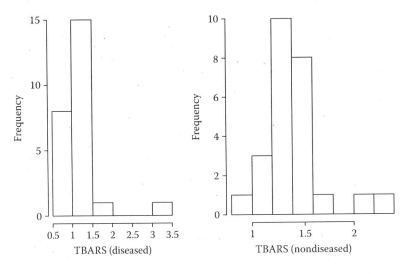

FIGURE 8.3
Histogram of measurements of TBARS in diseased (left) and healthy (right) individuals.

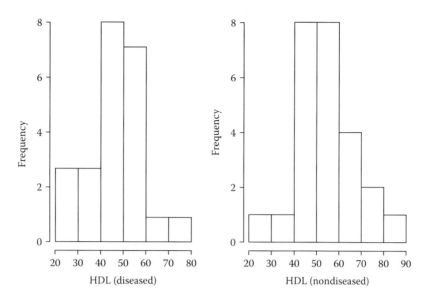

FIGURE 8.4
Histogram of measurements of HDL cholesterol levels in diseased (left) and healthy (right) individuals.

(the ith ordered value among X_i's) in the combined sample of X_i's and Y_j's, and S_j be the rank of Y_j's (the j th ordered value among Y_j's) in the combined sample of X_i's and Y_j's. Define

$$S_{10}^2 = \frac{1}{(m-1)n^2}\left[\sum_{i=1}^{m}(R_i - i)^2 - m\left(\frac{1}{m}\sum_{i=1}^{m}R_i - \frac{m+1}{2}\right)^2\right],$$

$$S_{01}^2 = \frac{1}{(n-1)m^2}\left[\sum_{j=1}^{n}(S_j - j)^2 - n\left(\frac{1}{n}\sum_{j=1}^{n}S_i - \frac{n+1}{2}\right)^2\right].$$

Then the estimated variance of this empirical estimator of the AUC is

$$S^2 = \left(\frac{mS_{01}^2 + nS_{10}^2}{m+n}\right)\bigg/\left(\frac{mn}{m+n}\right).$$

Based on the asymptotic normal distribution of the empirical estimator of the AUC, the p-value can be easily obtained and the 95% confidence interval of the AUC is $[\hat{A} - 1.96S, \hat{A} + 1.96S]$. The test for $H_0 : \beta = 0$ versus $H_1 : \beta \neq 0$ is based on the asymptotic distribution of the estimated coefficient β from the logistic regression fit (Hosmer and Lemeshow 2004). It should be noted that the test $H_0 : \beta = 0$ versus $H_1 : \beta \neq 0$ is one of association, which is a less stringent measure than prediction.

For the sample of TBARS, the p-value based on the asymptotic normality of the empirical AUC is 0.032, suggesting a significant discriminant ability of TBARS between the diseased and nondiseased populations. In this case, the p-value of the testing for the coefficient in the logistic regression is 0.077, concluding an insignificant discriminant ability of TBARS between the diseased and nondiseased populations. As for the sample of HDL, the p-value based on the asymptotic normality of the empirical AUC is 0.333, suggesting an insignificant discriminant ability of HDL between the diseased and nondiseased populations, while the p-value of the testing for the coefficient in the logistic regression is 0.037, concluding a significant discriminant ability of HDL between the diseased and nondiseased populations.

The R code to implement the procedures is presented below:

```
> # empirical AUC (Mann-Whitney stat)
> # returns p-value for H_0: AUC=1/2 versus H_1: AUC!=1/2
> AUC.pval<-function(x,y) {
+ m<-length(x)
+ n<-length(y)
+ x<-sort(x)
+ y<-sort(y)
+ rankall<-rank(c(x,y))
+ R<-rankall[1:m]
+ S<-rankall[-c(1:m)] # ranks of y
+
+ S10<-1/((m-1)*n^2)*(sum((R-1:m)^2)-m*(mean(R)-(m+1)/2)^2)
+ S01<-1/((n-1)*m^2)*(sum((S-1:n)^2)-n*(mean(S)-(n+1)/2)^2)
+ S2<-(m*S10+n*s2)/(m+n)
+
+ a<-wilcox.test(y,x)$statistic/(n*m)
+ AUC<-ifelse(a>=0.5,a,1-a) # empirical AUC
+ pval<- as.numeric(2*(1-pnorm(abs(AUC-0.5)/sqrt(S2/(m*n/(m+n))))))
+ return(pval)
+ }
>
> # logistic regression
> logistic.pval<-function(x,y){
+ if (!is.null(ncol(x))) {
+   Z<-rbind(x,y)
+   m<-nrow(x)
+   n<-nrow(y)
+ } else{
+   Z<-c(x,y)
+   m<-length(x)
+   n<-length(y)
+ }
+ q<-c(rep(0,m),rep(1,n))
+ newdata<-data.frame(cbind(q,Z))
+ glm.out = glm(q ~Z, family=binomial(logit), data=newdata)
+ return(summary(glm.out)$coef[-1,c(1,4)])
+ }
>
> # "tbars", AUC
> tbars.x<-c(1.350,1.143,1.043,1.209,1.034,1.509,1.509,1.336,1.085,1.117,
  1.256,1.440,1.139,1.531,1.171,0.930,0.928,1.374,1.719,0.970,0.950,
  1.324,1.509,1.509,0.918)
> tbars.y<-c(1.613,1.553,1.062,1.894,1.498,1.199,1.109,1.558,1.105,1.667,
  1.347,1.295,1.131,1.349,1.109,1.472,1.558,1.635,3.239,1.285,1.539,
  1.023,1.066,1.650,1.062)
> (AUC.p<-AUC.pval(tbars.x,tbars.y))
[1] 0.04486497
> (log.p<-logistic.pval(tbars.x,tbars.y)[2])
 Pr(>|z|)
0.06346792
>
> # "hdl", logistic
> hdl.x<-c(52.8,52.8,33.0,79.2,61.6,50.6,44.0,22.0,37.4,50.6,35.2,61.6,
  35.2,44.0,39.6,57.2,35.2,24.2,35.2,44.0,55.0,41.8,30.8,37.4,48.4)
> hdl.y<-c(50.6,35.2,50.6,70.4,28.6,83.6,52.8,39.6,37.4,30.8,33.0,44.0,
  44.0,74.8,72.6,74.8,46.2,57.2,68.2,57.2,33.0,66.0,85.8,85.8,41.8)
```

```
> (AUC.p<-AUC.pval(hdl.x,hdl.y))
[1] 0.06127496
> (log.p<-logistic.pval(hdl.x,hdl.y)[2])
 Pr(>|z|)
0.03493672
```

Example 8.4

In a manner similar to that of the previous example, we conducted 10,000 Monte Carlo simulations to evaluate the discriminant ability of the biomarkers in terms of testing for H_0 : AUC = 1/2 versus H_1: AUC ≠ 1/2 relative to the powers based on the logistic regression in terms of testing for the coefficient, β, H_0: $\beta = 0$ versus H_1: $\beta \neq 0$. In the simulations, we assume that both the case group X and the control group Y follow a lognormal distribution log N (μ, σ^2) with different μ's and a common σ^2, where $E(Y) = 3$, $E(X) = 3+\delta$, and δ ranges from 0 to 2.

Figure 8.5 demonstrates the experimental comparison of the Monte Carlo powers between the test based on the AUC for H_0: AUC = 1/2 versus H_1: AUC ≠ 1/2 (in black) and the test based on the logistic regression H_0: $\beta = 0$ versus H_1: $\beta \neq 0$ (in red) to detect the discriminant ability of the biomarkers at the 0.05 significance level, where the left and right panels correspond to sample sizes of 50 and 100, respectively. The tests are conducted based on the asymptotic distribution of the nonparametric estimator of the AUC and the estimator of logistic regression coefficient β described in Example 8.3. In these cases, the test based on the AUC demonstrates better discriminant ability of the biomarker than the test based on the logistic regression.

The R code to implement the procedures is presented below:

```
> # empirical AUC ( Mann-Whitney stat), returns p-value for H_0: AUC=1/2
  versus H_1: AUC!=1/2
> AUC.pval<-function(x,y) {
+ m<-length(x)
```

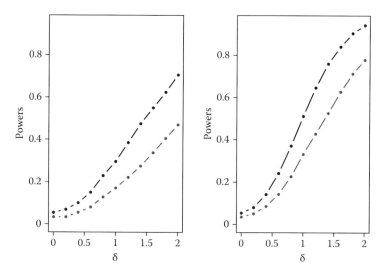

FIGURE 8.5
(See color insert.) Experimental comparisons based on the Monte Carlo powers related to the test based on the AUC concept, H_0: AUC = 1/2 vs. H_1: AUC ≠ 1/2 (in black), and the test based on the logistic regression concept, H_0: $\beta = 0$ vs. H_1: $\beta \neq 0$ (in red). The tests were performed in order to detect the discriminant ability of the biomarkers at the 0.05 significance level. The left and right panels correspond to sample sizes of 50 and 100, respectively.

```
+ n<-length(y)
+ x<-sort(x)
+ y<-sort(y)
+ rankall<-rank(c(x,y))
+ R<-rankall[1:m]
+ S<-rankall[-c(1:m)] # ranks of y
+
+ S10<-1/((m-1)*n^2)*(sum((R-1:m)^2)-m*(mean(R)-(m+1)/2)^2)
+ S01<-1/((n-1)*m^2)*(sum((S-1:n)^2)-n*(mean(S)-(n+1)/2)^2)
+ S2<-(m*S10+n*S01)/(m+n)
+
+ a<-wilcox.test(y,x)$statistic/(n*m)
+ AUC<-as.numeric(ifelse(a>=0.5,a,1-a)) # empirical AUC
+ pval<- 2*(1-pnorm(abs(AUC-0.5)/sqrt(S2/(m*n/(m+n)))))
+ return(pval)
+ }
>
> # logistic regression
> logistic.pval<-function(x,y){
+ if (!is.null(ncol(x))) {
+ Z<-rbind(x,y)
+ m<-nrow(x)
+ n<-nrow(y)
+ } else{
+ Z<-c(x,y)
+ m<-length(x)
+ n<-length(y)
+ }
+ q<-c(rep(0,m),rep(1,n))
+ newdata<-data.frame(cbind(q,Z))
+ glm.out = glm(q ~Z, family=binomial(logit), data=newdata)
+ return(summary(glm.out)$coef[-1,c(1,4)])
+ }
>
> MC<-10000
> alpha<-0.05
>
> Ex=3
> sigma2.x<-sigma2.y<-1
> delta.seq<-seq(0,2,.2)
> n.seq<-c(50,100)
>
> powers.all<-lapply(n.seq,function(n){
+ m<-n
+ powers<-sapply(delta.seq,function(delta){
+ Ey=Ex+delta
+ ux<-log(Ex)-0.5*sigma2.x
+ uy<-log(Ey)-0.5*sigma2.y
+ tmp<-sapply(1:MC,function(b){
+ x<-exp(rnorm(m,ux,sqrt(sigma2.x))) #x is lognormal
+ y<-exp(rnorm(n,uy,sqrt(sigma2.y))) #y is lognormal
+ pvals<-c(logistic.pval(x,y)[2]<alpha,AUC.pval(x,y)<alpha)
+ names(pvals)<-c("logistic","AUC")
+ return(pvals)
+ })
+ pow.delta<-apply(tmp,1,mean)
+ return(pow.delta)
+ })
+ colnames(powers)<-delta.seq
+ return(powers)
+ })
```

```
>
> names(powers.all)<-paste0("m=n=",n.seq)
> powers.all
$'m=n=50'
          0    0.2    0.4    0.6    0.8    1    1.2    1.4    1.6    1.8    2
logistic 0.0326 0.0332 0.0548 0.0796 0.1273 0.1695 0.2208 0.2743 0.3371 0.4046 0.4692
AUC      0.0540 0.0687 0.0998 0.1494 0.2286 0.2955 0.3845 0.4738 0.5499 0.6237 0.7055
$'m=n=100'
          0    0.2    0.4    0.6    0.8    1    1.2    1.4    1.6    1.8    2
logistic 0.0350 0.0501 0.0850 0.1423 0.2272 0.3317 0.4277 0.5252 0.6270 0.7122 0.7781
AUC      0.0538 0.0796 0.1414 0.2419 0.3710 0.5107 0.6464 0.7595 0.8397 0.9042 0.9422
```

Note that in the case where both the case group X and the control group Y follow a lognormal distribution $\log N (\mu,\sigma^2)$ with a common value for μ, and we vary the values for σ^2 between the case group and the control group, the AUC does not allow us to detect any significant difference between the two groups. This is because a simple log transformation of observed data points shows that the AUC equals 0.5 in this case. We refer the reader to Section 8.3.1 for the computation of the AUC under normal assumptions.

8.4.3 Remark

Medical diagnoses usually involve the classification of patients into two or more categories. When subjects are categorized in a binary manner, that is, nondiseased and diseased, the ROC curve methodology is an important statistical tool for evaluating the accuracy of continuous diagnostic tests, and the AUC is one of the common indices used for overall diagnostic accuracy. In many situations, the diagnostic decision is not limited to a binary choice. For example, a clinical assessment, NPZ-8, of the presence of HIV-related cognitive dysfunction (AIDS dementia complex [ADC]) would discriminate between patients exhibiting clinical symptoms of ADC (combined stages 1–3), subjects exhibiting minor neurological symptoms (ADC stage 0.5), and neurologically unimpaired individuals (ADC stage 0) (Nakas and Yiannoutsos 2004). For such disease processes with three stages, binary statistical tools such as the ROC curve and AUC need to be extended. In this case of three ordinal diagnostic categories, the ROC surface and the volume under the surface can be applied to assess the accuracy of tests. For details, we refer the reader to, for example, Nakas and Yiannoutsos (2004) and Kang and Tian (2013). In contrast, the logistic regression can be easily generalized, for example, the multinomial logistic regression, to deal with multiclass problems.

8.5 Best Combinations Based on Values of Multiple Biomarkers

In practice, different biomarkers' levels are usually associated with disease in various magnitudes and in different directions. For example, low levels of high-density lipoprotein (HDL) cholesterol and high levels of thiobarbituric acid reactive substances (TBARS), biomarkers of oxidative stress and antioxidant status, are indicators of coronary heart disease (Schisterman et al. 2001). When multiple biomarkers are available, it is of great interest to seek a combination of biomarkers to improve diagnostic accuracy (Liu et al. 2011). Pepe (2003) provided detailed considerations of best combinations of biomarkers that improve the classification accuracy. Due to the simplicity in practical applications, we will attend to the best linear combination (BLC) of biomarkers, such that the combined score achieves the maximum AUC or the maximum treatment effect over all possible linear combinations. Consider a study with d continuous-scale biomarkers yielding measurements $\mathbf{X}_i = (X_{1i}, ..., X_{di})^T$, $i = 1, ..., n$, on n diseased patients, and measurements $\mathbf{Y}_j = (Y_{1j}, ..., Y_{dj})$, $j = 1, ..., m$, on m nondiseased patients, respectively. It is of interest to construct effective one-dimensional combined scores of biomarker measurements, that is, $X(\mathbf{a}) = \mathbf{a}^T\mathbf{X}$ and $Y(\mathbf{a}) = \mathbf{a}^T\mathbf{Y}$, such that the AUC based on these scores is maximized over all possible linear combinations of biomarkers. Define $A(\mathbf{a}) = \Pr(X(\mathbf{a})>Y(\mathbf{a}))$; the statistical problem is to estimate the maximum AUC defined as $A = A(\mathbf{a}_0)$, where the vector $\mathbf{a}_0$ consists of the BLC coefficients satisfying $\mathbf{a}_0 = \arg\max_{\mathbf{a}} A(\mathbf{a})$. For simplicity, we assume that the first component of the vector $\mathbf{a}$ equals 1 (Pepe et al. 2006). For example, in the case of two biomarkers, i.e. $d = 2$, the AUC can be defined as $A(a) = \Pr(X_1 + aX_2 > Y_1 + aY_2)$.

8.5.1 Parametric Method

Assuming $\mathbf{X}_i \sim N(\mathbf{\mu}_X, \Sigma_X)$, $i = 1, ..., n$, and $\mathbf{Y}_j \sim N(\mathbf{\mu}_Y, \Sigma_Y)$, $j = 1, ..., m$, Su and Liu (1993) derived the BLC coefficients $\mathbf{a}_0 \propto \Sigma_C^{-1}\mathbf{\mu}$ and the corresponding optimal AUC as $\Phi(\omega^{1/2})$, where $\mathbf{\mu} = \mathbf{\mu}_X - \mathbf{\mu}_Y$, $\Sigma_C = \Sigma_X + \Sigma_Y$, $\omega = \mathbf{\mu}^T\Sigma_C^{-1}\mathbf{\mu}$, and Φ is the standard normal cumulative distribution function.

Based on Su and Liu's point estimator, we can derive the confidence interval estimation for the BLC-based AUC under multivariate normality assumptions (Reiser and Faraggi 1997).

Example 8.5: Optimal combination of biomarkers via ROC methods

Let's revisit the study described in Section 8.4 where the data sets are presented in Figure 8.3 and consider the combination of thiobarbituric acid reactive substances (TBARS) and high-density lipoprotein (HDL). We would like to compare the best linear combination given by Su and Liu (1993) and the logistic regression. In this case, the BLC coefficients provided by Su and Liu (1993) are (1, 0.0337), while the logistic coefficients (the first coefficient is scaled to 1 to be comparable to Su and Liu's BLC) are (1, 0.0281), which are close to each other.

The R code to implement the procedures is presented below:

```
> ## BLC
> data.x<-cbind(tbars.x,hdl.x)
> data.y<-cbind(tbars.y,hdl.y)
>
> # Su and Liu based on MVN
> A.analyt<-function(mu.x,mu.y,Sigma.x,Sigma.y)
+ {
+ sig.inv<-solve(Sigma.x+Sigma.y)
+ A <- pnorm(sqrt(t(mu.x-mu.y)%*%sig.inv%*%(mu.x-mu.y)))
+ a <- sig.inv%*%(mu.x-mu.y)
+ return(list(BLC=a/a[1],AUC=as.numeric(A)))
+ }
> (AUC.BLC<-A.analyt(mu.x=colMeans(data.x),mu.y=colMeans(data.y), Sigma.
    x=cov(data.x),Sigma.y=cov(data.y)) )
$BLC
         [,1]
tbars.x 1.00000000
hdl.x 0.03373123
$AUC
[1] 0.7238904
```

```
> # logistic
> log.BLC<-logistic.pval(data.x,data.y)
> log.BLC[,"Estimate"]/log.BLC[1,"Estimate"] # set the first one to be 1
 Ztbars.x Zhdl.x
1.00000000 0.02807472
```

Note that the implementation of logistic regression based on several biomarkers does not aim to maximize the AUC; its objective is to maximize the likelihood function.

However, we challenge the reader, for example, via the Monte Carlo simulations, to compare the AUC based on BLC described in this section with the AUC based on the linear combinations of biomarkers obtained from logistic regression.

8.5.2 Nonparametric Method

Chen et al. (2015) proposed using kernel functions to develop the empirical likelihood (EL)–based confidence interval estimation of the BLC-based maximum AUC, via construction of the empirical likelihood ratio (ELR) test statistic for testing the hypothesis H_0: $A = A_0$ versus H_1: $A \neq A_0$, where $A = A(a_0)$.

Let k be a symmetric kernel function and define $K_h(x) = \int_{-\infty}^{x/h} k(u)\,du$, $v_i(\mathbf{a}) = m^{-1} \sum_{j=1}^{m} K_h(\mathbf{a}^T \mathbf{X}_i - \mathbf{a}^T \mathbf{Y}_j)$, $i = 1, ..., n$, where h is the bandwidth parameter. Regarding the kernel estimation, we refer the reader to the textbook of Silverman (1986). Let $\mathbf{p} = (p_1, p_2, ..., p_n)^T$ be a probability weight vector, $\sum_{i=1}^{n} p_i = 1$, and $p_i \geq 0$ for all $i = 1, ..., n$. The EL for the BLC-based AUC evaluated at the true value A_0 of AUC can be defined as

$$L(A_0) = \sup\left\{\prod_{i=1}^{n} p_i : \sum_{i=1}^{n} p_i = 1, \sum_{i=1}^{n} p_i v_i(\hat{\mathbf{a}}_0) = A_0\right\},$$

where $\hat{\mathbf{a}}_0$ satisfies $\sum_{i=1}^{n} p_i \,\partial v_i(\mathbf{a})/\partial \mathbf{a}\big|_{\mathbf{a}=\hat{\mathbf{a}}_0} = 0$. One can show (using Lagrange multipliers) that

$$p_i = \frac{1}{n}\frac{1}{1 + \lambda\left(v_i(\hat{\mathbf{a}}_0) - A_0\right)}, \quad i = 1, ..., n,$$

where the Lagrange multiplier λ is the root of

$$\frac{1}{n}\sum_{i=1}^{n}\frac{v_i(\hat{\mathbf{a}}_0)}{1 + \lambda\left(v_i(\hat{\mathbf{a}}_0) - A_0\right)} = A_0.$$

Under the alternative hypothesis, we have just the constraint $\sum_{i=1}^{n} p_i = 1$, and hence $L(A_0) = (1/n)^n$ at $p_i = 1/n$. Therefore, the empirical log-likelihood ratio test statistic is

$$l(A_0) = 2\log ELR(A_0) = 2\sum_{i=1}^{n}\log(1 + \lambda(v_i(\hat{\mathbf{a}}_0) - A_0)).$$

We define $\hat{\mathbf{a}}_K = \arg\max_{\mathbf{a}} A_{m,n}^K(\mathbf{a})$, where $A_{m,n}^K(\mathbf{a}) = n^{-1} \sum_{i=1}^{n} v_i(\mathbf{a})$. Under some general conditions (for details see Chen et al. 2015), the asymptotic distribution of $l(A_0)$ under $H_0 : A = A_0$ is a scaled chi-square distribution with one degree of freedom, that is,

$$\gamma(A_0)l(A_0) \xrightarrow{d} \chi_1^2, \text{ as } n,m \to \infty,$$

where

$$\gamma(A_0) = \frac{m\hat{\sigma}^2}{(m+n)s^2}, \; \hat{\sigma}^2 = n^{-1}\sum_{i=1}^{n}(v_i(\hat{\mathbf{a}}_K) - n^{-1}\sum_{j=1}^{n}v_j(\hat{\mathbf{a}}_K))^2, \; s^2 = \frac{m\hat{\sigma}_{10}^2 + n\hat{\sigma}_{01}^2}{m+n},$$

$$\sigma_{10}^2 = \text{Cov}(K_h(\mathbf{a}_0^T\mathbf{X}_1 - \mathbf{a}_0^T\mathbf{Y}_1), K_h(\mathbf{a}_0^T\mathbf{X}_1 - \mathbf{a}_0^T\mathbf{Y}_2)),$$

$$\sigma_{01}^2 = \text{Cov}(K_h(\mathbf{a}_0^T\mathbf{X}_1 - \mathbf{a}_0^T\mathbf{Y}_1), K_h(\mathbf{a}_0^T\mathbf{X}_2 - \mathbf{a}_0^T\mathbf{Y}_1)),$$

and $\hat{\sigma}_{10}^2$, $\hat{\sigma}_{01}^2$ are the corresponding estimates.

Based on the asymptotic distribution of the statistic $l(A_0)$, the $100(1-\alpha)\%$ empirical likelihood–based confidence interval for the maximum AUC can be constructed as

$$R_\alpha = \left\{ A_0 : \gamma(A_0)l(A_0) \leq \chi_1^2(1-\alpha) \right\},$$

where $\chi_1^2(1-\alpha)$ is the $(1-\alpha)$th quantile of the chi-square distribution with one degree of freedom. It gives a confidence interval with asymptotically correct coverage probability $1-\alpha$, that is, $\Pr(A_0 \in R_\alpha) = 1-\alpha + o(1)$. R code related to the problem described above can be found at the following web domain: http://www.sciencedirect.com/science/article/pii/S0167947314002710.

8.6 Notes Regarding Treatment Effects

Many clinical and biomedical studies evaluate treatment effects based on multiple biomarkers that commonly consist of pre- and post-treatment measurements. Some biomarkers can show significant positive treatment effects, while other biomarkers can reflect no effects or even negative effects of the treatments, giving rise to the necessity to develop methodologies that may correctly and efficiently evaluate the treatment effects based on multiple biomarkers as a whole. In the setting of pre- and post-treatment measurements of multiple biomarkers, Vexler et al. (2014a) proposed applying a ROC curve methodology based on the best combination of biomarkers maximizing the AUC-type criterion among all possible linear combinations. The likelihood ratio test was used to compare two treatment groups (e.g., case and control) based on the AUC-type criterion computed with respect to the best linear combinations of biomarkers' values. We present their work in this section.

8.6.1 Best Linear Combination of Markers

Without loss of generality and with respect to our practical examples, suppose two biomarkers are involved in a study to analyze treatment effects. Let X_{1i}, X_{2i} be the pre- and post-treatment measurements of one biomarker, respectively, regarding the ith ($i = 1, ..., n$) patient for a certain treatment. Let Y_{1i}, Y_{2i} be the pre- and post-treatment measurements of another biomarker, respectively, with respect to the ith ($i = 1, ..., n$) patient. Assume that $(X_1, X_2, Y_1, Y_2)^T$ (here T stands for the transpose operation) follows a multivariate normal distribution with the mean vector $\mu = (\mu_{X_1}, \mu_{X_2}, \mu_{Y_1}, \mu_{Y_2})^T$ and the covariance matrix $\Sigma = (\sigma_{hl})$, $1 \le h \le 4$, $1 \le l \le 4$. To represent a simple measure of treatment effects, we are interested in reducing dimensionality by constructing an effective linear combination of biomarkers with values X's and Y's. This implies that we derive certain optimal linear coefficients (λ_1, λ_2) so that for groups of marker values (X_1, Y_1) and (X_2, Y_2), the one-dimensional random variables $U_1 = \lambda_1 X_1 + \lambda_2 Y_1$ and $U_2 = \lambda_1 X_2 + \lambda_2 Y_2$ can be presented. This linear combination of measurements of biomarkers dominates all the other possible linear combinations in the sense that it provides a maximum of the AUC-type measure $\Pr(U_1 < U_2)$ for all λ_1 and λ_2. Thus, the optimal $\lambda° = (\lambda_1°, \lambda_2°)^T$ maximizes the AUC-type measure, denoted by A, where

$$A(\lambda_1, \lambda_2) = \Pr(\lambda_1 X_1 + \lambda_2 Y_1 < \lambda_1 X_2 + \lambda_2 Y_2) = \Pr(\lambda_1 X_1 - \lambda_1 X_2 + \lambda_2 Y_1 - \lambda_2 Y_2 < 0)$$

over all possible values of λ_1 and λ_2, that is, $(\lambda_1°, \lambda_2°) = \arg \max\limits_{\lambda_1, \lambda_2} A(\lambda_1, \lambda_2)$.

Under the assumption of multivariate normality of the biomarker measurements' distribution, $(\lambda_1, -\lambda_1, \lambda_2, -\lambda_2) (X_1, X_2, Y_1, Y_2)^T$ follows the normal distribution with mean $\lambda_1 \Delta\mu_X + \lambda_2 \Delta\mu_Y$ and variance $\delta_1 \lambda_1^2 = 2\delta_2 \lambda_1 \lambda_2 + \delta_3 \lambda_2^2$, where $\Delta\mu_X = \mu_{X_1} - \mu_{X_2}$, $\Delta\mu_Y = \mu_{Y_1} - \mu_{Y_2}$, and $\delta_1 = \sigma_{11} + \sigma_{22} - 2\sigma_{12}$, $\delta_2 = \sigma_{13} - \sigma_{14} - \sigma_{23} + \sigma_{24}$, $\delta_3 = \sigma_{33} + \sigma_{44} - 2\sigma_{34}$. Then, the corresponding AUC-type measure has the form of

$$\Phi\left(-\frac{\lambda_1 \Delta\mu_X + \lambda_2 \Delta\mu_Y}{\sqrt{\delta_1 \lambda_1^2 + 2\delta_2 \lambda_1 \lambda_2 + \delta_3 \lambda_2^2}} \right),$$

where Φ is a standard normal cumulative distribution function. The best linear combination can be defined by maximizing the AUC-type measure and obtaining values of $(\lambda_1^0, \lambda_2^0)$ shown in the following proposition.

Proposition 8.1

The best linear combination coefficients are

$$(\lambda_1^0, \lambda_2^0) \propto (\Delta\mu_X, \Delta\mu_Y) \begin{pmatrix} -\delta_3 & \delta_2 \\ \delta_2 & -\delta_1 \end{pmatrix} = (-\Delta\mu_X \delta_3 + \Delta\mu_Y \delta_2, \Delta\mu_X \delta_2 - \Delta\mu_Y \delta_1).$$

Given the best linear combination coefficients derived in Proposition 8.1, the maximized AUC-type measure has the form

$$\Phi\left(\frac{\delta_3 \Delta\mu_X^2 + \delta_1 \Delta\mu_Y^2 - 2\delta_2 \Delta\mu_X \Delta\mu_Y}{\sqrt{\delta_1 \delta_3^2 \Delta\mu_X^2 + \delta_3 \delta_1^2 \Delta\mu_Y^2 - \delta_3 \delta_2^2 \Delta\mu_X^2 - \delta_1 \delta_2^2 \Delta\mu_Y^2 - 2\delta_1 \delta_2 \delta_3 \Delta\mu_X \Delta\mu_Y + 2\delta_2^3 \Delta\mu_X \Delta\mu_Y}} \right).$$

If biomarkers are mutually independent, that is, $X = (X_1, X_2)$ and $Y = (Y_1, Y_2)$ are independent, the best linear combination coefficients are $(\lambda_1^0, \lambda_2^0) \propto (\Delta\mu_X, \Delta\mu_Y) \begin{pmatrix} -\delta_3 & 0 \\ 0 & -\delta_1 \end{pmatrix}$, that is,

proportional to the weighted change in the mean vector $(-\delta_3 \Delta\mu_X, -\delta_1 \Delta\mu_Y)$.

In a special case of independent pre- and post-treatment measurements of biomarkers, which is an analogy to the statement of a case-control study, we have the same result as that proposed by Su and Liu (1993). This result is formalized in the following proposition.

Proposition 8.2

If pre- and post-treatment measurements are independent for both markers, that is, X_1 is independent of X_2, and Y_1 is independent of Y_2, the best linear combination coefficients are $\left(\lambda_1^0, \lambda_2^0\right) \propto \left(-\Delta\mu_X\delta_3 + \Delta\mu_Y\delta_2, \Delta\mu_X\delta_2 - \Delta\mu_Y\delta_1\right)$. Thus, $\left(\lambda_1^0, \lambda_2^0\right)^T \propto \left(\Sigma_{post} + \Sigma_{pre}\right)^{-1}\left(\mu_{post} - \mu_{pre}\right)$, where

$$\mu_{pre} = \left(\mu_{X_1}, \mu_{Y_1}\right)^T, \ \mu_{post} = \left(\mu_{X_2}, \mu_{Y_2}\right)^T, \ \Sigma_{pre} = \begin{pmatrix} \sigma_{11} & \sigma_{13} \\ \sigma_{31} & \sigma_{33} \end{pmatrix}, \ \Sigma_{post} = \begin{pmatrix} \sigma_{22} & \sigma_{24} \\ \sigma_{42} & \sigma_{44} \end{pmatrix}.$$

Thus, we propose to use the maximized AUC-type measure in the context of the best linear combinations to depict the total treatment effects based on pre- and post-treatment measurements of biomarkers. The total treatment effect $\Pr(\lambda_1 X_1 + \lambda_2 Y_1 < \lambda_1 X_2 + \lambda_2 Y_2)$ has value in the form of the maximized AUC-type measure defined above.

8.6.2 Maximum Likelihood Ratio Tests

In this section, we propose the maximum likelihood ratio test for comparing treatment effects based on best linear combinations of pre- and post-treatment measurements of biomarkers. To this end, we modify the technique proposed in Vexler et al. (2008a).

Let X_{rki} represent the pre- ($r = 1$) and post-treatment ($r = 2$) measurements of a biomarker (X) for the ith ($i = 1, ..., n_k$) patient in the kth group, $k = 1$ for the new therapy group and $k = 2$ for the control group, respectively. Likewise, let Y_{jki} represent the pre- ($r = 1$) and post-treatment ($r = 2$) measurements of another biomarker (Y) for the ith ($i = 1, ..., n_k$) patient in the kth group, $k = 1$ for the new therapy group and $k = 2$ for the control group, respectively. Assume biomarker measurements for the new therapy group $v_{1i} = (X_{11i}, X_{21i}, Y_{11i}, Y_{21i})^T$ ($i = 1, ..., n_1$) and biomarker measurements for the control group $v_{2j} = (X_{11j}, X_{21j}, Y_{11j}, Y_{21j})^T$ ($j = 1, ..., n_1$) follow a multivariate normal distribution with the mean vector $\mu_k = (\mu_{1k}, \mu_{2k}, \mu_{3k}, \mu_{4k})^T = E(v_{k1}) = (E(X_{1k1}), E(X_{2k1}), E(Y_{1k1}), E(Y_{2k1}))^T$ and with the covariance matrix $\Sigma_k = E\left((v_{k1} - E(v_{k1}))(v_{k1} - E(v_{k1}))^T\right) = (\sigma_{hlk})$, $1 \le h \le 4, 1 \le l \le 4, k = 1, 2$. Let A_1 and A_2 denote the maximized AUC-type measures for the new therapy group and the control group, respectively. In this section, for the comparison of the treatment effects for the new therapy group and the control group based on paired observations, we formally consider testing hypothesis

$$H_0: A_1 = A_2 \text{ versus } H_1: A_1 \ne A_2.$$

In Section 8.6.1, we presented the form of the maximized AUC-type measures, which can be applied in both groups. Thus, $A_k = \Phi\left(\dfrac{N_k}{\sqrt{D_k}}\right)$ can be expressed as a function of μ_k and Σ_k, where

$$N_k = (\mu_{1k} - \mu_{2k})^2 (\sigma_{33k} - 2\sigma_{34k} + \sigma_{44k}) + (\mu_{3k} - \mu_{4k})^2 (\sigma_{11k} - 2\sigma_{12k} + \sigma_{22k})$$
$$- 2(\mu_{1k} - \mu_{2k})(\mu_{3k} - \mu_{4k})(\sigma_{13k} - \sigma_{14k} - \sigma_{23k} + \sigma_{24k})$$

$$D_k = 2(\mu_{1k} - \mu_{2k})(\mu_{3k} - \mu_{4k})(\sigma_{13k} - \sigma_{14k} + \sigma_{23k} + \sigma_{24k})^3 - (\mu_{1k} - \mu_{2k})^2 (\sigma_{33k} - 2\sigma_{34k} + \sigma_{44k})$$
$$\times (\sigma_{13k} - \sigma_{14k} - \sigma_{23k} + \sigma_{24k})^2 - (\mu_{3k} - \mu_{4k})^2 (\sigma_{11k} - 2\sigma_{12k} + \sigma_{22k})(\sigma_{13k} - \sigma_{14k} - \sigma_{23k} + \sigma_{24k})^2$$
$$+ (\mu_{1k} - \mu_{2k})^2 (\sigma_{11k} - 2\sigma_{12k} + \sigma_{22k})(\sigma_{33k} - 2\sigma_{34k} + \sigma_{44k})^2 + (\mu_{3k} - \mu_{4k})^2 (\sigma_{11k} - 2\sigma_{12k} + \sigma_{22k})^2$$
$$\times (\sigma_{33k} - 2\sigma_{34k} + \sigma_{44k}) - 2(\mu_{1k} - \mu_{2k})(\mu_{3k} - \mu_{4k})(\sigma_{11k} - 2\sigma_{12k} + \sigma_{22k})(\sigma_{33k} - 2\sigma_{34k} + \sigma_{44k})$$
$$\times (\sigma_{13k} - \sigma_{14k} - \sigma_{23k} + \sigma_{24k})$$

Therefore, the hypothesis $H_0: A_1 = A_2$ versus $H_1: A_1 \neq A_2$ is equivalent to

$$H_0: \frac{N_1}{\sqrt{D_1}} = \frac{N_2}{\sqrt{D_2}} \quad \text{vs.} \quad H_1: \frac{N_1}{\sqrt{D_1}} \neq \frac{N_2}{\sqrt{D_2}}.$$

Under the null hypothesis, μ_{11} can be represented as a function of the remaining set of parameters, say, $\mu_{11} = h(\cdot) = h(\mu_{21}, \mu_{31}, \mu_{41}, \mu_2, \Sigma_1, \Sigma_2)$, for a certain function h. We show the exact form of the function h in the appendix. Thus, in a simple case, when all the parameters are known, we can utilize the classical most powerful likelihood ratio method for testing H_0. To this end, the likelihood functions under H_1 and H_0 can be presented correspondingly as

$$L_1\left(\mu_1, \mu_2, \Sigma_1, \Sigma_2\right) = \prod_{i=1,\ldots,n_1} \phi\left(v_{1i}; \mu_1, \Sigma_1\right) \prod_{j=1,\ldots,n_2} \phi\left(v_{2j}; \mu_2, \Sigma_2\right),$$

$$L_0\left(\mu_{21}, \mu_{31}, \mu_{41}, \mu_2, \Sigma_1, \Sigma_2\right) = \prod_{\substack{i=1,\ldots,n_1 \\ j=1,\ldots,n_2}} \phi\left(v_{1i}; \left(h, \mu_{21}, \mu_{31}, \mu_{41}\right)^T, \Sigma_1\right) \phi\left(v_{2j}; \mu_2, \Sigma_2\right),$$

where $\phi(\cdot)$ denotes the multivariate normal density function known as

$$\phi\left(v; \mu, \Sigma\right) = \left(2\pi\right)^{-2} \left|\Sigma\right|^{-\frac{1}{2}} e^{-\frac{1}{2}(v-\mu)^T \Sigma^{-1}(v-\mu)}.$$

Therefore, the classical likelihood ratio test statistic is

$$\Lambda = \prod_{i=1,\ldots,n_1} \frac{\phi\left(v_{1i}; \mu_1, \Sigma_1\right)}{\phi\left(v_{1i}; \left(h, \mu_{21}, \mu_{31}, \mu_{41}\right)^T, \Sigma_1\right)}.$$

When the parameters are unknown, we can apply the maximum likelihood ratio to be the test statistic

$$\Lambda = \frac{\sup\limits_{\mu_1, \mu_2, \Sigma_1, \Sigma_2} L_1\left(\mu_1, \mu_2, \Sigma_1, \Sigma_2\right)}{\sup\limits_{\mu_{21}, \mu_{31}, \mu_{41}, \mu_2, \Sigma_1, \Sigma_2} L_0\left(\mu_{21}, \mu_{31}, \mu_{41}, \mu_2, \Sigma_1, \Sigma_2\right)}$$

$$= \frac{\sup\limits_{\mu_1, \Sigma_1} \prod_{i=1,\ldots,n_1} \phi\left(v_{1i}; \mu_1, \Sigma_1\right) \sup\limits_{\mu_2, \Sigma_2} \prod_{j=1,\ldots,n_2} \phi\left(v_{2j}; \mu_2, \Sigma_2\right)}{\sup\limits_{\mu_{21}, \mu_{31}, \mu_{41}, \mu_2, \Sigma_1, \Sigma_2} \prod_{\substack{i=1,\ldots,n_1 \\ j=1,\ldots,n_2}} \phi\left(v_{1i}; \left(h, \mu_{21}, \mu_{31}, \mu_{41}\right)^T, \Sigma_1\right) \phi\left(v_{2j}; \mu_2, \Sigma_2\right)}.$$

The maximum likelihood estimators under H_1 have closed-form solutions. The maximum log-likelihood under H_1 is

$$2\left(\log\left(2\pi\right) + 1\right)\left(n_1 + n_2\right) + \frac{n_1}{2} \log\left|\hat{\Sigma}_1\right| + \frac{n_2}{2} \log\left|\hat{\Sigma}_2\right|,$$

where

$$\hat{\Sigma}_1 = \frac{1}{n_1} \sum_{i=1}^{n_1} \left(v_{1i} - \frac{1}{n_1} \sum_{i=1}^{n_1} v_{1i} \right) \left(v_{1i} - \frac{1}{n_1} \sum_{i=1}^{n_1} v_{1i} \right)^T,$$

$$\hat{\Sigma}_2 = \frac{1}{n_2} \sum_{j=1}^{n_2} \left(v_{2j} - \frac{1}{n_2} \sum_{j=1}^{n_2} v_{2j} \right) \left(v_{2j} - \frac{1}{n_2} \sum_{j=1}^{n_2} v_{2j} \right)^T.$$

Under H_0, in order to calculate the maximum likelihood, one can use the numerical approach without specifying the closed forms of the estimators of the unknown parameters.

8.6.2.1 Remark Regarding Numerical Calculations

Note that statistical software packages such as R, SAS, or SPlus allow us to numerically perform the minimization of $-\log(L_0 (\mu_{21}, \mu_{31}, \mu_{41}, \mu_2, \Sigma_1, \Sigma_2))$ without using closed forms of the estimators of the unknown parameters. The basic procedure *optim* in R (R Development Core Team 2014) can be carried out with respect to minimizing the negative log-likelihood under H_0, and the procedure *multiroot* helps find this minimization. The related R codes are available from the authors upon request.

In this setting, we reject the null hypothesis if $\Lambda > \Lambda_\alpha$, where the threshold Λ_α corresponds to the Type I error rate α. Following Wilks's theorem (e.g., Lehmann 1998), under H_0, the statistic $2\ln\Lambda$ asymptotically has a χ_1^2-distribution. Thus, the threshold Λ_α can be easily obtained from $Pr(\Lambda > \Lambda_\alpha)$ as $n_1, n_2 \to \infty$. Moreover, the proposed test is asymptotically locally most powerful (e.g., see Choi et al. 1996).

8.7 Supplement

8.7.1 ROC

1. Lee and Wolfe (1976) proposed a two-sample distribution-free procedure for testing equal locations under a stochastic ordering restriction. The test statistic M is an estimator of $Pr(X \leq Y)$ based on maximum likelihood estimators of stochastically ordered distribution functions. Some properties of the M-test were developed and critical values were provided for selected sample sizes. A Monte Carlo power study indicated that the M-test is more effective (for shift alternatives) than the Mann–Whitney–Wilcoxon test when the form of the underlying distribution is heavy-tailed, but the Mann–Whitney–Wilcoxon is preferred for moderate-tailed distributions.

2. Murtaugh (1995) explored properties of ROC curves for markers that are measured repeatedly, through space or time, for each subject. The true underlying response, positive or negative, of each subject is assumed to be constant across marker measurements and is determined from assessment of some gold standard. A marker-based test is considered positive when at least one of a subject's marker values exceeds a designated cutoff. If subjects with positive and negative

underlying responses differ in the number of marker measurements per subject, the ROC curve for a noninformative marker is bowed above or below the diagonal line representing the null curve for a marker that is measured just once per subject. If subjects with negative responses tend to have more measurements than those with positive responses, the ROC curve for even an informative marker may lie beneath the curve for the same marker measured once per subject. The form of the ROC curve for a marker used in this way will be strongly influenced by the strength of the correlation of measurements within subjects.

3. Song (1997) extended the procedure of DeLong et al. (1988) to a Wald test for general situations of diagnostic testing. The method of analyzing jackknife pseudovalues by treating them as data is extremely useful when the number of area measures to be tested is quite small. The Wald test based on covariances of multivariate multisample U-statistics is compared with two approaches of analyzing pseudovalues, the univariate mixed-model analysis of variance (ANOVA) for repeated measurements and the three-way factorial ANOVA. Monte Carlo simulations demonstrated that the three tests give good approximation to the nominal size at the 5% levels for large sample sizes, but the paired *t*-test using ROC areas as data lacks the power of the other three tests, and Hanley and McNeil's (1982) method is inappropriate for testing diagnostic accuracies. The Wald statistic performs better than the ANOVAs of pseudovalues. Jackknifing schemes of multiple deletions where different structures of normal and diseased distributions are accounted for appear to perform slightly better than simple multiple-deletion schemes, but no appreciable power difference is apparent, and deletion of too many cases at a time may sacrifice power. These methods have important applications in diagnostic testing in ROC studies of radiology and of medicine in general. The method was illustrated with sample data from an experiment in radiology.

4. Leisenring and Pepe (1998) proposed a new regression method that allows for direct assessment of covariate effects on likelihood ratios for binary diagnostic tests. This may be particularly useful in assessing how factors that are under the control of the clinician can be altered to maximize the predictive ability of the test. Similarly, patient characteristics that influence the ability of the test to discriminate between diseased and nondiseased subjects may be identified using the regression model. The regression method is flexible in that it can accommodate clustered data arising from a variety of study designs. The authors illustrated the method with data from an audiology study.

5. Lloyd (1998) proposed a kernel smoothing estimator for the ROC curve and showed his estimator has better mean squared error than the empirical ROC curve estimator. However, Lloyd's estimator involves two bandwidths and has a boundary problem. In addition, his choice of bandwidths is ad hoc. Peng and Zhou (2004) proposed another kernel smoothing estimator that involves only one bandwidth, which is asymptotically optimal, and does not have the boundary problem.

6. Shapiro (1999) reviewed statistical methodology for assessing laboratory diagnostic test accuracy and interpreting individual test results, with an emphasis on diagnostic tests that yield a continuous measurement. The author presented a summary of basic concepts and terminology, a brief discussion of study design and methods for assessing the accuracy of a single diagnostic test, and a comparison of the accuracy of two or more diagnostic tests and interpreting individual test results.

7. Venkatraman (2000) developed a permutation test in an earlier paper (Venkatraman and Begg 1996) to test the equality of receiver operating characteristic curves based on continuous paired data. The authors extended the underlying concepts to develop a permutation test for continuous unpaired data, and studied its properties through simulations.

8. Lloyd (2000) described a family of regression models for analyzing empirical data on a test's performance, which often come in the form of observed true positive and false positive relative frequencies under varying conditions. The underlying ROC curves are specified by a quality parameter Δ and a shape parameter μ and are guaranteed to be convex provided $\Delta > 1$. Both the position along the ROC curve and the quality parameter Δ are modeled linearly with covariates at the level of the individual. The shape parameter μ enters the model through the link functions $\log(p^\mu) - \log(1-p^\mu)$ of a binomial regression and is estimated either by search or from an appropriate constructed variate. The method was illustrated with the following applications: a meta-analysis of independent studies of the same diagnostic test based on some data of Moses et al. (1993), and the so-called vigilance data, where ROC curves differ across subjects and modeling of the position along the ROC curve was of primary interest.

9. Pepe (2000a) presented an interpretation for each point on the ROC curve being a conditional probability of a test result from a random diseased subject exceeding that from a random nondiseased subject. This interpretation gives rise to new methods for making inference about ROC curves. It was shown that inference can be achieved with binary regression techniques applied to indicator variables constructed from pairs of test results, one component of the pair being from a diseased subject and the other from a nondiseased subject. Within the generalized linear model (GLM) binary regression framework, ROC curves can be estimated, and a new semiparametric estimator can be highlighted. Covariate effects can also be evaluated with the GLM models. The methodology was applied to a pancreatic cancer data set where the regression framework was used to compare two different serum biomarkers. Asymptotic distribution theory was developed to facilitate inference and provide insight into factors influencing variability of estimated model parameters.

10. Pepe (2000b) discussed issues of cost, disease prevalence, and consequences of misdiagnosis that will enter into the ultimate evaluation of test usefulness. The following major statistical challenges for evaluating diagnostic tests in general and for applying ROC methodology were discussed: (a) inference for a ROC curve in settings where a definitive gold standard assessment of disease status, D, is not available (e.g., infection with *Chlamydia trachomatis* can be assessed only imprecisely with standard bacterial culture techniques); (b) the role of ROC curves in determining how to combine different sources of information to optimize diagnostic accuracy, since in practice test results may be much more complicated, involving several components rather than a simple numeric value; (c) the sensible incorporation of the time aspect into ROC analysis where disease status is often not a fixed entity, but rather can evolve over time; and (d) alternatives to the ROC curve for describing test accuracy and generalizing the notions of predictive values to continuous tests. For binary outcomes, two ways of describing test accuracy are to report (a) true and false positive rates and (b) positive and negative predictive values. ROC curves can be thought of as generalizing the former to continuous tests; that is, ROC curves generalize the binary test notions of true positive and false positive rates to continuous tests.

11. Mahalanobis distances can be used, often in a disguised form, to compare two multivariate normal populations in many statistical problems. Assuming a common covariance matrix, the overlapping coefficient (Bradley 1985), optimal error rates (Rao and Dorvlo 1985), and generalized ROC criterion (Reiser and Faraggi 1997) are all monotonic functions of the Mahalanobis distance. Approximate confidence intervals for all of these have appeared in the literature on an ad hoc basis. Reiser (2001) provided a unified approach to obtaining an effectively exact confidence interval for the Mahalanobis distance and all the above measures.

12. Logistic regression is often used to find a linear combination of covariates that best discriminates between two groups or populations. The ROC curve is a good way of assessing the performance of the resulting score, but using the same data both to fit the score and to calculate its ROC leads to an overoptimistic estimate of the performance that the score would give if it were to be validated on a sample of future cases. Copas and Corbett (2002) studied the extent of the overestimation of the performance by ROC that the score resulting from the logistic regression would give if it were to be validated on a sample of future cases. The authors suggested a shrinkage correction for the ROC curve itself and for the area under the curve. The correction is consistent with Efron's (1983, 1986a) formula for the bias in the error rate of a binary prediction rule. The following two medical examples were discussed: the study of prognosis in breast cancer (Berwick et al. 1996), where the aim was to see whether clinical characteristics measured before surgery could be effective in discriminating in advance between patients who did and did not respond to surgery, and the case-control study of melanoma reported in Berwick et al. (1996), where the aim was to study how the risk of the disease can be assessed in terms of measurable risk factors.

13. Qin and Zhang (2003) explored a semiparametric approach by assuming a density ratio model for disease and disease-free densities. This model has a natural connection with the logistic regression model. This semiparametric approach was shown to be more robust than a fully parametric approach and is more efficient than a fully nonparametric approach. Two real examples demonstrated that the ROC curve estimated by the semiparametric method is much smoother than that estimated by the nonparametric method.

14. Hall et al. (2004) studied methods for constructing confidence intervals and confidence bands for estimators of receiver operating characteristics, focusing on the way in which smoothing should be implemented, when estimating either the characteristic itself or its variance. The authors showed that substantial undersmoothing is necessary if coverage properties are not to be impaired. A theoretical analysis of the problem suggested an empirical, plug-in rule for bandwidth choice, optimizing the coverage accuracy of interval estimators. The performance of this approach was explored. The preferred technique was based on asymptotic approximation, rather than a more sophisticated approach using the bootstrap, since the latter requires a multiplicity of smoothing parameters, all of which must be chosen in nonstandard ways. It was shown that the asymptotic method can give very good performance.

15. Zhou and Qin (2005) proposed two new intervals for the sensitivity of a continuous-scale diagnostic test at a fixed level of specificity. The authors conducted simulation studies to compare the relative performance of these two

intervals with the best existing Efron's bias-corrected acceleration (BCa) bootstrap interval, proposed by Platt et al. (2000). The simulation results showed that the newly proposed intervals are better than the BCa bootstrap interval in terms of coverage accuracy and interval length.

16. Liu J.P. (2006) proposed using the standardized difference for assessing equivalence or noninferiority in diagnostic accuracy based on paired areas under ROC curves between two diagnostic procedures. The bootstrap technique was suggested for both the nonparametric method and the standardized difference approach. A simulation study was conducted empirically to investigate the size and power of the four methods for various combinations of distributions, data types, sample sizes, and different correlations. Simulation results demonstrated that the bootstrap procedure of the standardized difference approach not only adequately control the Type I error rate at the nominal level but also provides equivalent power under both symmetrical and skewed distributions. The methods were illustrated with the data where two radiologists used three-dimensional magnetic resonance angiography (MRA) to evaluate the degree of arterial atherosclerotic stenosis of 65 carotid arteries (left and right) in 36 patients (Obuchowski 1997).

17. O'Malley and Zou (2006) developed a Bayesian multivariate hierarchical transformation model (BMHTM) for the ROC analysis based on clustered continuous diagnostic outcome data with covariates. Two special features of this model are that it incorporates nonlinear monotone transformations of the outcomes and that multiple correlated outcomes may be analyzed. The mean, variance, and transformation components are all modeled parametrically, enabling a wide range of inferences. The general framework was illustrated by focusing on two problems: (a) analysis of the diagnostic accuracy of a covariate-dependent univariate test outcome requiring a Box–Cox transformation within each cluster to map the test outcomes to a common family of distributions, and (b) development of an optimal composite diagnostic test using multivariate clustered outcome data. In the second problem, the composite test was estimated using discriminant function analysis and compared to the test derived from logistic regression analysis where the gold standard is a binary outcome. The proposed method was illustrated on prostate cancer biopsy data from a multicenter clinical trial.

18. Brumback et al. (2006) adapted recently developed methods for the ROC curve regression analysis to extend the Mann–Whitney test to accommodate covariate adjustment and evaluation of effect modification. This approach naturally extends use of the Mann–Whitney statistic in a fashion that is analogous to how linear models extend the t-test. The authors illustrated the methodology with data from clinical trials of a therapy for cystic fibrosis.

19. Fawcett (2006) presented an introduction to ROC graphs and a guide for using them in research. He demonstrated that ROC graphs are useful for organizing classifiers and visualizing their performance. Although ROC graphs are apparently simple, the author noted that there are some common misconceptions and pitfalls when using them in practice.

20. Zou et al. (2007) reviewed the measures of accuracy—sensitivity, specificity, and AUC—and illustrated how they can be applied using the evaluation of a hypothetical new diagnostic test as an example.

21. Vexler et al. (2008b) associated the additive measurement errors and pooling design (see Chapter 15) into one stated problem. The integrated approach creates an opportunity to investigate new fields, for example, a subject of pooling errors, issues regarding pooled data affected by measurement errors. To be specific, the authors consider the stated problem in the context of the ROC curve analysis, which is the well-accepted tool for evaluating the ability of a biomarker to discriminate between two populations. The paper considers a wide family of biospecimen distributions. In addition, applied assumptions, which are related to distribution functions of biomarkers, are mainly conditioned by the reconstructing problem. The authors proposed and examined maximum likelihood techniques based on the following data: a biomarker with measurement error, pooled samples, and pooled samples with measurement error. The obtained methods were illustrated by applications to real data studies.

22. Nachar (2008) presented a summary, applications, and the explanation of the logic underlying the Mann–Whitney U-test. Moreover, the forces and weaknesses of the Mann–Whitney U-test were mentioned. The author showed that one major limit of the Mann–Whitney U-test was that the Type I error or alpha (α) is amplified in a situation of heteroscedasticity.

23. Branscum et al. (2008) developed a novel semiparametric modeling framework involving mixtures of Pólya trees for screening data with the dual purpose of diagnosing infection or disease status and assessing the accuracy of continuous diagnostic measures. In this framework, the authors obtained predictive probabilities of disease based on continuous diagnostic test outcomes in conjunction with other information, including relevant covariates and results from one or more independent binary diagnostic tests. An example would be the modeling of a serum enzyme-linked immunosorbent assay (ELISA) procedure for detecting antibodies to an infectious agent when used in conjunction with culture for antigen detection. It also characterized measures of diagnostic performance of continuous tests by estimating the ROC and AUC, primarily when such extra information is available. When true disease status is unknown, parametric and nonparametric analyses require sufficient separation between the distributions of outcome values for the diseased and nondiseased populations. However, this overlap becomes less problematic when information in the form of an informative prior that is based on real (preferably data-based) scientific input or additional information is available. The additional information can be used to distinguish diseased from nondiseased individuals. The authors presented an example using simulated data that illustrates this point and an example involving data from an animal health survey for Johne's disease, where the performance of a serum ELISA was evaluated using additional information obtained from fecal culture. Issues related to identifiability and partial identifiability were also discussed.

24. Janes and Pepe (2009) proposed the covariate-adjusted receiver operating characteristic curve, a measure of covariate-adjusted classification accuracy. Nonparametric and semiparametric estimators were proposed, asymptotic distribution theory was provided, and finite sample performance was investigated. The method was illustrated with an example of the age-adjusted discriminatory accuracy of prostate-specific antigen as a biomarker for prostate cancer.

25. Seshan et al. (2013) demonstrated that both the test statistic and its estimated variance are seriously biased when predictions from nested regression models

are used as data inputs for the test, and examined in detail the reasons for these problems. Although it is possible to create a test reference distribution by resampling that removes these biases, Wald or likelihood ratio tests remain the preferred approach for testing the incremental contribution of a new marker.

26. Bantis et al. (2014) studied parametric and nonparametric approaches for the construction of confidence intervals for the pair of sensitivity and specificity proportions that correspond to the Youden index-based optimal cutoff point. These approaches result in the anticipated coverage under different scenarios for the distributions of healthy and diseased subjects. The authors found that a parametric approach based on a Box–Cox transformation to normality often works well. For biomarkers following more complex distributions, a nonparametric procedure using log spline density estimation can be used.

8.7.2 AUC

1. Hanley and McNeil (1982) provided a representation and interpretation of the AUC obtained by the "rating" method, or by mathematical predictions based on patient characteristics. It was shown that in such a setting, the area represents the probability that a randomly chosen diseased subject is (correctly) rated or ranked with greater suspicion than a randomly chosen nondiseased subject. Moreover, this probability of a correct ranking is the same quantity that is estimated by the already well-studied nonparametric Wilcoxon statistic. These two relationships were exploited in the following aspects: (a) to provide rapid closed-form expressions for the approximate magnitude of the sampling variability, that is, standard error that one uses to accompany the area under a smoothed ROC curve; (b) to guide in determining the size of the sample required to provide a sufficiently reliable estimate of this area; and (c) to determine how large sample sizes should be to ensure that one can statistically detect differences in the accuracy of diagnostic techniques.

2. Halperin et al. (1987) reviewed the problem of obtaining a distribution-free confidence interval for the probability (p) that one random variable is less than another independent random variable based on the two-sample uncensored Wilcoxon–Mann–Whitney statistic. The pivotal quantities used by Sen (1967) and Govindarajulu (1968) were modified to take into account that the variance of estimated p depends on p. A number of simulations were conducted to compare the various methods. The results suggest that the proposed modification is superior in the sense that over the entire range of p, the modification generally yields values of coverage probability much closer to nominal coverage than the methods of Sen (S) and Govindarajulu (G). The coverage values for the S and G methods were shown to be very close to each other; both share the characteristics for one-sided lower confidence limits of being conservative for small values of p and nonconservative (sometimes extremely so) for large values of p. One-sided upper limits have coverages that are essentially the mirror image of lower-limit coverages. The contrasts between the modified method and the S and G methods diminish in magnitude as sample size increases, but are still nontrivial for a sample size of 80. The authors concluded tentatively that the modified procedure can be preferable to that of Sen and Govindarajulu

and can be used when the sample size in both groups is equal to or greater than 20. An example illustrating the use of their modified pivotal quantity and comparing it with the S and G results was presented.

3. When two or more empirical curves are constructed based on tests performed on the same individuals, statistical analysis on differences between curves must take into account the correlated nature of the data. DeLong et al. (1988) presented a nonparametric approach to the analysis of areas under correlated ROC curves, by using the theory on generalized U-statistics to generate an estimated covariance matrix.

4. Wieand et al. (1989) studied a broad class of parametric and nonparametric statistics for comparing two diagnostic markers. One can compare the sensitivities of these diagnostic markers over restricted ranges of specificity by selecting an appropriate statistic from this class. As special cases, one can compare AUC or one can compare the sensitivities at a fixed common specificity. The authors recommended a comparison based on an average of sensitivities over a restricted high level of specificities. Test procedures and confidence intervals were based on asymptotic normality. These procedures were applicable for paired data, in which both diagnostic markers were performed on each subject, and for unpaired data. The procedures may be used to compare two real functions of multiple diagnostic markers, as well as to compare individual markers. Molodianovitch et al. (2006) extended Wieand's parametric test using the Box–Cox power family of transformations to nonnormal situations. These three test procedures were compared in terms of significance level and power by means of a large simulation study. Overall, the authors found that transforming to normality is to be preferred. The method was illustrated with an example of two pancreatic cancer serum biomarkers.

5. In order to compare the partial AUC within a specific range of specificity for two correlated ROC curves, Zhang et al. (2002) proposed a nonparametric method based on Mann–Whitney U-statistics. The estimation of AUC, along with its estimated variance and covariance, was simplified by a method of grouping the observations according to their cutoff point values. The method was used to evaluate alternative logistic regression models that predict whether a subject has incident breast cancer based on information in Medicare claims data.

6. Faraggi and Reiser (2002) discussed and compared estimation procedures for the AUC, based on the following aspects: (a) the Mann–Whitney statistic, (b) kernel smoothing, (c) normal assumptions, and (d) empirical transformations to normality. These were compared in terms of bias and root mean squared error in a large variety of situations by means of an extensive simulation study. The authors found that transforming to normality usually is to be preferred, except for bimodal cases where kernel methods can be effective.

7. Magni et al. (2002) proposed and evaluated a nonparametric Bayesian scheme for AUC estimation in population studies with arbitrary sampling protocols. In the stochastic model representing the whole population, the individual plasma concentration curves and the mean population curve were described by random walk processes, allowing the application of the method to the reconstruction of any kind of regular curves. Population and individual AUC estimation were performed by numerically computing the posterior expectation through a Markov chain Monte Carlo algorithm.

8. Claeskens et al. (2003) derived empirical likelihood confidence regions for the comparison distribution of two populations whose distributions are to be tested for equality using random samples. Another application they considered was for ROC curves, which are used to compare measurements of a diagnostic test from two populations. The authors investigated the smoothed empirical likelihood method for estimation in this context, and empirical likelihood–based confidence intervals were obtained by means of Wilks's theorem. Confidence bands were constructed based on a bootstrap approach. The method was illustrated with a simulation study and the data set analyzed by Wieand et al. (1989) on the accuracy of a carbohydrate antigenic determinant (CA19-9) in detecting pancreatic cancer.

9. Kotz et al. (2003) devoted work to a seemingly very simple topic: estimation of the probabilities of the type $\Pr(X < Y)$, and so forth, and their extensions. However, in spite of their apparent simplicity, this set of probabilistic models, usually referred as the stress–strength models, are of substantial interest and usefulness in various subareas of engineering (most prominently in reliability theory), psychology, genetics, and clinical trials, not to mention purely statistical problems connected with the well-known Mann–Whitney tests. The author presented the point estimation as well as the interval estimation of $\Pr(X < Y)$.

10. Cook et al. (2004) found that the AUC based on longitudinal growth curve models can be used to improve the prediction of young adult blood pressure from childhood measures. Quadratic random effects models over unequally spaced repeated measures were used to compute the area under the curve separately within the age periods 5–14 and 20–34 years in the Bogalusa Heart Study. This method adjusts for the uneven age distribution and captures the underlying or average blood pressure, leading to improved estimates of correlation and risk prediction. Tracking correlations were computed by race and gender, and were approximately 0.6 for systolic, 0.5–0.6 for K4 diastolic, and 0.4–0.6 for K5 diastolic blood pressure. The AUC can also be used to regress young adult blood pressure on childhood blood pressure and childhood and young adult body mass index (BMI). In these data, while childhood blood pressure and young adult BMI were generally directly predictive of young adult blood pressure, childhood BMI was negatively correlated with young adult blood pressure when childhood blood pressure was in the model. In addition, racial differences in young adult blood pressure were reduced, but not eliminated, after controlling for childhood blood pressure, childhood BMI, and young adult BMI, suggesting that other genetic or lifestyle factors contribute to this difference.

11. Ma and Huang (2005) proposed a novel method for biomarker selection and classification for microarray data using a sigmoid approximation to AUC as the objective function for classification and the threshold gradient descent regularization method for estimation and biomarker selection. Tuning parameter selection based on the V-fold cross-validation technique (Efron 1983) and predictive performance evaluation were also investigated. It was demonstrated that the proposed approach yields parsimonious models with excellent classification performance by a simulation study, colon data, and estrogen data.

12. Bandos et al. (2005) developed an exact nonparametric statistical procedure for comparing two ROC curves in paired design settings. The test, which is based on all permutations of the subject-specific rank ratings, is formally a test for the equality of ROC curves that is sensitive to the alternatives of AUC differences.

The operating characteristics of the proposed test were evaluated using extensive simulations over a wide range of parameters. The proposed procedure can be easily implemented in experimental ROC data sets. For small samples and for underlying parameters that are common in experimental studies in diagnostic imaging, the test possesses good operating characteristics and is more powerful than the conventional nonparametric procedure for AUC comparisons. The authors also derived an asymptotic version of the test that uses an exact estimate of the variance in the permutation space and provides a good approximation even when the sample sizes are small. This asymptotic procedure is a simple and precise approximation to the exact test and is useful for large sample sizes where the exact test may be computationally burdensome.

13. Walter (2005) extended the idea of using the partial AUC to the summary ROC curves in meta-analysis. Theoretical and numerical results described the variation in the partial AUC and its standard error as a function of the degree of interstudy heterogeneity and of the extent of truncation applied to the ROC space. A scaled partial area measure was proposed to restore the property that the summary measure should range from 0 to 1. The results suggested several disadvantages of the partial AUC measures. In contrast to earlier findings with the full AUC, the partial AUC is rather sensitive to heterogeneity. Comparisons between tests are more difficult, especially if an empirical truncation process is used. The partial area lacks a useful symmetry property enjoyed by the full AUC. Although the partial AUC may sometimes have clinical appeal, on balance use of the full AUC is preferred.

14. Zhang (2006) proposed a semiparametric Wald statistic to test whether a diagnostic test is capable of discriminating between diseased and nondiseased subjects based on the ROC curve area under a two-sample semiparametric density ratio model. The proposed Wald test was constructed on the basis of the maximum semiparametric likelihood estimator of the ROC curve area. The proposed test statistic has an asymptotic chi-square distribution under the null hypothesis and an asymptotic noncentral chi-square distribution under local alternatives to the null hypothesis. The author presented some results on a simulation study and on the analysis of two data sets.

15. Qin and Zhou (2006) proposed an empirical likelihood (EL) approach for the inference on the AUC. The authors defined an EL ratio for the AUC and showed that its limiting distribution is a scaled chi-square distribution. Then an EL-based confidence interval for the AUC using the scaled chi-square distribution was obtained. This EL inference for the AUC can be extended to stratified samples, and the resulting limiting distribution is a weighted sum of independent chi-square distributions. Additionally, the authors conducted simulation studies to compare the relative performance of the proposed EL-based interval with the existing normal approximation-based intervals and bootstrap intervals for the AUC.

16. He et al. (2006) developed a method for three-class ROC analysis based on decision theory, where the objects were classified by making the decision that provided the maximal utility relative to the other two. By making assumptions about the magnitudes of the relative utilities of incorrect decisions, the authors found a decision model that maximized the expected utility of the decisions when using log-likelihood ratios as decision variables. This decision model consists of a two-dimensional decision plane with log-likelihood ratios as the axes and a decision structure that separates the plane into three regions. Moving the decision structure

over the decision plane, which corresponds to moving the decision threshold in two-class ROC analysis, and computing the true class 1, 2, and 3 fractions allowed them to define a three-class ROC surface. The authors showed that the resulting three-class ROC surface shares many features with the two-class ROC curve; that is, using the log-likelihood ratios as the decision variables results in maximal expected utility of the decisions, and the optimal operating point for a given diagnostic setting (set of relative utilities and disease prevalences) lies on the surface. The volume under the three-class surface (VUS) serves as a figure of merit to evaluate different data acquisition systems or image processing and reconstruction methods when the assumed utility constraints are relevant.

17. Vexler et al. (2008a) considered comparing the areas under correlated ROC curves of diagnostic biomarkers whose measurements are subject to a limit of detection (LOD), a source of measurement error from instruments' sensitivity in epidemiological studies. The authors proposed and examined the likelihood ratio tests with operating characteristics that are easily obtained by classical maximum likelihood methodology.

18. Pencina et al. (2008) addressed the choice of measures of performance of prediction models by introducing two new measures, one based on integrated sensitivity and specificity and the other on reclassification tables. These new measures offer incremental information over the AUC. The authors discussed the properties of these new measures and contrasted them with the AUC, and developed simple asymptotic tests of significance. The use of these measures was illustrated with an example from the Framingham Heart Study. It is suggested that scientists consider these types of measures in addition to the AUC when assessing the performance of newer biomarkers.

19. Zhou (2008) made statistical inference about $\Pr(X < Y)$, where X and Y are two independent continuous random variables, the so-called stress–strength model, through the Edgeworth expansions and the bootstrap approximations of the studentized Wilcoxon–Mann–Whitney statistics. Finite sample accuracy of the confidence intervals was assessed through a simulation study. Two real data sets were analyzed to illustrate the methods, including the data set studied by Wieand et al. (1989) on the accuracy of a carbohydrate antigenic determinant (CA19-9) in detecting pancreatic cancer and a study on assessing the accuracy of cerebrospinal fluid CK-BB isoenzyme measured within 24 hours of injury as a means of predicting the outcome of severe head trauma (Hans et al. 1985).

20. For independent X and Y in the inequality $\Pr(X \leq Y + \mu)$, Clarkson et al. (2009) provided sharp lower bounds for unimodal distributions having finite variance and sharp upper bounds assuming symmetric densities bounded by a finite constant. The lower bounds depend on a result of Dubins (1962) about extreme points, and the upper bounds depend on a symmetric rearrangement theorem of Riesz (1930).

21. Harrell's c-index or concordance c has been widely used as a measure of separation of two survival distributions. In the absence of censored data, Koziol and Jia (2009) considered the c-index estimates of the Mann–Whitney parameter $\Pr(X > Y)$, which has been repeatedly utilized in various statistical contexts. In the presence of randomly censored data, the c-index no longer estimates $\Pr(X > Y)$, a parameter that involves the underlying censoring distributions. This is in contrast to Efron's (1967) maximum likelihood estimator of the Mann–Whitney parameter, which is recommended in the setting of random censorship.

22. Rezaei et al. (2010) developed the estimation of $R = \Pr(Y < X)$ when X and Y are two independent generalized Pareto distributions with different parameters. The maximum likelihood estimator and its asymptotic distribution were obtained. An asymptotic confidence interval of R was constructed using the asymptotic distribution. Assuming that the common scale parameter is known, MLE, UMVUE, Bayes estimation of R, and the confidence interval were obtained. The ML estimator of R, asymptotic distribution, and Bayes estimation of R in the general case were also studied. Monte Carlo simulations were performed to compare the different proposed methods.

23. Cross-validation is a typical strategy for estimating the classification performance of inferred predictive models, but it is difficult when working with small data sets. Through extensive simulation studies, Airola et al. (2011) noted that when the AUC is used as the summary measure of the diagnostic accuracy, many standard approaches to cross-validation suffer from extensive bias or variance. It was demonstrated that leave-pair-out cross-validation is almost unbiased for conditional AUC estimation, and its deviation variance is as low as that of the best alternative approaches.

24. Recently, the concept of generalized treatment effect, defined as $\Pr(X > Y)$, where X and Y denote continuous outcome variables for treatment arm and control arm, respectively, has been proposed as an appropriate measure of treatment effect in clinical trials with parallel design. Compared to the mean difference, the generalized treatment effect has many advantages; for example, it is a scaleless measure and it does not change under monotonic transformations. Tian et al. (2012) investigated the problem of testing equality of generalized treatment effects among several clinical trials. The proposed approach follows the same vein as the generalized variable method for testing the equality of several lognormal means proposed by Li (2009). Numerical study demonstrated that the proposed test has excellent Type I error control for clinical trials with small to medium sample sizes. A robustness study showed that the proposed method performs reasonably for categorical data. The authors illustrated the proposed approach using the data set given in Eddy (1989), which consists of eight randomized parallel clinical trials studying the effectiveness of a drug called amlodipine.

25. Feng et al. (2012) adopted the approach of the generalized propensity score, which is the conditional probability of receiving a particular level of the treatment given the pre-treatment variables, and developed a statistical methodology based on the generalized propensity score in order to estimate treatment effects in the case of multiple treatments. Two methods were discussed and compared: propensity score regression adjustment and propensity score weighting. The authors used these methods to assess the relative effectiveness of individual treatments in the multiple-treatment IMPACT clinical trial, where the patients were randomly allocated to the intervention arm that received collaborative care or to the control arm that received conventional primary care. The results revealed that both methods perform well when the sample size is moderate or large.

26. Gupta et al. (2013) developed large sample confidence intervals of the dependence and reliability $R = P(X > Y)$ parameters from a bivariate lognormal distribution with equal lognormal means. The parameter R provides a general measure of difference between the two populations and has applications in many areas. The performance of these confidence intervals was examined by extensive simulation studies.

The results were illustrated with a data set containing 56 assay pairs of cyclosporine, where the results were obtained by taking 56 blood samples from organ transplant recipients and assaying an aliquot of each sample by a standard approved method (high-performance liquid chromatography [HPLC]) and an alternative method (radioimmunoassay [RIA]) (Hawkins 2002).

27. Many researchers believe that a change in AUC is a poor metric because it increases only slightly with the addition of a marker with a large odds ratio. Because it is not possible on purely statistical grounds to choose between the odds ratio and AUC, Baker et al. (2014) invoked decision analysis, which incorporates costs and benefits. For example, a timely estimate of the risk of later nonelective operative delivery can help a woman in labor decide if she wants an early elective cesarean section to avoid greater complications from possible later nonelective operative delivery.

28. A basic risk prediction model for later nonelective operative delivery involves only antepartum markers. Because adding intrapartum markers to this risk prediction model increases AUC by 0.02, the authors questioned whether this small improvement is worthwhile. A key decision-analytic quantity is the risk threshold, here the risk of later nonelective operative delivery at which a patient would be indifferent between an early elective cesarean section and usual care. For a range of risk thresholds, the authors found that an increase in the net benefit of risk prediction requires collecting intrapartum marker data on 68–124 women for every correct prediction of later nonelective operative delivery. Because data collection is noninvasive, this test trade-off of 68–124 is clinically acceptable, indicating the value of adding intrapartum markers to the risk prediction model.

29. An empirical likelihood method of interval estimation of the AUC is not advisable in the case of right-censored data due to severe computational issues. Toward this end, Chrzanowski (2014) proposed an extension of a so-called weighted empirical likelihood (WEL) method for interval estimation of AUC. The author defined the WEL ratio and showed that it has a limiting scaled chi-square distribution, which allows us to construct a confidence interval for the AUC. The author conducted a simulation study to compare the performance of the proposed WEL-based interval with the one based on the already existing plug-in method.

8.7.3 Combinations of Markers

1. Bock et al. (1987) studied the behavior of the tail probabilities of weighted averages of certain independently and identically distribution random variables as the weights vary. The authors showed that the upper and lower tails are smallest when all the weights are equal. The results were applied to exponential, chi-square, gamma, and Weibull random variables.

2. Pepe and Thompson (2000) proposed a distribution-free rank-based approach for maximizing the area or partial area under the ROC curve based on linear combinations of markers and compared it with logistic regression and classic linear discriminant analysis (LDA). It was shown that the latter method optimizes the area under the ROC curve when test results have a multivariate normal distribution for diseased and nondiseased populations. Simulation studies suggested that the proposed nonparametric method is efficient when data are multivariate normal. The distribution-free method was generalized to a smooth

distribution-free approach in the following aspects: (a) to accommodate some reasonable smoothness assumptions, (b) to incorporate covariate effects, and (c) to yield optimized partial areas under the ROC curve. This latter feature is particularly important since it allows one to focus on a region of the ROC curve that is of most relevance to clinical practice. Neither logistic regression nor LDA necessarily maximizes partial areas. The approaches were illustrated on two cancer data sets, one involving serum antigen markers for pancreatic cancer and the other involving longitudinal prostate-specific antigen data.

3. Kramar et al. (2001) presented a computer program by using the generalized ROC criteria based on the BLC of the test for which the area under the ROC curve is maximal, as well as its confidence interval, obtained from the noncentral *F*-distribution. Quantified marker values are assumed to follow a multivariate normal distribution, but not necessarily with equal variances for two populations. Other options include Box–Cox variable transformations, Q-Q plots, and interactive graphics associated with changes in sensitivity and specificity as a function of the cutoff. The authors provided an example to illustrate the usefulness of data transformation and how a linear combination of markers can significantly improve discriminative power. This finding highlights potential difficulties with methods that reject individual markers based on univariate analyses.

4. Prabhakar and Jain (2002) proposed a scheme for classifier combination at the decision level that stresses the importance of classifier selection during combination. The proposed scheme is optimal (in the Neyman–Pearson sense) when sufficient data are available to obtain reasonable estimates of the joint densities of classifier outputs. Four different fingerprint-matching algorithms are combined using the proposed scheme to improve the accuracy of a fingerprint verification system. Experiments conducted on a large fingerprint database (close to 2700 fingerprints) confirmed the effectiveness of the proposed integration scheme. An overall matching performance increase of close to 3% was achieved. The authors further showed that a combination of multiple impressions or multiple fingers improves the verification performance by more than 4% and 5%, respectively. Analysis of the results provided some insight into the various decision-level classifier combination strategies.

5. Cooke and Peake (2002) provided a simple algorithm for finding the optimal ROC curve for a linear discriminant between two point distributions, given only information about the classes' means and covariances. The method made no assumptions concerning the exact type of distribution and was shown to provide the best possible discrimination for any physically reasonable measure of the classification error. This very general solution was shown to specialize in the results obtained in other papers that assumed multidimensional Gaussian distributed classes, or minimized the maximum classification error. Some numerical examples were provided that show the improvement in classification of this method over previously used methods.

6. McIntosh and Pepe (2002) considered how to combine multiple disease markers for optimal performance of a screening program. The authors showed that the risk score, defined as the probability of disease given data on multiple markers, is the optimal function in the sense that the ROC curve is maximized at every point, by virtue of the Neyman–Pearson lemma. This contrasts with the corresponding optimality result of the classic decision theory, which is set in a Bayesian framework and is based on minimizing an expected loss function associated with decision errors.

The result is optimally defined from a strictly frequentist point of view and does not rely on the notion of associating costs with misclassifications. The implication for data analysis is that binary regression methods can be used to yield appropriate relative weightings of different biomarkers, at least in large samples. The authors proposed some modifications to standard binary regression methods for application to the disease screening problem. A flexible biologically motivated simulation model for cancer biomarkers was presented, and the authors evaluated their methods by application to it. An application to real data concerning two ovarian cancer biomarkers was also presented. The results were equally relevant to the more general medical diagnostic testing problem, where results of multiple tests or predictors are combined to yield a composite diagnostic test. Moreover, the methods justified the development of clinical prediction scores based on binary regression.

7. Thompson (2003) considered the assessment of the overall diagnostic accuracy of a sequence of tests (e.g., repeated screening tests). The complexity of diagnostic choices with two or more continuous tests was illustrated, and different approaches to reducing the dimensionality were presented and evaluated. For instance, in practice, when a single test is used repeatedly in routine screening, the same screening threshold is typically used at each screening visit. One possible alternative is to adjust the threshold at successive visits according to individual-specific characteristics. Such possibilities represent a particular slice of a ROC surface, corresponding to all possible combinations of test thresholds. The author focused on the development and examples of the setting where an overall test is defined to be positive if any of the individual tests are believed to be positive. The ideas developed were illustrated by an example of application to screening for prostate cancer using prostate-specific antigen.

8. In order to examine methods for combining quantitative results for serum carbohydrate-deficient transferrin (CDT), gamma-glutamyltransferase (GGT), and aspartate aminotransferase (AST), and refining these by inclusion of patient characteristics, Chen et al. (2003b) developed clinical rules for combining the results based on the data from 1684 subjects, recruited from the general population, abstainer groups, and alcohol treatment centers (participants in the five-nation WHO/ISBRA study of biological markers of alcohol use). It was concluded that combining biochemical markers enhances detection of problem drinking in men but not in women. Information on clinical variables increases the ability to correctly detect problem drinking.

9. Hsu et al. (2004) showed how the method of multiple comparison with the best (MCB) for normal error general linear models can be adapted to compare diagnostic tools in terms of AUCs of their ROC curves. MCB of AUCs of ROC curves was illustrated by comparing diagnostic variables for predicting the need for emergency cesarean section, and for predicting the onset of juvenile myopia.

10. Liu et al. (2005) considered combining multiple biomarkers to improve diagnostic accuracy by maximizing sensitivity over a range of specificity. The authors first presented a simpler proof for the main theorem of Su and Liu (1993) and further investigated some other optimal properties of their linear combinations. Alternative linear combinations were derived that have higher sensitivity over a range of high (or low) specificity. The methods were illustrated using data from a study evaluating biomarkers for coronary heart disease.

11. Khurd and Gindi (2005) considered quantifying performance on decision tasks involving location uncertainty using the localization ROC (LROC) methodology and derived decision strategies that maximize the area under the LROC curve, A_{LROC}. The authors showed that these decision strategies minimize Bayes risk under certain reasonable cost constraints. The detection–localization task was modeled as a decision problem in three increasingly realistic ways. In the first two models, the authors treated location as a discrete parameter having finitely many values resulting in an $(L+1)$ class classification problem. In the first simple model, it does not include search tolerance effects, and in the second, more general, model, it does. In the third and most general model, location is treated as a continuous parameter and search tolerance effects are included. In all cases, the essential proof that the observer maximizes A_{LROC} was obtained with a modified version of the Neyman–Pearson lemma. A separate form of proof was used to show that in all three cases, the decision strategy minimizes the Bayes risk under certain reasonable cost constraints.

12. Pepe et al. (2006) considered an alternative objective function—the area under the empirical receiver operating characteristic curve (AUC). The authors noted that it yields consistent estimates of parameters in a generalized linear model for the risk score, but does not require specifying the link function. Like logistic regression, it yields consistent estimation with case-control or cohort data. Simulation studies suggested that AUC-based classification scores have performance comparable with that of logistic likelihood-based scores when the logistic regression model holds. Analysis of data from a proteomics biomarker study showed that performance can be far superior to that of logistic regression–derived scores when the logistic regression model does not hold. Model fitting by maximizing the AUC rather than the likelihood should be considered when the goal is to derive a marker combination score for classification or prediction.

13. Vexler et al. (2006b) considered the linear separation of two continuous multivariate distributions. Under mild conditions, the optimal linear separation exists uniquely. A kernel-smoothed approach was proposed to estimate the optimal linear combination and the corresponding separation measure. The proposed method yields consistent estimators, allowing the construction of confidence intervals.

14. Ma and Huang (2007) studied a ROC-based method for effectively combining multiple markers for disease classification and proposed a sigmoid AUC (SAUC) estimator that maximizes the sigmoid approximation of the empirical AUC. The SAUC estimator is computationally affordable, $n^{1/2}$ consistent, and achieves the same asymptotic efficiency as the AUC estimator. Inference based on the weighted bootstrap was investigated. The authors proposed Monte Carlo methods to assess the overall prediction performance and the relative importance of individual markers. Finite sample performance was evaluated using simulation studies and two public data sets.

15. Under the framework of a ROC curve, Gao et al. (2008) presented a method to estimate an optimum linear combination maximizing sensitivity at a fixed specificity while assuming a multivariate normal distribution in diagnostic tests. The method was applied to a real-world study where the accuracy of two biomarkers was evaluated in the diagnosis of pancreatic cancer. The performance of the method was also evaluated by simulation studies.

16. Tian et al. (2009) considered the problem of comparing the discriminatory abilities between two groups of biomarkers, focusing on confidence interval estimation of the difference between paired AUCs based on optimally combined markers under the assumption of multivariate normality. Simulation studies demonstrated that the generalized variable approach provided confidence intervals with satisfying coverage probabilities at finite sample sizes. This method can also easily provide p-values for hypothesis testing. Application to analysis of a subset of data from a study on coronary heart disease illustrated the utility of the method in practice.

17. Qin and Zhang (2010) considered the best combination of multiple diagnostic tests, and studied semiparametric likelihood estimation of the optimal ROC and the AUC. The authors presented a bootstrap procedure along with some results on simulation and on analysis of two real data sets.

18. Based on the smoothly clipped absolute deviation (SCAD) penalty and the area under the ROC curve (AUC), Lin et al. (2011) proposed a new method for selecting and combining biomarkers for disease classification and prediction. The proposed estimator for the combination of the biomarkers has an oracle property; that is, the estimated combination of the biomarkers performs as well as it would have had the biomarkers significantly associated with the outcome been known in advance, in terms of discriminative power. The estimator is computationally feasible, $n^{1/2}$ consistent, and asymptotically normal. Simulation studies showed that the proposed method performs better than existing methods. The authors illustrated the proposed methodology in the acoustic startle response study.

19. Perkins et al. (2011) developed asymptotically unbiased estimators, via the maximum likelihood technique, of the area under the ROC curve of BLC of two bivariate normally distributed biomarkers affected by LODs. Confidence intervals for the AUC were developed. Point and confidence interval estimates were scrutinized by simulation study, recording bias and root mean squared error and coverage probability, respectively. An example using polychlorinated biphenyl (PCB) levels to classify women with and without endometriosis illustrated the potential benefits of the methods.

20. B. Yu et al. (2011) proposed a method of combining multiple diagnostic tests in the absence of a golden standard, assuming that the test values and their classification accuracies are dependent on covariates. Simulation studies were performed to examine the performance of the combination method. The proposed method was applied to data from a population-based aging study to compare the accuracy of three screening tests for kidney function and to estimate the prevalence of moderate kidney impairment.

21. Wang and Li (2012) considered ROC analysis for bivariate marker measurements, focusing on extensions of tools and rules from univariate marker to bivariate marker settings for evaluating the predictive accuracy of markers using a tree-based classification rule. Using an and-or classifier, a ROC function, together with a weighted ROC function (WROC) and their conjugate counterparts, was proposed for examining the performance of bivariate markers. The proposed functions evaluate the performance of and-or classifiers among all possible combinations of marker values, and are ideal measures for understanding the predictability of biomarkers in a target population. Specific features of ROC and WROC functions and other related statistics are discussed in comparison with those familiar properties for the univariate marker. Nonparametric methods were developed for estimating

ROC-related functions' (partial) AUC and concordance probability. With emphasis on the average performance of markers, the proposed procedures and inferential results were useful for evaluating marker predictability based on a single or bivariate marker (or test) measurements with different choices of markers, and for evaluating different and-or combinations in classifiers. The inferential results developed extended to multivariate markers with a sequence of arbitrarily combined and-or classifiers.

8.8 Appendix

8.8.1 General Form of the AUC

By the definition of the AUC (area under the ROC curve) and the fact that F and G are cumulative distribution functions of X and Y, respectively, the AUC can be expressed as

$$\int_0^1 ROC(t)dt = \int_0^1 (1 - F(G^{-1}(1-t)))dt = \int_{-\infty}^{\infty} (1 - F(w))dG(w)$$

$$= 1 - \int_{-\infty}^{\infty} F(w)dG(w) = 1 - \Pr(X \le Y) = \Pr(X > Y).$$

8.8.2 Form of the AUC under the Normal Data Distribution Assumption

Assume $X \sim N(\mu_1, \sigma_1^2)$ and, for the nondiseased population, $Y \sim N(\mu_2, \sigma_2^2)$. Note that X and Y are independent. Consequently, we can obtain

$$A = \Pr(X > Y) = \Pr(X - Y > 0) = 1 - \Pr\left\{ \frac{(X-Y)-(\mu_1-\mu_2)}{\sqrt{\sigma_1^2 + \sigma_2^2}} \le -\frac{\mu_1 - \mu_2}{\sqrt{\sigma_1^2 + \sigma_2^2}} \right\}$$

$$= 1 - \Phi\left(-\frac{\mu_1 - \mu_2}{\sqrt{\sigma_1^2 + \sigma_2^2}} \right) = \Phi\left(\frac{\mu_1 - \mu_2}{\sqrt{\sigma_1^2 + \sigma_2^2}} \right).$$

8.8.3 Form of the Function h Associating μ_{11} with, μ_{21}, μ_{31}, μ_{41}, μ_2, Σ_1, Σ_2 under H_0

Based on the equation under the null hypothesis $\dfrac{N_1}{\sqrt{D_1}} = \dfrac{N_2}{\sqrt{D_2}}$ and assuming that higher values indicate better performance, that is, $A = \Pr$(combined pre-treatment biomarker values < combined post-treatment biomarkersvalues), the root of the equation under the null hypothesis for μ_{11} is

$$\mu_{11} = \mu_{21} + \frac{\left(\Delta_{\mu_{Y1}} (\sigma_{13} - \sigma_{14} - \sigma_{23} + \sigma_{24}) - \left((\Delta_{\mu_{Y1}}^2 - M(\sigma_{33} - 2\sigma_{34} + \sigma_{44}))S \right)^{\frac{1}{2}} \right)}{(\sigma_{33} - 2\sigma_{34} + \sigma_{44})},$$

where

$$\Delta_{\mu_{Y1}} = \mu_{31} - \mu_{41}, \ M = N_2^2/D_2,$$

$$S = \sigma_{13}^2 - 2\sigma_{13}\sigma_{14} - 2\sigma_{13}\sigma_{23} + 2\sigma_{13}\sigma_{24} + \sigma_{14}^2 + 2\sigma_{14}\sigma_{23} - 2\sigma_{14}\sigma_{24}$$
$$+ \sigma_{23}^2 - 2\sigma_{23}\sigma_{24} + \sigma_{24}^2 - \sigma_{11}\sigma_{33} + 2\sigma_{11}\sigma_{34} + 2\sigma_{12}\sigma_{33} - 4\sigma_{12}\sigma_{34}$$
$$- \sigma_{11}\sigma_{44} - \sigma_{22}\sigma_{33} + 2\sigma_{12}\sigma_{44} + 2\sigma_{22}\sigma_{34} - \sigma_{22}\sigma_{44}.$$

Assuming that lower values indicate better performance, that is, $A = \text{Pr}(\text{combined pre-treatment biomarker values} > \text{combined post-treatment biomarker values})$, the root of the equation under the null hypothesis for μ_{11} is

$$\mu_{11} = \mu_{21} + \frac{\left(\Delta_{\mu_{Y1}} (\sigma_{13} - \sigma_{14} - \sigma_{23} + \sigma_{24}) + \left(\left(\Delta_{\mu_{Y1}}^2 - M(\sigma_{33} - 2\sigma_{34} + \sigma_{44}) \right) S \right)^{1/2} \right)}{(\sigma_{33} - 2\sigma_{34} + \sigma_{44})}.$$

9

Nonparametric Comparisons of Distributions

9.1 Introduction

Parametric methods for comparing distributions, whose justification in probability is based on specific distributional assumptions, may lead to loss of efficiency when the distributional assumptions are violated or may lead to biased tests. For example, t-tests are known to be biased in terms of controlling the Type I error rate in the case of skewed data and are often less efficient than other tests given nonnormal data. As an alternative, nonparametric procedures based on functions of the ranks of the sample observations, or similarly based on empirical distribution function estimators, are in general asymptotically or exactly unbiased and are robustly more efficient than their parametric counterparts. In this chapter, we introduce several commonly used nonparametric tests for comparison of distributions, including the Wilcoxon rank-sum test and the Kolmogorov–Smirnov test, as well as novel density-based empirical likelihood (EL) ratio tests based on two samples and paired data. Multiple-group comparison methodology is also introduced.

9.2 Wilcoxon Rank-Sum Test

As a nonparametric analogue to the two-sample t-test, the Wilcoxon rank-sum test (also called the Mann–Whitney U-test or the Mann–Whitney–Wilcoxon test) can be used primarily when investigators do not want to, or cannot, assume that data distributions are known. The test itself is highly efficient and robust across a variety of parametric assumptions compared to the t-test. The key assumption for using the Wilcoxon rank-sum test is the idea of exchangeability of the observations under the null hypothesis; that is, the distribution functions for the two groups being tested are equivalent under the null hypothesis. This assumption may be generally assumed to be true in the randomized experimental setting, but may not be assumed in certain nonrandomized settings. If this assumption is not met, the Wilcoxon test might be biased.

In terms of the mechanics of the test, suppose that we have two samples of observations, containing independent and identically distributed (i.i.d.) measurements $X_1, ..., X_m$ and i.i.d. measurements $Y_1, ..., Y_n$, respectively. In practical applications, we often want to test the hypothesis that two populations are the same in the context of no location shift. Assume that $X_1, ..., X_m \sim F(x - u)$, $Y_1, ..., Y_n \sim F(y - v)$, that all $m + n$ observations are independent, and that $F(\cdot)$ is symmetric about zero; we are interested in testing $H_0: \Delta = v - u = 0$ against $H_1: \Delta = v - u > 0$. Let R_i be the rank of Y_i among all $m + n$ observations, where the rank refers to the ordinal number of the corresponding observation among a pre-ordered data set in ascending order. The Mann–Whitney statistic is $W = \sum_{i=1}^{n} R_i - n(n+1)/2 = \sum_{i=1}^{m} \sum_{j=1}^{n} I(X_i < Y_j)$, where $I(\cdot)$ is the indicator function. The decision-making rule is to reject H_0 for large values of W.

Since the indicator $I(X < Y) = I(F(X) < F(Y))$, it is clear that under H_0, when the random variables $F(X)$, $F(Y)$ are independent and uniformly $[0,1]$ distributed, the test statistic W is distributed independently of the distributions for X and Y. Thus, the Wilcoxon test is exact and its critical values can be evaluated by using the methods introduced in Chapter 16.

In cases of relatively large samples, it follows from one-sample U-statistics theory that, under the null hypothesis, W is asymptotically normal (Hettmansperger and McKean 1978), that is,

$$\frac{W - mn/2}{\sqrt{mn(m+n+1)/12}} \xrightarrow{d} N(0,1).$$

Therefore, a cutoff value for the α-level test can be found as

$$K_\alpha = mn/2 + 1/2 + z_\alpha \sqrt{mn(m+n+1)/12},$$

where the additional $1/2$ is added for a continuity correction.

The Wilcoxon rank-sum test has greater efficiency than the t-test given nonnormal distributions, and it is nearly as efficient as the t-test given normal distributions (e.g., Lehmann and Romano 2006).

Example 9.1: Two Group Comparison Using the Wilcoxon Rank-Sum Statistics

We consider the data of high-density lipoprotein (HDL) cholesterol measurements described in Figure 4.1 in Chapter 4 and conduct a Wilcoxon rank-sum test for examining a location shift between the two groups.

The function `wilcox.test` in R conducts the two-sample Wilcoxon test for equality on means. Note that the alternative can be revised to less or greater in terms of a one-sided test.

```
> X<-c (37.4, 70.4, 52.8, 46.2, 74.8, 96.8, 41.8, 55.0, 83.6, 63.8,
63.8, 52.8, 46.2, 37.4, 50.6, 74.8, 46.2, 39.6, 70.4, 30.8, 74.8, 61.6,
30.8, 74.8, 52.8)
> Y<-c (44.0, 35.2, 110.0, 63.8, 44, 26.4, 52.8, 30.8, 39.6, 44, 48.4,
39.6, 55, 52.8, 50.6, 39.6, 35.2, 55, 57.2, 37.4, 30.8, 46.2, 50.6, 44,
44)
> wilcox. test (X,Y)

        Wilcoxon rank sum test with continuity correction

data: X and Y
W = 432, p-value = 0.02065
alternative hypothesis : true location shift is not equal to 0
```

For these HDL cholesterol data, the p-value of the Wilcoxon rank-sum test is 0.02065. Thus, we reject the null hypothesis at the 0.05 significance level and conclude a significant difference in the location between the two groups.

9.3 Kolmogorov–Smirnov Two-Sample Test

The Kolmogorov–Smirnov test is a known procedure for comparing distributions of populations, where the test statistic is constructed using the empirical distribution function estimators from the respective samples.

Given two random samples $X_1, X_2, ..., X_m$ and $Y_1, Y_2, ..., Y_n$, each of size m and n from continuous populations F_X and F_Y, respectively, assume we would like to test $H_0: F_X(x) = F_Y(x)$ for all x versus $H_1: F_X(x) \neq F_Y(x)$ for some x. The respective empirical distribution function estimators of F_X and F_Y, denoted by $F_m(x)$ and $F_n(x)$, are given as $F_m(x) = m^{-1} \sum_{i=1}^{m} I(X_i \leq x)$ and $F_n(x) = n^{-1} \sum_{i=1}^{n} I(Y_i \leq x)$. Note that in a combined ordered arrangement of the $m + n$ sample observations, $F_m(x)$ and $F_n(x)$ are the respective proportions of X and Y observations that do not exceed a specified value for x.

If the null hypothesis $H_0: F_Y(x) = F_X(x)$ for all x is true, the population distribution functions are identical and the two samples come from equivalent populations. The empirical distribution functions for X and Y are unbiased estimates of their respective population cumulative distribution functions. Thus, taking into account sampling variability, two empirical distributions should be reasonably close to each other under H_0; otherwise, the data suggest that H_0 is not true and therefore should be rejected. This is the intuitive logic behind most two-sample tests. The problem is defining what is a reasonable absolute distance measure between the two empirical cumulative distribution functions (Gibbons and Chakraborti 2010). The two-sided Kolmogorov–Smirnov two-sample test statistic, denoted by $D_{m,n}$, is based on the maximum absolute difference between the two empirical distributions:

$$D_{m,n} = \max_x \left| F_m(x) - F_n(x) \right|.$$

Note that, here, only the magnitudes rather than the directions of the deviations are considered. We reject H_0 if $D_{m,n} \geq c_\alpha$ for pre-specified threshold c_α, where $\Pr(D_{m,n} \geq c_\alpha \mid H_0) \leq \alpha$. The p-value is $\Pr(D_{m,n} \geq D_0 \mid H_0)$, where D_0 denotes the observed value of the two-sample Kolmogorov–Smirnov test statistic. The Kolmogorov–Smirnov two-sample test is exact.

For the asymptotic null distribution, Smirnov (1939a, 1939b) proved that as m and n go to infinity in such a way that m/n remains constant, we have

$$\lim_{m,n \to \infty} \Pr\left(\sqrt{\frac{mn}{m+n}} D_{m,n} \leq d \right) = L(d),$$

where

$$L(d) = 1 - 2 \sum_{i=1}^{\infty} (-1)^{i-1} e^{-2i^2 d^2}.$$

9.4 Density-Based Empirical Likelihood Ratio Tests

In this section, we introduce exact density-based empirical likelihood ratio (LR) tests for composite hypotheses related to treatment effects in order to provide efficient tools that compare study groups proposed by Vexler et al. (2012a).

9.4.1 Hypothesis Setting and Test Statistics

To test for equality of the distribution of a new therapy group and a control therapy group based on paired observations $\{Z_{11},...,Z_{1m_1}\}$ and $\{Z_{21},...,Z_{1m_2}\}$, one may consider the hypotheses

$$H_{N0}: F_{Z_1} = F_{Z_2} = F_Z \text{ vs. } H_A: F_{Z_1} \neq F_{Z_2},$$

where Z_{ij} denotes a within-pair difference of subject j from sample i, $i = 1, 2; j = 1, ..., n_i$, $\{Z_{11},...,Z_{1m_1}\}$ and $\{Z_{21},...,Z_{2m_2}\}$ consist of i.i.d. observations from populations Z_1 and Z_2 with distribution functions $F_{Z_1}(\cdot)$ and $F_{Z_2}(\cdot)$, respectively. In contexts of treatment evaluations, Z_{ij} can be defined to be the difference of measurements between pre- and post-treatment. We consider different hypotheses simultaneously for the symmetry of F_{Z_1} and/or F_{Z_2} (detecting a treatment effect into groups) as well as for the equivalence $F_{Z_1} = F_{Z_2}$. We refer to the nonparametric literature to connect the term "treatment effect" with tests for symmetry (e.g., Wilcoxon, 1945). Note that the Kolmogorov–Smirnov test is a known procedure to compare distributions of populations, whereas the standard testing procedures such as paired t-test, the sign test, and the Wilcoxon signed rank test can be applied to the symmetric problem, i.e., to test for $H_0: F_Z(z) = 1 - F_Z(-z)$. Comparisons between distributions of new therapy and control groups as well as detecting treatment effects may be based on multiple hypotheses tests. To this end, one can create relevant tests, combining, for example, the Kolmogorov–Smirnov test and the Wilcoxon signed rank test. The use of the classical procedures commonly requires complex considerations to combine the known nonparametric tests. Alternatively, we will develop a direct distribution-free method for analyzing the two-sample problems. The proposed method can be easily applied to test nonparametrically for different composite hypotheses. The proposed approach approximates nonparametrically most powerful Neyman–Pearson-test rules.

To incorporate evaluation of the treatment effect on each therapy group, we point out three tests related to the null hypothesis: (1) the equality of the distributions of two therapy groups, and (2) no treatment effect in each group. This can be presented by H_0: (1) $F_{Z_1} = F_{Z_2} = F_Z$, and (2) $F_Z(z) = 1 - F_Z(-z)$, for all $z \in (-\infty, \infty)$. Against H_0, we can set up three different alternative hypotheses, H_{A1}, H_{A2}, and H_{A3}, where

1. H_{A1}: Not H_0, that is, $F_{Z_1} \neq F_{Z_2}$ or $F_{Z_1}(z_1) \neq 1 - F_{Z_1}(-z_1)$ or $F_{Z_2}(z_2) \neq 1 - F_{Z_2}(-z_2)$.

2. H_{A2}: There is a treatment effect in one therapy group, while there is no treatment effect in the other.

3. H_{A3}: One asserts that both therapy groups have the same treatment effect. In this case, because the distributions of two groups are assumed to be identical under H_0 and H_{A3}, a one-sample test for symmetry can be applied.

Cases 1–3 are formally noted in Table 9.1.

Let Tests 1–3 refer to the hypothesis tests for the composite hypotheses H_0 versus H_{A1}, H_0 versus H_{A2}, and H_0 versus H_{A3}, respectively. We then develop test statistics for Tests 1–3, which will be shown to be exact.

9.4.1.1 Test 1: H_0 versus H_{A1}

Consider the scenario where one is interested in testing for $H_0: F_{z_1} - F_{z_2} = F_Z$, $F_Z(z) = 1 - F_Z(-z)$, for all $z \in (-\infty, \infty)$ versus H_{A1}.

TABLE 9.1

Hypotheses of Interest to Be Tested Based on Paired Data

Null Hypothesis	vs.	Alternative Hypothesis
$H_{N0}: F_{Z_1} = F_{Z_2} = F_Z$		$H_A: F_{Z_1} \neq F_{Z_2}$
		$H_{A1}: F_{Z_1} \neq F_{Z_2}$ or $F_{Z_i}(z_i) \neq 1 - F_{Z_i}(-z_i)$, for $i = 1$ or 2
$H_0: F_{Z_1} = F_{Z_2} = F_Z; F_Z(z) = 1 - F_Z(-z),$		(i.e., not H_0)
for all $z \in (-\infty, \infty)$		$H_{A2}: F_{Z_1} \neq F_{Z_2}; F_{Z_1}(z_1) \neq 1 - F_{Z_1}(-z_1); F_{Z_2}(z_2) = 1 - F_{Z_2}(-z_2)$
		$H_{A3}: F_{Z_1} = F_{Z_2} = F_{H_{A3},Z}; F_{H_{A3},Z}(z) \neq 1 - F_{H_{A3},Z}(-z)$

The likelihood ratio test statistic based on observations Z_{ij}, $i = 1, 2; j = 1, \ldots, n_i$, is given by

$$LR_{H_{A1}} = \frac{\prod_{j=1}^{n_1} f_{Z_1}(Z_{1j}) \prod_{j=1}^{n_2} f_{Z_2}(Z_{2j})}{\prod_{j=1}^{n_1} f_Z(Z_{1j}) \prod_{j=1}^{n_2} f_Z(Z_{2j})} = \prod_{j=1}^{n_1} \frac{f_{Z_1,j}}{f_{ZZ_1,j}} \prod_{j=1}^{n_1} \frac{f_{Z_2,j}}{f_{ZZ_2,j}},$$

where $f_{Z_i}, i = 1, 2,$ are density functions related to $F_{Z_i}, i = 1, 2; f_Z$ is a density function related to a symmetric distribution $F_Z; f_{Z_1,j} = f_{Z_1}(Z_{1(j)}), f_{Z_2,j} = f_{Z_2}(Z_{2(j)}), f_{ZZ_1,j} = f_Z(Z_{1(j)}),$ and $f_{ZZ_2,j} = f_Z(Z_{2(j)});$ and $Z_{1(1)} \leq Z_{1(2)} \leq \cdots \leq Z_{1(n_1)}, Z_{2(1)} \leq Z_{2(2)} \leq \cdots \leq Z_{2(n_2)}$ are the order statistics based on $\{Z_{11}, \ldots, Z_{1n_1}\}$ and $\{Z_{21}, \ldots, Z_{2n_2}\}$, respectively.

The nonparametric test statistic is developed by modifying the maximum empirical likelihood (see Chapter 6 for details) concept to directly obtain estimated values of $f_{Z_1j}, j = 1, \ldots, n_1$, maximizing $\prod_{j=1}^{n_1} f_{Z_1,j}$ subject to an empirical constraint. This constraint controls estimated values of $f_{Z_1j}, j = 1, \ldots, n_1$, preserving the main property of the density function f_{Z_1} under the complex structure of the tested hypothesis. To obtain the associated empirical constraint, one may use the fact that the values of f_{Z_1j} should be restricted by the equation $\int f_{Z_1}(u) du = 1$. By applying the mean value theorem to approximate the constraint $\int f_{Z_1}(u) du = 1$ (Gurevich and Vexler 2011; Vexler and Gurevich 2010b; Vexler and Yu 2011; Vexler et al. 2011b), for all positive integer $m \leq n/2$, we have

$$(2m)^{-1} \sum_{j=1}^{n_1} \int_{Z_{1(j-m)}}^{Z_{1(j+m)}} f_{Z_1}(u) du = (2m)^{-1} \sum_{j=1}^{n_1} \int_{Z_{1(j-m)}}^{Z_{1(j+m)}} f_{Z_1}(u) \frac{f_Z(u)}{f_Z(u)} du$$

$$\cong (2m)^{-1} \sum_{j=1}^{n_1} \frac{f_{Z_1,j}}{f_{ZZ_1,j}} \int_{Z_{1(j-m)}}^{Z_{1(j+m)}} f_Z(u) du \tag{9.1}$$

$$\cong (2m)^{-1} \sum_{j=1}^{n_1} \frac{f_{Z_1,j}}{f_{ZZ_1,j}} \left(F_Z\left(Z_{1(j+m)}\right) - F_Z\left(Z_{1(j-m)}\right) \right).$$

Because under the null hypothesis H_0 the distribution function $F_Z = F_{Z_1} = F_{Z_2}$ is assumed to be symmetric, the idea presented by Schuster (1975) can be adapted to evaluate $\left(F_Z\left(Z_{1(j+m)}\right) - F_Z\left(Z_{1(j-m)}\right)\right)$ at (9.1) by using the following estimator, which is denoted as $\eta_{m,j}$:

$$\eta_{m,j} = \left(F_{n_1+n_2}\left(Z_{1(j+m)}\right) - F_{n_1+n_2}\left(Z_{1(j-m)}\right)\right), \tag{9.2}$$

where $F_{n_1+n_2}(u) = \dfrac{1}{2(n_1+n_2)} \sum_{i=1}^{2} \sum_{j=1}^{n_i} \left[I\left(Z_{ij} \le u\right) + I\left(-Z_{ij} \le u\right)\right]$, $I(\cdot)$ is the indicator function. Note that for all integers $m \le 0.5n_1$, we have

$$(2m)^{-1} \sum_{j=1}^{n_1} \int_{Z_{1(j-m)}}^{Z_{1(j+m)}} f_{Z_1}(u)du = \int_{Z_{1(1)}}^{Z_{1(n_1)}} f_{Z_1}(u)du - \sum_{r=1}^{m-1} \frac{(m-r)}{2m}\left[\int_{Z_{1(m-r)}}^{Z_{1(n_1-r+1)}} f_{Z_1}(u)du + \int_{Z_{1(r)}}^{Z_{1(r+1)}} f_{Z_1}(u)du\right],$$

$$\tag{9.3}$$

where $Z_{1(j-m)} = Z_{1(1)}$ if $j - m \le 1$ and $Z_{1(j+m)} = Z_{1(n_1)}$ if $j + m \ge n_1$, and $\int_{Z_{1(1)}}^{Z_{1(n_1)}} f_{Z_1}(u)du \le \int_{-\infty}^{\infty} f(u)du = 1$. Equation 9.3 demonstrates that

$$(2m)^{-1} \sum_{j=1}^{n_1} \int_{Z_{1(j-m)}}^{Z_{1(j+m)}} f_{Z_1}(u)du \le 1, \text{ and } (2m)^{-1} \sum_{j=1}^{n_1} \int_{Z_{1(j-m)}}^{Z_{1(j+m)}} f_{Z_1}(u)du \approx 1$$

when $m/n_1 \to 0$ as $m, n_1 \to \infty$. By replacing the distribution functions in (9.3) by their empirical counterparts based on $F_{n_1}(u) = n_1^{-1} \sum_{j=1}^{n_1} I\left(Z_{1j} \le u\right)$, the empirical version of Equation 9.3 then has the form

$$(2m)^{-1} \sum_{j=1}^{n_1} \int_{Z_{1(j-m)}}^{Z_{1(j+m)}} f_{Z_1}(u)du \cong F_{n_1}\left(Z_{1(n_1)}\right) - F_{n_1}\left(Z_{1(1)}\right)$$

$$- \sum_{r=1}^{m-1} \frac{(m-r)}{2m}\left[F_{n_1}\left(Z_{1(n_1-r+1)}\right) - F_{n_1}\left(Z_{1(n_1-r)}\right) + F_{n_1}\left(Z_{1(r+1)}\right) - F_{n_1}\left(Z_{1(r)}\right)\right]. \tag{9.4}$$

This leads to

$$(2m)^{-1} \sum_{j=1}^{n_1} \int_{Z_{1(j-m)}}^{Z_{1(j+m)}} f_{Z_1}(u)du \cong 1 - (m+1)(2n_1)^{-1}. \tag{9.5}$$

Now, by Equations 9.1, 9.2, and 9.5, the resulting empirical constraint for values of $f_{Z_{1,j}}$ is

$$(2m)^{-1} \sum_{j=1}^{n_1} \frac{f_{Z_{1,j}}}{f_{ZZ_{1,j}}} \eta_{m,j} \cong 1 - (m+1)(2n_1)^{-1}. \tag{9.6}$$

To find values of $f_{Z_{1,j}}$ that maximize the likelihood $\prod_{j=1}^{n_1} f_{Z_{1,j}}$, provided the condition (9.6) holds, we formalize the Lagrange function as

$$\sum_{j=1}^{n_1} \log f_{Z_{1,j}} + \lambda_1 \left[1 - (m+1)(2n_1)^{-1} \sum_{j=1}^{n_1} \frac{f_{Z_{1,j}}}{f_{ZZ_{1,j}}}\right],$$

where λ_1 is a Lagrange multiplier. Maximizing the equation above, the values of $f_{Z_1,j}, \ldots, f_{Z_1,n_1}$ have the form

$$f_{Z_1,j} = \frac{m(2n_1 - m - 1)}{n_1^2 \eta_{m,j}} f_{ZZ_1,j}, \quad j = 1, \ldots, n_1,$$

where $Z_{1(j-m)} = Z_{1(1)}$ if $j - m \leq 1$ and $Z_{1(j+m)} = Z_{1(n_1)}$ if $j + m \geq n_1$.

As a consequence, the density-based EL estimator of the ratio $\prod_{j=1}^{n_1} f_{Z_1,j}/f_{ZZ_1,j}$ can be formulated by

$$V_{1,m,1} = \prod_{j=1}^{n_1} \frac{m(2n_1 - m - 1)}{n_1^2 \eta_{m,j}}.$$

One can show that properties of the statistic $V_{1,m,1}$ strongly depend on the selection of the values for the integer parameter m. A similar problem also arises in the well-known goodness-of-fit tests based on sample entropy (Vasicek 1976; Vexler and Gurevich 2010b; Vexler et al. 2011b). Attending to this issue, we eliminate the dependence on the integer parameter m. Toward this end, we use the maximum EL concept in a manner similar to the arguments proposed in Vexler and Gurevich (2010b), Gurevich and Vexler (2011), and Vexler et al. (2011b). Thus, the modified test statistic can be written as

$$V_{1,1} = \min_{n_1^{0.5+\delta} \leq m \leq n_1^{1-\delta}} \prod_{j=1}^{n_1} \frac{m(2n_1 - m - 1)}{n_1^2 \eta_{m,j}}, \quad \delta \in (0, 1/4). \tag{9.7}$$

Likewise, the approximation to the likelihood ratio $\prod_{j=1}^{n_2} f_{Z_2,j}/f_{ZZ_2,j}$ is

$$V_{2,2} = \min_{n_2^{0.5+\delta} \leq k \leq n_2^{1-\delta}} \prod_{j=1}^{n_2} \frac{k(2n_2 - k - 1)}{n_2^2 \phi_{k,j}}, \quad \delta \in (0, 1/4), \tag{9.8}$$

where $\phi_{k,j} = \left(F_{n_1+n_2} \left(Z_{2(j+k)} \right) - F_{n_1+n_2} \left(Z_{2(j-k)} \right) \right)$, $F_{n_1+n_2}$ is defined in (9.2).

Finally, we can obtain the test statistic for Test 1 in the form of

$$V_{n_1 n_2}^{H_{A1}} = \prod_{i=1}^{2} V_{i,i} = \min_{n_1^{0.5+\delta} \leq m \leq n_1^{1-\delta}} \prod_{j=1}^{n_1} \frac{m(2n_1 - m - 1)}{n_1^2 \eta_{m,j}} \min_{n_2^{0.5+\delta} \leq k \leq n_2^{1-\delta}} \prod_{j=1}^{n_2} \frac{k(2n_2 - k - 1)}{n_2^2 \phi_{k,j}},$$

which approximates the likelihood ratio $LR_{H_{A1}}$. Consequently, the decision rule is to reject H_0 if

$$\log \left(V_{n_1 n_2}^{H_{A1}} \right) > C^{H_{A1}}, \tag{9.9}$$

where $C^{H_{A1}}$ is a test threshold. (Similarly to Canner [1975], we will arbitrarily define $\eta_{m,j} = 1/(n_1 + n_2)$ or $\phi_{k,j} = 1/(n_1 + n_2)$, if $\eta_{m,j} = 0$ or $\phi_{k,j} = 0$, respectively.)

Proposition 9.1 in Section 9.4.2 demonstrates that the proposed test statistic $\log \left(V_{n_1 n_2}^{H_{A1}} \right)$ in (9.9) is asymptotically consistent. The upper and lower bounds for the integer parameters m and k in the definitions of (9.7) and (9.8) were selected to provide the asymptotic consistency.

Note that to test the composite hypotheses H_0 versus H_{A1}, a complex consideration regarding a reasonable combination of the Kolmogorov–Smirnov test and the Wilcoxon signed-rank test can be applied. Alternatively, the test (9.9) uses measurements from the therapy groups, in an approximate Neyman–Person manner, providing a simple procedure to evaluate the treatment effect on each therapy group.

9.4.1.2 Test 2: H_0 versus H_{A2}

Our goal is to test for

$$H_0: F_{Z_1} = F_{Z_2} = F_Z, F_Z(z) = 1 - F_Z(-z), \text{ for all } z \in (-\infty, \infty),$$

$$\text{vs. } H_{A2}: F_{Z_1} \neq F_{Z_2}, F_{Z_1}(z_1) \neq 1 - F_{Z_1}(-z_1), F_{Z_2}(z_2) = 1 - F_{Z_2}(-z_2).$$

In a manner similar to that of the development of the density-based EL approximation to the ratio $\prod_{j=1}^{n_1} f_{Z_1,j}/f_{ZZ_1,j}$, the EL ratio related to test for H_0 versus H_{A2} can be derived as

$$V_{1,1} = \min_{n_1^{0.5+\delta} \leq m \leq n_1^{1-\delta}} \prod_{j=1}^{n_1} \frac{m(2n_1 - m - 1)}{n_1^2 \eta_{m,j}}, \quad \delta \in (0, 1/4), \tag{9.10}$$

where $\eta_{m,j}$ are defined in (9.2). Consider the density-based EL approximation to the corresponding ratio $\prod_{j=1}^{n_2} f_{Z_2,j}/f_{ZZ_2,j}$. The empirical constraint for values of $f_{Z_2,j}$ can be constructed based on the symmetric property of F_{Z_2}. By analogy with Equations 9.1 through 9.6, one can show that the resulting empirical constraint on values of $f_{Z_2,j}$ in Test 2 has the form

$$(2k)^{-1} \sum_{j=1}^{n_2} \frac{f_{Z_2,j}}{f_{ZZ_2,j}} \phi_{k,j} = \Lambda_{n_2}^k, \tag{9.11}$$

where $\phi_{k,j}$ are defined in (9.8) and

$$\Lambda_{n_2}^k = (2n_2)^{-1} \left\{ \sum_{j=1}^{n_2} \left[I\left(-Z_{2j} \leq Z_{2(n_2)}\right) - I\left(-Z_{2j} \leq Z_{2(1)}\right) \right] + n_2 - 1 \right.$$

$$- \sum_{r=1}^{k-1} \frac{(k-r)}{2k} \sum_{j=1}^{n_2} \left[I\left(-Z_{2j} \leq Z_{2(n_2-r+1)}\right) - I\left(-Z_{2j} \leq Z_{2(n_2-r)}\right) \right.$$

$$\left. + I\left(-Z_{2j} \leq Z_{2(r+1)}\right) - I\left(-Z_{2j} \leq Z_{2(r)}\right) \right] - \frac{(k-1)}{2} \right\}. \tag{9.12}$$

Then the corresponding Lagrange function can be formulated by

$$\sum_{j=1}^{n_2} \log f_{Z_2,j} + \lambda_2 \left[\Lambda_{n_2}^k - (2k)^{-1} \sum_{j=1}^{n_2} \frac{f_{Z_2,j}}{f_{ZZ_2,j}} \phi_{k,j} \right], \tag{9.13}$$

where λ_2 is a Lagrange multiplier. Maximizing the equation above, the values of $f_{Z_2,j}, \ldots, f_{Z_2,n_2}$ have the form of

$$f_{Z_2,j} = \frac{2k\Lambda_{n_2}^k}{n_2 \phi_{k,j}}, \quad j = 1, \ldots, n_2,$$

where $Z_{2(j-m)} = Z_{2(1)}$ if $j - k \leq 1$ and $Z_{2(j+k)} = Z_{2(n_2)}$ if $j + k \geq n_2$. Similar to (9.7) and (9.8), the density-based EL estimator of the ratio $\prod_{j=1}^{n_2} f_{Z_2,j} / f_{ZZ_2,j}$ can be presented as

$$\tilde{V}_{2,2} = \min_{n_2^{0.5+\delta} \leq k \leq n_2^{1-\delta}} \prod_{j=1}^{n_2} \frac{2k\Lambda_{n_2}^k}{n_2 \phi_{k,j}}, \quad \delta \in (0, 1/4). \tag{9.14}$$

Finally, taking into account (9.10) and (9.14), the test statistic for Test 2 can be constructed as

$$V_{n_1 n_2}^{HA2} = \min_{n_1^{0.5+\delta} \leq m \leq n_1^{1-\delta}} \prod_{j=1}^{n_1} \frac{m(2n_1 - m - 1)}{n_1^2 \eta_{m,j}} \min_{n_2^{0.5+\delta} \leq k \leq n_2^{1-\delta}} \prod_{j=1}^{n_2} \frac{2k\Lambda_{n_2}^k}{n_2 \phi_{k,j}}.$$

In this case, the decision rule developed for Test 2 is to reject the null hypothesis if

$$\log\left(V_{n_1 n_2}^{HA2}\right) > C^{HA2}, \tag{9.15}$$

where C^{HA2} is a test threshold.

9.4.1.3 Test 3: H_0 versus H_{A3}

Consider the following hypothesis of interest

$$H_0: F_{Z_1} = F_{Z_2} = F_Z, \ F_Z(z) = 1 - F_Z(-z), \quad \text{for all } z \in (-\infty, \infty),$$

$$\text{vs. } H_{A3}: F_{Z_1} = F_{Z_2} = F_{H_{A3}, Z}, F_{H_{A3}, Z}(z) \neq 1 - F_{H_{A3}, Z}(-z).$$

The corresponding likelihood ratio test statistic based on observations Z_{ij}, $i = 1, 2$; $j = 1, \ldots, n_i$, can be defined as

$$LR_{H_{A3}} = \frac{\prod_{i=1}^{2} \prod_{j=1}^{n_i} f_{H_{A3}, Z}(Z_{ij})}{\prod_{i=1}^{2} \prod_{j=1}^{n_i} f_Z(Z_{ij})} = \frac{\prod_{s=1}^{N} f_{H_{A3}, Z}(Z_{(s)})}{\prod_{s=1}^{N} f_Z(Z_{(s)})} = \prod_{s=1}^{N} \frac{f_{H_{A3}, s}}{f_{H_0, s}},$$

where $N = n_1 + n_2$; $f_{H_0, s} = f_Z\left(Z_{(s)}\right)$ and $f_{H_{A3}, s} = f_{H_{A3}, z}\left(Z_{(s)}\right)$ denote the density functions of observations Z under H_0 and H_{A3}, respectively, and $Z_{(s)}$ $s = 1, \ldots, N$, are the order statistics based on the pooled sample of $\{Z_{11}, \ldots, Z_{1n_1}\}$ and $\{Z_{21}, \ldots, Z_{2n_2}\}$ that are denoted by Z_s, $s = 1, \ldots, N$. Using the same technique as that used in Test 1 above, we derive values of $f_{H_{A3}, s}, s = 1, \ldots, N$, that maximize the log-likelihood $\sum_{s=1}^{N} \log\left(f_{H_{A3}, s}\right)$ given a constraint, empirical form of $\int f_{H_{A3}}(u) du$. The proposed test statistic for Test 3 is

$$V_N^{HA3} = \min_{N^{0.5+\delta} \leq m \leq N^{1-\delta}} \prod_{s=1}^{N} \frac{m(2N - m - 1)}{N^2 w_{m,s}}, \tag{9.16}$$

where $\omega_{m,s} = (2N)^{-1} \sum_{s=1}^{N} [I(Z_s \leq Z_{(s+m)}) + I(-Z_s \leq Z_{(s+m)}) - I(Z_s \leq Z_{(s-m)}) - I(-Z_s \leq Z_{(s-m)})]$ and $\delta \in (0, 1/4)$.

Thus, the decision rule for Test 3 is to reject the null hypothesis if

$$\log\left(V_N^{HA3}\right) > C^{HA3}, \tag{9.17}$$

where C^{HA3} is a test threshold.

9.4.2 Asymptotic Consistency and Null Distributions of the Tests

In this section, we present the following propositions to demonstrate the asymptotic consistency and the null distributions of the tests described in Section 9.4.1:

Proposition 9.1

Let $f_{Z_i}(Z)$ be the density function with the expectations $E(\log f_{Z_i}(Z_{i1})) < \infty$ and $E(\log f_{Z_i}(-Z_{i1})) < \infty$, $i = 1, 2$. Let $f_i(u) = (f_{Z_i}(u) + f_{Z_i}(-u))/2$. Then, under H_0, $(n_1 + n_2)^{-1} \log\left(V_{n_1 n_2}^{HA_t}\right) \xrightarrow{p} 0, t = 1, 2$, and under H_{A1} and H_{A2},

$$(n_1 + n_2)^{-1} \log\left(V_{n_1 n_2}^{HA_t}\right) \to -\frac{\gamma}{1+\gamma} E_{HA_t} \log\left\{\frac{\gamma}{1+\gamma} + \frac{\gamma}{1+\gamma}\left(\frac{f_2(Z_{11})}{f_1(Z_{11})}\right)\right\}$$
$$- \frac{\gamma}{1+\gamma} E_{HA_t} \log\left\{\frac{\gamma}{1+\gamma} + \frac{\gamma}{1+\gamma}\left(\frac{f_1(Z_{21})}{f_2(Z_{21})}\right)\right\} \geq 0,$$

$t = 1, 2$, as $n_1 \to \infty$, $n_2 \to \infty$, $n_1/n_2 \to \gamma > 0$, where γ is a constant.

The proof is shown in the appendix.

We then consider the testing problem H_0 versus H_{A3}.

Proposition 9.2

Let the pooled sample Z_s, $s = 1, \ldots, N$, have the density function f, with the expectations $E(\log f(Z_1)) < \infty$ and $E(\log f(-Z_1)) < \infty$. Then under H_0, $N^{-1} \log\left(V_N^{HA3}\right) \xrightarrow{p} 0$, and under H_{A3}, $N^{-1} \log\left(V_N^{HA3}\right) \xrightarrow{p} -E_{HA3} \log\left\{0.5 + 0.5 f(-Z_1)/f(Z_1)\right\} \geq 0$ as $N \to \infty$.

The proof of Proposition 9.2 is similar to that of Proposition 9.1.

In order to obtain critical values of the proposed tests, we employ the fact that the proposed test statistics are based on indicator functions $I(\cdot)$ and $I(Z_1 < Z_2) = I(F_Z(Z_1) < F_Z(Z_2))$ and $I(Z_1 < -Z_2) = I(F_Z(Z_1) < F_Z(-Z_2)) = I(F_Z(Z_1) < 1 - F_Z(Z_2))$, where the random variables $F_Z(Z_1)$ and $F_Z(Z_2)$ have the uniform distribution, $Unif[0, 1]$, under H_0. Thus, the distributions of the proposed test statistics are independent of the distributions of observations, and hence the critical values of the proposed tests can be exactly computed. For each proposed test, we conducted the following procedures to determine the critical values, C_α, of the null distributions. We first generated data of Z_1 and Z_2 from the standard normal distribution $N(0, 1)$ and then calculated the test statistics corresponding to each proposed test. For more details regarding the determination of the critical values, we refer the reader to Chapters 1 and 16. The computer codes to implement the procedure are provided in the appendix.

The construction of the two-sample density-based EL ratio tests, based on paired observations, employs approximations to the most powerful test statistics with respect to the stated problems, thus providing efficient nonparametric procedures. The two-sample density-based EL ratio tests are exact and simple to perform. Based on extensive Monte Carlo studies, Vexler et al. (2012a) confirmed powerful properties of the density-based EL ratio tests and showed that the density-based EL ratio tests outperform different tests with a structure based on the Wilcoxon signed-rank test or the Kolmogorov–Smirnov test, and outperform the parametric likelihood ratio tests when the underlying distributions are misspecified. For more discussions about the density-based EL ratio tests, we refer the reader to Vexler et al. (2012a).

9.5 Density-Based Empirical Likelihood Ratio Based on Paired Data

In this section, we introduce an empirical likelihood (EL) ratio approach for testing the equality of marginal distributions given that sampling is from a continuous bivariate population, as proposed by Vexler et al. (2013b). This test is exact and superior to the classic nonparametric procedures, which may break down completely or are frequently inferior to the density-based EL ratio test. This is particularly true in the cases where there is a nonconstant shift under the alternative or the data distributions are skewed.

In order to express the general framework for the statement of the test development process, let us first define (X_1, Y_1), ..., (X_n, Y_n) to be a random sample from a bivariate population with absolutely continuous joint distribution function $F_{XY}(x,y)$ with marginal distributions of X_i and Y_i given as $F_X(x)$ and $F_Y(y)$, respectively. Oftentimes, given this type of data, the general location testing problem consists of testing $H_0: \theta = 0$ versus $H_1: \theta \neq 0$ through the relationship $F_X(x) = F_Y(x - \theta)$. For example, in biomedical experiments θ may represent the mean or median difference between subject values measured pre- and post-treatment. Common statistical procedures for testing $H_0: \theta = 0$ versus $H_1: \theta \neq 0$ consist of the paired t-test, the sign test and the Wilcoxon signed-rank test. These tests are based on the n paired differences $Z_i = X_i - Y_i$ (e.g., Bhattacharya et al. 1982; Fellingham and Stocker 1964; Lam and Longnecker 1983). In the paired data case, the classical nonparametric Wilcoxon signed-rank procedure for testing $H_0: \theta = 0$ versus $H_1: \theta \neq 0$ is a permutation based method under the assumption that Z is symmetric about the parameter θ under the null hypothesis. Similarly, the sign test assumes symmetry under the null hypothesis and uses the binomial distribution with respect to generating the null distribution of the test statistic.

Let Z_1, ..., Z_n be i.i.d. random variables with corresponding distribution function F, where $Z_i = X_i - Y_i$. We begin by developing the basic methodology from which to construct the density-based EL ratio test statistic given the following null and alternative hypotheses:

$$H_0: F = F_{H_0}, F_{H_0}(u) = 1 - F_{H_0}(-u), \text{ for all } -\infty < u < \infty \text{ versus}$$

$$H_1: F = F_{H_1}, F_{H_1}(u) \neq 1 - F_{H_1}(-u), \text{ for some } -\infty < u < \infty.$$

(9.18)

The parametric likelihood ratio statistic based on $Z_1, \ldots, Z_n$ takes the form

$$LR = \frac{\prod\limits_{i=1}^{n} f_{H_1}(Z_i)}{\prod\limits_{i=1}^{n} f_{H_0}(Z_i)} = \frac{\prod\limits_{j=1}^{n} f_{H_1}(Z_{(j)})}{\prod\limits_{j=1}^{n} f_{H_0}(Z_{(j)})} = \frac{\prod\limits_{j=1}^{n} f_{H_1,j}}{\prod\limits_{j=1}^{n} f_{H_0,j}}, \tag{9.19}$$

where $f_{H_1}(u)$, $f_{H_0}(u)$ denote the density functions of Z under H_1 and H_0, respectively, $Z_{(1)} \le Z_{(2)} \le \ldots \le Z_{(n)}$ is the order statistic, and $f_{H_K,j} = f_{H_K}(Z_{(j)}), k = 0, 1, j = 1, \ldots, n$. In order to generate the nonparametric test for (9.18), we first estimate the values of $f_{H_1,j}, j = 1, \ldots, n$. This is accomplished via maximizing the log-likelihood $\sum_{j=1}^{n} \log\left(f_{H_1,j}\right)$ provided that $f_{H_1,j}, j = 1, \ldots, n$ satisfy an empirical constraint that is the empirical equivalent of $\int f_{H_1}(u)du = 1$ (e.g., see Vexler and Gurevich [2010b] for details). To formalize this constraint, we specify $Z_{(j)} = Z_{(1)}$ if $j \le 1$ and $Z_{(j)} = Z_{(n)}$ if $j \ge n$ and employ the relationship

$$\frac{1}{2m}\sum_{j=1}^{n}\int_{Z_{(j-m)}}^{Z_{(j+m)}} f_{H_1}(u)du = \int_{Z_{(1)}}^{Z_{(n)}} f_{H_1}(u)du - \sum_{l=1}^{m-1}\frac{m-l}{2m}\left(\int_{Z_{(n-l)}}^{Z_{(n-l+1)}} f_{H_1}(u)du + \int_{Z_{(l)}}^{Z_{(l+1)}} f_{H_1}(u)du\right), \tag{9.20}$$

for all integer $m \le \dfrac{n}{2}$,

which appears in Proposition 2.1 of Vexler and Gurevich (2010b). Since $\int_{Z_{(1)}}^{Z_{(n)}} f_{H_1}(u)du \le \int_{-\infty}^{\infty} f_{H_1}(u)du = 1$, Equation 9.20 implies the inequality that $(1/2m)\sum_{j=1}^{n}\int_{Z_{(j-m)}}^{Z_{(j+m)}} f_{H_1}(u)du \le 1$. In addition, based on previous work, one can expect that $(1/2m)\sum_{j=1}^{n}\int_{Z_{(j-m)}}^{Z_{(j+m)}} f_{H_1}(u)du \approx 1$ when $m/n \to 0$, as $m, n \to \infty$ (Vexler et al. 2011b).

Let $\hat{F}_{H_0}$ and $\hat{F}_{H_1}$ denote estimators of F_{H_0} and F_{H_1}, respectively. Applying the approximate analogue to the mean value integration theorem, the empirical approximations

$$\sum_{j=1}^{n}\int_{Z_{(j-m)}}^{Z_{(j+m)}} f_{H_1}(u)du = \sum_{j=1}^{n}\int_{Z_{(j-m)}}^{Z_{(j+m)}} \frac{f_{H_1}(u)}{f_{H_0}(u)} f_{H_0}(u)du$$

$$\approx \sum_{j=1}^{n}\frac{f_{H_1,j}}{f_{H_0,j}}\int_{Z_{(j-m)}}^{Z_{(j+m)}} f_{H_0}(u)du \approx \sum_{j=1}^{n}\frac{f_{H_1,j}}{f_{H_0,j}}\left(F_{H_0}(Z_{(j+m)}) - F_{H_0}(Z_{(j-m)})\right)$$

$$\approx \sum_{j=1}^{n}\frac{f_{H_1,j}}{f_{H_0,j}}\left(\hat{F}_{H_0}(Z_{(j+m)}) - \hat{F}_{H_0}(Z_{(j-m)})\right),$$

$$\int_{Z_{(1)}}^{Z_{(n)}} f_{H_1}(u)du \approx \hat{F}_{H_1}(Z_{(n)}) - \hat{F}_{H_1}(Z_{(1)}),$$

$$\left(\int_{Z_{(n-l)}}^{Z_{(n-l+1)}} f_{H_1}(u)\,du + \int_{Z_{(l)}}^{Z_{(l+1)}} f_{H_1}(u)\,du \right) \approx \left(\hat{F}_{H_1}(Z_{(n-l+1)}) - \hat{F}_{H_1}(Z_{(n-l)}) + \hat{F}_{H_1}(Z_{(l+1)}) - \hat{F}_{H_1}(Z_{(l)}) \right)$$

can be derived and applied directly to functions defined at (9.20). If we let $\hat{F}_{H_1}$ be the empirical distribution function in these approximations, we can record the empirical version of (9.20) having the following form:

$$\frac{1}{2m} \sum_{j=1}^{n} \frac{f_{H_1,j}}{f_{H_0,j}} \left(\hat{F}_{H_0}(Z_{(j+m)}) - \hat{F}_{H_0}(Z_{(j-m)}) \right) = \left(1 - \frac{1}{n} \right) - \frac{(m-1)}{2n}.$$

To define $\hat{F}_{H_0}$, the distribution-free estimation for a symmetric distribution proposed by Schuster (1975) is applied. Thus, we formulate the empirical constraint

$$\frac{1}{2m} \sum_{j=1}^{n} \frac{f_{H_1,j}}{f_{H_0,j}} \Delta_{jm} = 1 - \frac{(m+1)}{2n},$$

$$\Delta_{jm} := \frac{1}{2n} \sum_{i=1}^{n} \left(I(Z_i \le Z_{(j+m)}) + I(-Z_i \le Z_{(j+m)}) - I(Z_i \le Z_{(j-m)}) - I(-Z_i \le Z_{(j-m)}) \right) \qquad (9.21)$$

on $f_{H_1,j}$, $j = 1, \ldots, n$, where $I(\cdot)$ denotes the standard indicator function. In order to find values of $f_{H_1,j}$ that maximize the log-likelihood $\sum_{j=1}^{n} \log(f_{H_1,j})$ subject to the constraints at (9.21), we derive $\partial / \partial f_{H_1,i}$, $i = 1, \ldots, n$, from the Lagrange function given by

$$\Lambda_\lambda = \sum_{j=1}^{n} \log(f_{1j}) + \lambda \left(1 - \frac{m+1}{2n} - \frac{1}{2m} \sum_{j=1}^{n} \frac{f_{H_1,j}}{f_{H_0,j}} \Delta_{jm} \right)$$

with a Lagrange multiplier λ. It is straightforward to obtain that

$$f_{H_1,j} = f_{H_0,j} \frac{2m(1 - (m+1)(2n)^{-1})}{n\Delta_{jm}}, \quad j = 1, \ldots, n,$$

are the roots of the equation $\partial \Lambda_\lambda / \partial f_{H_0,j} = 0$ such that $f_{H_1,j}$, $j = 1, \ldots, n$, satisfy the constraints at (9.21). This implies that the empirical maximum likelihood approximation to the H_1-likelihood $\prod_{j=1}^{n} f_{H_1,j}$ can be presented as

$$\prod_{j=1}^{n} f_{H_0,j} \frac{2m(1 - (m+1)(2n)^{-1})}{n\Delta_{jm}}.$$

Therefore, the likelihood ratio given at (9.19) has the empirical form

$$V_{nm} = \prod_{j=1}^{n} \frac{2m(1 - (m+1)(2n)^{-1})}{n\Delta_{jm}}. \qquad (9.22)$$

Under mild conditions (see Vexler et al. [2013b] for details), the test statistic (9.22) can be modified slightly to be of the form

$$V_n = \min_m \prod_{j=1}^{n} \frac{2m(1-(m+1)(2n)^{-1})}{n\Delta_{jm}}. \tag{9.23}$$

Now to complete the construction of the test statistic, we note that $m/n \to 0$ as $m, n \to \infty$ is a necessary assumption. In accordance with the constraints at (9.20) and (9.21), the requirement $m/n \to 0$ as $m, n \to \infty$ reduces asymptotically the remainder terms

$$\sum_{l=1}^{m-1} \frac{m-l}{2m} \left(\int_{Z_{(n-l)}}^{Z_{(n-l+1)}} f_{H_1}(u)du + \int_{Z_{(l)}}^{Z_{(l+1)}} f_{H_1}(u)du \right) \text{ and } \frac{(m+1)}{2n},$$

respectively. Here, as mentioned above,

$$\sum_{l=1}^{m-1} \frac{m-l}{2m} \left(\int_{Z_{(n-l)}}^{Z_{(n-l+1)}} f_{H_1}(u)du + \int_{Z_{(l)}}^{Z_{(l+1)}} f_{H_1}(u)du \right) \approx \frac{(m+1)}{2n} \underset{m,n\to\infty}{\to} 0, \quad \text{if } m/n \to 0 \text{ as } m, n \to \infty$$

Thus, based on combining all of the results provided above, we propose the new test statistic taking the form

$$V_n = \min_{a(n) \le m \le b(n)} \prod_{j=1}^{n} \frac{2m(1-(m+1)(2n)^{-1})}{n\Delta_{jm}}, a(n) = n^{0.5+\delta}, b(n) = \min(n^{1-\delta}, n/2), \quad \delta \in (0, 1/4) \tag{9.24}$$

(Here, in a manner similar to that of Canner [1975], we arbitrarily define $\Delta_{jm} = 1/n$ if $\Delta_{jm} = 0$.) The V_n-test of the hypothesis (9.18) is a test with critical region

$$\log(V_n) > C, \tag{9.25}$$

where C is a test threshold. More specially, in this chapter we arrive at the practical value of $\delta = 0.1$. It is shown that the power of the test statistic at (9.24) does not differ substantially for values of $\delta \in (0, 1/4)$ given various alternatives.

9.5.1 Significance Level of the Proposed Test

It is important to note that the null distribution of the test statistic V_n is independent of the distribution of the observations $Z_1, \ldots, Z_n$. In order to substantiate this claim, we note that under H_0,

$$I(Z_i \le Z_j) = I\left(\Phi^{-1}\left(F_{H_0}(Z_i)\right) \le \Phi^{-1}\left(F_{H_0}(Z_j)\right)\right),$$

and

$$I(-Z_i \leq Z_j) = I(\Phi^{-1}(F_{H_0}(-Z_i)) \leq \Phi^{-1}(F_{H_0}(Z_j)))$$

$$= I(\Phi^{-1}(1 - F_{H_0}(Z_i)) \leq \Phi^{-1}(F_{H_0}(Z_j)))$$

$$= I(-\Phi^{-1}(F_{H_0}(Z_i)) \leq \Phi^{-1}(F_{H_0}(Z_j))), \text{ for } i \neq j \in [1, n],$$

where $\Phi^{-1}(x)$ denotes the inverse function of the standard normal cumulative distribution function $\Phi(x)$. This fact implies, via the construction of the test statistic V_n, that

$$\Pr_{H_0}(\log(V_n) > C) = \Pr_{X_1, \dots, X_n \sim Norm(0,1)}(\log(V_n) > C).$$

From this result, it is clear that the proposed test is exact and the corresponding critical values can be tabulated for fixed sample sizes based on Monte Carlo simulations. The generated values of the test statistic $\log(V_n)$ were used to determine the critical values C_α: $\Pr_{H_0}(\log(V_n) > C_\alpha) = \alpha$ of the null distribution of $\log(V_n)$ at the significance level α. For more details, we refer the reader to Chapter 16.

The consistency of the test defined at (9.25) is stated in the following proposition:

Proposition 9.3

Let $f(x)$ define a density function of the observations $Z_1, \dots, Z_n$ with the finite expectations $E(\log f(Z_1))$ and $E(\log(0.5 f(Z_1) + 0.5 f(-Z)))$. Then

$$\frac{1}{n}\log(V_n) \xrightarrow{p} -E\left(\log\left(0.5 + 0.5\frac{f(-Z_1)}{f(Z_1)}\right)\right), \quad \text{as } n \to \infty,$$

for all $0 < \delta < 1/4$ in the definition (9.24) of the statistic V_n.

For the proof of this proposition, we refer the reader to Appendix B of Vexler et al. (2013b).

It is obvious that the limiting value of $n^{-1}\log(V_n)$, the expectation $-E(\log(0.5 + 0.5 f(-Z_1) f(Z_1)^{-1}))$ stated in Proposition 9.1, has the forms of

$$-E_{H_0} \log\left(0.5 + 0.5 f_{H_0}(-Z_1)(f_{H_0}(Z_1))^{-1}\right) = 0$$

and

$$-E_{H_1}\left(\log\left(0.5 + 0.5 f_{H_1}(-Z_1)\left(f_{H_1}(Z_1)\right)^{-1}\right)\right) \geq -\log\left(0.5 + 0.5 E_{H_1}\left(f_{H_1}(-Z_1)\left(f_{H_1}(Z_1)\right)^{-1}\right)\right) \geq 0.$$

This implies that the test statistic $\log(V_n)$ is consistent.

In summary, the exact density-based empirical likelihood ratio test for paired data described in this section employs the EL concept in a nonparametric fashion in order to approximate a Neyman–Pearson-type parametric likelihood ratio test statistic given paired data. The benefit of using this approach is threefold: (1) we are able to construct an exact and robust nonparametric test, (2) the proposed technique is highly efficient given that it approximates well the optimal parametric likelihood ratio, and (3) the new test has consistently high power over a variety of alternative distributions, resulting in a large power gain in comparison to the classical procedures. For more discussions, we refer the reader to Vexler et al. (2013b).

9.6 Multiple-Group Comparison

The k-sample problem, as a natural extension of the two-sample problem, considers observations taken under a variety of different and independent conditions. Let $n_1, \ldots, n_k$ denote the respective sample sizes corresponding to the K-samples being compared, with a total sample size $N = \sum_{i=1}^{K} n_i$. Assume that the K-samples are represented by the vectors of observations given as $\{X_{11}, \ldots, X_{1n_1}\}, \ldots, \{X_{k1}, \ldots, X_{kn_k}\}$ from the corresponding distribution functions $F_{X_1}, \ldots, F_{X_k}$. We are interested in testing the hypothesis $H_0: F_{X_1} = \ldots = F_{X_k} = F_Z$ versus H_1: not all $F_{Xi} = F_{Xj}, i \neq j$. In this section, we introduce tests that are appropriate for comparing more than two groups, including the classical Kruskal–Wallis one-way analysis of variance and a novel and powerful density-based empirical likelihood procedure for testing the symmetry of data distributions and k-sample comparisons proposed by Vexler et al. (2014c).

9.6.1 Kruskal–Wallis One-Way Analysis of Variance

The Kruskal–Wallis one-way analysis of variance by ranks is a nonparametric method for testing whether two or more samples have the same underlying distribution (Kruskal and Wallis 1952). It extends the Wilcoxon rank-sum test to more than two groups. Since it is a nonparametric method, the Kruskal–Wallis test does not assume a normal distribution of the residuals, unlike the analogous one-way analysis of variance. As with the Wilcoxon rank-sum test, this is a permutation test, which requires the assumption of exchangeability under the null hypothesis assumption to be met in order for the test to be unbiased.

Note that under H_0 we can consider all the observations as a single sample of size N from the common population. Combining the N observations into a single ordered sequence from smallest to largest, if adjacent ranks are well distributed among the k-samples, which would be true for a random sample from a single population, the total sum of ranks would be divided proportionally according to sample size among the K-samples. Similar to the Wilcoxon rank-sum test described in Section 9.2, a reasonable test statistic can be based on a function of the differences between these observed and expected rank sums. Given K-samples, we denote the sum of ranks assigned to the elements in the ith sample by $W_i, i = 1, \ldots, K$. Then the Kruskal–Wallis test statistic is defined as

$$H = \frac{12}{N(N+1)} \sum_{i=1}^{K} \frac{1}{n_i} \left(W_i - \frac{n_i(N+1)}{2} \right)^2.$$

Let $\overline{W}_i = W_i/n_i$ denote the average rank sum for the ith sample. Since $\overline{W}_i$ is a sample mean, when n_i is large, based on the central limit theorem, we have

$$Z_i = \frac{\overline{W}_i - (N+1)/2}{\sqrt{(N+1)(N-n_i)/12n_i}} \xrightarrow{d} N(0,1).$$

Kruskal and Wallis demonstrated that under H_0, if n_i is relatively small, then

$$H = \sum_{i=1}^{K} \frac{N - n_i}{N} Z_i^2$$

has an asymptotical chi-square distribution with $K-1$ degrees of freedom. Therefore, the decision-making rule is to reject H_0 if $H \geq \chi^2_{\alpha, K-1}$, where $\chi^2_{\alpha, K-1}$ is the α-upper quantile of the chi-square distribution with $K-1$ degrees of freedom.

Rejecting the null hypothesis of the Kruskal–Wallis test implies that at least one sample stochastically dominates at least one other sample. The test does not identify where this stochastic dominance occurs or how many pairs of groups stochastic dominance obtains.

9.6.2 Density-Based Empirical Likelihood Procedures for K-Sample Comparisons

To outline the K-sample procedure in the empirical likelihood framework, we suppose that the data consist of K independent samples and we are interested in testing whether all K-samples are distributed identically in a nonparametric fashion. Assume that the K-samples are represented by the vectors of observations given as $\{X_{11}, ..., X_{1m_1}\}, ..., \{X_{K1}, ..., X_{Kn_K}\}$ from the corresponding distribution functions $F_{X_1}, ..., F_{X_K}$. We now want to test the hypothesis $H_0: F_{X_1} = ... = F_{X_K} = F_Z$ versus H_1: not all $F_{Xi} = F_{Xj}, i \neq j$. If the corresponding density functions are known, the LR statistic has the form $LR = \prod_{j=1}^{K} \prod_{i=1}^{n_j} f_{X_j}(X_{ji})/f_Z(X_{ji}) = \prod_{j=1}^{K} \prod_{i=1}^{n_j} f_{X_j,i}/f_{ZX_j,i}$, where $f_{X_j}(\cdot)$ denotes the density function of the jth sample under H_1, f_Z is the theoretical density function of observations under H_0. Let $X_{j(i)}, j = 1, ..., K$, be the order statistics per sample based on the observations $X_{j1}, ..., X_{jn_j}$. As before, we denote $f_{X_j}(X_{j(i)}) = f_{X_j,i}$ and $f_Z(X_{j(i)}) = f_{ZX_j,i}, j = 1, ..., K$. We apply the maximum EL method to obtain the density-based empirical likelihood (DBEL) ratio test statistic

$$V_{n_1 n_2 ... n_k} = \prod_{j=1}^{K} ELR_{X_j, n_j},$$

where the EL estimator of $\prod_{i=1}^{n_j} f_{X_j,i}/f_{ZX_j,i}$, for $j = 1, ..., K$ is

$$ELR_{X_j, n_j} = \min_{a_{nj} \leq m_j \leq b_{nj}} \prod_{i=1}^{n_j} \frac{2m_j}{n_j \left[F_{Z(N)}\left(X_{j(i+m_j)}\right) - F_{Z(N)}\left(X_{j(i-m_j)}\right) \right]},$$

$$a_l = l^{0.5+\delta}, \, b_l = \min(l^{1-\delta}, l/2), \, \delta \in (0, 1/4),$$

and the corresponding empirical distribution function under H_0 is given as

$$F_{Z(N)}(u) = \frac{1}{N}\sum_{j=1}^{K}\sum_{i=1}^{n_j} I\left(X_{ji} \le u\right), N = \sum_{j=1}^{K} n_j, X_{j(i)} = X_{j(1)}, \text{if } i \le 1, \text{ and } X_{j(i)} = X_{j(n_j)} \quad \text{if } i \ge n_j.$$

As in the two-group setting, we define $F_{Z(N)}(x) - F_{Z(N)}(y) = 1/N$ if $F_{Z(N)}(x) = F_{Z(N)}(y)$. The Type I error of the K-sample test can be monitored exactly by following the probability statement $\mathrm{Pr}_{H_0}(\log(V_{n_1 n_2 \dots n_k}) > C) = \mathrm{Pr}_{X_{11},\dots,X_{1n_1},\dots,X_{k1},\dots,X_{Kn_K} \sim unif[0,1]}(\log(V_{n_1 n_2 \dots n_k}) > C)$. Set a value of $\delta = 0.1$. The DBEL test statistic approximates nonparametrically the most powerful parametric LR test statistic; consequently, one can assume heuristically that the DBEL test also has good relative efficiency. For more details, we refer the reader to Vexler et al. (2014c).

9.7 Supplement

1. Fisher (1936a) proposed applying a combination technique to the results of the individual tests based on the probability integral transformation. When the hypothesis tested is true for all combined tests, it was shown that the logarithm of the product of the tail errors of the individual tests multiplied by 2 has a chi-square distribution with $2k$ degrees of freedom, where k is the number of the tests. However, Fisher's technique suffers from the following disadvantages: (a) it is exact only if the statistics of the combined tests have continuous distributions (Wallis 1942), and (b) change in the weights of the individual tests may lead to more complications in the procedure. Toward this end, Van Elteren (1960) studied two versions of the linear combinations of independent Wilcoxon's two-sample tests based on a linear combination of the statistics of the individual tests. One of them yields a test with a region of consistency that is independent of the proportion of the sample sizes, and the other has, in an important special case, the largest efficiency. The two versions of linear combinations are equivalent with the sum of the statistics in certain special cases. The obtained combined statistics were shown to be approximately normally distributed under the hypothesis tested, as either the individual statistics have approximately normal distribution or the number of the combined tests is large.

2. Let X and Y be independent random variables with distribution functions $F(x)$ and $G(y)$, respectively. In order to test equal locations under a stochastic ordering restriction, that is, H_0: $F(x) \equiv G(x)$ versus H_1: $F(x) \ge G(x)$ with strict inequality for at least one value of x, Lee and Wolfe (1976) proposed a two-sample distribution-free procedure via the test statistic M, which is an estimator of $\theta = \mathrm{Pr}(X \le Y) = \int_{-\infty}^{\infty} F(x)\,dG(x)$ based on maximum likelihood estimators of stochastically ordered distribution functions. The authors presented some properties of the M-test and critical values for certain sample sizes. Based on a Monte Carlo power study, it was shown that for shift alternatives, the M-test is more effective than the Mann–Whitney–Wilcoxon test when the form of the underlying distribution is heavy-tailed, while the Mann–Whitney–Wilcoxon performs better for moderate-tailed distributions.

3. When dealing with two-sample data, the Wilcoxon rank-sum test is commonly used to test the equality of the distributions, H_0: $F_1 = F_2$. However, the Wilcoxon rank-sum test statistic is sensitive to the hypothesis H_0: $F(y) = F(y - \Delta)$, where y is a continuous random variable and Δ denotes a location shift between two distributions of responses. Note that for categorical data, tied responses must be accommodated in the Wilcoxon test statistic and alternative hypotheses must be characterized, rather than by simple transformations of the data. When there are few distinct responses available to describe the shapes of the distributions and when the difference between distributions is not a location shift, tests that accommodate ordinal categorical data, for example, tests based on the omnibus Smirnov statistic, may be more powerful than the Wilcoxon test. In the scenarios of location shift and scale alternatives, Hilton (1996) made a comparison of the power of the exact tests based on the Wilcoxon statistic, O'Brien's generalized Wilcoxon statistic (O'Brien 1988), and the Smirnov statistic (Smirnov 1939a, 1939b). It was shown that all three tests can gain power as a function of the scale parameter, relying on its magnitude relative to the shift parameter. When the relative influence of the scale parameter increases, the O'Brien test is the most powerful. The author also compared the power of the asymptotic Wilcoxon test with its exact version and noted that if there exists a scale change, the asymptotic Wilcoxon test will either inflate or deflate the statistical power. The author investigated the following problems: (a) non–location shift differences between distributions in a study of maternal alcohol consumption during pregnancy and occurrence of malformation of their infants where the alcohol data were collected as average number of drinks per day in five categories (Graubard and Korn 1987), and (b) studies with bounded outcome scores where the responses fell into 21 categories, with high probabilities in the first and last categories (Lesaffre et al. 1993).

4. Leuraud and Benichou (2001) examined several tests, including one based on isotonic regression, the T-test based on contrasts, and a test based on adjacent contrasts (Dosemeci–Benichou test). The authors compared Type I error and the power of these tests and of the commonly used Mantel-extension test for overall trend. The authors studied one- and two-sided versions of the tests and considered the tests under the null hypothesis of no relationship between exposure and disease and under various alternative patterns of monotonic or nonmonotonic dose–response relationships. It was shown that Mantel-extension trend tests can lead to an incorrect conclusion of a monotonic dose–response relationship. The test based on isotonic regression tends to be too powerful in the case of nonmonotonic dose–response relationship patterns. The tests based on contrasts have more well-controlled Type I error, high power for monotonic alternatives, and low power for nonmonotonic alternatives. The author presented these results with case-control data on occupational risks of bladder cancer (Madure and Greenland 1992).

5. Baumgartner et al. (1998) proposed a nonparametric two-sample test. It was demonstrated that the test is at least as powerful as commonly used nonparametric tests, such as the Wilcoxon test. The Baumgartner–Weiß–Schindler statistic can be modified to identify the minimum effective dose. The modified statistic is very powerful and can be used in the step-down procedure instead of the Wilcoxon rank sum. Neuhäuser (2002) compared two step-down closed testing procedures based on the Wilcoxon and modified Baumgartner–Weiß–Schindler statistics in a Monte Carlo study. It was shown that in order to identify the minimum effective

dose, the procedure based on the Mann–Whitney or Wilcoxon test is less power-ful than that based on the modified Baumgartner–Weiß–Schindler statistic. The author illustrated the introduced methods with a data set with one control and three treatment groups (Neuhäuser et al. 1998).

6. Verbeke and Molenberghs (2003) studied the choice between one-sided and two-sided tests whenever inference for variance components is required, focusing on the random intercepts model: $Y_{ij} = x_{ij}^T \beta + b_i + \varepsilon_{ij}$, where Y_{ij} is the response for member $j = 1, \ldots, n_i$ of cluster $i = 1, \ldots, N$, x_{ij} is a vector of known covariate values, β is a vector of unknown regression coefficients, and $b_i \sim N(0, \tau^2)$ is a cluster-specific random effect, assumed to be independently distributed from the residual error components $\varepsilon_{ij} \sim N(0, \sigma^2)$. It was demonstrated that classical two-sided score test statistics cannot be used in this context, and one-sided counterparts could be used instead. The authors presented the construction of one-sided likelihood ratio and score tests for variance components, as well as the derivation of the corresponding asymptotic null distribution. The authors illustrated the use of score tests with a randomized longitudinal experiment in which 50 male Wistar rats were random-ized to either a control group or one of the two treatment groups where treatment consisted of a low or high dose of the drug Decapeptyl, which is an inhibitor for testosterone production in rats (Verdonck et al. 1998).

7. In order to compare two multivariate distributions, Rosenbaum (2005) proposed a test by using distances between observations. This test statistic is exactly distri-bution-free and has a known exact distribution. The construction of an optimal nonbipartite matching, that is, a matching of the observations into disjoint pairs to minimize the total distance within pairs, was based on the interpoint distances. Define the cross-match statistic as the number of pairs containing one observation from the first distribution and one from the second. It was shown that different distributions will exhibit few cross-matches. The test was shown to be consistent against all alternatives when comparing two discrete distributions with finite sup-port. The author further discussed a second exact distribution-free test that ranks the pairs and sums the ranks of the cross-matched pairs. The author illustrated the tests with a study of brain activation measured by functional magnetic resonance imaging during two linguistic tasks, comparing brains that are impaired by arte-riovenous abnormalities with normal controls (Lehéricy et al. 2002).

8. Li and Nie (2008) studied a class of partially nonlinear models with both a non-parametric component and a parametric component. Two procedures were developed to estimate the parameters in the parametric component. The authors established consistency and asymptotic normality of the corresponding estima-tors. For the nonparametric component in the partially nonlinear model, an esti-mation procedure and a generalized F-test procedure, as well as their asymptotic properties, were developed. Based on Monte Carlo simulation studies, finite sam-ple performance of the proposed inference procedures was confirmed to be good. The authors illustrated the use of their methods with an application in ecology.

9. Noting that psychological studies often involve small samples, Nachar (2008) inves-tigated several statistical tests to compare two independent groups that do not require large normally distributed samples, focusing on the Mann–Whitney U-test. The author reviewed the Mann–Whitney U-test and provided the logic underlying this test and its application. In addition, the author pointed out the Mann–Whitney U-test statistic may lead to an inflated Type I error in a situation of heteroscedasticity.

10. In a multivariate parallel two-sample group design, Frömke et al. (2008) proposed two nonparametric relevance-shifted multiple testing procedures on ratios, as extensions of existing procedures of multiplicity correction for point null hypotheses achieving exact control of the family-wise error rate. The first algorithm is a permutation-based algorithm, and it is appropriate for designs with a moderately large number of observations, while the second procedure is more appropriate in the case of limited sample sizes, where multiplicity is corrected according to a concept of data-driven order of hypotheses. The authors illustrated the methods with a subset of the microarray study where the entire data set consists of four subgroups of small, round, blue cell tumors (SRBCTs) of childhood (Khan et al. 2001).

11. Note that tests for comparing the locations of two independent populations are associated with different null hypotheses. Fagerland and Sandvik (2009a) examined the appropriateness of the practice of interpreting test results based on different null hypotheses as evidence for or against equality of means or medians. The authors investigated five frequently used tests: the two-sample T-test, the Welch U-test, the Yuen–Welch test, the Wilcoxon–Mann–Whitney test, and the Brunner–Munzel test. Based on simulation studies on a wide range of scenarios differing in skewness, skewness heterogeneity, variance heterogeneity, sample size, and sample size ratio, it was shown that small differences in distribution properties can alter test performance dramatically, therefore confounding the effort to present simple test recommendations. The authors suggested that though the Welch U-test cannot be considered an omnibus test for this problem, it can be used most frequently. The authors presented the comparison of the considered tests based on a study of hormone therapy (HT), where the goal is to examine whether different HT regimens have different effects on blood coagulation by randomizing 202 healthy women to either low-dose HT, conventional-dose (high-dose) HT, tibolone, or raloxifene (Eilertsen et al. 2006).

12. Zhang and Zhang (2009) investigated the Mann–Whitney U-test and the Kruskal–Wallis test, which are designed to detect whether two or more samples come from the same distribution or to test whether medians between comparison groups are different, under the assumption that the shapes of the underlying distributions are the same. The authors emphasized that the Mann–Whitney U-test and Kruskal–Wallis test should be used for comparisons of differences in medians instead of means.

13. Based on simulation studies, Fagerland and Sandvik (2009b) demonstrated that the problem of the Wilcoxon–Mann–Whitney (WMW) test, which is sensitive to differences in the shapes of the distributions, is more serious than was thought to be the case. Specifically, small differences in variances and moderate degrees of skewness may lead to large deviations from the nominal Type I error rate. When the two distributions have different degrees of skewness, the problem gets worse. The authors investigated the performance of the WMW test for a wide range of skewed distributions, including small and common deviations from the pure shift model. Taking the WMW test as a nonparametric version of the two-sample T-test, the authors explained the results by focusing on some undesirable properties of the rank transformation. The authors suggested examining the ranked samples to find sufficiently satisfactory and reasonable symmetry and variance homogeneity before interpreting the test results.

14. In order to test for the difference in location between two populations, Tabesh et al. (2010) proposed a powerful test statistic that requires few assumptions

and that reduces the bivariate problem to the univariate problem of sum or subtraction of measurements. The authors compared their test with Hotelling's T^2-test, the two-sample rank test, Mathur's test, and Cramer's test for multivariate two-sample problems. Based on Monte Carlo simulation techniques, it was shown that the method proposed by Tabesh et al. performs better in terms of power than any of its competitors under different conditions of underlying population distribution, such as normality or nonnormality, skewed or symmetric, and medium-tailed or heavy-tailed, and is equivalent to the rank test in certain distributions.

15. Biomedical and dental research often involves the analysis of repeated measures based typically on a small to moderate number of subjects. In such cases, nonparametric multivariate methods, which have weaker assumptions and are less sensitive to outliers, may be favored over parametric ones. Preisser et al. (2011) presented a thorough review of univariate and multivariate nonparametric hypothesis testing procedures to a longitudinal study. The goal of the study was to assess changes over time in 31 biomarkers measured from the gingival crevicular fluid in 22 subjects, where gingivitis was induced by temporarily withholding tooth brushing. In order to identify biomarkers inducing change, multivariate Wilcoxon signed-rank tests for a set of four summary measures based on area under the curve were introduced for each biomarker. Those multivariate tests for a set of summary measures for each biomarker were compared to their univariate counterparts. The authors considered multiple hypothesis testing methods focusing on the control of the false discovery rate or strong control of the family-wise error rate (see Chapter 14 for details regarding the false discovery rate and family-wise error rate).

9.7.1 *K*-Sample Comparison

1. For two samples of equal size n, Gnedenko and Korolyuk (1951) showed that the null distribution of the Kolmogorov–Smirnov statistic, $D_{2,n} = \sup_t \left| F_{2,n}(t) - F_{1,n}(t) \right|$, where $F_{i,n}(t)$ is the sample cumulative distribution function for the ith sample, $i = 1, \ldots K$, follows $\lim_{n \to \infty} \Pr\left\{ n^{1/2} D_{2,n} \geq \lambda \right\} = 2 \sum_{i=1}^{\infty} (-1)^{i+1} e^{-(i\lambda)^2}$. Gnedenko and Korolyuk's proof relies on the fact that in the null case (for two samples drawn from the same continuous distribution), $\Pr(D_{2,n} \geq l/n)$ equals the probability that the maximum deviation from the origin of a certain random walk in the line is at least l. David (1958) showed that the null distribution of the three-sample extension of $D_{2,n}$ can be derived by extending the geometric approach of Gnedenko and Korolyuk (1951) from the line to the plane and presented its small sample null distribution.

2. In order to test if a random sample $X_1, \ldots, X_m$, with empirical distribution $F_m(x)$, comes from a continuous population with completely specified distribution function $F_0(x)$, Anderson and Darling (1952, 1954) introduced the goodness-of-fit statistic $A_m^2 = m \int_{-\infty}^{\infty} \frac{\left\{ F_m(x) - F_0(x) \right\}^2}{F_0(x)\left\{ 1 - F_0(x) \right\}} dF_0(x)$. In order to test the homogeneity of samples, Scholz and Stephens (1987) extended an Anderson–Darling rank statistic to

two *K*-sample versions. The *K*-sample Anderson–Darling test is essentially a rank test, and therefore requires no restrictive parametric model assumptions. Two versions of test statistics were proposed, which are both essentially based on a doubly weighted sum of integrated squared differences between the empirical distribution functions of the individual samples and that of the pooled sample. These two versions of test statistics differ primarily in defining the empirical distribution function, while one weighting adjusts for the possibly different sample sizes and the other is inside the integration placing more weight on tail differences of the compared distributions. These tests are consistent against all alternatives. The authors derived the asymptotic null distributions for both continuous and discrete cases. The asymptotic distributions in the continuous case were shown to be the same with the $(K - 1)$–fold convolution of the asymptotic distribution for the Anderson–Darling one-sample statistic. Large sample approximation was investigated based on small sample Monte Carlo simulations for both versions of the statistic under different data settings and degrees of imbalances in sample size. These tests may be applied in a one-way analysis of variance to test for differences in the sampled populations without distributional assumptions or to justify the pooling of separate samples for increased sample size and power.

3. Given *K* random samples of equal size *n* with the common absolutely continuous distribution function, David (1958) proposed a geometric approach to *K*-sample Kolmogorov–Smirnov tests that resulted in the exact distribution of a three-sample test statistic. However, the distribution of David's test statistic is not simple. Kiefer (1959) investigated David's *K*-sample random variables and other *K*-sample analogues of the Kolmogorov–Smirnov test. Dwass (1960) and Conover (1965) investigated several *K*-sample Kolmogorov–Smirnov tests of the same nature. Conover suggested the appropriate test statistics to use in the following situations: (a) testing the null hypothesis that the *K*-samples were drawn from populations having identical distributions against the alternative hypothesis that at least one of the populations differs by location parameter, (b) dividing the *K*-samples into groups having similar location parameters, and (c) testing against the alternative hypothesis that the populations differ by only a scale parameter.

4. O'Brien (1984) studied five procedures for the comparison of two or more multivariate samples, including a nonparametric rank-sum test and a generalized least-squares test, ordinary least squares, Hotelling's T^2, and a Bonferroni per experiment error rate approach. The authors presented applications in which each variable represents a qualitatively different measure of response to treatment. The author examined testing the null hypothesis of no treatment difference with power directed toward alternatives in which at least one treatment is uniformly better than the others. The author derived a convenient expression for this procedure and evaluated its asymptotic relative efficiency with respect to the ordinary least-squares test. Based on simulations, it was shown that the nonparametric procedure provides relatively good power and accurate control over the size of the test. The generalized least-squares procedure may be useful with normally distributed data in moderate or large samples. The author illustrated the considered methods with a randomized trial comparing two therapies, experimental and conventional, for the treatment of diabetes, in which the objective of the study was to determine whether the experimental therapy resulted in better nerve function, as measured by 34 electromyographic variables, than the standard therapy.

5. In order to compare multiple outcomes, Huang et al. (2005) made an improvement on O'Brien (1984) rank-sum tests by accumulating evidence across comparisons on each individual outcome, that is, by replacing the ad hoc variance with the asymptotic variance of the test statistics. For the improved tests, the Type I error rate is controlled at the desired level and the power is increased when the differences between two groups in each outcome variable lie in the same direction. Nevertheless, when the differences are in opposite directions, one may lose power. To this end, Liu et al. (2010) studied an alternative test statistic by maximizing the individual rank-sum statistics. This method was shown to be able to control the Type I error rate and maintain power at a satisfactory level regardless of the direction of the differences. Based on simulation studies, it was shown that Liu's test has higher power than other tests in a certain alternative parameter space of interest. The method was illustrated with growth-related hormone data from the Growth and Maturation in Young Children with Autism or Autistic Spectrum Disorder Study.

9.8 Appendix

Proof of Proposition 9.1

Proof for Test 1

Consider the case of testing H_0 versus H_{A1} ($t = 1$) in Proposition 9.1. Toward this end, we define

$$V_{n_1 m}^* = \sum_{j=1}^{n_1} \left[\log\left(\frac{2m}{n_1 \eta_{m,j}} \right) + \log\left(1 - \frac{m+1}{2n_1} \right) \right],$$

$$V_{n_2 k}^{**} = \sum_{j=1}^{n_2} \left[\log\left(\frac{2k}{n_2 \varphi_{k,j}} \right) + \log\left(1 - \frac{k+1}{2n_2} \right) \right]. \tag{9.26}$$

Then the proposed test statistic at (9.9), $(n_1 + n_2)^{-1} \log\left(V_{n_1 n_2}^{H_{A1}} \right)$, can be expressed as

$$(n_1 + n_2)^{-1} \log\left(V_{n_1 n_2}^{H_{A1}} \right) = \min_{n_1^{0.5+\delta} \leq m \leq n_1^{1-\delta}} (n_1 + n_2)^{-1} V_{n_1 m}^* + \min_{n_2^{0.5+\delta} \leq k \leq n_2^{1-\delta}} (n_1 + n_2)^{-1} V_{n_2 k}^{**}. \tag{9.27}$$

We first investigate the first term of the right-hand side of Equation 9.27. To this end, we define the distribution function $Q(x)$ to be

$$Q(x) = (n_1 F_1(x) + n_2 F_2(x))/(n_1 + n_2),$$

where $F_1(x) = (F_{Z_1}(x) + 1 - F_{Z_1}(-x))/2$ and $F_2(x) = (F_{Z_2}(x) + 1 - F_{Z_2}(-x))/2$.

Also, an empirical distribution function is defined by

$$G_{m_1 + n_2}(x) = (n_1 G_{n_1}(x) + n_2 G_{n_2}(x))/(n_1 + n_2),$$

where

$$G_{n_1}(x) = \left(n_1^{-1} \sum_{j=1}^{n_1} I\left(Z_{1j} \le x\right) + n_1^{-1} \sum_{j=1}^{n_1} I\left(-Z_{1j} \le x\right) \right) \Big/ 2$$

and

$$G_{n_2}(x) = \left(n_2^{-1} \sum_{j=1}^{n_2} I\left(Z_{2j} \le x\right) + n_2^{-1} \sum_{j=1}^{n_2} I\left(-Z_{2j} \le x\right) \right) \Big/ 2$$

are the empirical distribution functions based on observations $Z_{11}, \ldots, Z_{1n_1}$ and $Z_{21}, \ldots, Z_{2n_2}$, respectively. Consequently, the first term of $V_{n_1 m}^*$ in (9.26) can be reformulated as

$$\frac{1}{n_1 + n_2} \sum_{j=1}^{n_1} \log\left(\frac{2m}{n_1 \eta_{m,j}} \right) = -\frac{1}{n_1 + n_2} \sum_{j=1}^{n_1} \log\left(\frac{n_1 \left[G_{n_1+n_2}\left(Z_{1(j+m)}\right) - G_{n_1+n_2}\left(Z_{1(j-m)}\right) \right]}{2m} \right)$$

$$= -\frac{1}{n_1 + n_2} \sum_{j=1}^{n_1} \log\left(\frac{Q\left(Z_{1(j+m)}\right) - Q\left(Z_{1(j-m)}\right)}{F_1\left(Z_{1(j+m)}\right) - F_1\left(Z_{1(j-m)}\right)} \right)$$

$$+ \frac{1}{n_1 + n_2} \sum_{j=1}^{n_1} \log\left(\frac{Q\left(Z_{1(j+m)}\right) - Q\left(Z_{1(j-m)}\right)}{G_{n_1+n_2}\left(Z_{1(j+m)}\right) - G_{n_1+n_2}\left(Z_{1(j-m)}\right)} \right)$$

$$- \frac{1}{n_1 + n_2} \sum_{j=1}^{n_1} \log\left(\frac{n_1 \left[F_1\left(Z_{1(j+m)}\right) - F_1\left(Z_{1(j+m)}\right) \right]}{2m} \right). \qquad (9.28)$$

The first term on the right-hand of Equation 9.28 can be expressed as

$$\frac{1}{n_1 + n_2} \sum_{j=1}^{n_1} \log\left(\frac{Q\left(Z_{1(j+m)}\right) - Q\left(Z_{1(j-m)}\right)}{F_1\left(Z_{1(j+m)}\right) - F_1\left(Z_{1(j-m)}\right)} \right) = \frac{1}{n_1 + n_2} \sum_{j=1}^{n_1} \log\left(\frac{Q\left(Z_{1(j+m)}\right) - Q\left(Z_{1(j-m)}\right)}{Z_{1(j+m)} - Z_{1(j-m)}} \right)$$

$$- \frac{1}{n_1 + n_2} \sum_{j=1}^{n_1} \log\left(\frac{F_1\left(Z_{1(j+m)}\right) - F_1\left(Z_{1(j-m)}\right)}{Z_{1(j+m)} - Z_{1(j-m)}} \right). \qquad (9.29)$$

The result shown in theorem 1 of Vasicek (1976) leads to

$$\frac{1}{n_1 + n_2} \sum_{j=1}^{n_1} \log\left(\frac{Q\left(Z_{1(j+m)}\right) - Q\left(Z_{1(j-m)}\right)}{Z_{1(j+m)} - Z_{1(j-m)}} \right) = \frac{n_1}{n_1 + n_2} \frac{1}{2m} \sum_{d=1}^{2m} S_d, \qquad (9.30)$$

where

$$S_d = \sum_{j=1}^{n_1} \log\left(\frac{Q(Z_{1(j+m)}) - Q(Z_{1(j-m)})}{Z_{1(j+m)} - Z_{1(j-m)}}\right)\left(F_1(Z_{1(j+m)}) - F_1(Z_{1(j-m)})\right), \quad j \equiv d \pmod{2m}.$$

Let $f_i(x) = dF_i(x)/dx = (f_{Z_i}(x) + f_{Z_i}(-x))/2$, $i = 1, 2$. Suppose $Z_{1(j-m)}$ and $Z_{1(j+m)}$ are within an interval in which

$$q(x) = dQ(x)/dx = n_1 f_1(x)/(n_1 + n_2) + n_2 f_2(x)/(n_1 + n_2)$$

is positive and continuous; then

$$q(Z_d') = \frac{Q(Z_{1(j+m)}) - Q(Z_{1(j-m)})}{Z_{1(j+m)} - Z_{1(j-m)}},$$

for some existing value $Z_d' \in (Z_{1(j-m)}, Z_{1(j+m)})$. (The assumption that $q(x)$ is positive and continuous when $x \in (Z_{1(j-m)}, Z_{1(j+m)})$ is used to simplify the proof, and this condition can be excluded; for example, see the proof scheme applied in Vasicek [1976].) It follows that S_d can be written as

$$S_d = \sum_{j=1}^{n_1} \log(q(Z_d'))\left(F_1(Z_{1(j+m)}) - F_1(Z_{1(j-m)})\right), \quad j \equiv d \pmod{2m}.$$

Let us define a density function $\bar{q}(x)$ that approximates $q(x)$ as follows:

$$\bar{q}(x) = \gamma f_1(x)/(1+\gamma) + f_2(x)/(1+\gamma).$$

For each $\varepsilon > 0$ and sufficiently large n_1 and n_2, $n_1/n_2 \to \gamma$ so that we have $(1-\varepsilon)\bar{q}(x) \le q(x) \le (1+\varepsilon)\bar{q}(x)$. It follows that for sufficiently large n_1 and n_2,

$$S_{d,(-\varepsilon)} \le S_d \le S_{d,\varepsilon},$$

where $S_{d,(-\varepsilon)} = \sum_{j=1}^{n_1} \log((1-\varepsilon)\bar{q}(Z_d'))\left(F_1(Z_{1(j+m)}) - F_1(Z_{1(j-m)})\right)$ and $S_{d,\varepsilon} = \sum_{j=1}^{n_1} \log((1+\varepsilon)\bar{q}(Z_d'))$ $\left(F_1(Z_{1(j+m)}) - F_1(Z_{1(j-m)})\right)$; that is, $S_{d,(-\varepsilon)}$ and $S_{d,\varepsilon}$ are Stieltjes sums of the functions $\log((1-\varepsilon)\bar{q}(Z_{11}))$ and $\log((1+\varepsilon)\bar{q}(Z_{11}))$, respectively, with respect to the measure F_1 over the sum of intervals of continuity of $f_1(x)$ and $f_2(x)$ in which $\bar{q}(x) > 0$.

Since in any interval in which $\bar{q}(x)$ is positive, $Z_{1(j+m)} - Z_{1(j-m)} \to 0$ as $n_1 \to \infty$ uniformly over $m \in [n_1^{0.5+\delta}, n_1^{1-\delta}]$, $\delta \in (0, 1/4)$, and uniformly over Z_1, $S_{d,(-\varepsilon)}$ converges in probability to

$$\int_{-\infty}^{\infty} \log((1-\varepsilon)\bar{q}(Z_{11}))dQ(Z_{11}) = E\{\log((1-\varepsilon)\bar{q}(Z_{11}))\} \text{ as } n_1 \to \infty.$$ Furthermore, this convergence is uniformly over j and $n_1^{0.5+\delta} \le m \le n_1^{1-\delta}$, $\delta \in (0, 1/4)$. Similarly, $S_{d,\varepsilon}$ converges in probability to $E\{\log((1+\varepsilon)\bar{q}(Z_{11}))\}$, uniformly over j, and $n_1^{0.5+\delta} \le m \le n_1^{1-\delta}$, $\delta \in (0, 1/4)$.

Therefore,

$$E\left\{\log\left((1-\varepsilon)\bar{q}\left(Z_{11}\right)\right)\right\} \le \frac{1}{2m}\sum_{t=1}^{2m}S_t \le E\left\{\log\left((1+\varepsilon)\bar{q}\left(Z_{11}\right)\right)\right\},$$

as $n_1 \to \infty$ uniformly over $n_1^{0.5+\delta} \le m \le n_1^{1-\delta}$, $\delta \in (0, 1/4)$.

Recalling from (9.30), we find

$$\left(n_1+n_2\right)^{-1}\sum_{j=1}^{n_1}\log\left(\frac{Q\left(Z_{1(j+m)}\right)-Q\left(Z_{1(j-m)}\right)}{Z_{1(j+m)}-Z_{1(j-m)}}\right) \xrightarrow{P} \frac{\gamma}{1+\gamma}E\left\{\log\left(\bar{q}\left(Z_{11}\right)\right)\right\}, \tag{9.31}$$

as $n_1 \to \infty$, $n_2 \to \infty$, $n_1/n_2 \to \gamma > 0$, uniformly over $n_1^{0.5+\delta} \le m \le n_1^{1-\delta}$, $\delta \in (0, 1/4)$.

Similarly, we have

$$\left(n_1+n_2\right)^{-1}\sum_{j=1}^{n_1}\log\left(\frac{F_1\left(Z_{1(j+m)}\right)-F_1\left(Z_{1(j-m)}\right)}{Z_{1(j+m)}-Z_{1(j-m)}}\right) \xrightarrow{P} \frac{\gamma}{1+\gamma}E\left\{\log\left(f_1\left(Z_{11}\right)\right)\right\}, \tag{9.32}$$

as $n_1 \to \infty$, $n_2 \to \infty$, $n_1/n_2 \to \gamma > 0$, uniformly over $n_1^{0.5+\delta} \le m \le n_1^{1-\delta}$, $\delta \in (0, 1/4)$.

Combining the results of (9.29), (9.31), and (9.32) yields

$$\left(n_1+n_2\right)^{-1}\sum_{j=1}^{n_1}\log\left(\frac{Q\left(Z_{1(j+m)}\right)-Q\left(Z_{1(j-m)}\right)}{F_1\left(Z_{1(j+m)}\right)-F_1\left(Z_{1(j-m)}\right)}\right)$$

$$\xrightarrow{P} \frac{\gamma}{1+\gamma}E\left(\log\left(\frac{\bar{q}\left(Z_{11}\right)}{f_1\left(Z_{11}\right)}\right)\right) = \frac{\gamma}{1+\gamma}E\log\left\{\frac{\gamma}{1+\gamma}+\frac{1}{1+\gamma}\left(\frac{f_2\left(Z_{11}\right)}{f_1\left(Z_{11}\right)}\right)\right\}, \tag{9.33}$$

as $n_1 \to \infty$, $n_2 \to \infty$, $n_1/n_2 \to \gamma > 0$, uniformly over $n_1^{0.5+\delta} \le m \le n_1^{1-\delta}$, $\delta \in (0, 1/4)$.

Now, we consider the second term on the right-hand side of the Equation 9.28. By theorem A in Serfling (2009), we know that for $0 \le \epsilon \le \delta/2$,

$$\Pr\left(\sup_{-\infty<x<\infty}\left|F_1(x)-F_{n_1}(x)\right|>n_1^{-0.5+\epsilon}\right) \to 0, \quad \text{as } n_1 \to \infty,$$

and

$$\Pr\left(\sup_{-\infty<x<\infty}\left|F_2(x)-F_{n_2}(x)\right|>n_2^{-0.5+\epsilon}\right) \to 0, \quad \text{as } n_2 \to \infty,$$

implying that $\Pr\left(\sup_{-\infty<x<\infty}\left|F_2(x)-F_{n_2}(x)\right|>\left(2n_1/\gamma\right)^{-0.5+\epsilon}\right) \to 0$ as $n_1 \to \infty$, $n_2 \to \infty$, $n_1/n_2 \to \gamma$.

Hence, $\Pr\left(\sup_{-\infty<x<\infty}\left|Q(x)-G_{m_1+n_2}(x)\right|>n_1^{-0.5+2\epsilon}\right) \to 0$ as $n_1 \to \infty$, $n_2 \to \infty$, for $0 \le \epsilon \le \delta/2$.

Now we consider the case when $\sup\limits_{-\infty < x < \infty} |Q(x) - G_{n_1+n_2}(x)| \leq n_1^{-0.5+2\epsilon}$. According to the definition of $G_{n_1+n_2}(x)$, we have the inequality

$$G_{n_1+n_2}\left(Z_{1(j+m)}\right) - G_{n_1+n_2}\left(Z_{1(j-m)}\right) \geq n_1 \left(n_1+n_2\right)^{-1} 2m(n_1)^{-1} = 2m/(n_1+n_2).$$

Thus, for the case of $\sup\limits_{-\infty < x < \infty} |Q(x) - G_{n_1+n_2}(x)| \leq n_1^{-0.5+2\epsilon}$, we have

$$\frac{1}{n_1+n_2} \sum_{j=1}^{n_1} \log\left(\frac{Q\left(Z_{1(j+m)}\right) - Q\left(Z_{1(j-m)}\right)}{G_{n_1+n_2}\left(Z_{1(j+m)}\right) - G_{n_1+n_2}\left(Z_{1(j-m)}\right)}\right)$$

$$\leq \frac{1}{n_1+n_2} \sum_{j=1}^{n_1} \log\left(\frac{G_{n_1+n_2}\left(Z_{1(j+m)}\right) - G_{n_1+n_2}\left(Z_{1(j-m)}\right) + n_1^{-0.5+\delta/2}}{G_{n_1+n_2}\left(Z_{1(j+m)}\right) - G_{n_1+n_2}\left(Z_{1(j-m)}\right)}\right)$$

$$\leq \frac{1}{n_1+n_2} \sum_{j=1}^{n_1} \log\left(1 + \frac{n_1^{-0.5+\frac{\delta}{2}}}{2m/(n_1+n_2)}\right) \leq \frac{1}{n_1+n_2} \sum_{j=1}^{n_1} \left(\frac{n_1^{-0.5+\delta/2}}{2n_1^{0.5+\delta}/(n_1+n_2)}\right) = \frac{1}{2n_1^{\delta/2}} \to 0,$$

for a sufficiently large n_1 and $m \in \left[n_1^{0.5+\delta}, n_1^{1-\delta}\right]$.

Also, note that

$$\frac{1}{n_1+n_2} \sum_{j=1}^{n_1} \log\left(\frac{Q\left(Z_{1(j+m)}\right) - Q\left(Z_{1(j-m)}\right)}{G_{n_1+n_2}\left(Z_{1(j+m)}\right) - G_{n_1+n_2}\left(Z_{1(j-m)}\right)}\right)$$

$$\geq \frac{1}{n_1+n_2} \sum_{j=1}^{n_1} \log\left(\frac{G_{n_1+n_2}\left(Z_{1(j+m)}\right) - G_{n_1+n_2}\left(Z_{1(j-m)}\right) - n_1^{-0.5+\delta/2}}{G_{n_1+n_2}\left(Z_{1(j+m)}\right) - G_{n_1+n_2}\left(Z_{1(j-m)}\right)}\right)$$

$$\geq \frac{1}{n_1+n_2} \sum_{j=1}^{n_1} \log\left(1 - \frac{n_1^{-0.5+\frac{\delta}{2}}}{2m/(n_1+n_2)}\right) \geq -\frac{1}{n_1+n_2} \sum_{j=1}^{n_1} \left(\frac{2n_1^{-0.5+\delta/2}}{2n_1^{0.5+\delta}/(n_1+n_2)}\right) = -\frac{1}{n_1^{\delta/2}} \to 0$$

for a sufficiently large n_1 and $m \in \left[n_1^{0.5+\delta}, n_1^{1-\delta}\right]$. Hence, we prove that the second term on the right-hand side of the equality (9.28) converges to zero in probability. That is,

$$\frac{1}{n_1+n_2} \sum_{j=1}^{n_1} \log\left(\frac{Q\left(Z_{1(j+m)}\right) - Q\left(Z_{1(j-m)}\right)}{G_{n_1+n_2}\left(Z_{1(j+m)}\right) - G_{n_1+n_2}\left(Z_{1(j-m)}\right)}\right) \xrightarrow{P} 0, \tag{9.34}$$

as $n_1 \to \infty$, $n_2 \to \infty$, $n_1/n_2 \to \gamma > 0$, uniformly over $n_1^{0.5+\delta} \leq m \leq n_1^{1-\delta}$.

Finally, using the result of lemma 1 of Vasicek (1976), the last term on the right-hand side of the equality of (9.28) also converges to zero in probability. That is,

$$-\left(n_1+n_2\right)^{-1}\sum_{j=1}^{n_1}\log\left(\frac{n_1\left[F_1\left(Z_{1(j+m)}\right)-F_1\left(Z_{1(j-m)}\right)\right]}{2m}\right)\overset{P}{\to}0, \tag{9.35}$$

as $n_1\to\infty$, $n_2\to\infty$, $n_1/n_2\to\gamma>0$, uniformly over $n_1^{0.5+\delta}\le m\le n_1^{1-\delta}$, $\delta\in(0,1/4)$.
  By (9.33) through (9.35), we show that

$$\left(n_1+n_2\right)^{-1}V_{n_1m}^{*}\overset{P}{\to}-\frac{\gamma}{1+\gamma}E\log\left\{\frac{\gamma}{1+\gamma}+\frac{1}{1+\gamma}\left(\frac{f_2(Z_{11})}{f_1(Z_{11})}\right)\right\}, \tag{9.36}$$

as $n_1\to\infty$, $n_2\to\infty$, $n_1/n_2\to\gamma>0$, uniformly over $n_1^{0.5+\delta}\le m\le n_1^{1-\delta}$, $\delta\in(0,1/4)$.
  Likewise, following the same procedure as shown in the proof of $V_{n_1m}^{*}$, we have

$$\left(n_1+n_2\right)^{-1}V_{n_2k}^{**}=\left(n_1+n_2\right)^{-1}\sum_{j=1}^{n_2}\left[\log\left(\frac{2k}{n_2\varphi_{k,j}}\right)+\log\left(1-\frac{k+1}{2n_2}\right)\right]$$

$$\overset{P}{\to}-\frac{1}{1+\gamma}E\log\left\{\frac{\gamma}{1+\gamma}\left(\frac{f_1(Z_{21})}{f_2(Z_{21})}\right)+\frac{1}{1+\gamma}\right\},$$

as $n_1\to\infty$, $n_2\to\infty$, $n_1/n_2\to\gamma>0$, uniformly over $n_2^{0.5+\delta}\le k\le n_2^{1-\delta}$, $\delta\in(0,1/4)$. Based on this and (9.36), it can be concluded that

$$\left(n_1+n_2\right)^{-1}\log\left(V_{n_1n_2}^{H_{A1}}\right)\overset{P}{\to}-\frac{\gamma}{1+\gamma}E\log\left\{\frac{\gamma}{1+\gamma}+\frac{1}{1+\gamma}\left(\frac{f_2(Z_{11})}{f_1(Z_{11})}\right)\right\}$$

$$-\frac{1}{1+\gamma}E\log\left\{\frac{\gamma}{1+\gamma}\left(\frac{f_1(Z_{21})}{f_2(Z_{21})}\right)+\frac{1}{1+\gamma}\right\},$$

as $n_1\to\infty$, $n_2\to\infty$, $n_1/n_2\to\gamma>0$.
  Hence, under H_0, we have

$$\frac{f_2(Z_{11})}{f_1(Z_{11})}=\frac{\left(f_{Z_2}(Z_{11})+f_{Z_2}(-Z_{11})\right)/2}{\left(f_{Z_1}(Z_{11})+f_{Z_1}(-Z_{11})\right)/2}=\frac{f_{Z_2}(Z_{11})}{f_{Z_1}(Z_{11})},$$

$$\frac{f_1(Z_{21})}{f_2(Z_{21})}=\frac{\left(f_{Z_1}(Z_{21})+f_{Z_1}(-Z_{21})\right)/2}{\left(f_{Z_2}(Z_{21})+f_{Z_2}(-Z_{21})\right)/2}=\frac{f_{Z_1}(Z_{21})}{f_{Z_2}(Z_{21})},$$

$$\left(n_1+n_2\right)^{-1}\log\left(V_{n_1n_2}^{H_{A1}}\right)\overset{P}{\to}-\frac{\gamma}{1+\gamma}E_{H_0}\log\left\{\frac{\gamma}{1+\gamma}+\frac{1}{1+\gamma}\left(\frac{f_{Z_2}(Z_{11})}{f_{Z_1}(Z_{11})}\right)\right\}$$

$$-\frac{1}{1+\gamma}E_{H_0}\log\left\{\frac{\gamma}{1+\gamma}\left(\frac{f_{Z_1}(Z_{21})}{f_{Z_2}(Z_{21})}\right)+\frac{1}{1+\gamma}\right\}=0,$$

and under H_{A1},

$$(n_1 + n_2)^{-1} \log\left(V_{n_1 n_2}^{H_{A1}}\right) \overset{p}{\to} -\frac{\gamma}{1+\gamma} E_{H_{A1}} \log\left\{\frac{\gamma}{1+\gamma} + \frac{1}{1+\gamma}\left(\frac{f_2(Z_{11})}{f_1(Z_{11})}\right)\right\}$$

$$-\frac{1}{1+\gamma} E_{H_{A1}} \log\left\{\frac{\gamma}{1+\gamma}\left(\frac{f_1(Z_{21})}{f_2(Z_{21})}\right) + \frac{1}{1+\gamma}\right\}$$

$$\geq -\frac{\gamma}{1+\gamma} \log\left\{\frac{\gamma}{1+\gamma} + \frac{1}{1+\gamma} E_{H_{A1}}\left(\frac{f_2(Z_{11})}{f_1(Z_{11})}\right)\right\}$$

$$-\frac{1}{1+\gamma} \log\left\{\frac{\gamma}{1+\gamma} E_{H_{A1}}\left(\frac{f_1(Z_{21})}{f_2(Z_{21})}\right) + \frac{1}{1+\gamma}\right\} \geq 0,$$

as $n_1 \to \infty$, $n_2 \to \infty$, $n_1/n_2 \to \gamma > 0$.

We complete the proof of Proposition 9.1 for the case of $t = 1$, that is, the consistency related to Test 1.

Proof for Test 2

Here, we will consider the case of $t = 2$. That is, we show that

$$(n_1 + n_2)^{-1} \log\left(V_{n_1 n_2}^{H_{A2}}\right) \overset{p}{\to} -\frac{\gamma}{1+\gamma} E \log\left\{\frac{\gamma}{1+\gamma} + \frac{1}{1+\gamma}\left(\frac{f_2(Z_{11})}{f_1(Z_{11})}\right)\right\}$$

$$-\frac{1}{1+\gamma} E \log\left\{\frac{\gamma}{1+\gamma}\left(\frac{f_1(Z_{21})}{f_2(Z_{21})}\right) + \frac{1}{1+\gamma}\right\},$$

as $n_1 \to \infty$, $n_2 \to \infty$, $n_1/n_2 \to \gamma > 0$.

It is clear that if one can show that $\log\left(\Lambda_{n_2}^k\right) \overset{p}{\to} 0$ as $n_2 \to \infty$, where $\Lambda_{n_2}^k$ is defined by (9.12), the rest of the proof is similar to the proof shown for the test statistic of the proposed Test 1, $\log\left(V_{n_1 n_2}^{H_{A1}}\right)$. To consider $\log\left(\Lambda_{n_2}^k\right)$ as $n_2 \to \infty$, we begin with a proof that

$$\tilde{F}_{Z_2}\left(Z_{2(n_2)}\right) - \tilde{F}_{Z_2}\left(Z_{2(1)}\right) = \frac{1}{2n_2} \sum_{j=1}^{n_2}\left[I\left(Z_{2j} \leq Z_{2(n_2)}\right) + I\left(-Z_{2j} \leq Z_{2(n_2)}\right)\right]$$

$$-\frac{1}{2n_2} \sum_{j=1}^{n_2}\left[I\left(Z_{2j} \leq Z_{2(1)}\right) + I\left(-Z_{2j} \leq Z_{2(1)}\right)\right] \overset{p}{\to} 1, \text{ as } n_2 \to \infty.$$

To this end, we apply theorem A of Serfling (2009), having that for $\epsilon \in$ (0, 1/2), $\sup_{-\infty < u < \infty}\left|\tilde{F}_{Z_2}(u) - F_{Z_2}(u)\right| = o\left(n_2^{-0.5+\epsilon}\right)$ as $n_2 \to \infty$. Thus, $\tilde{F}_{Z_2}\left(Z_{2(n_2)}\right) - \tilde{F}_{Z_2}\left(Z_{2(1)}\right) =$

$F_{Z_2}\left(Z_{2(n_2)}\right) - F_{Z_2}\left(Z_{2(1)}\right) + o\left(n_2^{-0.5+\epsilon}\right)$. It is obvious that $F_{Z_2}\left(Z_{2(n_2)}\right) \to 1$ and $F_{Z_2}\left(Z_{2(1)}\right) \to 0$ as $n_2 \to \infty$. Hence,

$$\tilde{F}_{Z_2}\left(Z_{2(n_2)}\right) - \tilde{F}_{Z_2}\left(Z_{2(1)}\right) \xrightarrow{p} 1 \text{ as } n_2 \to \infty. \tag{9.37}$$

Next, we will show that the part of $\Lambda_{n_2}^k$, $\sum_{r=1}^{k-1}(2k)^{-1}(k-r)\sum_{j=1}^{n_2}\left[\tilde{F}_{Z_2}\left(Z_{2(r+1)}\right) - \tilde{F}_{Z_2}\left(Z_{2(r)}\right)\right] \xrightarrow{p} 0$ as $n_2 \to \infty$. Let $\tilde{F}_{-Z_2}(u)$ denote the empirical distribution function of $-Z_2$ distributed with $\left(1 - F_{Z_2}(-u)\right)$ (Here the symmetry of the Z_2-distribution under H_0 and H_{A_2} is used.) Then

$$\sum_{r=1}^{k-1}\frac{(k-r)}{2k}\left[\tilde{F}_{Z_2}\left(Z_{2(r+1)}\right) - \tilde{F}_{Z_2}\left(Z_{2(r)}\right)\right]$$

$$= \frac{1}{2n_2}\sum_{r=1}^{k-1}\frac{(k-r)}{2k}\sum_{j=1}^{n_2}\left[I\left(Z_{2j} \le Z_{2(r+1)}\right) + I\left(-Z_{2j} \le Z_{2(r+1)}\right) - I\left(Z_{2j} \le Z_{2(r)}\right) - I\left(-Z_{2j} \le Z_{2(r)}\right)\right]$$

$$= \frac{(k-r)}{4n_2} + \sum_{r=1}^{k-1}\frac{(k-r)}{2k}\left[\tilde{F}_{-Z_2}\left(Z_{2(r+1)}\right) - \tilde{F}_{-Z_2}\left(Z_{2(r)}\right)\right]. \tag{9.38}$$

Since the first term of (9.38), $(4n_2)^{-1}(k-r)$, vanishes to zero as $n_2 \to \infty$, we focus on the remaining terms of Equation 9.38, which can be reorganized as follows:

$$\sum_{r=1}^{k-1}\frac{(k-r)}{2k}\left[\tilde{F}_{-Z_2}\left(Z_{2(r+1)}\right) - \tilde{F}_{-Z_2}\left(Z_{2(r)}\right)\right] = \sum_{r=1}^{k-1}\frac{(k-(r-1))}{2k}\tilde{F}_{-Z_2}\left(Z_{2(r)}\right) - \frac{k}{2k}\tilde{F}_{-Z_2}\left(Z_{2(1)}\right)$$

$$+ \frac{(k-(k-1))}{2k}\tilde{F}_{-Z_2}\left(Z_{2(k)}\right) - \sum_{r=1}^{k-1}\frac{(k-r)}{2k}\tilde{F}_{-Z_2}\left(Z_{2(r)}\right)$$

$$= \frac{1}{2k}\sum_{r=1}^{k-1}\tilde{F}_{-Z_2}\left(Z_{2(r)}\right) - \frac{1}{2}\tilde{F}_{-Z_2}\left(Z_{2(1)}\right) + \frac{1}{2k}\tilde{F}_{-Z_2}\left(Z_{2(k)}\right). \tag{9.39}$$

In respect to the empirical distribution function, $\tilde{F}_{-Z_2}(u)$, which appears in (9.39), again by virtue of theorem A of Serfling (2009), we have that for $\epsilon \in (0, 1/2)$,

$$\sum_{r=1}^{k-1}\frac{(k-r)}{2k}\left[\tilde{F}_{-Z_2}\left(Z_{2(r+1)}\right) - \tilde{F}_{-Z_2}\left(Z_{2(r)}\right)\right]$$

$$= \frac{1}{2k}\sum_{r=1}^{k-1}F_{-Z_2}\left(Z_{2(r)}\right) - \frac{1}{2}F_{-Z_2}\left(Z_{2(1)}\right) + \frac{1}{2k}F_{-Z_2}\left(Z_{2(k)}\right) + o\left(n_2^{-0.5+\epsilon}\right). \tag{9.40}$$

Clearly, $F_{-Z_2}\left(Z_{2(1)}\right)/2 \to 0$ and $F_{-Z_2}\left(Z_{2(k)}\right)/2k \to 0$ as $n_2 \to \infty$. Now, we prove that the first item of (9.40) converges to zero in probability as $n_2 \to \infty$.

Since the distribution of $Z_{21}, \ldots, Z_{2n_2}$ is symmetric under H_0 and the statistic $\Lambda_{n_2}^k$ is based on $I\left(-Z_{2j} \leq Z_{2(r)}\right)$ under H_0 and H_{A_2}, the distribution of $Z_{21}, \ldots, Z_{2n_2}$ can be taken as the uniform distribution on the interval $[-1, 1]$. Thus, we obtain $F_{-Z_2}\left(Z_{2(r)}\right) = \left(1 + Z_{2(r)}\right)/2$, where $U_{(r)} = \left(1 + Z_{2(r)}\right)/2$ is the rth-order statistic based on a standard uniformly distributed, $Unif[0, 1]$, random variable. Since

$$E\left\{(2k)^{-1} \sum_{r=1}^{k-1} U_{(r)}\right\} = \frac{k(k-1)}{4k(n_2+1)} \to 0, \quad \text{as } n_2 \to \infty,$$

applying Chebyshev's inequality yields $(2k)^{-1} \sum_{r=1}^{k-1} U_{(r)} \overset{p}{\to} 0$ as $n_2 \to \infty$.

Combining (9.38) through (9.40), we conclude that

$$\sum_{r=1}^{k-1} \frac{(k-r)}{2k}\left[\tilde{F}_{Z_2}\left(Z_{2(r+1)}\right) - \tilde{F}_{Z_2}\left(Z_{2(r)}\right)\right] \overset{p}{\to} 0 \quad \text{as } n_2 \to \infty. \tag{9.41}$$

Similarly, one can show that

$$\sum_{r=1}^{k-1} \frac{(k-r)}{2k}\left[\tilde{F}_{Z_2}\left(Z_{2(n_2-r+1)}\right) - \tilde{F}_{Z_2}\left(Z_{2(n_2-r)}\right)\right] \overset{p}{\to} 0 \quad \text{as } n_2 \to \infty \tag{9.42}$$

The results of (9.37), (9.41), and (9.42) complete the proof of $\log\left(\Lambda_{n_2}^k\right) \overset{p}{\to} 0$ as $n_2 \to \infty$.

9.8.1 R Code to Conduct Two-Sample Density-Based Empirical Likelihood Ratio Test

```
#Test for H0: X~Y; H1 not H0
# define sample size
n1<-10 #Sample size of X
n2<-30 #Sample size of Y
delta<-0.1
MC<-10000 #Number Number of Monte Carlo repetitions/ If do not need it
MC<-1
#set.seed(6666) ###set seed to make sure the generated samples to be the
  same

finalts<-c()
for(i in 1:MC){
x<-rnorm(n1,1,1) #Generated values of X, Y under H0/ x,y can be taken
# from your data
y<-rnorm(n2,0,0.5) #
z<-c(x,y)
sx<-sort(x)
sy<-sort(y)
sz<-sort(z)
```

```
#################################################
#######obtain test statistic of sample 1#########
#################################################
m<-c(round(n1^(delta+0.5)):min(c(round((n1)^(1-delta)),round(n1/2))))
  ###generate a vector of "m"
a<-replicate(n1,m)    ###store repeated values of a vector "m"
rm<-as.vector(t(a))   ###transpose the previous length(m)*n1 matrix and
  # make it to be a vector
#rm<-rep(m, each = n1) ###repeat a vector of "m" n1 times
L<-c(1:n1)- rm    ###order from (1-m) to (n1-m)
LL<-replace(L, L <= 0, 1 ) ###replace value<=0 with 1 when (1-m)<=0
U<-c(1:n1)+ rm    ###order from (1+m) to (n1+m)
UU<-replace(U, U > n1, n1) ###replace value>n1 with n1 when (n1+m)>n1
xL<-sx[LL] ###obtain x(i-m)
xU<-sx[UU] ###obtain x(i+m)
F<-ecdf(z)(xU)-ecdf(z)(xL) ###empirical distribution function
##The empirical distribution function would be set up to the reciprocal
  # of the total sample size when it equals to zero
F[F==0]<-1/(n1+n2)
### a (n1*length(m)) vector of (2*m)/(n1*empirical distribution function)
I<-2*rm/ ( n1*F )
ux<-array(I, c(n1,length(m))) # make previous vector a n1 * length(m)
  # matrix
tstat1<-log(min(apply(ux,2,prod))) #get a test statistic of sample 1
#################################################
#######obtain test statistic of sample 2#########
#################################################
m<-c(round(n2^(delta+0.5)):min(c(round((n2)^(1-delta)),round(n2/2))))
  ###generate a vector of "m"
a<-replicate(n2,m)    ###store repeated values of a vector "m"
rm<-as.vector(t(a))    ###transpose the previous length(m)*n2 matrix and
  # make it to be a vector
#rm<-rep(m, each = n2)   ###repeat a vector of "m" n2 times
L<-c(1:n2)- rm   ###order from (1-m) to (n2-m)
LL<-replace(L, L <= 0, 1 )   ###replace value<=0 with 1 when (1-m) <=0
U<-c(1:n2)+ rm   ###order from (1+m) to (n1+m)
UU<-replace(U, U > n2, n2)   ###replace value>n1 with n1 when (n1+m)>n1
yL<-sy[LL] ###obtain y(i-m)
yU<-sy[UU] ###obtain y(i+m)
F<-ecdf(z)(yU)-ecdf(z)(yL) ###empirical distribution function
F[F==0]<-1/(n1+n2) ###The empirical distribution function would be set up
  # to the reciprocal of the total # sample size when it equals to zero
I<-2*rm/ ( n2*F ) ### a (n2*length(m)) vector of (2*m)/(n2*empirical
  # distribution function)
uy<-array(I, c(n2,length(m))) # make previous vector a n2 * length(m)
  # matrix
tstat2<-log(min(apply(uy,2, prod))) #get a test statistic of sample 2
finalts[i]<-tstat1+tstat2 # final test statistic
}
# MC mean
mean(1*(finalts>=12.64385))
# obtain the critical value
quantile(finalts,0.95)
```

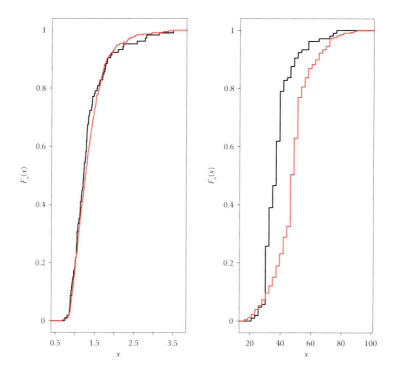

FIGURE 3.7
EDF of the data of TBARS measurements (left) and HDL measurements (right) for the diseased (black) and nondiseased (red) groups, respectively.

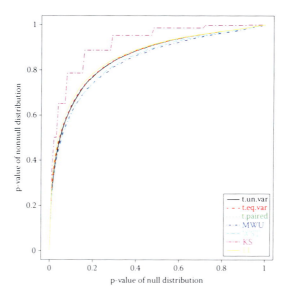

FIGURE 3.14
P–P plot for comparisons among empirical power of seven tests for equality of means where $X \sim N(1, \sqrt{5})$, $Y \sim N(2,1)$ and the sample size is 25. The tests considered include the two-sample t-test with unpooled variances (t.un.var) or pooled variances (t.eq.var), the paired two-sample t-test (t.paired), the Mann–Whitney U-test (MWU), the Wilcoxon signed-rank test (WST), the Kolmogorov–Smirnov test (KS), and the empirical likelihood test (EL).

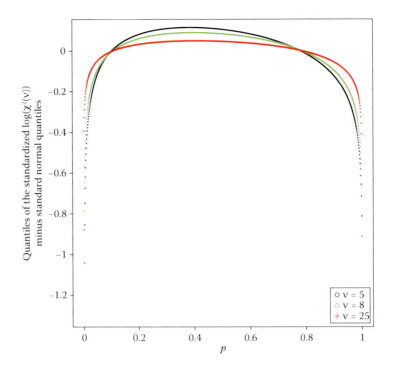

FIGURE 3.15
Difference in quantiles of standardized $\log \chi^2(v)$ ($v = 5, 8, 25$) and the standard normal quantiles versus p.

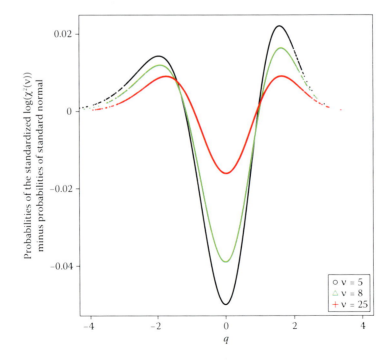

FIGURE 3.16
Difference in probabilities of the standardized $\log \chi^2(v)$ ($v = 5, 8, 25$) and the standard normal quantiles versus q.

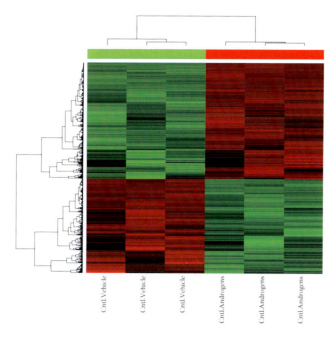

FIGURE 3.20
Heat map generated from microarray data reflecting gene expression values in the control siRNA transfection group with two different treatments: vehicle or androgens.

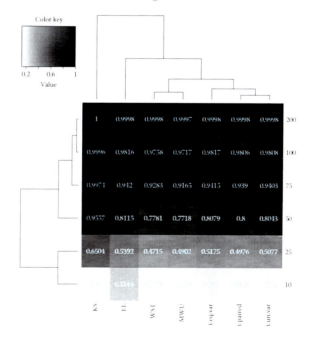

FIGURE 3.21
Grayscale heat map for comparisons among the empirical powers of several tests for equality of means where $X \sim N (1,\sqrt{5})$, $Y \sim N (2,1)$ with various sample sizes ($n = 10, 25, 50, 75, 100, 200$) at the 0.05 significance level. The tests considered include the two-sample t-test with unpooled variances (t.un.var) or pooled variances (t.eq.var), the paired two-sample t-test (t.paired), the Mann–Whitney U-test (MWU), the Wilcoxon signed-rank test (WST), the Kolmogorov–Smirnov test (KS) and the empirical likelihood test (EL).

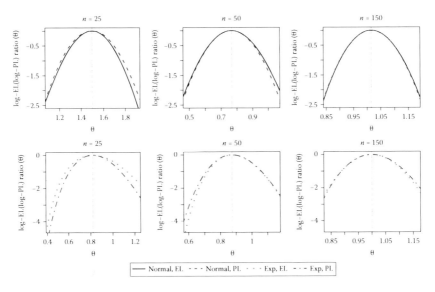

FIGURE 6.1

The log-empirical likelihood ratios and the log-likelihood ratios based on samples of sizes $n = 25, 50, 150$, where the black solid line and the red dashed line represent the log-empirical likelihood ratios and the log-likelihood ratios when the underlying distribution is normal, respectively, while the green dotted line and the blue dot-dash line represent the log-empirical likelihood ratio and the log-likelihood ratio when the underlying distribution is exponential, respectively.

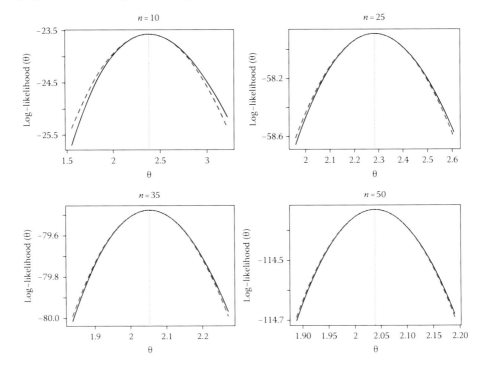

FIGURE 7.1

Plot of log-likelihood (black solid line) and its quadratic approximation (red dashed line) versus the shape parameter θ based on samples of sizes $n = 10, 25, 35, 50$ from a gamma distribution with a true shape parameter of $\theta_0 = 2$ and a known scale parameter of 2.

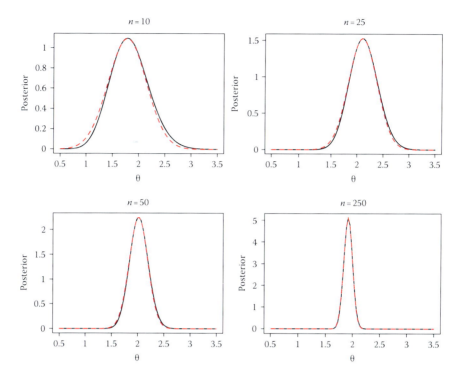

FIGURE 7.2
Plot of the posterior function (black solid line) and its normal approximation (red dashed line) versus the shape parameter θ. The prior is based on a uniform distribution function. The samples are from a gamma distribution with a true shape parameter of $\theta_0 = 2$ and a known scale parameter of 2. $n = 10, 25, 50, 250$.

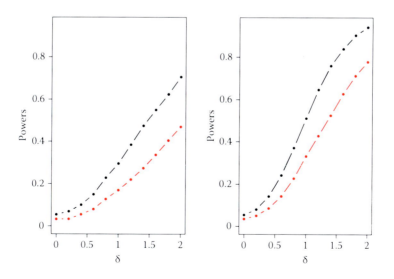

FIGURE 8.5
Experimental comparisons based on the Monte Carlo powers related to the test based on the AUC concept, $H_0 :$ AUC $= 1/2$ vs. $H_1 :$ AUC $\neq 1/2$ (in black), and the test based on the logistic regression concept, $H_0 : \beta = 0$ vs. $H_1 : \beta \neq 0$ (in red). The tests were performed in order to detect the discriminant ability of the biomarkers at the 0.05 significance level. The left and right panels correspond to sample sizes of 50 and 100, respectively.

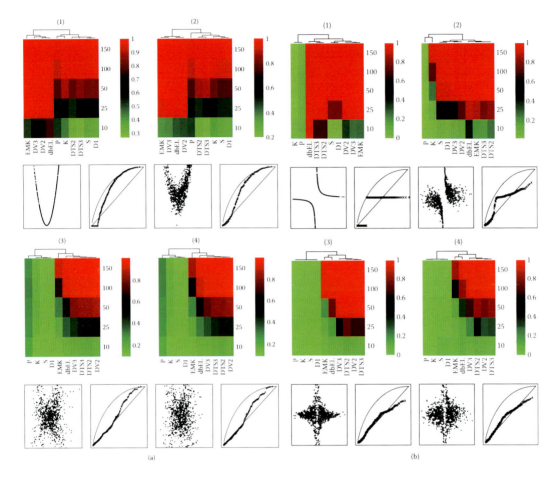

FIGURE 10.5

Graphical summarization and the comparison of the powers of the considered tests at the 0.05 significance level, based on data with the dependence structure M3 (LinearQuadratic) in the left panel (a) and M5 (Reciprocal with $k = 1$) in the right panel. (b), as well as various types of random effects that correspond to one of the subpanels. In each subpanel (1–4), the top level is the heat map and the bottom level shows the scatterplot (left panel) and K-plot (right panel). The following random effects schemes are considered: (1) $X = X_0$, $Y = Y_0$; (2) $X = X_0$, $Y = Y_0 + \varepsilon_A$; (3) $X = X_0$, $Y = \varepsilon_M Y_0$; and (4) $X = X_0$, $Y = \varepsilon_M Y_0 + \varepsilon_A$, where the random effects ε_A and $\varepsilon_M \sim N(0, 1)$. For M3 (LinearQuadratic), the measures of MIC (AUK) for each type of random effect are (1) 1 (0.664), (2) 0.664 (0.639), (3) 0.276 (0.534), and (4) 0.271 (0.533). For M5 (Reciprocal with $k = 1$), the measures of MIC (AUK) for each type of random effect are (1) 1 (0.438), (2) 0.69 (0.522), (3) 0.32 (0.471), and (4) 0.278(0.483).

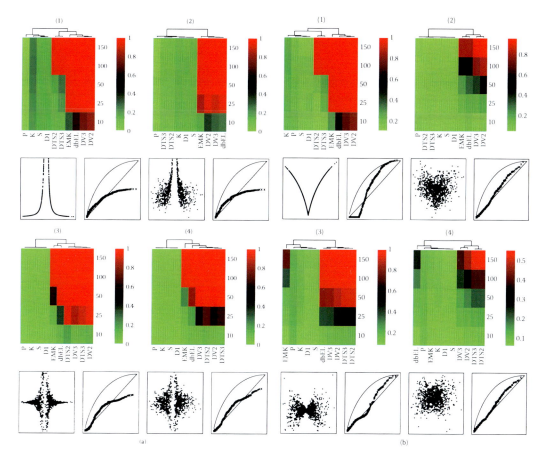

FIGURE 10.6

Graphical summarization and the comparison of the powers of the considered tests at the 0.05 significance level, based on data with the dependence structure M6 (Reciprocal with $k = 2$) in the left panel (a) and M8 (Logarithm) in the right panel. (b), as well as various types of random effects that correspond to one of the subpanels. In each subpanel (1–4), the top level is the heat map and the bottom level shows the scatterplot (left panel) and K-plot (right panel). The following random effects schemes are considered: (1) $X = X_{()}$, $Y = Y_{()}$; (2) $X = X_{()}$, $Y = Y_{()} + \varepsilon_A$; (3) $X = X_{()}$, $Y = \varepsilon_M Y_{()}$; and (4) $X = X_{()}$, $Y = \varepsilon_M Y_{()} + \varepsilon_A$, where the random effects ε_A and $\varepsilon_m \sim N(0, 1)$. For M6 (Reciprocal with $k = 2$), the measures of MIC (AUK) for each type of random effect are (1) 1 (0.407), (2) 0.756 (0.416), (3) 0.429 (0.458), and (4) 0.379 (0.473). For M8 (Logarithm), the measures of MIC (AUK) for each type of random effect are (1) 1 (0.576), (2) 0.281 (0.526), (3) 0.277 (0.519), and (4) 0.237 (0.511).

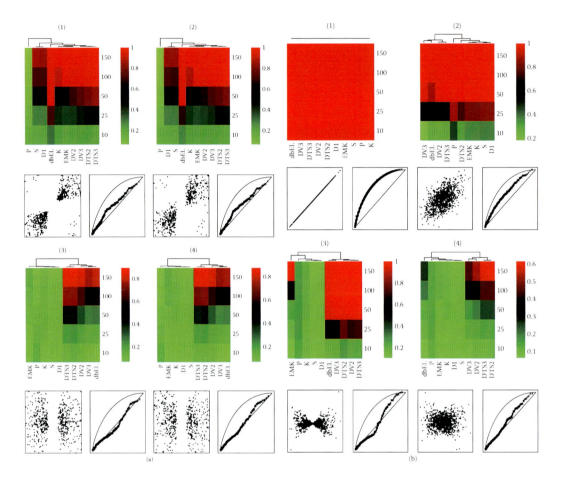

FIGURE 10.7

Graphical summarization and the comparison of the powers of the considered tests at the 0.05 significance level, based on data with the dependence structure M24 (Reciprocal-Normal) in the left panel (a) and M1 (Linear) in the right panel. (b) and various types of random effects that correspond to one of the subpanels. In each subpanel (1–4), the top level is the heat map and the bottom level shows the scatterplot (left panel) and K-plot (right panel). The following random effects schemes are considered: (1) $X = X_0$, $Y = Y_0$; (2) $X = X_0$, $Y = Y_0 + \varepsilon_A$; (3) $X = X_0$, $Y = \varepsilon_M Y_0$; and (4) $X = X_0$, $Y = \varepsilon_M Y_0 + \varepsilon_A$, where the random effects ε_A and $\varepsilon_m \sim N(0, 1)$. For M24 (Reciprocal-Normal), the measures of MIC (AUK) for each type of random effect are (1) 0.522 (0.571), (2) 0.506 (0.569), (3) 0.241 (0.512), and (4) 0.241 (0.512). For M1 (Linear), the measures of MIC (AUK) for each type of random effect are (1) 1 (0.75), (2) 0.405 (0.619), (3) 0.305 (0.522), and (4) 0.237 (0.511).

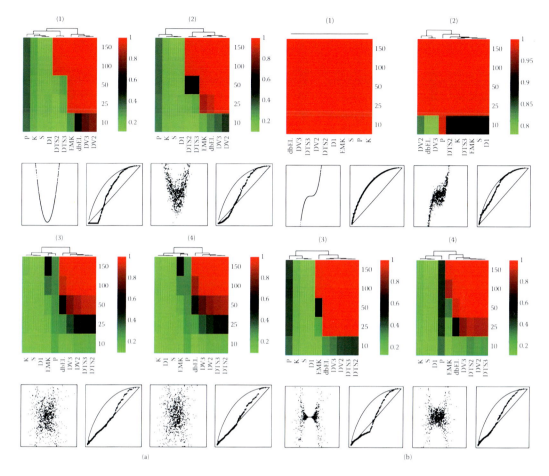

FIGURE 10.8

Graphical summarization and the comparison of the powers of the considered tests at the 0.05 significance level, based on data with the dependence structure M2 (Quadratic) in the left panel (a) and M4 (Cubic) in the right panel. (b) and various types of random effects that correspond to one of the subpanels. In each subpanel (1–4), the top level is the heat map and the bottom level shows the scatterplot (left panel) and K-plot (right panel). The following random effects schemes are considered: (1) $X = X_0$, $Y = Y_0$; (2) $X = X_0$, $Y = Y_0 + \varepsilon_A$; (3) $X = X_0$, $Y = \varepsilon_M Y_0$; and (4) $X = X_0$, $Y = \varepsilon_M Y_0 + \varepsilon_A$, where the random effects ε_A and $\varepsilon_m \sim N(0, 1)$. For M2 (Quadratic), the measures of MIC (AUK) for each type of random effect are (1) 1 (0.576), (2) 0.636 (0.563), (3) 0.244 (0.52), and (4) 0.242 (0.519). For M4 (Cubic), the measures of MIC (AUK) for each type of random effect are (1) 1 (0.75), (2) 0.708 (0.703), (3) 0.484 (0.529), and (4) 0.305 (0.526).

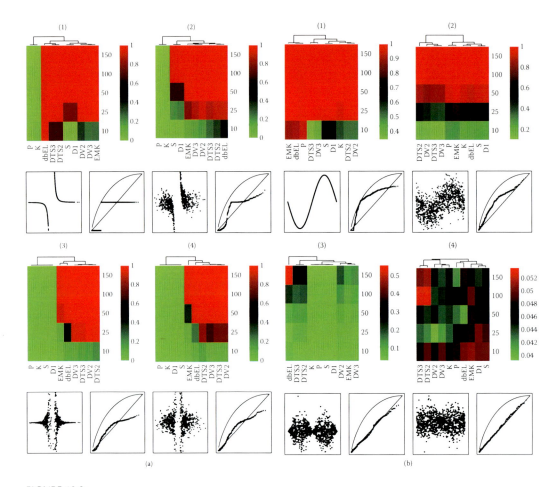

(a)

(b)

FIGURE 10.9

Graphical summarization and the comparison of the powers of the considered tests at the 0.05 significance level, based on data with the dependence structure M7 (Reciprocal with $k = 3$) in the left panel (a) and M9′ ($\sin(\pi X)$ where $X \sim Uniform[-2, 2]$) in the right panel. (b) and various types of random effects that correspond to one of the subpanels. In each subpanel (1–4), the top level is the heat map and the bottom level shows the scatterplot (left panel) and K-plot (right panel). The following random effects schemes are considered: (1) $X = X_0$, $Y = Y_0$; (2) $X = X_0$, $Y = Y_0 + \varepsilon_A$; (3) $X = X_0$, $Y = \varepsilon_M Y_0$; and (4) $X = X_0$, $Y = \varepsilon_M Y_0 + \varepsilon_A$, where the random effects ε_A and $\varepsilon_m \sim N(0, 1)$. For M7 (Reciprocal with $k = 3$), the measures of MIC (AUK) for each type of random effect are (1) 1 (0.438), (2) 0.708 (0.48), (3) 0.488 (0.452), and (4) 0.445 (0.469). For M9′ ($\sin(\pi X)$ where $X \sim Uniform[-2, 2]$), the measures of MIC (AUK) for each type of random effect are (1) 1.000 (0.397), (2) 0.391 (0.443), (3) 0.242 (0.501), and (4) 0.237 (0.503).

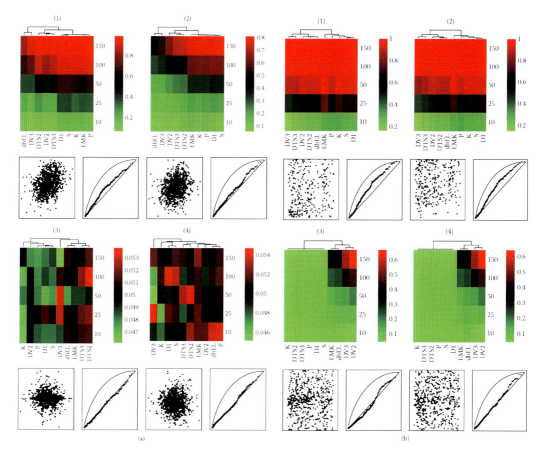

FIGURE 10.12
Graphical summarization and the comparison of the powers of the considered tests at the 0.05 significance level, based on data with the dependence structure M14 (Morgenstern) in the left panel (a) and M15 (Plackett) in the right panel. (b) and various types of random effects that correspond to one of the subpanels. In each subpanel (1–4), the top level is the heat map and the bottom level shows the scatterplot (left panel) and K-plot (right panel). The following random effects schemes are considered: (1) $X = X_0$, $Y = Y_0$; (2) $X = X_0$, $Y = Y_0 + \varepsilon_A$; (3) $X = X_0$, $Y = \varepsilon_M Y_0$; and (4) $X = X_0$, $Y = \varepsilon_M Y_0 + \varepsilon_A$, where the random effects ε_A and $\varepsilon_m \sim N(0, 1)$. For M14 (Morgenstern), the measures of MIC (AUK) for each type of random effect are (1) 0.298 (0.568), (2) 0.265 (0.55), (3) 0.238 (0.504), and (4) 0.238 (0.504). For M15 (Plackett), the measures of MIC (AUK) for each type of random effect are (1) 0.455 (0.622), (2) 0.42 (0.616), (3) 0.257 (0.519), and (4) 0.256 (0.519).

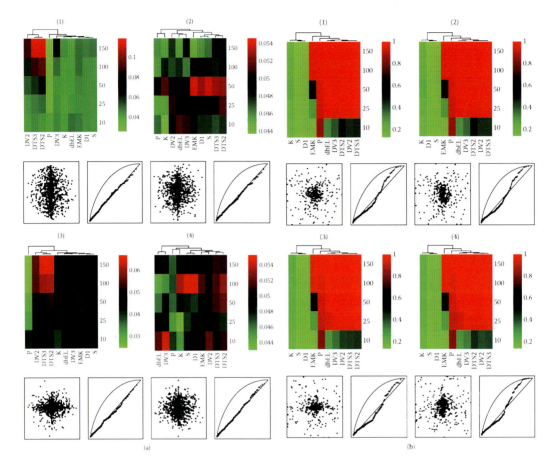

FIGURE 10.13

Graphical summarization and the comparison of the powers of the considered tests at the 0.05 significance level, based on data with the dependence structure M16 (PearsonII) in the left panel (a) and M17 (PearsonVII) in the right panel. (b) and various types of random effects that correspond to one of the subpanels. In each subpanel (1–4), the top level is the heat map and the bottom level shows the scatterplot (left panel) and K-plot (right panel). The following random effects schemes are considered: (1) $X = X_0, Y = Y_0$; (2) $X = X_0, Y = Y_0 + \varepsilon_A$; (3) $X = X_0, Y = \varepsilon_M Y_0$; and (4) $X = X_0, Y = \varepsilon_M Y_0 + \varepsilon_A$, where the random effects ε_A and $\varepsilon_m \sim N(0, 1)$. For M16 (PearsonII), the measures of MIC (AUK) for each type of random effect are (1) 0.237 (0.5), (2) 0.237 (0.503), (3) 0.238 (0.502), and (4) 0.237 (0.503). For M17 (PearsonVII), the measures of MIC (AUK) for each type of random effect are (1) 0.463 (0.532), (2) 0.459 (0.532), (3) 0.425 (0.531), and (4) 0.42 (0.53).

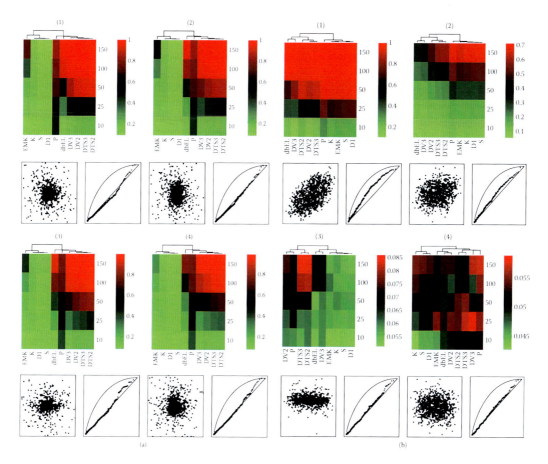

FIGURE 10.14

Graphical summarization and the comparison of the powers of the considered tests at the 0.05 significance level, based on data with the dependence structure M18 (Cauchy) in the left panel (a) and M19 (EP) in the right panel. (b) and various types of random effects that correspond to one of the subpanels. In each subpanel (1–4), the top level is the heat map and the bottom level shows the scatterplot (left panel) and K-plot (right panel). The following random effects scheme are considered: (1) $X = X_{()}$, $Y = Y_{()}$; (2) $X = X_{()}$, $Y = Y_{()} + \varepsilon_A$; (3) $X = X_{()}$, $Y = \varepsilon_M Y_{()}$; and (4) $X = X_{()}$, $Y = \varepsilon_M Y_{()} + \varepsilon_A$, where the random effects ε_A and $\varepsilon_m \sim N(0, 1)$. For M18 (Cauchy), the measures of MIC (AUK) for each type of random effect are (1) 0.245 (0.522), (2) 0.241 (0.52), (3) 0.24 (0.519), and (4) 0.238 (0.518). For M19 (EP), the measures of MIC (AUK) for each type of random effect are (1) 0.37 (0.6), (2) 0.256 (0.545), (3) 0.237 (0.505), and (4) 0.237 (0.504).

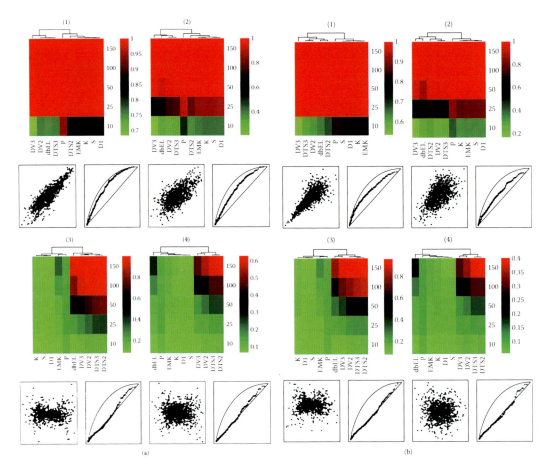

FIGURE 10.15

Graphical summarization and the comparison of the powers of the considered tests at the 0.05 significance level, based on data with the dependence structure M20 (Gumbel) in the left panel (a) and M21 (Clayton) in the right panel. (b) and various types of random effects that correspond to one of the subpanels. In each subpanel (1–4), the top level is the heat map and the bottom level shows the scatterplot (left panel) and K-plot (right panel). The following random effects schemes are considered: (1) $X = X_0$, $Y = Y_0$; (2) $X = X_0$, $Y = Y_0 + \varepsilon_A$; (3) $X = X_0$, $Y = \varepsilon_M Y_0$; and (4) $X = X_0$, $Y = \varepsilon_M Y_0 + \varepsilon_A$, where the random effects ε_A and $\varepsilon_m \sim N(0, 1)$. For M20 (Gumbel), the measures of MIC (AUK) for each type of random effect are (1) 0.693 (0.692), (2) 0.426 (0.629), (3) 0.242 (0.52), and (4) 0.237 (0.513). For M21 (Clayton), the measures of MIC (AUK) for each type of random effect are (1) 0.642 (0.646), (2) 0.403 (0.602), (3) 0.241 (0.506), and (4) 0.238 (0.505).

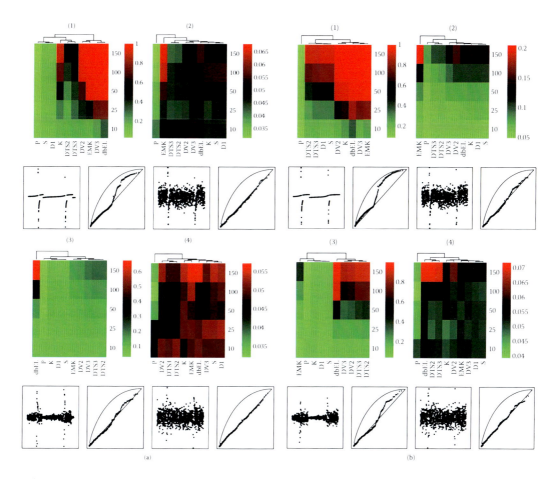

FIGURE 10.16

Graphical summarization and the comparison of the powers of the considered tests at the 0.05 significance level, based on data with the dependence structure M24 (DDF1) in the left panel (a) and M25 (DDF2) in the right panel. (b) and various types of random effects that correspond to one of the subpanels. In each subpanel (1–4), the top level is the heat map and the bottom level shows the scatterplot (left panel) and K-plot (right panel). The following random effects schemes are considered: (1) $X = X_0$, $Y = Y_0$; (2) $X = X_0$, $Y = Y_0 + \varepsilon_A$; (3) $X = X_0$, $Y = \varepsilon_M Y_0$; and (4) $X = X_0$, $Y = \varepsilon_M Y_0 + \varepsilon_A$, where the random effects ε_A and $\varepsilon_m \sim N(0, 1)$. For M24 (DDF1), the measures of MIC (AUK) for each type of random effect are (1) 0.909 (0.576), (2) 0.248 (0.509), (3) 0.245 (0.508), and (4) 0.237 (0.505). For M25 (DDF2), the measures of MIC (AUK) for each type of random effect are (1) 0.941 (0.628), (2) 0.255 (0.524), (3) 0.271 (0.519), and (4) 0.237 (0.506).

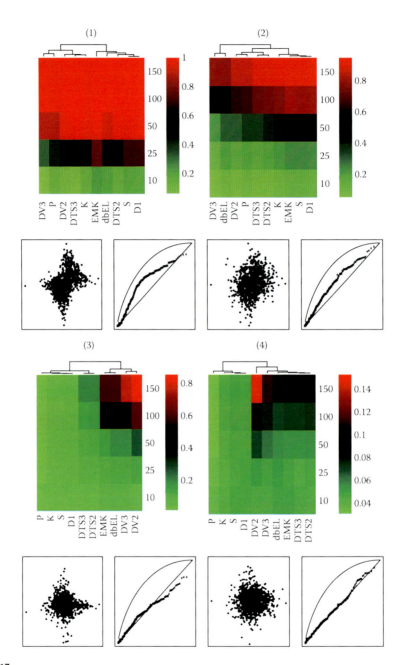

FIGURE 10.17

Graphical summarization and the comparison of the powers of the considered tests at the 0.05 significance level, based on data with the dependence structure M25 (CondN) and various types of random effects that correspond to one of the subpanels. In each subpanel (1–4), the top level is the heat map and the bottom level shows the scatterplot (left panel) and K-plot (right panel). The following random effects schemes are considered: (1) $X = X_{()}, Y = Y_{()}$; (2) $X = X_{()}, Y = Y_{()} + \varepsilon_A$; (3) $X = X_{()}, Y = \varepsilon_M Y_{()}$; and (4) $X = X_{()}, Y = \varepsilon_M Y_{()} + \varepsilon_A$, where the random effects ε_A and $\varepsilon_m \sim N(0, 1)$. The measures of MIC (AUK) for each type of random effect are (1) 0.425 (0.567), (2) 0.292 (0.55), (3) 0.268 (0.478), and (4) 0.242 (0.494).

10

Dependence and Independence: Structures, Testing, and Measuring

10.1 Introduction

In statistical analyses of medical data, exploring dependence between variables plays a fundamental role. For example, it is important to detect and quantify the dependence between disease status and a variety of potential predictors to determine significant risk factors. In genetic epidemiology, genomewide association studies are commonly conducted in order to examine the dependence between common genetic variants, for example, single-nucleotide polymorphisms, and traits like major diseases. The study of dependence was developed extensively at the beginning of the nineteenth century by Beeton et al. (1900) under multivariate normal assumptions and was most often referred to as the theory of correlation (Kendall and Stuart 1979). Since that time, various nonparametric tests have been proposed with the exchangeable, although not always technically correct, usage of the terms *correlation* and *dependence*. Let $F_X(x)$ and $F_Y(y)$ denote the marginal distribution functions of X and Y, respectively, and let $F_{XY}(x, y) = \Pr(X \leq x, Y \leq y)$ be the joint distribution function of the (X, Y) pairs. For the purpose of this chapter, we define dependence to be the case where the bivariate distribution function $F_{XY}(x, y) \neq F_X(x)F_Y(y)$ for some $(x, y) \in \Re \times \Re$.

Classical dependence measures, such as the Pearson, Spearman, and Kendall rank correlation coefficients, and their accompanying tests of independence, technically target only specific subsets of dependence structures. For example, Pearson's correlation coefficient (Pearson 1920) measures the degree of the linear correlation, while the Spearman correlation coefficient (Spearman 1904) focuses on a monotone relationship between two random variables, both of which may fail in the broader sense when the underlying dependence structure is nonmonotone (Embrechts et al. 2002). Furthermore, Pearson and Spearman correlation coefficients may not be well suited for measuring dependence across several well-known cases, for example, in the models $Y = 1/X$ or $Y = \varepsilon/X^k$, $k = 1, 2$, where ε is a random variable and X, Y are dependent in an inverse manner. In the second case, $E(XY)$ may not even exist. The Kendall rank correlation coefficient quantifies the concordance in ranks between pairs of random variables (Kendall 1938, 1948) but shows relatively low power in many cases compared to the Pearson and Spearman correlation coefficients (Mudholkar and Wilding 2003). Herein lies the difficulty of interpreting the classical correlation coefficients as general dependence measures. Kendall and Stuart (1979) claimed that "in general, the problem of joint variation is too complex to be comprehended in a single coefficient p. 308."

In practice, the dependence structure may be more complex than those detectable by classical correlation coefficients. For example, in dose–response studies, the dependence between the change in effect on an organism's metabolism and levels of exposure (or doses) of a stressor (e.g., amount of a drug) may be described by a polynomial (Harrell et al. 1996) or U-shaped curve (May and Bigelow 2005). More recently, emphasis has been placed on developing methods that go beyond the limitations of classical approaches toward capturing a broad spectrum of dependence structures. For example, rank-based tests of independence are proposed against a wide class of alternatives assuming an exponential family of distributions, which have great power stability and are sensitive to both grade linear correlation and grade correlations of higher-order polynomials (Kallenberg and Ledwina 1999). Einmahl and McKeague (2003) proposed a test of independence based on the empirical likelihood (EL) methodology (Owen 1990; see Chapter 6 for details), which has greater power than the corresponding Cramer–von Mises-type statistics. Vexler et al. (2014e) developed a highly efficient nonparametric likelihood ratio test that has very favorable and robust power properties against linear and nonmonotone forms of dependence.

Once the existence of dependence is established, it is important to quantify dependence in an informative and interpretable fashion. A wide range of dependence measures have been developed in addition to those classical correlation coefficients described above. For example, Hoeffding's (1948) D measure describes nonlinear dependence. The maximal information coefficient (MIC) provides scores similar to those of different dependence structures with equal noise (Reshef et al. 2011). In practice, it is also desirable to visualize the dependence structure. In contrast with formal tests that provide at best a single piece of information about a single form of association, graphical tools provide a rich source of information about dependence (Fisher and Switzer 2001). A traditional scatterplot of the raw data is widely used as a graphical tool for examining dependence between two variables. However, when we visualize dependence structures via a scatterplot, the null model of independence is a random scatter of points and is difficult to characterize. In order to manifest independence in a characteristic manner, Genest and Boies (2003) proposed a Kendall plot (K-plot) by adapting the concept of a probability plot (Wilk and Gnanadesikan 1968) to aid in the detection of dependence. The K-plot has many advantages, including the property of invariance with respect to monotone transformations of the marginal distributions, easy interpretation, and extendibility to the multivariate context. In a manner similar to that of the receiver operating characteristic (ROC) curve methodology (Pepe 1997; Vexler et al. 2008b), Vexler et al. (2015a) proposed a dependence measure by calculating the area under the K-plot (AUK). The proposed AUK measure, in conjunction with the scatterplot and the K-plot, provides a consistent unification of quantification and a graphical presentation of dependence.

It should be emphasized that when random effects exist in the model structure, they should be accounted for when examining dependence. Random effects, which may arise from a variety of sources, such as instrumentation specificity or biological variations, are common in practice and should be considered to avoid inconsistent or invalid statistical inference. For instance, Gu et al. (2012) investigated the inconsistency in results of different studies in the association between lung cancer and two polymorphisms, rs1051730 and rs8034191, and suggested considering random effects to address heterogeneity and publication bias. Furthermore, Rakovski et al. (2011) showed that the power of testing dependence of DNA methylation between patient groups can be improved when the random effects due to sampling variation are taken into account.

With a variety of tests and measures of dependence available, an inevitable question may arise regarding how to choose an appropriate one. In the statistical literature, comparisons of powers of tests of independence are rarely performed (Kallenberg and Ledwina 1999). Toward this end, Vexler et al. (2015a) suggested comparing powers of several classical methods and some more nonparametric approaches under a variety of complex dependence structures, focusing on their usefulness in practice. The following aspects were investigated at the interface between statistical methodology and areas of application: (1) suggesting the choice of nonparametric test of independence to use under different dependence structures, as illustrated via scatterplots; (2) pointing out situations where classical methods may break down; (3) demonstrating the influence various random effects may have on the test of independence; (4) showing an efficient way to visualize comparisons of powers of different tests; and (5) adding additional situations to classically described scenarios, such as some particular forms of heteroscedasticity. In this chapter, we present the results of Vexler et al. (2015a), with which practitioners can choose an efficient test of independence.

This chapter is organized as follows. Section 10.2 presents various tests of independence. Dependence measures that can be applied in general cases are presented in Section 10.3. Section 10.4 considers various sorts of dependence structures. In Section 10.5, we conduct simulation studies to compare powers of the tests of independence. Application of tests and measures of dependence to real data examples are discussed in Section 10.6. Section 10.7 presents a broader discussion on choosing appropriate tests of independence.

10.2 Tests of Independence

Assume we obtain a random sample of n independent and identically distributed (i.i.d.) pairs of observations $(X_1, Y_1), \ldots, (X_n, Y_n)$ from a continuous bivariate population. Let $F_X(x)$ and $F_Y(y)$ denote the marginal distribution functions of X and Y, respectively, and let $F_{XY}(x, y) = \Pr(X \leq x, Y \leq y)$ denote the joint distribution function of the (X, Y) pairs. The hypothesis testing for bivariate independence between X and Y can be formally stated as

$$H_0: F_{XY}(x,y) = F_X(x)F_Y(y), \text{ for all } (x,y) \in \Re \times \Re$$

against $H_a: F_{XY}(x,y) \neq F_X(x)F_Y(y)$ for some $(x,y) \in \Re \times \Re$. Throughout this chapter, we use the following notations. Let R_i and S_i denote the rank of X_i and Y_i, $i = 1, \ldots, n$, respectively, and F_{Xn}, F_{Yn}, and F_n be the empirical distribution functions corresponding to F_X, F_Y, and F_{XY}, respectively.

10.2.1 Classical Methods

In this section, we review three well-known correlation coefficients and related testing procedures for independence. Tests of independence under assumed specific model assumptions, for example, bivariate normality, are conducted via H_0: no correlation against H_a: nonzero correlation coefficient. To test a corresponding positive or negative dependence between X and Y, a one-sided test alternative can be constructed in a standard manner similarly.

Pearson's correlation coefficient was developed to measure the linear dependence between a pair of variables (X, Y) under bivariate normality assumptions. It is defined in terms of moments as $\rho = \rho(X, Y) = \sigma_{XY}/(\sigma_X \sigma_Y)$, where σ_{XY} represents the covariance of X and Y, and $\sigma_X \sigma_Y > 0$ denote the standard deviation of X and Y, respectively. By applying the Cauchy–Schwarz inequality to the σ_{XY}, it can be obtained that $-1 \leq \rho \leq 1$, where $\rho = 1$ indicates a perfect increasing linear relationship and $\rho = -1$ shows a perfect decreasing linear relationship. Spearman's rank correlation coefficient ρs is Pearson's correlation between ranks of X and Y, that is, $\rho s = \rho s(X, Y) = \rho(F_X(X), F_Y(Y))$, $-1 \le \rho s \le 1$. It accesses the monotonic relationship between two variables. Kendall's rank correlation coefficient has the form of $\tau = \Pr((X_1 - X_2) (Y_1 - Y_2) > 0) - \Pr((X_1 - X_2) (Y_1 - Y_2) < 0)$, $-1 \le \tau \le 1$. It measures the strength of monotonic dependence. Under those specific dependence structures, the null hypothesis of independence can be rejected for large values of the absolute values of corresponding correlation coefficients. For details regarding estimators of correlation coefficients described above, as well as the asymptotic distribution, we refer the reader to see Balakrishnan and Lai (2009).

10.2.1.1 Pearson Correlation Coefficient

The estimator of the Pearson correlation coefficient ρ is obtained by replacing the population moments with their sample counterparts and given as

$$ r = \frac{\sum_{i=1}^{n}\left(X_i - \bar{X}\right)\left(Y_i - \bar{Y}\right)}{\sqrt{\sum_{i=1}^{n}\left(X_i - \bar{X}\right)^2 \sum_{i=1}^{n}\left(Y_i - \bar{Y}\right)^2}}, -1 \le r \le 1, \bar{X} = \frac{1}{n}\sum_{i=1}^{n}X_i, \bar{Y} = \frac{1}{n}\sum_{i=1}^{n}Y_i. $$

Under bivariate normality assumptions and in the large sample setting, the test statistic $t = \left((n-2)/(1-r^2)\right)^{1/2} r$ has an asymptotic t-distribution with $n - 2$ degrees of freedom under the null hypothesis (Cox and Hinkley 1974). Accordingly, we reject H_0 if $|t| \ge t_{\alpha/2, n-2}$, where $t_{\alpha/2, n-2}$ is the $(1 - \alpha/2)$th quantile of the t-distribution with $n - 2$ degrees of freedom.

In practice, it is not uncommon to deal with heavy-tailed distributions whose second moment does not exist (i.e., is infinite), for example, Student's t-distribution with degrees of freedom equal to 2 or 1. For example, many financial time series data sets have heavy tails and tend to correspond to distributions that do not possess finite second moments or higher (Embrechts 2002; Kendall and Stuart 1961; Spearman 1904). In this case, the Pearson correlation is not defined. Another limitation of the Pearson correlation is that it is invariant only with respect to linear transformations of the variables, but not with respect to strictly increasing nonlinear transformations. Furthermore, zero correlation only requires $cov(X, Y) = 0$, whereas independence requires $cov(f_1(X), f_2(Y)) = 0$ for any functions f_1 and f_2. Therefore, independence implies zero correlation, but not vice versa, manifesting a drawback of using the correlation as a measure of dependence. For example, if the random variable X is symmetrically distributed about 0, and $Y = X^2$, then $\rho = 0$ but X and Y are perfectly dependent. Only in the specific case where X and Y are from a bivariate normal distribution does zero correlation imply independence.

These limitations and robustness considerations have motivated the development of rank-based correlation measures, alternative measures of dependence, which are considered in the next subsection.

10.2.1.2 Spearman's Rank Correlation Coefficient

Testing of independence based on Spearman's rank correlation coefficient, ρ_s, is equivalent to testing $H_0: \rho_s = 0$ versus $H_a: \rho_s \ne 0$. The estimator of Spearman's rank correlation coefficient ρ_s is given as

$$ r_s = 1 - 6\sum_{i=1}^{n}\left(R_i - S_i\right)^2 \Big/ \left(n(n^2 - 1)\right). $$

Note that if there are tied X values or tied Y values, each observation in the tied group is assigned with the average of the ranks associated with the tied group.

At the significance level α, we reject H_0 if $|r_s| \geq r_{s,\alpha/2}$, where $r_{s,\alpha/2}$ can be found by *qSpearman* (Wheeler 2009) in R (R Development Core Team 2014). For large sample sizes, one can also conduct the test based on the asymptotic t-distribution of the Pearson correlation coefficient between the ranked variables.

10.2.1.3 Kendall's Rank Correlation Coefficient

Testing of independence based on Kendall's rank correlation coefficient τ is equivalent to testing $H_0: \tau = 0$ versus $H_a: \tau \neq 0$. The Kendall statistic is defined as

$$K = \sum_{i=1}^{n} \sum_{j=i+1}^{n} \text{sgn}\left\{ \left(Y_j - Y_i\right)\left(X_j - X_i\right)\right\},$$

where $\text{sgn}\{x\} = 1$ if $x > 0$, 0 if $x = 0$, and -1 if $x < 0$. Accordingly, at the significance level α, an exact test can be conducted, and we reject H_0 if $\bar{K} \geq k_{\alpha/2}$, where $\bar{K} = K/\left(n(n-1)/2\right)$ and $k_{\alpha/2}$ can be found by *qKendall* in R (Kendall 1961). Alternatively, the test can be conducted based on the asymptotic standard normal distribution of the standardized $K^* = (n(n-1)(2n+5)/18)^{-1/2} K$ under H_0. The null hypothesis is rejected if $|K^*| \geq z_{\alpha/2}$, where $z_{\alpha/2}$ is the $100(1 - \alpha/2)$th quantile of the standard normal distribution.

Note that although the rank correlation measures ρ_s and τ are invariant under monotonic transformations and can capture perfect monotone dependence, they are not simple functions of moments and therefore are more computationally involved.

10.2.2 Data-Driven Rank Tests

In order to take into account not only linear correlation but also correlations of higher-order polynomials of random variables, Kallenberg and Ledwina (1999) used approximations to the joint distribution of $(F_X(X), F_Y(Y))$ via Fourier coefficients to propose data-driven rank tests of independence between X and Y. In this case, the joint distribution of $(F_X(X), F_Y(Y))$, called the copula function (Schweizer and Wolff 1981) or the grade representation (Kendall and Buckland 1957), is assumed to be in an exponential family, which is defined with growing dimension and with sufficient statistics in terms of Legendre polynomials. Then the test of independence converges to the powerful maximum likelihood ratio hypothesis testing regarding parameters in a Neyman–Pearson (1992) manner. Note that two random variables X and Y are independent if and only if $\text{cov}(g(X), h(Y)) = 0$ for all functions g and h ranging over a separating class of functions (Breiman 1968). By means of Legendre polynomial approximations to functions g and h, the data-driven approach, which essentially originates from Neyman and is the basis for the smooth tests, provides tests with very high power levels where the degree of the polynomials involved is determined by the data. Define $X^* = F_X(X)$ and $Y^* = F_Y(Y)$.

First, consider the joint distribution $\Pr(X^* < x^*, Y^* < y^*)$ of (X^*, Y^*) in an exponential family restricted to the "diagonal." Within the exponential families that are restricted to the diagonal, the joint distribution of (X^*, Y^*) has the form

$$h(x^*, y^*) = c(\theta) \exp\left\{ \sum_{j=1}^{k} \theta_j b_j(x^*) b_j(y^*) \right\},$$

where b_j denotes the jth orthonormal Legendre polynomial, $\theta = (\theta_1, \ldots, \theta_k)^T$, and $c(\theta)$ is a normalizing constant. In the diagonal case, the joint distribution of (X^*, Y^*) is symmetric in x^* and y^* and contains only elements $\theta_j b_j(x^*)b_j(y^*)$, that is, products of the parameter θ_j and Legendre polynomials with the same order in both variables. It is of particular interest if the correlation of $\{X^*\}^r$ and $\{Y^*\}^s$ is the same as that of $\{X^*\}^s$ and $\{Y^*\}^r$. For most symmetric distributions used in practice, restriction to the diagonal models is sufficient. The null hypothesis of independence corresponds to $\theta = 0$. If F_X and F_Y are known, the score test for testing $\theta = 0$ against $\theta \neq 0$ is given by rejecting large values of $\left\{ n^{-\frac{1}{2}} \sum_{i=1}^{n} b_r\left(F_X(X_i)\right) b_s\left(F_Y(Y_i)\right) \right\}^2$.

When F_X and F_Y are unknown, by replacing the unknown distribution functions F_X and F_Y with their corresponding empirical distribution functions and then applying a correction for continuity, smooth test statistics can be obtained in the form

$$T_k = \sum_{j=1}^{k} V(j, j), \text{ with } V(r, s) = \left\{ n^{-\frac{1}{2}} \sum_{i=1}^{n} b_r\left(\frac{R_i - 1/2}{n}\right) b_s\left(\frac{S_i - 1/2}{n}\right) \right\}^2.$$

According to the modified Schwarz's rule (similar to the one presented in Inglot et al. [1997]), a diagonal test statistic $TS2 = T_{S2}$ can be obtained where the order is chosen as

$$S2 = \text{argmin}_k \{T_k - k \log(n) \geq T_j - j \log(n), 1 \leq j, k \leq d(n)\},$$

and $d(n)$ is a sequence of numbers, $d(n) \to \infty$ as $n \to \infty$. To simplify notation, Kallenberg and Ledwina (1999) gave the test statistic only in the case of $d(n) = 2$. The null hypothesis is rejected for large values of the diagonal test statistic $TS2$.

On the other hand, in the more general "mixed" product case without assuming the aforementioned symmetry, we consider k-dimensional exponential families always containing $b_1(x^*)b_1(y^*)$ with the index $(1, 1)$, and $k - 1$ other products $b_i(x^*)b_j(y^*)$ with the index (i, j), $i, j = 1, \ldots d(n)$, $(i, j) \neq (1, 1)$. Consider the one-dimensional model $[(1, 1)]$, the two-dimensional models $[(1, 1), (i, j)]$ with $i, j = 1, \ldots d(n)$, $(i, j) \neq (1, 1)$, the three-dimensional models $[(1, 1), (i, j), (k, l)]$ with $i, j, k, l = 1, \ldots, d(n)$, all pairs being different, and so on. For example, $[(1, 1), (2, 1), (2, 3)]$ refers to the exponential family

$$c(\theta)\exp\{\theta_1 b_1(x^*)b_1(y^*) + \theta_2 b_2(x^*)b_1(y^*) + \theta_3 b_2(x^*)b_3(y^*)\},$$

with $c(\theta)$ a normalizing constant. Let Λ denote a set of indices, $T_\Lambda = \sum_{(r,s)\in\Lambda} V(r, s)$, and $|\Lambda|$ denote the cardinality of Λ. We search for a model

$$\Lambda^* = \text{argmax}_\Lambda \{T_\Lambda - |\Lambda| \log(n)\}.$$

Then we reject H_0 for large values of the mixed statistic $V = T_{\Lambda^*}$. If Λ^* is not unique, the first among those Λ^*s that have the smallest cardinality is chosen.

Remark 10.1

Under exponential families of data distributions, it is most probable that model-free tests of independence have less power than the data-driven rank tests (Kallenberg and Ledwina 1999). However, many familiar classes of distributions are nonexponential families (Klauer 1986). A concrete example is the reciprocal-normal-type distribution, which can be generated using the R command 1/mvrnorm(n, mu, Sigma), where mu is the mean vector and Sigma is a positive definite symmetric matrix specifying the covariance matrix of the variables. Furthermore, by virtue of the structures of the tests, to be consistent, the data-driven rank test requires that $E_{H_1} b_j(F_X(X)) b_s(F_Y(Y)) \neq 0$ for some j and s.

For example, when $X_i \sim Uniform[0, 1]$ and $Y_i = \arg\min_z \left\{ \left(\sum_{j=1}^{2} b_j(X) b_j(z) \right)^2 \right\}$, $i = 1, \ldots n$, the

data-driven rank tests of independence may render low power performance. We will show the comparison of the powers of various tests of independence via Monte Carlo simulations in Section 10.5.

R codes for obtaining the data-driven rank test statistic and the critical values are presented below:

```
# some basic functions #
funs<-list(b1<-function(x) sqrt(3)*(2*x-1),
b2<-function(x) sqrt(5)*(6*x^2-6*x+1),
b3<-function(x) sqrt(7)*(20*x^3-30*x^2+12*x-1),
b4<-function(x) 3*(70*x^4-140*x^3+90*x^2-20*x+1) )
DataDriven.ts<-function(x,y,d.n){
n<-length(x)
R<-rank(x)
S<-rank(y)
V_rs<-function(r,s) sum(funs[[r]]((R-1/2)/n)*funs[[s]]((S-1/2)/n))^2/n
######### test TS2 ###############
## eq(4): order k (first smooth test statistics)
T_k<-function(k) sum(sapply(1:k,function(j) V_rs(j,j)))
## choice of the order k is done by the modified Schwarz's rule
S2_d.n <- sapply(1:d.n,function(k) T_k(k)-k*log(n))
S2<- which.max(S2_d.n)[1]
TS2<-T_k(S2)
######### test V ###############
## the SECOND data-driven smooth test stat V
## consider one and two dimension models for now
if (d.n==1) V<-V_rs(1,1) else {
rs_all<-expand.grid(1:d.n,1:d.n)
V_all=apply(rs_all,1,function(x) c(x[1],x[2],V_rs(x[1],x[2])))
other.max=max(V_all[-1])
V<-ifelse(other.max<log(n),V_all[1],V_all[1]+other.max)
}
return(cbind(TS2,V))
}

############ get critival value ###############
# mc: The number of the Monte Carlo simulations
DataDriven.crit<-function(n,alpha,d.n,mc){
x <- matrix(rnorm(n*mc), nrow =n)
y <- matrix(rnorm(n*mc), nrow =n)
# Obtain the test statistic value following Eq. (5) (after taking log)
vt <- sapply(seq_len(mc), function(j) {
DataDriven.ts(x[,j],y[,j],d.n=d.n)
})
```

```
crit<-apply(vt,1,function(ts) as.numeric(quantile(ts, 1-alpha)))
names(crit)<-c("TS2","V")
return(crit )
}

# an example
# DataDriven.crit(n,alpha,d.n)
```

10.2.3 Empirical Likelihood–Based Method

In this section, we consider the empirical likelihood (EL) $L(\tilde{F}) = \prod_{i=1}^{n} \tilde{P}\{(X_i, Y_i)\}$, where $\tilde{P}\{\cdot\}$ is the probability measure corresponding to the distribution function $\tilde{F}$. As a pioneer of nonparametric likelihood-based tests of independence, Einmahl and McKeague (2003) constructed a very powerful test statistic by integrating the localized EL over variables. To this end Einmahl and McKeague (2003) considered the maximum EL ratio

$$R(x,y) = \sup\left\{L(\tilde{F}) : \tilde{F}(x,y) = \tilde{F}_1(x)\tilde{F}_2(y)\right\}/\sup\left\{L(\tilde{F})\right\},$$

demonstrating that the local log-EL ratio test statistic is

$$\log R(x,y) = nP_n(A_{11})\log\frac{F_{Xn}(x)F_{Yn}(y)}{P_n(A_{11})} + nP_n(A_{12})\log\frac{F_{Xn}(x)\left(1-F_{Yn}(y)\right)}{P_n(A_{12})}$$

$$+ nP_n(A_{21})\log\frac{\left(1-F_{Xn}(x)\right)F_{Yn}(y)}{P_n(A_{21})} + nP_n(A_{22})\log\frac{\left(1-F_{Xn}(x)\right)\left(1-F_{Yn}(y)\right)}{P_n(A_{22})},$$

$$F_{Xn}(x) = \frac{1}{n}\sum_{i=1}^{n} I(X_i \le x), \quad F_{Yn}(y) = \frac{1}{n}\sum_{i=1}^{n} I(Y_i \le y).$$

for $(x, y) \in \mathbf{R}^2$. Here P_n is the empirical probability measure, and $A_{11} = (-\infty, x] \times (-\infty, y]$, $A_{12} = (-\infty, x] \times (y, \infty)$, $A_{21} = (x, \infty) \times (-\infty, y]$, $A_{22} = (x, \infty) \times (y, \infty)$, and $0 \log(\cdot/0) = 0$. Note that the unrestricted likelihood in the denominator is maximized by setting $\tilde{F}$ as the corresponding empirical joint distribution function. Based on the constraint of independence, the supremum in the numerator is attained by the product of corresponding empirical marginal distributions. The distribution-free test statistic T_n is then constructed by integrating the local log-EL ratio over variables $(x, y) \in \mathbf{R}^2$, where

$$T_n = -2\int_{-\infty}^{\infty}\int_{-\infty}^{\infty} \log R(x,y)dF_{Xn}(x)dF_{Yn}(y).$$

We reject H_0 for large values of T_n.

Clearly T_n is distribution-free and its null distribution can be approximated easily by using the Monte Carlo method. If F_X and F_Y are continuous, then under H_0, the limit distribution of T_n is given by

$$T_n \xrightarrow{D} \int_0^1\int_0^1 \frac{W_0^2(u,v)}{uv(1-u)(1-v)}dudv,$$

where W_0 is a four-sided tied-down Wiener process on $[0, 1]^2$.

R codes for obtaining the empirical likelihood–based test statistic and the critical values are presented below.

```
############# test statistics value for EMK ####################
EMcK.ts<-function(x,y){
Fn.x<-ecdf(x)
Fn.y<-ecdf(y)
n<-length(x)
zz<-expand.grid(x,y)
logR<-apply(zz,1,function(xy){
u<-xy[1]
v<-xy[2]
f1n<-Fn.x(u) #f1n<-sum( (x<=u) )/n
f2n<-Fn.y(v) #f2n<-sum( (y<=v) )/n
pa11<-sum((x<=u)*(y<=v))/n
pa12<-sum((x<=u)*(y>v))/n
pa21<-sum((x>u)*(y<=v))/n
pa22<-sum((x>u)*(y>v))/n
if (pa11!=0) {a<-pa11*log( (f1n*f2n)/pa11 )} else {a<-0}
if (pa12!=0) {b<-pa12*log( (f1n*(1-f2n))/pa12 )} else {b<-0}
if (pa21!=0) {c<-pa21*log( ((1-f1n)*f2n)/pa21 )} else {c<-0}
if (pa22!=0) {d<-pa22*log( ((1-f1n)*(1-f2n))/pa22 )} else {d<-0}
return(n*(a+b+c+d))
})
Tn<-(-(2*sum(logR))/(n^2))
return(Tn)
}


############ get crital value ##############

# mc: The number of the Monte Carlo simulations
EMcK.crit<-function(n,alpha,mc){
x <- matrix(rnorm(n*mc), nrow =n)
y <- matrix(rnorm(n*mc), nrow =n)
# Obtain the test statistic value following Eq. (5) (after taking log)
vt <- sapply(seq_len(mc), function(j) {
EMcK.ts(x[,j],y[,j])
})
return( as.numeric(quantile(vt, 1-alpha)))
}
```

10.2.4 Density-Based Empirical Likelihood Ratio Test

In Section 10.2.1, the EL approaches were introduced. In this section, we present a distribution-free test statistic via the density-based EL method proposed by Vexler et al. (2014e), which approximates the parametric Neyman–Pearson statistic, to test the null hypothesis of bivariate independence against a wide class of alternatives. The density-based EL test statistic is

$$VT_n = \prod_{i=1}^{n} n^{1-\beta_2} \tilde{\Delta}_i \left([0.5n^{\beta_2}], [0.5n^{\beta_2}] \right),$$

where the function $[x]$ denotes the nearest integer to x,

$$\tilde{\Delta}_i(m,r) = \left(F_{Xn}(X_{(C_i+r)}) - F_{Xn}(X_{(C_i-r)}) \right)^{-1} \left(F_n(X_{(C_i+r)}, Y_{(i+m)}) - F_n(X_{(C_i-r)}, Y_{(i+m)}) \right.$$

$$\left. - F_n(X_{(C_i+r)}, Y_{(i-m)}) + F_n(X_{(C_i-r)}, Y_{(i-m)}) + n^{-\beta_1} \right),$$

C_i is an integer number such that $X_{(C_i)} = X_{t(i)}$, where $X_{t(i)}$ is the concomitant (David and Nagaraja 2003) of the ith order statistic $Y_{(i)}$; $X_{(C_i+r)} = X_{(n)}$ if $C_i + r > n$, $X_{(c_i-r)} = X_{(1)}$ if $C_i - r < 1$; and $\beta_1 \in (0, 0.5)$, $\beta_2 \in (0.75, 0.9)$.

The power of the density-based empirical likelihood test does not depend significantly on values of $\beta_1 \in (0, 0.5)$ and $\beta_2 \in (0.75, 0.9)$ under various alternative distributions applied to the hypothesis of bivariate independence; see Vexler et al. (2014e) for more details. The null hypothesis is rejected if $\log(VT_n) > C_\alpha$, where C_α is an α-level test threshold. It follows that

$$\text{Pr}_{H_0}\left(\log(VT_n) > C_\alpha\right) = \text{Pr}_{\{X_i\}_{i=1}^n, \{Y_i\}_{i=1}^n \sim Uniform[0,1]}\left(\log(VT_n) > C_\alpha \mid H_0\right).$$

Note that the term $n^{-\beta_1}$, $0 < \beta_1 < 0.5$, ensures the consistency of the density-based empirical likelihood ratio test. This test is exact, and the critical values for the proposed test can be accurately approximated using Monte Carlo techniques.

R codes for obtaining the density-based empirical likelihood ratio test statistic and the critical values were presented in Vexler et al. (2014e) and are omitted here.

Remark 10.2

The data-driven techniques, the EL-based method, and the density-based EL ratio test described above are all exact. Their critical values can be calculated numerically using Monte Carlo techniques. For example, the critical values of the density-based EL ratio test can be determined by drawing 50,000 independent samples of $X_1, \ldots, X_n \sim Uniform[0, 1]$ and $Y_1, \ldots, Y_n \sim Uniform[0, 1]$ and then calculating the $1 - \alpha$ quantile of generated values of the test statistic $\log(VT_n)$ at each sample size n, where α is the significance level.

10.3 Indices of Dependence

Indices of dependence indicate how closely the variables X and Y are related in some particular manner. Among these indices, classical correlation coefficient–based measures of dependence, especially Pearson's correlation coefficient, are by far the most prominent. These classical measures of dependence are geared toward specific dependence structures (Balakrishnan and Lai 2009). However, more complex forms of dependence lie outside the scope of these measures. In order to capture more general dependence structures, we introduce the maximal information coefficient (Reshef et al. 2011) and propose a novel measure of dependence based on the Kendell plot (Genest and Boies 2003).

10.3.1 Classical Measures of Dependence

The classical correlation coefficient–based measures of dependence, as was discussed in detail in Section 10.2, are widely used but can only work well for linear or monotone dependence structures.

Hoeffding's (1948) measure of dependence, D, is a rank-based dependence measure that detects more general departures from independence. It approximates a weighted sum over observations of chi-square statistics for 2×2 classification tables by setting each set of (X_i, Y_i), $i = 1, \ldots, n$, values as cut points. Hoeffding's D is defined as

$$D = 30\left[(n-2)(n-3)\sum_{i=1}^{n}\prod_{j=1}^{2}(Q_i - j) + \sum_{i=1}^{n}\prod_{j=1}^{2}(R_i - j)(S_i - j) - 2(n-2)D_*\right]\left(\prod_{i=0}^{4}(n-i)\right)^{-1},$$

where R_i is the rank of X_i, S_i is the rank of Y_i, the bivariate rank Q_i is $1 + \sum_{j \neq i} I\{X_j < X_i, Y_j < Y_i\}$, $i = 1, \ldots, n$, and $D_* = \sum_{i=1}^{n}(R_i - 2)(S_i - 2)(Q_i - 1)$. A point that is tied on both X and Y contributes $1/4$ to Q_i. A point that is tied on only the X value or Y value contributes $1/2$ to Q_i if the other value is less than the corresponding value for the ith point.

Without ties in the data set, Hoeffding's D measure of dependence is on the interval $[-0.5, 1]$, with 1 indicating perfect dependence. However, when ties occur, Hoeffding's D measure may result in a smaller value (Hollander et al. 2013). These traditional dependence measures can be difficult (1) to decide when a particular value indicates association strong enough for a given purpose, and (2) in a given situation, for weighing the losses involved in obtaining more strongly associated variables against the gains (Elffers 1980). Therefore, it is suggested to use functions of these traditional dependence measures that can be interpreted as the probability of making a wrong decision in certain situations, for example, the cube of correlation coefficient, correlation ratio, maximal correlation (sup correlation), and monotone correlations, as well as concordance measures such as the Gini index and Blomqvist's β; we refer the reader to see Balakrishnan and Lai (2009) for more details.

10.3.2 Maximal Information Coefficient

The maximal information coefficient (MIC) (Reshef et al. 2011) is a measure of pairwise dependence defined by constructing a grid to create bins on the scatterplot of (X, Y) variables and encapsulating dependence within the grid. It can detect general dependence structures.

For a grid G among all grids up to a maximal grid resolution, dependent on the sample size n, let $I_G = \sum_{(x,y) \in G} p(x,y)\log\dfrac{p(x,y)}{p(x)p(y)}$ denote the mutual information of the probability distribution induced on the boxes of G, where the probability of a box $p(x, y)$ is the proportion of data points falling inside the bin box. Define the characteristic matrix $M = (m_{x,y})$. For every ordered pair of integers (x, y), the maximum normalized mutual information achieved by any $x \times y$ grids G is $m_{x,y} = \max_G \{I_G/\text{logmin}\{x, y\}\}$. Normalizing by logmin $\{x, y\}$ ensures modified values between 0 and 1, in addition to a fair comparison between grids of different dimensions and therefore across different distributions. Then MIC is defined to be $\max_{xy < B(n)} \{m_{x,y}\}$, where $B(n)$ is a function of sample size and usually set to be $n^{0.6}$.

The value of MIC is between 0 for independence and 1 for a noiseless functional relationship. The MIC measure focuses on equitability; that is, relationships with similar noise levels may result in similar scores regardless of the type of relationship. However, MIC works only for bivariate data and may fail to detect some important scenarios, for example, linear dependence with a certain amount of noisy data due to discrepancy in the concept of equitability (Simon and Tibshirani 2014). The results represented in this chapter related to the calculation of MIC are obtained via the function `mine` in the R package *minerva*.

10.3.3 Area under the Kendall Plot

Genest and Boies (2003) proposed a Kendall plot (K-plot) as a graphical tool to detect dependence, which adopts the concept of the probability plot (P-P plot). Similar to the standard P-P plot, in which a lack of linearity indicates nonnormality of the distribution of a random variable, the K-plot is close to a straight line in the independent bivariate case. The amount of curvature in the K-plot is characteristic of the strength of dependence in the data. Similar to data-driven rank tests that express the dependence via Fourier coefficients of the copula function, the K-plot essentially characterizes the underlying dependence structure based on the copula function. It plots the Kendall function $K(w) = \Pr\{F_{XY}(X,Y) < w\}$ versus $\Pr(UV \le w)$, where U and V are independent uniform random variables on the interval [0, 1]. Here F_{XY} denotes the joint cumulative distribution function of (X,Y). The K-plot has the property of invariance with respect to monotone transformations of marginal distributions and can be extended to the multivariate context.

Vexler et al. (2015a) proposed a new index of dependence that borrows strength from the K-plot in $[0, 1] \times [0, 1]$ space (Genest and Boies 2003). To this end, we use principles related to the receiver operating characteristic (ROC) curve analysis that are extensively used in biostatistical literature. The ROC curves graphically represent differences between two distributions, for example, the cumulative distribution functions F_X and F_Y of two populations. The ROC curve $R(t)$ can be defined as $R(t) = 1 - F_X(F_Y^{-1}(1-t))$, where $t \in [0, 1]$. Accordingly, the area under the ROC curve (AUC), which can be calculated by $\int_0^1 R(t)dt$, is defined as an indicator of a distance between two distributions (Bamber 1975; Vexler et al. 2008b). It is a convenient way to compare two distributions based on the ROC curve since it places tests on the same scale where they can be compared for accuracy. For several details regarding the ROC methodology, see Chapter 8. In analogy to the AUC, Vexler et al. (2015a) proposed the area under the K-plot (AUK) as an index of dependence, which we will present in this section.

Consider a bivariate sample (X_i, Y_i), $i = 1, \ldots, n$; we define a random variable H_i as

$$H_i = \hat{H}_n(X_i, Y_i) = \frac{1}{n-1} \sum_{j \ne i} I\{X_j \le X_i, Y_j \le Y_i\},$$

where $I\{\cdot\}$ is the indicator function. Note that the empirical distribution function $\hat{H}_n$ converges to H as $n \to \infty$, where $H = F_{XY}$ is the bivariate cumulative distribution function of (X, Y). Order the H_i to get $H_{(1)} \le \ldots \le H_{(n)}$ and define $K(w) = \Pr(H(X,Y) \le w)$. Under H_0: $F_{XY} = F_X F_Y$, we can obtain $K_0(w) = \Pr(UV \le w) = w - w \log(w)$, $w \in [0, 1]$, where U and V are independent uniform random variables on the interval [0, 1]. Then by definition of the density of an order statistic, the expectation of the ith-order statistic in a random sample of size n from the distribution K_0 of the H_i under the null hypothesis of independence can be expressed as

$$W_{i:n} = n \binom{n-1}{i-1} \int_0^1 w \{K_0(w)\}^{i-1} \{1 - K_0(w)\}^{n-i} dK_0(w),$$

A K-plot can be obtained via plotting the pairs $(W_{i:n}, H_{(i)})$, $1 \leq i \leq n$. For a large enough sample, the K-plot will be a plot of $K^{-1}\{K_0(w)\}$ versus w, $w \in [0, 1]$. The area under the K-plot (AUK) is $1 - \int_0^1 K(w)dK_0(w)$, that is, $1 + \int_0^1 K(w)\log(w)dw$.

In the case of an unknown joint distribution of (X, Y), the empirical cumulative distribution function can be used and the corresponding empirical area under the K-plot can be estimated. The following propositions provide a way to consider the AUK in light of the AUC analysis well addressed in the statistical literature. Define U and V to be independent uniformly distributed random variables between 0 and 1.

Proposition 10.1

Suppose continuous random variables X and Y are distributed according to a bivariate distribution function H. Then

$$\text{AUK} = \Pr\{UV < H(X, Y)\} = E\{H(X, Y) - H(X, Y)\log(H(X, Y))\}.$$

Proof. Based on the definition, we have

$$\text{AUK} = 1 - \int_0^1 \Pr\{H(X,Y) < t\}\, d\Pr\{UV < t\} = \Pr\{UV < H(X,Y)\}$$

$$= E(\Pr\{UV < H(X,Y) \mid H(X,Y)\}) = E(H(X,Y) - H(X,Y)\log H(X,Y)).$$

Proposition 10.1 shows a simple method for expressing the AUK. It is very useful both for direct evaluations and for simulations. This proposition presents a result that is similar to that obtained regarding the AUC (see Chapter 8 for details). Suppose, for example, that a random sample (X_i, Y_i), $i = 1, \ldots, n$, has been drawn from a bivariate distribution H. By virtue of Proposition 10.1, we can estimate the AUK in a nonparametric manner via the statistic

$$\overline{\text{AUK}} = \frac{1}{n}\sum_{i=1}^n \left\{\hat{H}(X_i, Y_i) - \hat{H}(X_i, Y_i)\log(\hat{H}(X_i, Y_i))\right\},$$

where we replace the distribution function H by its empirical estimator $\hat{H}$. The form of $\overline{\text{AUK}}$, the estimator of AUK, is much simpler than that which can be obtained directly by using the definition of the AUK.

Schriever (1987) defined the "more associated ordering" for bivariate distributions. By virtue of Proposition 10.1, we have $\text{AUK} = \iint J(H(x,y))dH(x,y)$, where the function $J(u) = u - u\log(u)$ increases and is upper convex for $u \in [0, 1]$. Then Example 3.2 in Schriever (1987) can be directly adapted to show that the proposed AUK-based measure preserves more concordant ordering for dependence. We refer the reader to see Schriever (1987) for details regarding the ordering for dependence.

In the context of the Fréchet-Hoeffding copula bounds (Balakrishnan and Lai 2009), it is clear that we have AUK = 0 when $\tau = -1$, and AUK = 3/4 when $\tau = 1$. The well-known Fréchet-Hoeffding results regarding copula bounds (Fréchet 1951) implies the following proposition.

Proposition 10.2

For any continuous random variables X and Y distributed according to a bivariate distribution function $H(x, y)$, the measurements AUK satisfy $0 \le \text{AUK} \le 3/4$, where the case with $(X, Y = X)$ provides AUK to reach the upper bound $3/4$ and $(X, Y = -X)$ leads to the lower bound zero.

Proof. By virtue of the Fréchet-Hoeffding upper bound, we have

$$\Pr\{H(X, Y) < t\} \ge \Pr\{\min(F_X(X), F_Y(Y)) < t\} \ge \Pr\{F_X(X) < t\} = t$$

It is clear that $\Pr\{H(X, Y) < t\} \le 1$. Then

$$0 \le \text{AUK} = \int_0^1 \Pr\{H(X,Y) > t\} d(t - t\log(t)) \le \int_0^1 (1 - t)(-\log(t)) dt = 3/4.$$

The range of AUK is $[0, 3/4]$. In the case $(X, Y = X)$, we have $H(x, y) = \Pr(X < x, X < y)$ and $H(X, Y) = H(X, X)$. Thus, $\Pr\{H(X, Y) > t\} = \Pr\{F_X(X) > t\}$ and

$$\text{AUK} = \int_0^1 \Pr\{F_X(X) > t\} d(t - t\log(t)) = \int_0^1 (1 - t)d(-\log(t)) = 3/4$$

In the case $(X, Y = -X)$, we have $H(x, y) = \Pr(X < x, -X < y)$ and $H(X, Y) = H(X, -X)$, which leads to $\Pr\{H(X, Y) > t\} = 0$ and $\text{AUK} = 0$.

The R codes to implement the Kendall plot and the computation of the AUK measure of dependence are presented below:

```
####### to obtain AUK based on the definition #######
# x and y two samples to be tested for independence
# plot: Logical; whether the Kendall plot is presented.
# installing package 'CDVine' for the first time:
if (!require('CDVine')) install.packages('CDVine')
require(CDVine)

get.AUK<-function(x,y,plot = TRUE){
tmp <- BiCopKPlot(x,y,PLOT=FALSE)
if (plot == TRUE) BiCopKPlot(x,y,PLOT=TRUE)
W <- c(0,tmp$W.in,1)
H <- c(0,tmp$Hi.sort,1)
idx <- 2:length(W)
area <- as.double(((W[idx]-W[idx-1])%*%(H[idx]+H[idx-1])))/2
return(min(area,0.75))
}
###### to obtain AUK.bar based on Proposition 1 in Section 7 of SM
######
get.AUK.bar<-function(x,y,plot = TRUE){
get.H<-function(u1,u2) mean(1*(x<u1)&(y<u2))
get.H.V<-Vectorize(get.H)
G<-get.H.V(x,y)
```

```
GlogG<-array(0,length(x)*length(y))
GlogG[G!=0]<-G[G!=0]*log(G[G!=0])
area <- mean(G-GlogG)
return(min(area,0.75))
}
# an example
x=rnorm(300)
y=x+3
get.AUK(x,y,plot=TRUE)
get.AUK.bar(x,y,plot=TRUE)
```

10.4 Structures of Dependence

Researchers within the earlier scientific literature, for example, Reshef et al. (2011) and Johnson (2013), thoroughly addressed the examination of a variety of dependence structures. Included in the coverage were linear, quadratic, cubic, reciprocal, logarithmic, trigonometric, and bivariate distributions, such as bivariate normal distributions, bivariate Pearson distribution families, bivariate normal offset distributions, bivariate Morgenstern distributions, bivariate Plackett distributions, bivariate Cauchy distributions, bivariate exponential power distribution families, copula families, and the reciprocal-normal distribution, among others. In this section, details about these dependence structures as well as random effects–type dependencies will be presented.

10.4.1 Basic Structures

Regression analysis is one of the commonly used techniques that provide an estimate of the formulaic dependence between variables. For example, we can consider $Y = f(X) + \varepsilon$ in general, where the function $f(X) = E(Y|X)$ describes the formulaic dependence between X and Y and ε represents an unobserved random effect with mean zero conditioned on the variable X.

Linear dependence: Linear dependence is very common in our everyday life. For example, the average weights for humans in the population of American women ages 30–39 can be expected to be linearly dependent on their height. The simple linear model $Y = \alpha + \beta X + \varepsilon$ can be applied, where the linear dependence $f(X) = \alpha + \beta X$ between X and Y is considered (Edwards 1976).

Quadratic dependence: In many settings, linear dependence between X and Y may not hold. For example, in the field of chemistry, it is often found that the yield of a chemical synthesis improves by increasing amounts for each unit increase in temperature at which the synthesis takes place. In this case, a quadratic dependence between X and Y can be assumed and a quadratic model can be proposed in the form of $Y = f(X) + \varepsilon$, where the conditional expectation of Y is a quadratic function of X and $f(X) = \beta_0 + \beta_1 X + \beta_k X^2$. The test of independence is conducted via the null hypothesis H_0: $\beta_1 = 0$, $\beta_2 = 0$. In general, we can consider a polynomial regression model $Y = \beta_0 + \beta_1 X + \dots + \beta_k X^k + \varepsilon$, where the dependence between X and Y is modeled as a kth- (k is a positive integer) order polynomial and ε is a random effect with mean zero conditioned on X.

Reciprocal dependence: In the case when the variable Y descends to a floor or ascends to a ceiling as the variable X increases (e.g., approaches an asymptote), a reciprocal dependence between X and Y can be expected. For example, in economics, the marginal utility of each homogeneous unit decreases as the supply of units increases. In this case, a reciprocal model can be considered, where $f(X) = 1/X^k$ and the order k is a positive integer.

Logarithmic dependence: Let us next consider logarithmic growth, for example, a phenomenon whose size or cost can be described as a logarithm function of some input. For example, in microbiology, bacterial growth can be modeled as a logarithm function of the number of colony forming units. In this case, a linear-log model can be specified, where $f(X) = \alpha + \beta \log(X)$. This model is also commonly used in econometrics, for example, the dependence of consumption spending on income. Note that any logarithm base can be used since they are convertible by multiplying the function by a fixed constant.

Trigonometric dependence: Trigonometric models can be applied in modeling periodic phenomena. For example, tidal experts and meteorologists use sine waves to help predict tides. Electromagnetic radiation also can be modeled with sine waves. There are many familiar trigonometric functions and different trigonometric models can be considered, for example, the sinusoidal with non-Fourier frequency $Y = \sin(9\pi x)$. In particular, we have two-dimensional spirals for curves winding around a fixed center point at a continuously increasing or decreasing distance, which are common in plants and in some animals. For example, chambers of the shell in the nautilus (a cephalopod mollusc) are arranged in a logarithmic spiral (Maor and King 1994). Given a modern understanding of fractals, a growth spiral can be viewed as a special case of self-similarity (Ball 2011). Two-dimensional spirals can be described via polar coordinates. For example, the above-mentioned logarithmic spiral can be described in parametric form as $X(\theta) = a \exp(b\theta)\cos(\theta)$ and $Y(\theta) = a \exp(b\theta)\sin(\theta)$, with the angle θ and real numbers a, b.

Bivariate distributions: Knowledge of the marginal distributions is known to be inadequate in terms of determining the joint distribution function. Instead of modeling $E(Y|X)$ as a function of X to consider the dependence structure between X and Y, we can consider the joint distribution of (X, Y) directly. A variety of joint distribution functions have been developed (Johnson 2013; Johnson et al. 2004; Mardia 1970).

The bivariate (or multivariate, for more than two random variables) normal distribution is the most useful joint distribution in probability. Assume that $(X, Y)^T$ follow the bivariate normal distribution with the mean vector $(\mu_X, \mu_Y)^T$ and the covariance matrix $\begin{pmatrix} \sigma_X^2 & \rho\sigma_X\sigma_Y \\ \rho\sigma_X\sigma_Y & \sigma_Y^2 \end{pmatrix}$, where ρ is the correlation between X and Y, and σ_X, $\sigma_Y > 0$ denote the standard deviations of X and Y, respectively. The conditional expectation of Y given X is $\mu_Y + \rho(X - \mu_X)\sigma_Y/\sigma_X$. In this case, Pearson's correlation coefficient ρ is fully informative about the joint dependence between X and Y, and zero correlation is equivalent to independence. Note that the bivariate normal distribution is a special case of elliptical distributions. For other elliptical distributions, such as bivariate Pearson II and Pearson VII distributions, which share some properties of the bivariate normal distributions, the dependence structure is also fully determined by the correlation matrix (Kai-Tai and Yao-Ting 1990). When the data exhibit skewness, the multivariate skew-normal distribution may be considered, where the marginal densities are scalar skew-normal (Azzalini and Dalla Valle 1996).

Generalizing the multivariate normal distribution by adding a "nonnormality" parameter $\kappa > 0$, multivariate exponential power distributions can be presented (Johnson 2013). The parameter κ represents the kurtosis departure from the multivariate normal distribution. As a special case, the multivariate normal distribution is derived when $\kappa = 2$.

Plackett's distribution (Johnson 2013) can include a full range of dependence from completely negative through independence to completely positive. With normal marginals, it shares considerable similarity to the bivariate normal distribution, especially when the correlation parameter in the bivariate normal distribution $\rho = -\cos(\pi\phi^{1/2}/(1 + \phi^{1/2}))$, where the parameter ϕ governs the dependence between Plackett distributed $(X, Y)^T$'s.

Weak dependence properties are presented in the Morgenstern distribution (Johnson 2013). The bivariate distribution function of (X, Y) is $F_{XY}(x, y) = F_X(x)F_Y(y)(1 + \alpha((1 - F_X(x))((1 - F_Y(y))))$, $0 \leq x, y \leq 1$, and the parameter $-1 \leq \alpha \leq 1$ controls the dependence structure between X and Y. In particular, for uniform marginals, the Pearson's correlation coefficient is $\rho = \alpha/3$, implying $|\rho| \leq 1/3$. The maximum is $1/\pi$ for normal marginals and $1/4$ for exponential marginals.

Note that the joint distributions can also be determined by the incorporation of marginal and conditional specifications. It is possible to construct distributions where the two conditional densities $f_{X|Y}(x|y)$ and $f_{Y|X}(y|x)$ are each normal, and yet the joint distribution is not bivariate normal; a simple example is the joint density function $f_{X,Y}(x, y) = C\exp\{-(x^2 + y^2 + 2xy(x + y + xy))\}$, where $C > 0$ is the normalizing constant. It may be verified that $E(Y|X = x) = -x^2/(1 + 2x + 2x^2)$ and $\mathrm{var}(Y|X = x) = 1/(2 + 4x + 4x^2)$.

10.4.2 Random Effects–Type Dependence

Random effects are common in practice and should be considered to avoid inconsistent or invalid statistical inference. For example, the sample Pearson's correlation coefficient calculated from a small sample may be totally misleading if not viewed in the context of its likely sampling error (Balakrishnan and Lai 2009). Random effects can represent different types of measurement error (ME), which may arise from a variety of sources, for example, instrumentation specificity, biological variations, or questionnaire-based self-report data. For example, the observed response may be formulated as $Y = \log(|X + \varepsilon|)$, where measurements of X contain additive random effect ε, or formulated as $Y = \log(|X + \varepsilon_X|) + \varepsilon_Y$, where both X and Y contain additive random effects ε_X and ε_Y, respectively.

Standard regression procedures assume that the predictor variables are measured without error, and random effects inherent in the model are associated with the response variable only. For example, commonly, in terms of regression models, additive random effects are considered in the form $Y = Y_0 + \varepsilon$, where Y is the observed variable, $Y_0 = f(X)$ is the true value, and ε is a random variable with mean zero and independent of X.

In the case when predictor variables are measured with errors, a common situation in practice, estimation based on the standard assumption of no error leads to bias or inconsistency of statistical inferences. In this case, models that account for random effects in both predictor variables and response variables, for example, errors-in-variables models, should be applied. In the two-variable case involving X and Y, random effects in either variable will result in conservative inferences in view of attenuated correlations in magnitude (Johnston and DiNardo 1963) and will reduce the power of the test of independence in linear models (Cochran 1968). Various models and designs are developed to tackle the errors-in-variables issue. For example, the simple linear errors-in-variables model considers additive random effects in both the predictor variable and the response variable, that is, $Y = \alpha + \beta X_0 + \varepsilon_Y$ and $X = X_0 + \varepsilon_X$, where X_0 and Y_0 are the unobserved true values for X and Y, respectively.

To illustrate, we show the scatterplots ($n = 1000$) of observed (X, Y) in Figure 10.1 for some dependence structures with no random effects and with additive normally distributed random effects with mean 0 and variance 0.25 or 2. In Figure 10.1, each row corresponds to the true values of $(X_0, Y_0)^T$ (M3) the polynomial-type dependence with the order $k = 2$ (abbreviated as LinearQuadratic); (M4) Cubic; (M5) Reciprocal with the order $k = 1$; (M6) Reciprocal with the order $k = 2$; (M8) Logarithm $Y_0 = \log(1 + |X_0|)$; and (M9) sinusoidal $Y_0 = \sin(\pi X_0)$; see Table 10.2 for more details. Each column in both panels of Figure 10.1 displays various random effects, where (a) represents the case of no random effect in either X or Y, that is, $X = X_0$, $Y = Y_0$; (b) and (b') show the case where X has no random effect and Y has additive effects, that is, $X = X_0$, $Y = Y_0 + \varepsilon_Y$ with the variance of noise var(ε_Y) assumed to be 0.25 (shown in (b)) or 2 (shown in (b')), respectively; (c) and (c') show the case where Y has no random effect and X has additive random effects, that is, $Y = Y_0$, $X = X_0 + \varepsilon_X$ with the variance of noise var(ε_X) assumed to be 0.25 or 2, respectively; (d) and (d') show the case where both X and Y have additive random effect, that is, $X = X_0 + \varepsilon_X$, $Y = Y_0 + \varepsilon_Y$, with the variance of noise var(ε_X) = var(ε_Y) assumed to be 0.25 or 2, respectively. Note that in Figure 10.1, scatterplots with different random effects are shown in the same scale for each type of dependence structures.

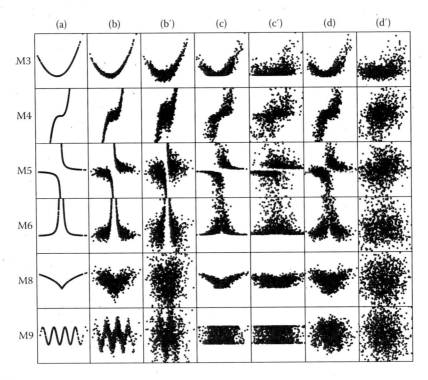

FIGURE 10.1
Scatterplots ($n = 1000$) of measurements of (X, Y) under different dependence structures with normally distributed random effects with mean 0, where the unobserved true values of X_0 and Y_0 can be formulated as $Y_0 = f(X_0)$. Each row corresponds to each of the following structures: M3, the polynomial dependence with the order $k = 2$ (abbreviated as LinearQuadratic); M4, cubic; M5, reciprocal with the order $k = 1$; M6, reciprocal with the order $k = 2$; M8, logarithm $Y_0 = \log(1 + |X_0|)$; and M9, sinusoidal $Y_0 = \sin(\pi X_0)$. Each column of both panels displays various random effects schemes: (a) $X = X_0$, $Y = Y_0$; (b and b') $X = X_0$, $Y = Y_0 + \varepsilon_Y$, with the variance of noise var(ε_Y) assumed to be 0.25 or 2, respectively; (c and c') $Y = Y_0$, $X = X_0 + \varepsilon_X$, with the variance of noise var(ε_X) assumed to be 0.25 or 2, respectively; and (d and d') $X = X_0 + \varepsilon_X$, $Y = Y_0 + \varepsilon_Y$, with the variance of noise var(ε_X) = var(ε_Y) assumed to be 0.25 or 2, respectively.

It can be observed that not only the variance of random effects, but also the type of random effects affect the dependence structure. In addition, Table 10.1 shows the corresponding MIC and AUK measures of dependence with $n = 1000$. We further show measures of MIC and AUK for sample size $n = 100$ under various dependence structures and random effects in Section 10.5. Note that the MIC can range from 0 for the independence case to 1 for the perfect dependence case, while the AUK can range from 0 for the perfect negatively dependent case to 0.75 for the perfect positively dependent case, where the value 0.5 indicates independence. When the variance of random effects increases, the MIC decreases, showing comparatively weaker dependence, while the AUK measures only vary by a small amount, showing a lightly weaker dependence.

Similar to Figure 10.1, Figure 10.2 shows the scatterplots ($n = 1000$) of observed (X, Y) for some other dependence structures with no random effects and with additive normally distributed random effects with mean 0 and variance 0.25 or 2. In Figure 10.2, each row corresponds to the true values of $(X_0, Y_0)^T$, and each column in both panels displays various random effects. Note that in Figure 10.2, scatterplots with different random effects are shown in the same scale for each type of dependence structures. It can be observed that not only the variance of random effects, but also the type of random effects affect the dependence structure.

In addition, we present the scatterplots ($n = 1000$) of several bivariate distributions described in Section 10.4.1. In Figure 10.3, each row represents the bivariate distributions of the true values of (X_0, Y_0). Here we consider additive random effects only in Y since X and Y are exchangeable for most considered bivariate distributions. Each column of Figure 10.3 represents the case $X = X_0$, $Y = Y_0 + \varepsilon_Y$, where the random effects $\varepsilon_Y \sim N(0, \sigma^2)$ and $\sigma^2 = 0.25, 0.5, 1$, and 2, from left to right. In such a case, the presence of additive random effects in one variable of bivariate distributions does not change the dependence structure as much as the case where one variable is simply a function of the other variable, as shown in Figure 10.2.

TABLE 10.1

Dependence Measures of MIC and AUK under Different Dependence Structures and Normally Distributed Random Effects with Mean 0, Where the Unobserved True Values of the Predictor Variable X_0 and the Response Variable Y_0 Can Be Formulated as $Y_0 = f(X_0)$

Structure	Measures	a	b	b′	c	c′	d	d′
M3	MIC[0,1]	1	0.814	0.497	0.591	0.234	0.541	0.202
(LinearQuadratic)	AUK[0,0.75]	0.664	0.652	0.63	0.633	0.587	0.628	0.578
M4	MIC[0,1]	1	0.807	0.623	0.753	0.427	0.608	0.307
(Cubic)	AUK[0,0.75]	0.75	0.717	0.69	0.708	0.649	0.693	0.616
M5	MIC[0,1]	1	0.904	0.501	0.745	0.375	0.583	0.162
(Inverse)	AUK[0,0.75]	0.404	0.488	0.523	0.492	0.525	0.523	0.539
M6	MIC[0,1]	1	0.842	0.699	0.567	0.221	0.497	0.169
(Inverse2)	AUK[0,0.75]	0.377	0.38	0.395	0.431	0.472	0.422	0.476
M8	MIC[0,1]	1	0.32	0.185	0.589	0.207	0.28	0.124
(log)	AUK[0,0.75]	0.582	0.537	0.512	0.557	0.53	0.542	0.507
M9	MIC[0,1]	1	0.572	0.25	0.21	0.125	0.166	0.129
(sin)	AUK[0,0.75]	0.492	0.484	0.492	0.498	0.511	0.495	0.493
M10	MIC[0,1]	0.373	0.15	0.136	0.193	0.125	0.135	0.136
(Spiral)	AUK[0,0.75]	0.491	0.498	0.505	0.495	0.51	0.5	0.501

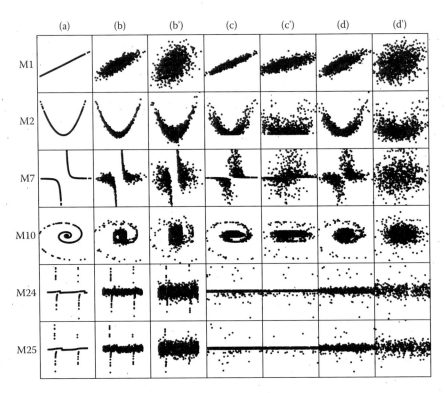

FIGURE 10.2
Scatterplots ($n = 1000$) of measurements of (X, Y) under different dependence structures with normally distributed random effects with mean 0, where the unobserved true values of X_0 and Y_0 can be formulated as $Y_0 = f(X_0)$. Each row corresponds to each of the following structures: M1, linear; M2, quadratic; M7, reciprocal with order $k = 3$; M10, spirals; M24, DDF1; and M25, DDF2. Each column displays various random effects schemes: (a) $X = X_0$, $Y = Y_0$; (b and b') $X = X_0$, $Y = Y_0 + \varepsilon_Y$, with the variance of noise var(ε_Y) assumed to be 0.25 or 2, respectively; (c and c') $Y = Y_0$, $X = X_0 + \varepsilon_X$, with the variance of noise var(ε_X) assumed to be 0.25 or 2, respectively; and (d and d') $X = X_0 + \varepsilon_X$, $Y = Y_0 + \varepsilon_Y$, with the variance of noise var(ε_X) = var(ε_Y) assumed to be 0.25 or 2, respectively.

Instead of the additive random effect, the true value could also be modified proportionally, for example, exposure by chemicals or radiation. In such cases, the multiplicative random effect can be assumed, that is, $Y = \varepsilon Y_0$, where Y and Y_0 are the observed and unobserved truth variables, respectively, and the multiplicative noise ε is a random variable independent of X. Similarly, the random effect of X can also be present. As a concrete example, we consider the reciprocal dependence $f(X) = 1/X$ and the multiplicative random effects in the response variable. The dependence between X and Y can be formulated as $Y = \varepsilon/X$, where var($Y|X$) = var(ε)/X^2. Also, in the model $Y = \alpha + \beta X + \varepsilon/X$, the random effect affects the signal in a proportionally inverse manner. In such cases, random effects cause heteroscedasticity, a common situation in areas such as epidemiological studies (Kulathinal et al. 2002), and extended least-squares or weighted least-squares techniques are often used for estimation (Peck et al. 1984). Another example would be generalized linear mixed models (Wood 2013). In a special case of generalized linear mixed models, $Y = \alpha + \gamma X + \varepsilon$, where γ is a random variable independent of X and the random error ε, both additive and multiplicative random effects are considered.

In order to illustrate the impact of various types of random effects, we provide the scatterplots ($n = 1000$) from several bivariate distributions, including additive and

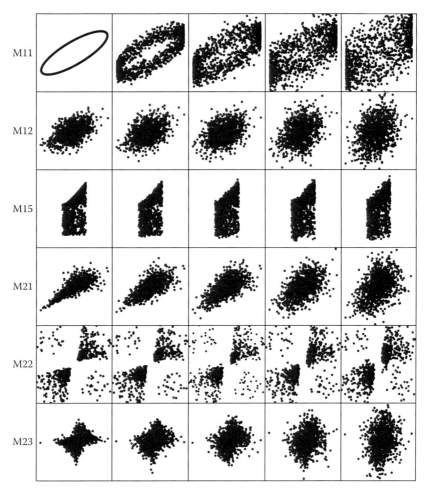

FIGURE 10.3
Scatterplots ($n = 1000$) of dependence structures of (X, Y) that can be represented via bivariate distributions with additive random effects of mean 0. Each row represents the bivariate distributions where the true values of $(X_0, Y_0)^T$ follow M11, ellipse; M12, bivariate normal distribution with correlation 0.5; M15, bivariate Plackett distribution with $\phi = 3.5$; M21, two marginally normal distributions coupled with the Clayton copula; M22, reciprocal-normal-type distribution; and M23, normal conditional distributions. Each column represents $X = X_0$, $Y = Y_0 + \varepsilon_Y$, where the random effects $\varepsilon_Y \sim N(0, \sigma^2)$ and $\sigma^2 = 0.25, 0.5, 1$, and 2, from left to right.

multiplicative random effects in Figure 10.4. Each row represents the bivariate distributions, and each column displays various random effects schemes in the same scale for each type of bivariate distribution. It can be seen that the shapes of the scatterplots are heavily affected by the types of random effects, even when the variance of random effects is relatively small. Note that parameters of the bivariate distributions can be affected by random effects. For example, when measurements of X and Y consist of multiplicative random effects γ, which follow the normal distribution with mean a and variance 1, and the underlying true values $(X_0, Y_0)^T \sim \mathrm{MVN}_2(\mu, \Sigma)$, the mean parameter of the observed measurements $(X, Y)^T$ is $a\mu$, and the corresponding covariance matrix is impacted by the random effects.

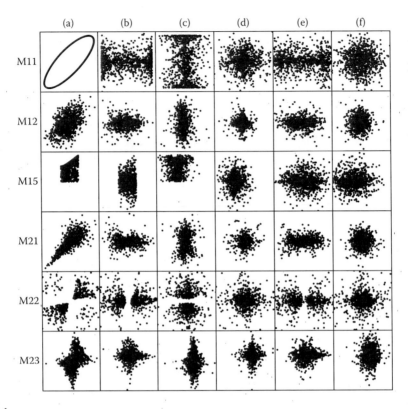

FIGURE 10.4

Scatterplots ($n = 1000$) of bivariate dependence structures with additive and multiplicative random effects. Each row represents the bivariate distributions where the true values of $(X_0, Y_0)^T$ follow: M11, ellipse; M12, bivariate normal distribution with correlation 0.5; M15, bivariate Plackett distribution with $\phi = 3.5$; M21, two marginally normal distributions coupled with the Clayton copula; M22, reciprocal-normal-type distribution; and M23, normal conditional distributions. Each column displays the following random effects schemes in the same scale for each type of bivariate distribution: (a) $X = X_0$, $Y = Y_0$; (b) $X = X_0$, $Y = \varepsilon_{Y_M} Y_0$; (c) $Y = Y_0$, $X = \varepsilon_{X_M} X_0$; (d) $X = \varepsilon_{X_M} X_0$, $Y = \varepsilon_{Y_M} Y_0$; (e) $X = X_0 + \varepsilon_{X_A}$, $Y = \varepsilon_{Y_M} Y_0$; and (f) $X = \varepsilon_{X_M} X_0 + \varepsilon_{X_A}$, $Y = \varepsilon_{Y_M} Y_0 + \varepsilon_{Y_A}$, where all random effects $\varepsilon_{jk} \sim N(0, 0.25)$, $j = X$ or Y, $k = A$ or M.

10.5 Monte Carlo Comparisons of Tests of Independence

We conducted an extensive Monte Carlo study in order to compare the power of tests of independence under different dependence structures and various random effects at the 0.05 significance level. Classical methods, such as Pearson's product–moment correlation coefficient (P), Kendall's tau (K), and Spearman's rho (S), as well as nonparametric tests, including the empirical likelihood–based hypothesis testing (EMK), data-driven rank tests TS and V in the cases $d(n) = 1, 2, 3$, and the density-based empirical likelihood ratio test (dbEL) described in Section 10.2, were evaluated. Without loss of generality, in the density-based empirical likelihood ratio test, we set $\beta_1 = 0.45$ and $\beta_2 = 0.8$, respectively.

We attended to general forms of dependence (Johnson 2013; Reshef et al. 2011), which have been commonly pointed out with respect to bivariate data, including linear dependence, nonlinear dependence, and bivariate distributions, as shown in Table 10.2. The estimates of indices of dependence based on samples of sizes 1000 are given in Table 10.3.

TABLE 10.2

Dependence Structures

Designs	Models/Description	
	X	$f(X)$
Linear		
M1 (Linear)	$N(0,2)$	$0.5X$
Nonlinear		
M2 (Quadratic)	$N(0,2)$	$2 + X^2$
M3 (LinearQuadratic)	$N(0,2)$	$2 + X + X^2$
M4 (Cubic)	$N(0,2)$	X^3
M5 (Reciprocal $k = 1$)	$N(0,2)$	$1/X$
M6 (Reciprocal $k = 2$)	$N(0,2)$	$1/X^2$
M7 (Reciprocal $k = 3$)	$N(0,2)$	$1/X^3$
M8 (Logarithm)	$N(0,2)$	$\log(1 + |X|)$
M9 ($\sin(\pi x)$)	$N(0,2)$	$\sin(\pi X)$
M9' ($\sin(\pi X)$)	$Uniform[-2, 2]$	$\sin(\pi X)$
M10 (Spiral)	$\exp(0.2\pi\theta)\cos(\pi\theta)$	$\exp(0.2\pi\theta)\sin(\pi\theta)$, where $\theta \sim N(0,2)$

Bivariate Distributions

M11 (Ellipse) — An ellipse of a 95% probability region for MVN

$$\mathrm{MVN}_2\left(\mathbf{0}, \begin{pmatrix} 1 & .8 \\ .8 & 1 \end{pmatrix}\right)$$

M12 (Normal) — Bivariate normal distribution $\mathrm{MVN}_2\left(\mathbf{0}, \begin{pmatrix} 1 & .5 \\ .5 & 1 \end{pmatrix}\right)$

M13 (NormOffset) — Bivariate NormOffset distribution

M14 (Morg) — Bivariate Morgenstern distribution with $\alpha = 1$

M15 (Plackett) — Bivariate Plackett distribution with $\phi = 3.5$

M16 (PearsonII) — Bivariate Pearson type II distribution with $\mu = \mathbf{0}$, $\Sigma = \mathbf{I}$ and $m = 1.1$

M17 (PearsonVII) — Bivariate Pearson type VII distribution with $\mu = \mathbf{0}$, $\Sigma = \mathbf{I}$ and $m = 1.1$

M18 (Cauchy) — Bivariate Cauchy distribution

M19 (EP) — Bivariate exponential power distribution

M20 (Gumbel) — Two marginally normal distributions coupled with the Gumbel copula

M21 (Clayton) — Two marginally normal distributions coupled with the Clayton copula

M22 (RecipN) — Reciprocal-normal-type distribution

M23 (CondN) — Conditional distributions are each normal and $f_{X,Y}(x, y) = C\exp\{-(x^2 + y^2 + 2xy(x + y + xy))\}$

M24 (DDF1) — Unif[0,1]

$$\arg\min_z \left(\sum_{j=1}^2 b_j(X)\, b_j(z)\right)^2$$

M25 (DDF2) — Unif[0,1]

$$\arg\min_z \left(b_1(X)b_1(z) + 0.3 b_1(X)b_2(z) + 0.5 b_2(X)b_1(z) + b_2(X)b_2(z)\right)^2$$

Motivated by the necessity to consider random effect–type dependencies between two sets of observations, we investigate comparisons of the above-mentioned tests of independence of X and Y via the Monte Carlo simulations, under the representative cases where X has no random effect and Y has the following scenarios: (1) no random effect in Y, (2) an additive random effect in Y, (3) a multiplicative random effect in Y, and (4) both additive and multiplicative random effects in Y. All random effects are assumed to follow the normal distribution with mean 0 and variance σ_ε^2; see Table 10.4 for details. For instance,

TABLE 10.3

Indices of Dependence, including Pearson Correlation Coefficient, Spearman's Rank Correlation Coefficient, Kendall's Rank Correlation Coefficient, the MIC Measure, and the AUK Measure

Structures [Range]; (Measure under H_0)	Pearson [−1,1];(0)	Spearman [−1,1];(0)	Kendall [−1,1];(0)	MIC [0,1];(0)	AUK [0, 0.75];(0.5)
M1	1.000	1.000	1.000	1.000	0.750
M2	−0.000	0.001	0.001	1.000	0.578
M3	0.447	0.383	0.443	1.000	0.664
M4	0.781	1.000	1.000	1.000	0.750
M5	0.028	−0.000	0.498	1.000	0.404
M6	−0.000	−0.001	−0.001	1.000	0.377
M7	0.000	−0.000	0.498	1.000	0.419
M8	0.000	0.001	0.001	1.000	0.582
M9	0.001	0.004	0.005	1.000	0.590
M10	−0.099	−0.025	−0.015	0.373	0.491
M11	0.800	0.592	0.785	0.623	0.625
M12	0.500	0.333	0.482	0.267	0.603
M13	−0.001	−0.001	−0.001	1.000	0.386
M14	0.319	0.223	0.333	0.205	0.566
M15	0.452	0.356	0.487	0.392	0.622
M16	0.000	0.000	0.000	0.142	0.496
M17	−0.018	0.000	0.001	0.447	0.533
M18	0.005	−0.000	−0.000	0.159	0.523
M19	0.500	0.333	0.491	0.279	0.599
M20	0.858	0.667	0.848	0.610	0.691
M21	0.775	0.600	0.785	0.549	0.644
M22	0.000	0.079	0.102	0.248	0.525
M23	0.361	0.290	0.476	0.333	0.560

Note: The Pearson correlation coefficient, Spearman's rank correlation coefficient, and Kendall's rank correlation coefficient can range from −1 for the perfect negative dependence case to 1 for the perfect dependence case, where 0 stands for the independence case. The MIC measure can range from 0 for the independence case to 1 for the perfect dependence case, while the AUK can range from 0 for the perfect negatively dependent case to 0.75 for the perfect positive dependence case, where the value 0.5 indicates independence.

TABLE 10.4

Random Effects Schemes Considered for the Monte Carlo Comparison of Tests of Independence between X and Y, where X_0 and Y_0 Are Unobserved True Values

Scenario	X	Y
(1)	$X = X_0$	$Y = Y_0$
(2)	$X = X_0$	$Y = Y_0 + \varepsilon_A$
(3)	$X = X_0$	$Y = \varepsilon_M Y_0$
(4)	$X = X_0$	$Y = \varepsilon_M Y_0 + \varepsilon_A$

Note: The additive random effects ε_A and multiplicative random effects ε_M follow the $N(0,1)$ distribution.

when $f(X) = 1/X$, as considered in M5 in Table 10.2, the case that X has no random effect and Y has both additive and multiplicative random effects (as described in scenario 4 in Table 10.4) leads to the model $Y = \varepsilon_M/X + \varepsilon_A$.

Figures 10.5a through 10.17 show powers of different methods via graphs under different alternative relationships assuming $\sigma_\varepsilon^2 = 1$, over 10,000 simulations at the 5% nominal significance level for sample sizes $n = 10, 25, 50, 100$, where the MIC and AUK, indices of

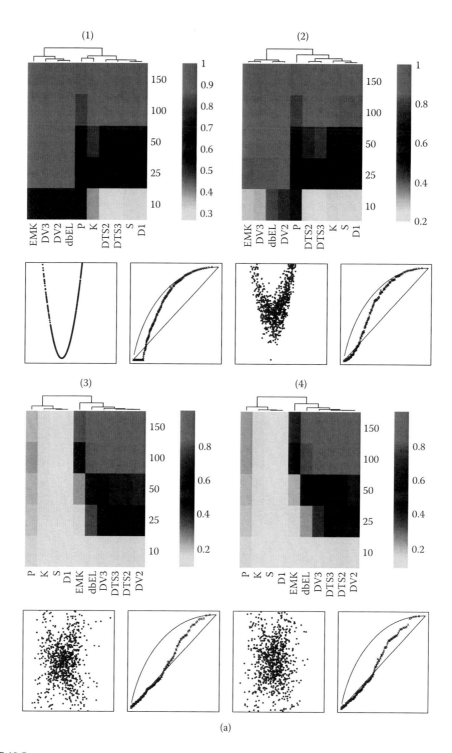

(a)

FIGURE 10.5

(See color insert.) Graphical summarization and the comparison of the powers of the considered tests at the 0.05 significance level, based on data with the dependence structure M3 (LinearQuadratic) in the left panel (a) and M5 (Reciprocal with $k = 1$) in the right panel. *(Continued)*

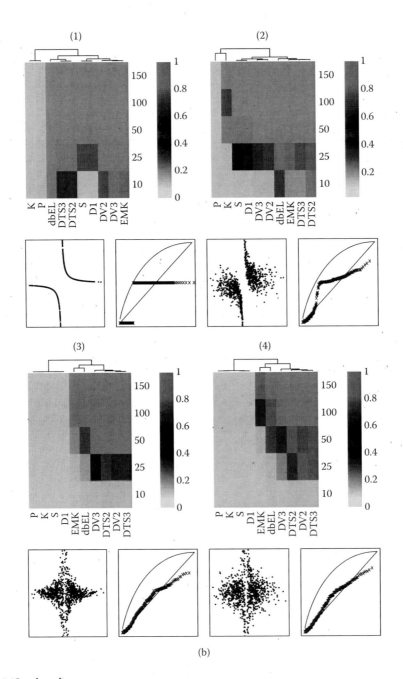

FIGURE 10.5 (Continued)
Graphical summarization and the comparison of the powers of the considered tests at the 0.05 significance level, based on data with the dependence structure M3 (LinearQuadratic) in the left panel (b), as well as various types of random effects that correspond to one of the subpanels. In each subpanel (1–4), the top level is the heat map and the bottom level shows the scatterplot (left panel) and K-plot (right panel). The following random effects schemes are considered: (1) $X = X_0$, $Y = Y_0$; (2) $X = X_0$, $Y = Y_0 + \varepsilon_A$; (3) $X = X_0$, $Y = \varepsilon_M Y_0$; and (4) $X = X_0$, $Y = \varepsilon_M Y_0 + \varepsilon_A$, where the random effects ε_A and $\varepsilon_M \sim N(0, 1)$. For M3 (LinearQuadratic), the measures of MIC (AUK) for each type of random effect are (1) 1 (0.664), (2) 0.664 (0.639), (3) 0.276 (0.534), and (4) 0.271 (0.533). For M5 (Reciprocal with $k = 1$), the measures of MIC (AUK) for each type of random effect are (1) 1 (0.438), (2) 0.69 (0.522), (3) 0.32 (0.471), and (4) 0.278 (0.483).

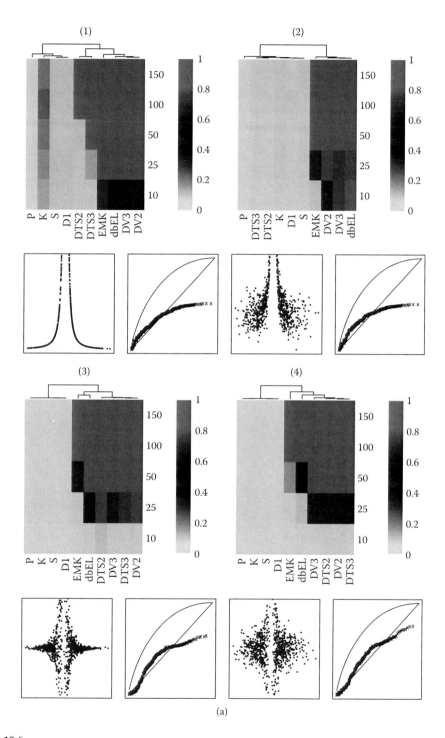

FIGURE 10.6
(See color insert.) Graphical summarization and the comparison of the powers of the considered tests at the 0.05 significance level, based on data with the dependence structure M6 (Reciprocal with $k = 2$) in the left panel (a) and M8 (Logarithm) in the right panel. *(Continued)*

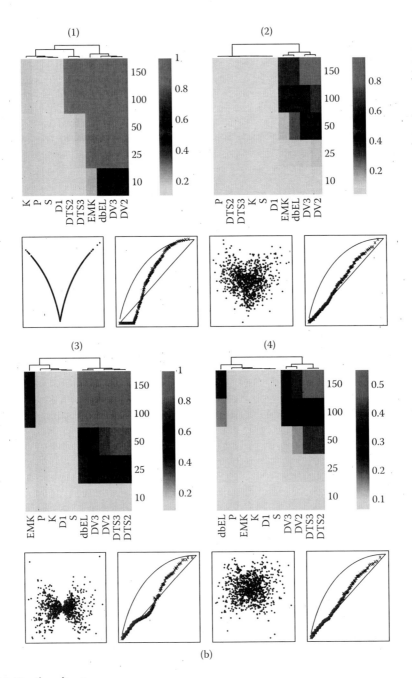

FIGURE 10.6 (Continued)

Graphical summarization and the comparison of the powers of the considered tests at the 0.05 significance level, based on data with the dependence structure M6 (Reciprocal with $k = 2$) in the left panel (b), as well as various types of random effects that correspond to one of the subpanels. In each subpanel (1–4), the top level is the heat map and the bottom level shows the scatterplot (left panel) and K-plot (right panel). The following random effects schemes are considered: (1) $X = X_0$, $Y = Y_0$; (2) $X = X_0$, $Y = Y_0 + \varepsilon_A$; (3) $X = X_0$, $Y = \varepsilon_M Y_0$; and (4) $X = X_0$, $Y = \varepsilon_M Y_0 + \varepsilon_A$, where the random effects ε_A and $\varepsilon_m \sim N(0, 1)$. For M6 (Reciprocal with $k = 2$), the measures of MIC (AUK) for each type of random effect are (1) 1 (0.407), (2) 0.756 (0.416), (3) 0.429 (0.458), and (4) 0.379 (0.473). For M8 (Logarithm), the measures of MIC (AUK) for each type of random effect are (1) 1 (0.576), (2) 0.281 (0.526), (3) 0.277 (0.519), and (4) 0.237 (0.511).

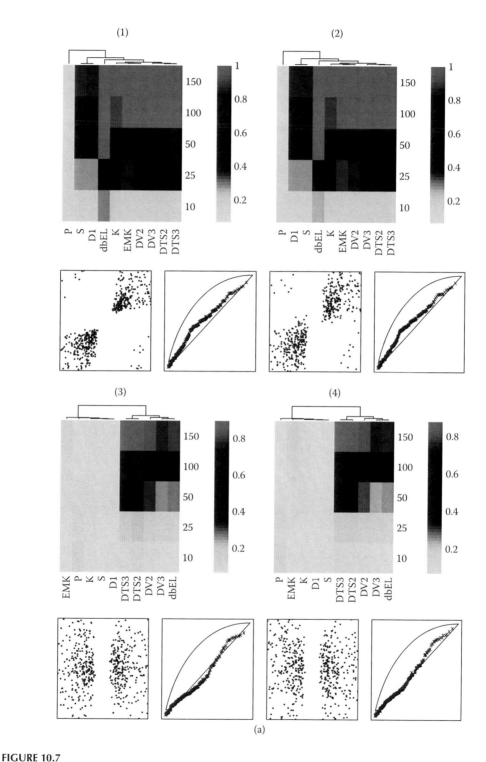

FIGURE 10.7

(See color insert.) Graphical summarization and the comparison of the powers of the considered tests at the 0.05 significance level, based on data with the dependence structure M24 (Reciprocal-Normal) in the left panel (a) and M1 (Linear) in the right panel. *(Continued)*

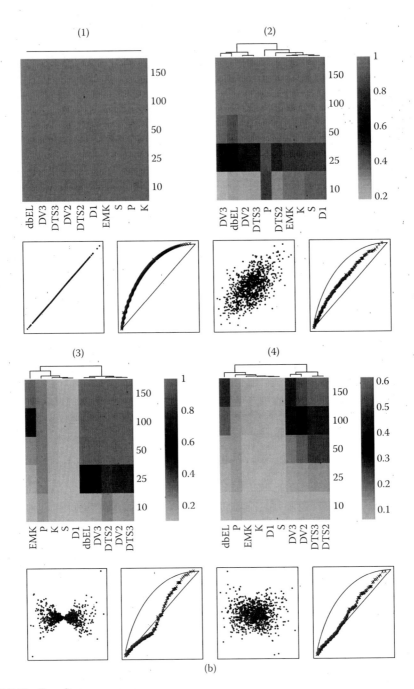

FIGURE 10.7 (Continued)
Graphical summarization and the comparison of the powers of the considered tests at the 0.05 significance level, based on data with the dependence structure M24 (Reciprocal-Normal) in the left panel (b) and various types of random effects that correspond to one of the subpanels. In each subpanel (1–4), the top level is the heat map and the bottom level shows the scatterplot (left panel) and K-plot (right panel). The following random effects schemes are considered: (1) $X = X_0, Y = Y_0$; (2) $X = X_0, Y = Y_0 + \varepsilon_A$; (3) $X = X_0, Y = \varepsilon_M Y_0$; and (4) $X = X_0, Y = \varepsilon_M Y_0 + \varepsilon_A$, where the random effects ε_A and $\varepsilon_m \sim N(0, 1)$. For M24 (Reciprocal-Normal), the measures of MIC (AUK) for each type of random effect are (1) 0.522 (0.571), (2) 0.506 (0.569), (3) 0.241 (0.512), and (4) 0.241 (0.512). For M1 (Linear), the measures of MIC (AUK) for each type of random effect are (1) 1 (0.75), (2) 0.405 (0.619), (3) 0.305 (0.522), and (4) 0.237 (0.511).

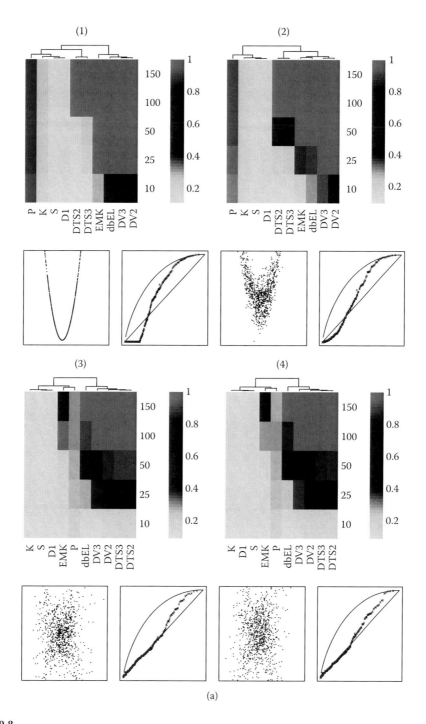

FIGURE 10.8
(See color insert.) Graphical summarization and the comparison of the powers of the considered tests at the 0.05 significance level, based on data with the dependence structure M2 (Quadratic) in the left panel (a) and M4 (Cubic) in the right panel. *(Continued)*

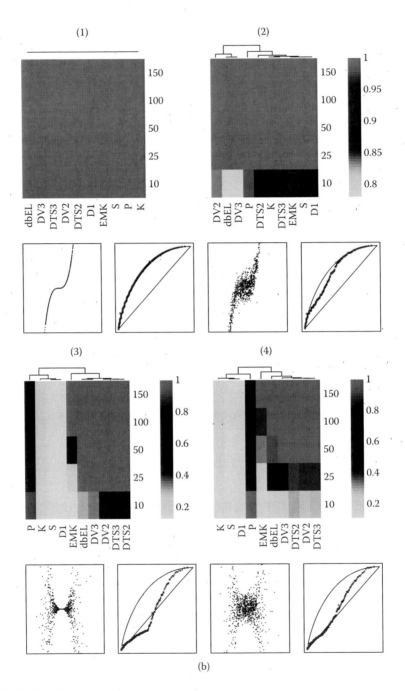

(b)

FIGURE 10.8 (Continued)
Graphical summarization and the comparison of the powers of the considered tests at the 0.05 significance level, based on data with the dependence structure M2 (Quadratic) in the left panel (b) and various types of random effects that correspond to one of the subpanels. In each subpanel (1–4), the top level is the heat map and the bottom level shows the scatterplot (left panel) and K-plot (right panel). The following random effects schemes are considered: (1) $X = X_0$, $Y = Y_0$; (2) $X = X_0$, $Y = Y_0 + \varepsilon_A$; (3) $X = X_0$, $Y = \varepsilon_M Y_0$; and (4) $X = X_0$, $Y = \varepsilon_M Y_0 + \varepsilon_A$, where the random effects ε_A and $\varepsilon_m \sim N(0, 1)$. For M2 (Quadratic), the measures of MIC (AUK) for each type of random effect are (1) 1 (0.576), (2) 0.636 (0.563), (3) 0.244 (0.52), and (4) 0.242 (0.519). For M4 (Cubic), the measures of MIC (AUK) for each type of random effect are (1) 1 (0.75), (2) 0.708 (0.703), (3) 0.484 (0.529), and (4) 0.305 (0.526).

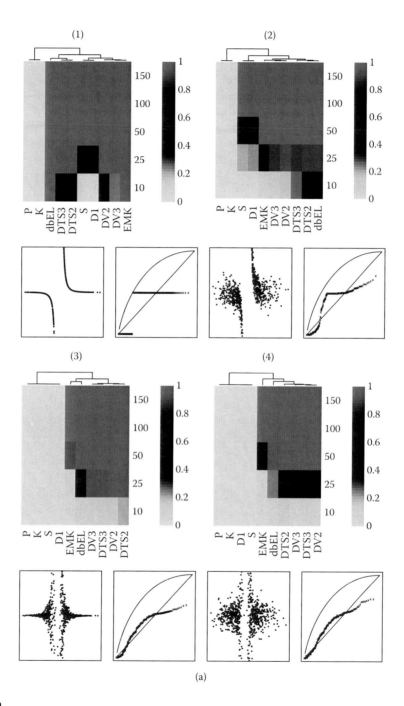

FIGURE 10.9
(See color insert.) Graphical summarization and the comparison of the powers of the considered tests at the 0.05 significance level, based on data with the dependence structure M7 (Reciprocal with $k = 3$) in the left panel (a) and M9' ($\sin(\pi X)$ where $X \sim Uniform[-2, 2]$) in the right panel. *(Continued)*

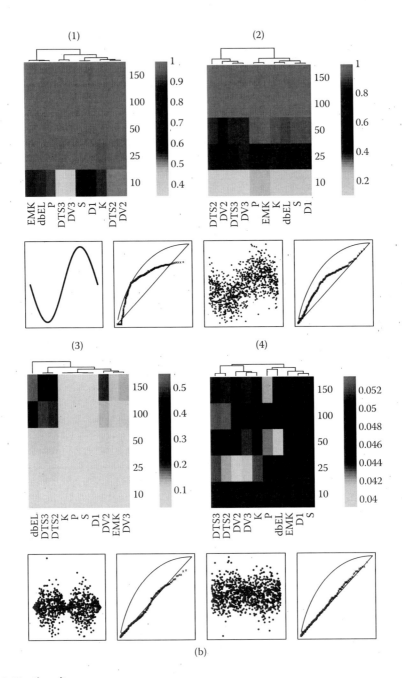

FIGURE 10.9 (Continued)
Graphical summarization and the comparison of the powers of the considered tests at the 0.05 significance level, based on data with the dependence structure M7 (Reciprocal with $k = 3$) in the left panel (b) and various types of random effects that correspond to one of the subpanels. In each subpanel (1–4), the top level is the heat map and the bottom level shows the scatterplot (left panel) and K-plot (right panel). The following random effects schemes are considered: (1) $X = X_0$, $Y = Y_0$; (2) $X = X_0$, $Y = Y_0 + \varepsilon_A$; (3) $X = X_0$, $Y = \varepsilon_M Y_0$; and (4) $X = X_0$, $Y = \varepsilon_M Y_0 + \varepsilon_A$, where the random effects ε_A and $\varepsilon_m \sim N(0, 1)$. For M7 (Reciprocal with $k = 3$), the measures of MIC (AUK) for each type of random effect are (1) 1 (0.438), (2) 0.708 (0.48), (3) 0.488 (0.452), and (4) 0.445 (0.469). For M9' ($\sin(\pi X)$ where $X \sim Uniform[-2, 2]$), the measures of MIC (AUK) for each type of random effect are (1) 1.000 (0.397), (2) 0.391 (0.443), (3) 0.242 (0.501), and (4) 0.237 (0.503).

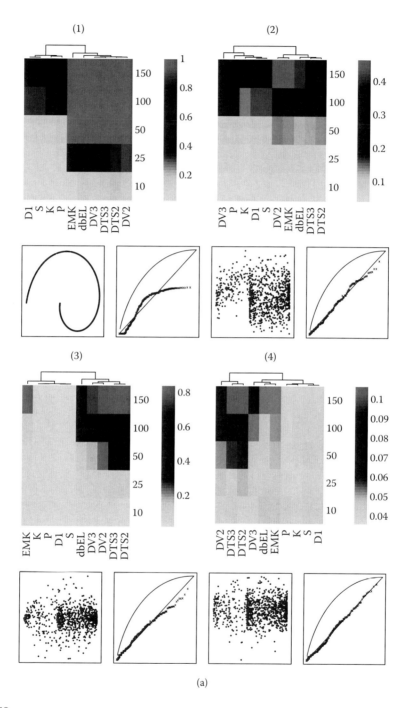

FIGURE 10.10

Graphical summarization and the comparison of the powers of the considered tests at the 0.05 significance level, based on data with the dependence structure M10 (Spiral) in the left panel (a) and M11 (ellipse) in the right panel. *(Continued)*

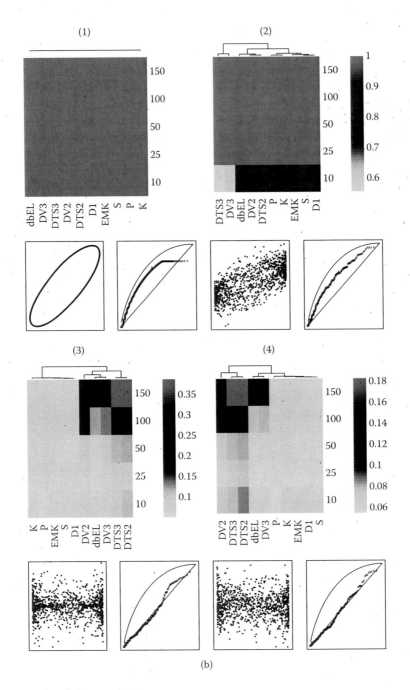

FIGURE 10.10 (Continued)
Graphical summarization and the comparison of the powers of the considered tests at the 0.05 significance level, based on data with the dependence structure M11 (Spiral) in the left panel (b) and various types of random effects that correspond to one of the subpanels. In each subpanel (1–4), the top level is the heat map and the bottom level shows the scatterplot (left panel) and K-plot (right panel). The following random effects schemes are considered: (1) $X = X_0$, $Y = Y_0$; (2) $X = X_0$, $Y = Y_0 + \varepsilon_A$; (3) $X = X_0$, $Y = \varepsilon_M Y_0$; and (4) $X = X_0$, $Y = \varepsilon_M Y_0 + \varepsilon_A$, where the random effects ε_A and $\varepsilon_m \sim N(0, 1)$. For M11 (Spiral), the measures of MIC (AUK) for each type of random effect are (1) 0.287 (0.508), (2) 0.241 (0.512), (3) 0.239 (0.512), and (4) 0.237 (0.509). For M11 (ellipse), the measures of MIC (AUK) for each type of random effect are (1) 0.64 (0.628), (2) 0.558 (0.63), (3) 0.235 (0.51), and (4) 0.237 (0.508).

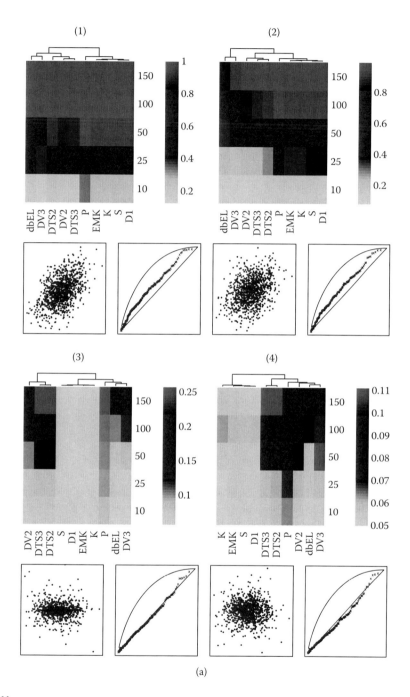

FIGURE 10.11

Graphical summarization and the comparison of the powers of the considered tests at the 0.05 significance level, based on data with the dependence structure M12 (Normal with $\rho = 0.5$) in the left panel (a) and M13 (NormOffset) in the right panel. *(Continued)*

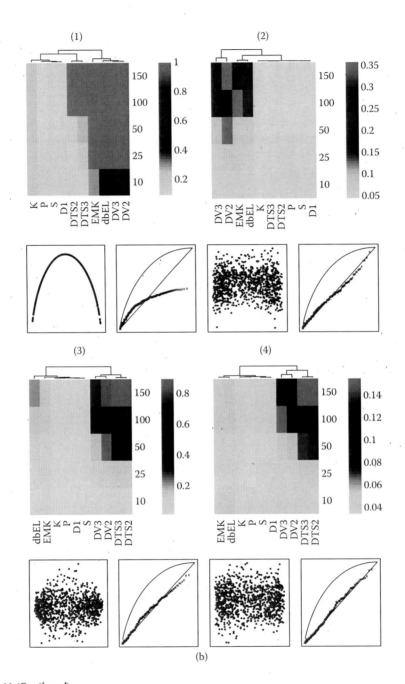

FIGURE 10.11 (Continued)
Graphical summarization and the comparison of the powers of the considered tests at the 0.05 significance level, based on data with the dependence structure M12 (Normal with $\rho = 0.5$) in the left panel (b) and various types of random effects that correspond to one of the subpanels. In each subpanel (1–4), the top level is the heat map and the bottom level shows the scatterplot (left panel) and K-plot (right panel). The following random effects schemes are considered: (1) $X = X_0$, $Y = Y_0$; (2) $X = X_0$, $Y = Y_0 + \varepsilon_A$; (3) $X = X_0$, $Y = \varepsilon_M Y_0$; and (4) $X = X_0$, $Y = \varepsilon_M Y_0 + \varepsilon_A$, where the random effects ε_A and $\varepsilon_m \sim N(0, 1)$. For M12 (Normal with $\rho = 0.5$), the measures of MIC (AUK) for each type of random effect are (1) 0.359 (0.603), (2) 0.295 (0.574), (3) 0.238 (0.508), and (4) 0.237 (0.506). For M13 (NormOffset), the measures of MIC (AUK) for each type of random effect are (1) 1 (0.406), (2) 0.246 (0.491), (3) 0.238 (0.492), and (4) 0.237 (0.5).

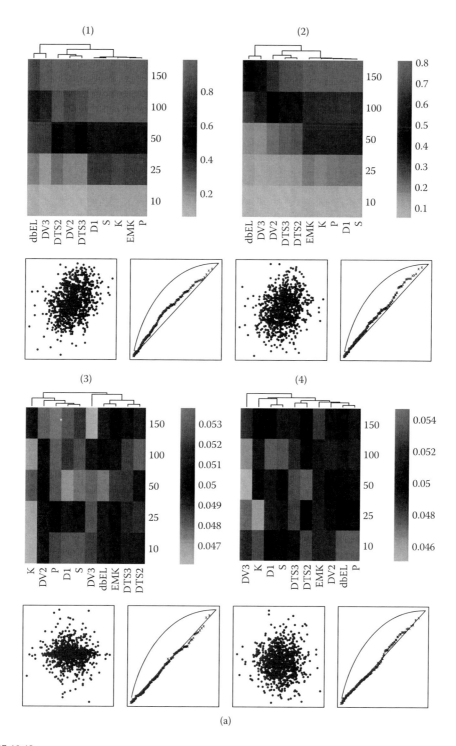

FIGURE 10.12
(See color insert.) Graphical summarization and the comparison of the powers of the considered tests at the 0.05 significance level, based on data with the dependence structure M14 (Morgenstern) in the left panel (a) and M15 (Plackett) in the right panel. *(Continued)*

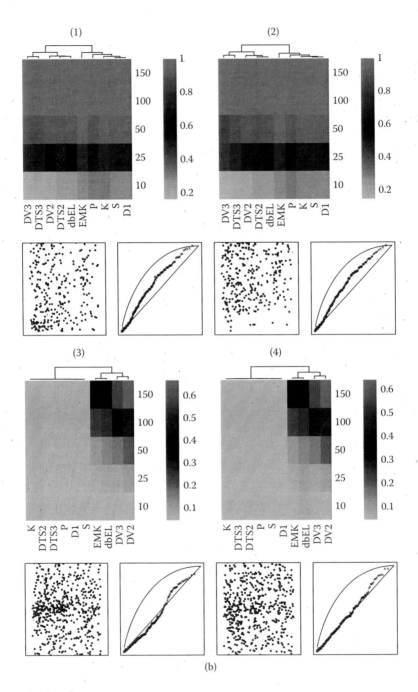

FIGURE 10.12 (Continued)
Graphical summarization and the comparison of the powers of the considered tests at the 0.05 significance level, based on data with the dependence structure M14 (Morgenstern) in the left panel (b) and various types of random effects that correspond to one of the subpanels. In each subpanel (1–4), the top level is the heat map and the bottom level shows the scatterplot (left panel) and K-plot (right panel). The following random effects schemes are considered: (1) $X = X_0$, $Y = Y_0$; (2) $X = X_0$, $Y = Y_0 + \varepsilon_A$; (3) $X = X_0$, $Y = \varepsilon_M Y_0$; and (4) $X = X_0$, $Y = \varepsilon_M Y_0 + \varepsilon_A$, where the random effects ε_A and $\varepsilon_m \sim N(0, 1)$. For M14 (Morgenstern), the measures of MIC (AUK) for each type of random effect are (1) 0.298 (0.568), (2) 0.265 (0.55), (3) 0.238 (0.504), and (4) 0.238 (0.504). For M15 (Plackett), the measures of MIC (AUK) for each type of random effect are (1) 0.455 (0.622), (2) 0.42 (0.616), (3) 0.257 (0.519), and (4) 0.256 (0.519).

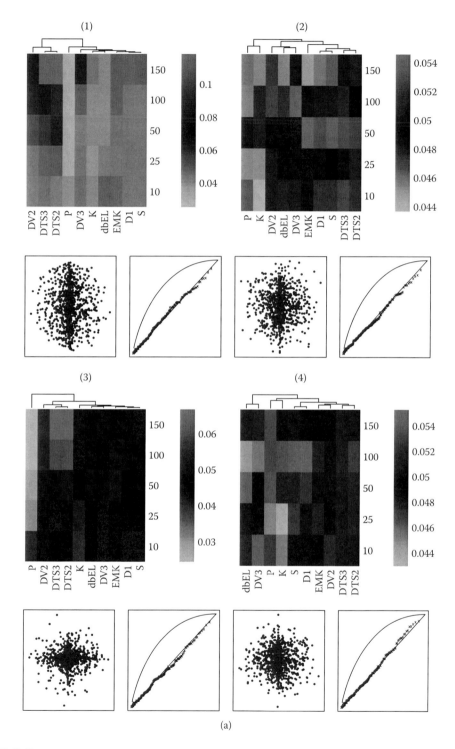

FIGURE 10.13
(See color insert.) Graphical summarization and the comparison of the powers of the considered tests at the 0.05 significance level, based on data with the dependence structure M16 (PearsonII) in the left panel (a) and M17 (PearsonVII) in the right panel. *(Continued)*

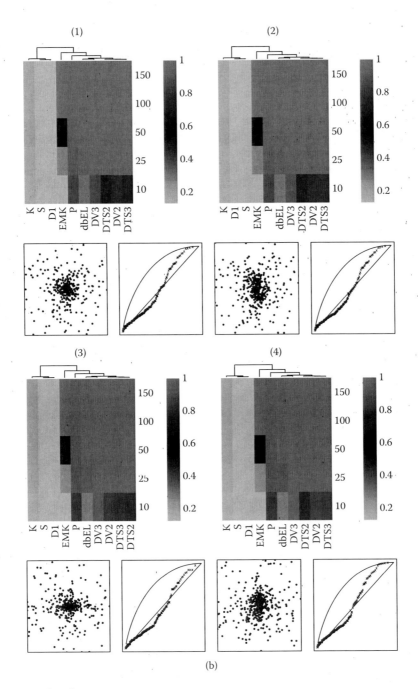

(b)

FIGURE 10.13 (Continued)
Graphical summarization and the comparison of the powers of the considered tests at the 0.05 significance level, based on data with the dependence structure M16 (PearsonII) in the left panel (b) and various types of random effects that correspond to one of the subpanels. In each subpanel (1–4), the top level is the heat map and the bottom level shows the scatterplot (left panel) and K-plot (right panel). The following random effects schemes are considered: (1) $X = X_0$, $Y = Y_0$; (2) $X = X_0$, $Y = Y_0 + \varepsilon_A$; (3) $X = X_0$, $Y = \varepsilon_M Y_0$; and (4) $X = X_0$, $Y = \varepsilon_M Y_0 + \varepsilon_A$, where the random effects ε_A and $\varepsilon_m \sim N(0, 1)$. For M16 (PearsonII), the measures of MIC (AUK) for each type of random effect are (1) 0.237 (0.5), (2) 0.237 (0.503), (3) 0.238 (0.502), and (4) 0.237 (0.503). For M17 (PearsonVII), the measures of MIC (AUK) for each type of random effect are (1) 0.463 (0.532), (2) 0.459 (0.532), (3) 0.425 (0.531), and (4) 0.42 (0.53).

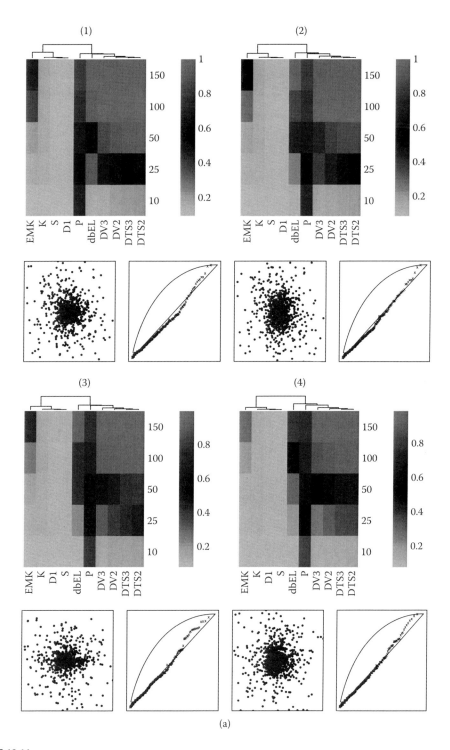

FIGURE 10.14

(See color insert.) Graphical summarization and the comparison of the powers of the considered tests at the 0.05 significance level, based on data with the dependence structure M18 (Cauchy) in the left panel (a) and M19 (EP) in the right panel. *(Continued)*

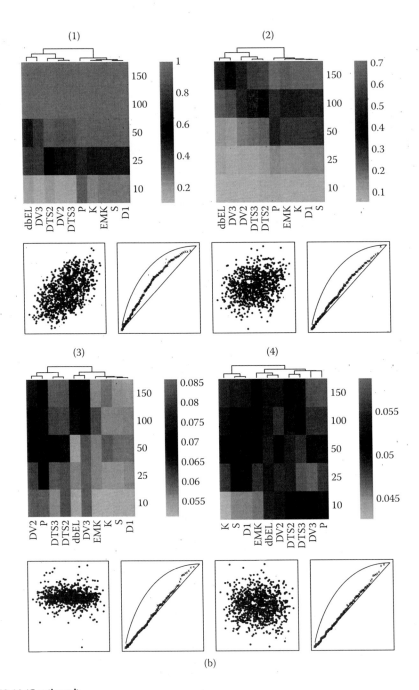

(b)

FIGURE 10.14 (Continued)
Graphical summarization and the comparison of the powers of the considered tests at the 0.05 significance level, based on data with the dependence structure M18 (Cauchy) in the left panel (b) and various types of random effects that correspond to one of the subpanels. In each subpanel (1–4), the top level is the heat map and the bottom level shows the scatterplot (left panel) and K-plot (right panel). The following random effects scheme are considered: (1) $X = X_0$, $Y = Y_0$; (2) $X = X_0$, $Y = Y_0 + \varepsilon_A$; (3) $X = X_0$, $Y = \varepsilon_M Y_0$; and (4) $X = X_0$, $Y = \varepsilon_M Y_0 + \varepsilon_A$, where the random effects ε_A and $\varepsilon_m \sim N(0, 1)$. For M18 (Cauchy), the measures of MIC (AUK) for each type of random effect are (1) 0.245 (0.522), (2) 0.241 (0.52), (3) 0.24 (0.519), and (4) 0.238 (0.518). For M19 (EP), the measures of MIC (AUK) for each type of random effect are (1) 0.37 (0.6), (2) 0.256 (0.545), (3) 0.237 (0.505), and (4) 0.237 (0.504).

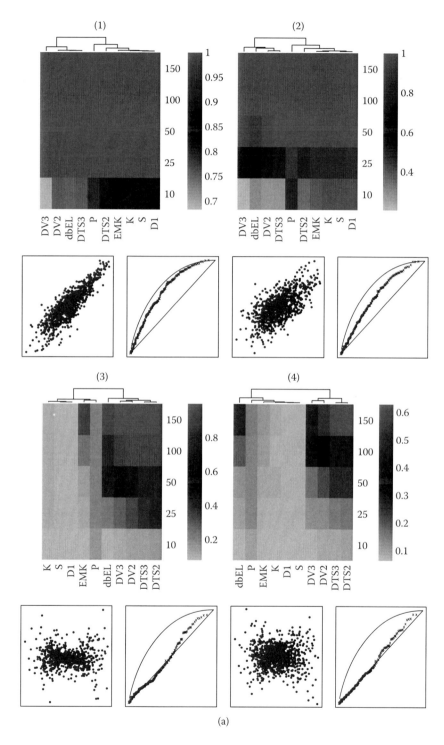

FIGURE 10.15

(See color insert.) Graphical summarization and the comparison of the powers of the considered tests at the 0.05 significance level, based on data with the dependence structure M20 (Gumbel) in the left panel (a) and M21 (Clayton) in the right panel.

(Continued)

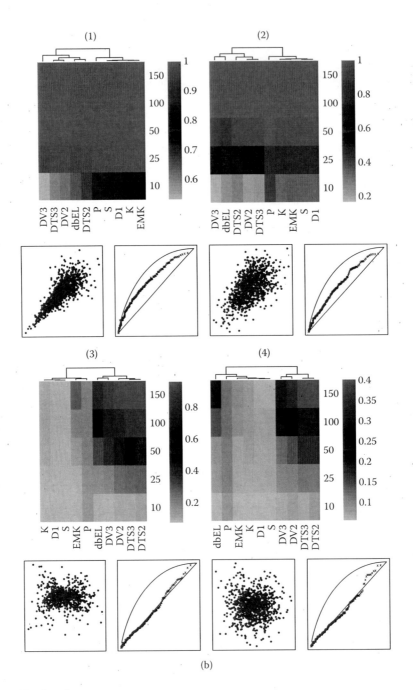

FIGURE 10.15 (Continued)
Graphical summarization and the comparison of the powers of the considered tests at the 0.05 significance level, based on data with the dependence structure M20 (Gumbel) in the left panel (b) and various types of random effects that correspond to one of the subpanels. In each subpanel (1–4), the top level is the heat map and the bottom level shows the scatterplot (left panel) and K-plot (right panel). The following random effects schemes are considered: (1) $X = X_0$, $Y = Y_0$; (2) $X = X_0$, $Y = Y_0 + \varepsilon_A$; (3) $X = X_0$, $Y = \varepsilon_M Y_0$; and (4) $X = X_0$, $Y = \varepsilon_M Y_0 + \varepsilon_A$, where the random effects ε_A and $\varepsilon_m \sim N(0, 1)$. For M20 (Gumbel), the measures of MIC (AUK) for each type of random effect are (1) 0.693 (0.692), (2) 0.426 (0.629), (3) 0.242 (0.52), and (4) 0.237 (0.513). For M21 (Clayton), the measures of MIC (AUK) for each type of random effect are (1) 0.642 (0.646), (2) 0.403 (0.602), (3) 0.241 (0.506), and (4) 0.238 (0.505).

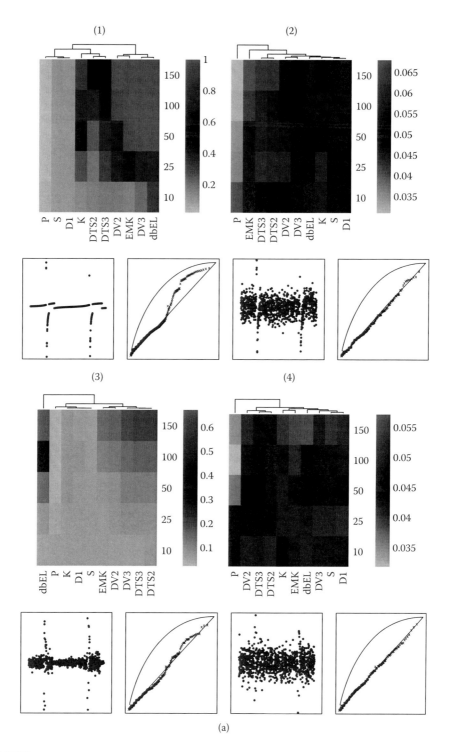

FIGURE 10.16
(See color insert.) Graphical summarization and the comparison of the powers of the considered tests at the 0.05 significance level, based on data with the dependence structure M24 (DDF1) in the left panel (a) and M25 (DDF2) in the right panel. *(Continued)*

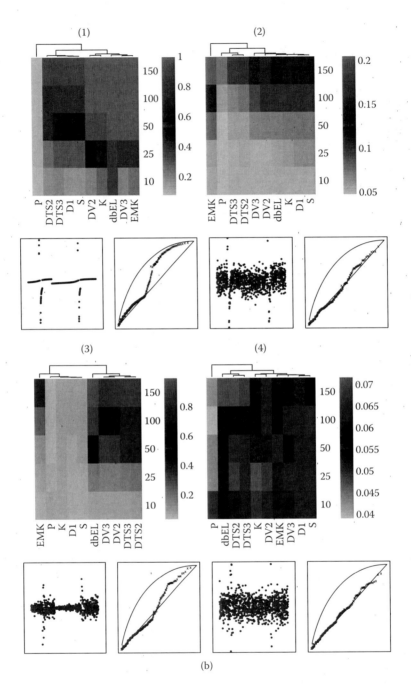

FIGURE 10.16 (Continued)
Graphical summarization and the comparison of the powers of the considered tests at the 0.05 significance level, based on data with the dependence structure M24 (DDF1) in the left panel (b) and various types of random effects that correspond to one of the subpanels. In each subpanel (1–4), the top level is the heat map and the bottom level shows the scatterplot (left panel) and K-plot (right panel). The following random effects schemes are considered: (1) $X = X_0$, $Y = Y_0$; (2) $X = X_0$, $Y = Y_0 + \varepsilon_A$; (3) $X = X_0$, $Y = \varepsilon_M Y_0$; and (4) $X = X_0$, $Y = \varepsilon_M Y_0 + \varepsilon_A$, where the random effects ε_A and $\varepsilon_m \sim N(0, 1)$. For M24 (DDF1), the measures of MIC (AUK) for each type of random effect are (1) 0.909 (0.576), (2) 0.248 (0.509), (3) 0.245 (0.508), and (4) 0.237 (0.505). For M25 (DDF2), the measures of MIC (AUK) for each type of random effect are (1) 0.941 (0.628), (2) 0.255 (0.524), (3) 0.271 (0.519), and (4) 0.237 (0.506).

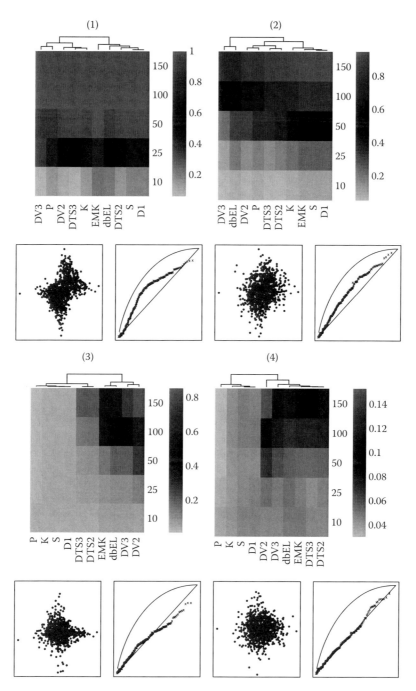

FIGURE 10.17
(See color insert.) Graphical summarization and the comparison of the powers of the considered tests at the 0.05 significance level, based on data with the dependence structure M25 (CondN) and various types of random effects that correspond to one of the subpanels. In each subpanel (1–4), the top level is the heat map and the bottom level shows the scatterplot (left panel) and K-plot (right panel). The following random effects schemes are considered: (1) $X = X_0$, $Y = Y_0$; (2) $X = X_0$, $Y = Y_0 + \varepsilon_A$; (3) $X = X_0$, $Y = \varepsilon_M Y_0$; and (4) $X = X_0$, $Y = \varepsilon_M Y_0 + \varepsilon_A$, where the random effects ε_A and $\varepsilon_m \sim N(0, 1)$. The measures of MIC (AUK) for each type of random effect are (1) 0.425 (0.567), (2) 0.292 (0.55), (3) 0.268 (0.478), and (4) 0.242 (0.494).

dependence, are also presented in the captions corresponding to the different dependence structures and random effects. Each figure can be divided into six subpanels corresponding to scenarios 1–4 described in Table 10.4. In each subpanel, the top level is the heat map and the bottom level shows the scatterplot and K-plot. A heat map manifests itself with comparisons of powers, with column names presenting tests for dependence considered and row names presenting sample sizes. A dendrogram at the top side of the heat map clusters tests for dependence considered. A grayscale color bar shows the magnitude of powers on the right of the heat map. It can easily tell what methods perform the best and how similar methods are. As an example, in Table 10.5, we summarize considered tests based on powers in descending order at the 0.05 significance level for different sample sizes n for the M5 (reciprocal with order $k = 1$) and M9 ($\sin(\pi X)$) dependence structures, considered the above-mentioned random effects 1–4 described in Table 10.4. For each dependence structure and sample size, considered tests of independence are clustered in three clusters. Within each cluster, results are ordered in descending order in terms of powers, as shown in parentheses. Between clusters, results are ordered in descending order in terms of powers, separated by >. For example, in the case of $Y = 1/X$ with additive random effects, when the sample size is 50, dbEL, EMK, and data-driven tests of statistics $TS2$ and V with $d(n) = 2, 3$ have the high power to detect dependence, while the Pearson and Kendall tests break down, as can also be seen in Figure 10.5b.

10.6 Data Examples

10.6.1 TBARS

In this section, we illustrate the practical application and comparisons of different tests of independence with data from a study related to thiobarbituric acid reactive substances (TBARS). TBARS are commonly used to summarize the antioxidant status process of an individual in laboratory research (Armstrong 1994), but their use as a discriminant factor between individuals with and without myocardial infarction (MI) disease is still controversial (Schisterman et al. 2001). In the study investigating the discriminant ability of TBARS with regard to MI disease, dependencies between TBARS and other antioxidant status related to MI disease are evaluated. The sampling frame for adults between the ages of 35 and 65 was the New York State Department of Motor Vehicles driver's license rolls. Also, a randomly selected elderly sample (ages 65–79) from the Health Care Financing Administration database was taken (Schisterman et al. 2001). Participants provided a 12-hour fasting blood specimen for biochemical analysis. A number of antioxidants were examined from fresh blood samples at baseline, including TBARS, high-density lipoprotein (HDL) cholesterol, and vitamin E (a fat-soluble antioxidant vitamin). We implemented tests of independence between TBARS and HDL cholesterol, with a random sample of 100 individuals with MI disease. Figure 10.18 presents the scatterplot of the TBARS data and the K-plot. The estimates of MIC and AUK measures are 0.210 and 0.484, respectively.

In accordance with ideas introduced by Stigler (1977), we organized a jackknife-type procedure to examine different tests of independence, including Pearson's product–moment correlation coefficient (P), Kendall's tau (K), Spearman's rho (S), the empirical likelihood–based hypothesis testing (EMcK) method (Einmahl and McKeague 2003), data-driven rank tests (Kallenberg and Ledwina 1999), and the density-based empirical likelihood ratio

TABLE 10.5

Summarization of Different Tests Based on Powers in Descending Order at the 0.05 Significance Level for Different Sample Sizes n under Dependence Structures and Different Random Effects

Designs (RE)		n	Clustering of the Test Powers (Order within/between Clusters)
M3:	$f(X) = 2 + X + X^2$		
	(1)	25	(EMK, DV2, DV3, dbEL) > (K, P) > (D1, S, DTS3, DTS2)
		50	(EMK, DV2, DV3, dbEL) > (K, DTS3) > (S, D1, DTS2, P)
		100	(EMK, DV2, DTS3, DV3, dbEL, DTS2) > (K, D1, S) > (P)
	(2)	25	(DV2, DV3, dbEL, EMK) > (P) > (K, DTS3, D1, S, DTS2)
		50	(EMK, DV2, DV3, dbEL) > (DTS3, DTS2) > (K, P, S, D1)
		100	(EMK, DV2, DV3, dbEL) > (DTS3, DTS2) > (K, D1, S, P)
	(3)	25	(DV2, DTS2, DTS3, DV3) > (dbEL, P) > (EMK, K, D1, S)
		50	(DV2, DTS2, DTS3, DV3, dbEL) > (EMK, P) > (K, S, D1)
		100	(DV2, DV3, DTS2, DTS3, dbEL) > (EMK) > (P, K, D1, S)
	(4)	25	(DV2, DTS2, DTS3, DV3) > (dbEL, P) > (EMK, K, D1, S)
		50	(DV2, DTS2, DTS3, DV3) > (dbEL) > (EMK, P, K, S, D1)
		100	(DV2, DTS2, DTS3, DV3, dbEL) > (EMK) > (P, K, D1, S)
M5:	$f(X) = 1/X$		
	(1)	25	(EMK, DV2, DV3, dbEL, DTS2, DTS3) > (S, D1) > (P, K)
		50	(EMK, DV2, DV3, dbEL, DTS2, DTS3, S, D1) > (P) > (K)
		100	(S, EMK, D1, DTS2, DV2, DTS3, DV3, dbEL) > (P) > (K)
	(2)	25	(dbEL, EMK, DTS2, DTS3, DV2, DV3, D1, S) > (K) > (P)
		50	(dbEL, EMK, DV2, DV3, DTS2, DTS3) > (S, D1) > (K, P)
		100	(EMK, DTS2, DV2, DTS3, DV3, dbEL, S, D1) > (K) > (P)
	(3)	25	(DTS2, DTS3, DV2, DV3) > (dbEL) > (EMK, D1, S, K, P)
		50	(DTS2, DTS3, DV2, DV3, dbEL) > (EMK) > (S, D1, K, P)
		100	(DTS2, DV2, DTS3, DV3, dbEL) > (EMK) > (D1, S, K, P)
	(4)	25	(DTS2, DTS3, DV2) > (DV3) > (dbEL, EMK, D1, S, K, P)
		50	(DTS2, DTS3, DV2, DV3) > (dbEL) > (EMK, S, D1, K, P)
		100	(DTS2, DTS3, DV2, DV3, dbEL) > (EMK) > (D1, S, K, P)
M9:	$f(X) = \sin(\pi X)$		
	(1)	25	(DV3, EMK) > (dbEL, DV2) > (K, DTS2, D1, S, DTS3, P)
		50	(EMK, dbEL) > (DV3) > (DV2, K, DTS3, DTS2, S, D1, P)
		100	(EMK, dbEL) > (DV3) > (DV2, K, DTS3, DTS2, D1, S, P)
	(2)	25	(DV3, EMK, dbEL) > (DV2, D1, DTS2, P, S) > (DTS3, K)
		50	(dbEL) > (EMK, DV3) > (DV2, DTS3, DTS2, K, S, D1, P)
		100	(dbEL) > (EMK) > (DV3, DV2, DTS3, DTS2, D1, S, K, P)
	(3)	25	(DTS3, DV3, DTS2) > (DV2, D1, dbEL) > (S, P, EMK, K)
		50	(DTS2, DTS3, EMK, DV3) > (P, S, D1, DV2, K) > (dbEL)
		100	(DTS2, EMK, DTS3) > (DV2, DV3, D1, P, S, K) > (dbEL)
	(4)	25	(EMK, DTS2) > (D1, DTS3, P, S) > (dbEL, DV2, K, DV3)
		50	(DV3) > (EMK, DV2, K, dbEL, DTS3) > (DTS2, S, D1, P)
		100	(K, D1, DV2, DTS3) > (S, EMK, DTS2, DV3) > (dbEL, P)

Note: The dependence structures are M3 ($f(X) = 2 + X + X^2$), M5 ($f(X) = 1/X$), and M9 ($f(X) = \sin(\pi X)$). (1) represents no random effect in Y; (2) represents additive random effects in Y; (3) represents multiplicative random effects in Y; (4) represents both additive and multiplicative random effects in Y. For each dependence structure and sample size, considered tests for independence are in three clusters. Within each cluster, results are ordered in descending order in terms of powers, as shown in parentheses. Between clusters, results are ordered in descending order in terms of powers, separated by the symbol >.

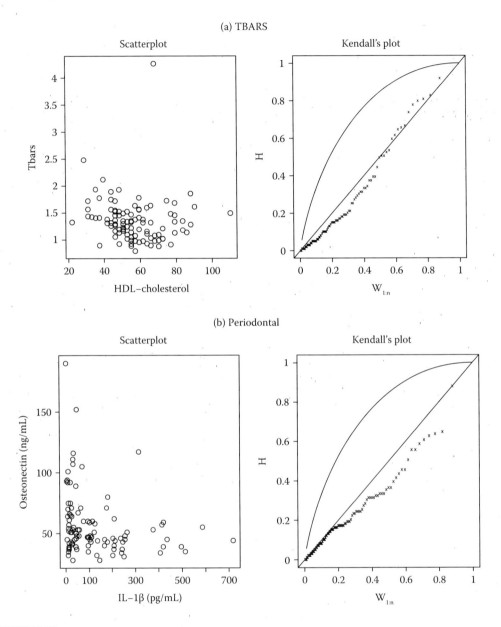

FIGURE 10.18

Panels (a) and (b) display the scatterplot (left side of each panel) and K-plot (right of each panel) based on the TBARS and the periodontal data, respectively.

test (dbEL) (Vexler et al. 2014e). The strategy was that a sample with sizes n_{sub} = 20, 30, 50, 70, and 100 was randomly selected from the data to be tested for independence at the 5% level of significance. For each test of independence, we repeated this strategy 1000 times calculating the mean of p-values. As shown in Table 10.6, this jackknife-type procedure showed that the EL-based hypothesis testing method and density-based EL ratio test have a stable power property and diagnose dependency faster than other methods with respect to the sample size. The EL-based hypothesis testing method and density-based EL ratio test start

TABLE 10.6

p-Values of the Tests of Independence in a Jackknife-Type Procedure Based on the TBARS Data and the Periodontal Data

Method	TBARS Data						Periodontal Data					
	20	30	50	60	70	100	20	30	50	70	85	100
P	0.426	0.438	0.432	0.422	0.392	0.245	0.318	0.244	0.124	0.056	0.031	0.016
K	0.343	0.266	0.134	0.090	0.053	0.007	0.294	0.209	0.093	0.028	0.009	0.002
S	0.356	0.287	0.155	0.109	0.067	0.010	0.305	0.219	0.098	0.031	0.010	0.002
EMK	0.301	0.222	0.100	0.059	0.032	0.003	0.306	0.223	0.103	0.033	0.011	0.002
DTS1	0.355	0.288	0.156	0.109	0.065	0.010	0.304	0.220	0.099	0.030	0.011	0.003
DV1	0.355	0.288	0.156	0.109	0.065	0.010	0.304	0.220	0.099	0.030	0.011	0.003
DTS2	0.380	0.322	0.189	0.139	0.095	0.028	0.316	0.236	0.117	0.048	0.023	0.008
DV2	0.489	0.431	0.238	0.167	0.080	0.006	0.539	0.488	0.358	0.227	0.077	0.010
DTS3	0.384	0.330	0.196	0.145	0.100	0.034	0.319	0.244	0.124	0.052	0.027	0.014
DV3	0.432	0.387	0.236	0.165	0.097	0.014	0.472	0.467	0.387	0.268	0.114	0.022
dbEL	0.346	0.264	0.133	0.080	0.044	0.001	0.344	0.257	0.171	0.093	0.045	0.013

to detect the dependence based on small samples, for example, $n_{sub} = 70$. Among those classical correlation-based methods, Kendall's rank correlation test can be recommended. The Pearson's product–moment correlation test completely fails.

10.6.2 Periodontal Disease

As an example, we consider a cross-sectional study (Ng et al. 2007) that evaluated the association between radiographic evidence of alveolar bone loss and the concentration of host-derived bone resorptive factor interleukin 1 beta (IL-1β) and markers of bone turnover (osteonectin) in stimulated human whole saliva collected from 100 untreated dental patients. In order to investigate candidate salivary biomarkers associated with alveolar bone loss, researchers are often interested in testing the independence between IL-1β and osteonectin to establish a biological linkage. Figure 10.19 presents the scatterplot of the data and the K-plot. The estimates of MIC and AUK measures are 0.287 and 0.429, respectively. In a manner similar to that described in the TBARS data, a jackknife-type procedure is conducted to examine different tests of independence with randomly selected subsamples of the sample sizes $n_{sub} = 20, 30, 50, 70, 85,$ and 100, repeating 1000 times. As shown in Table 10.7, among those classical correlation-based methods, Kendall's rank correlation test and Spearman's correlation test can be recommended. All methods but the data-driven testing using the U-statistic with $d(n) = 2, 3$ can detect the dependence starting from $n_{sub} = 85$.

10.6.3 VEGF Expression

The gynecologic oncology group study evaluated the association between the relative expression of the N-terminally truncated isoform and debulking status and the relative expression of vascular endothelial growth factor (VEGF) and VEGF receptor 1 based on 60 cases (Jewell et al. 2009). It is of great interest to test the independence between VEGF expression and VEGF receptor 1. Figure 10.19 presents the scatterplot of the data containing VEGF and VEGF receptor 1 expression measurements and the K-plot. The estimates of MIC and AUK measures are 0.706 and 0.687, respectively. In this data set,

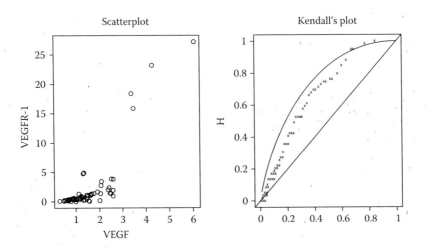

FIGURE 10.19

Scatterplot (left) and K-plot (right) based on the data containing VEGF expression and VEGF receptor 1 measurements.

TABLE 10.7

p-Values of the Tests of Independence Obtained via a Jackknife-Type Procedure Based on the Data Containing VEGF Expression and VEGF Receptor 1 Measurements

Method	Sample Size									
	10	11	12	13	14	15	16	17	18	19
P	0.059	0.045	0.038	0.032	0.025	0.019	0.015	0.012	0.009	0.007
S	0.057	0.044	0.034	0.025	0.020	0.014	0.011	0.008	0.006	0.003
K	0.050	0.037	0.028	0.020	0.015	0.011	0.008	0.006	0.004	0.002
EMK	0.054	0.040	0.030	0.022	0.017	0.012	0.009	0.006	0.004	0.003
DTS1	0.057	0.043	0.034	0.025	0.020	0.015	0.011	0.009	0.006	0.004
DV1	0.057	0.043	0.034	0.025	0.020	0.015	0.011	0.009	0.006	0.004
DTS2	0.077	0.059	0.047	0.037	0.031	0.024	0.018	0.014	0.010	0.007
DV2	0.122	0.095	0.079	0.065	0.053	0.036	0.029	0.024	0.015	0.011
DTS3	0.084	0.067	0.054	0.043	0.037	0.028	0.022	0.017	0.013	0.009
DV3	0.145	0.116	0.098	0.081	0.064	0.046	0.035	0.029	0.021	0.015
dbEL	0.082	0.064	0.051	0.038	0.029	0.021	0.016	0.010	0.007	0.005

measurements of VEGF expression and VEGF receptor 1 are highly dependent. In a similar manner described in the TBARS data, a jackknife-type procedure is conducted to examine different tests of independence with randomly selected subsamples of the sample size ranging from 10 to 19, repeating 5000 times. As shown in Table 10.7, among those classical correlation-based methods, Kendall's rank correlation performs the best. Except for the data-driven test using the U-statistic with $d(n) = 2, 3$, all methods can detect the dependence starting from $n_{sub} = 15$. Figure 10.20 displays measures of dependence, including AUK and MIC, as well as p-values obtained via a jackknife-type procedure, based on the data containing VEGF expression and VEGF receptor 1 measurements. It can be noted that the MIC measure of dependence slightly decreases as the sample size increases, demonstrating an inferior performance compared to the AUK measure of dependence.

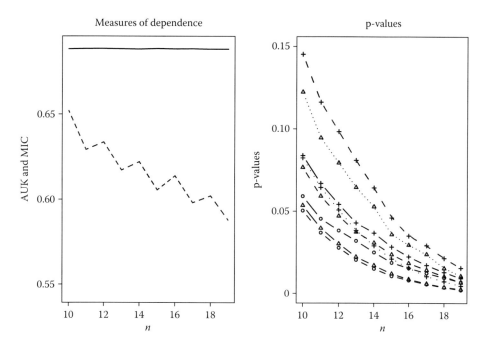

FIGURE 10.20

Measures of dependence (left panel) including AUK (black solid line) and MIC (gray dashed line), as well as p-values obtained via a jackknife-type procedure (right panel) based on the data containing VEGF expression and VEGF receptor 1 measurements: P (—○—), K (– – ○ – –), S (· · · ○ · · ·), EMK (—Δ—), DTS2 (– – Δ – –), DV2 (· · · Δ · · ·), DTS3 (—+—), DV3 (– – + – –), and dbEL (· · · + · · ·).

10.7 Discussion

In the set of the classical tests of dependence, including Pearson's correlation, Spearman's rank correlation, and Kendall's rank correlation, it is clear that Kendall's test demonstrates good power properties across most of the evaluated scenarios and practical examples; Pearson's test is very good for linear dependencies. However, in the nonmonotonic dependence structure, classical correlation-based tests tend to break down. Moreover, the correlation-based dependence measures calculated from a small sample may be totally misleading if not viewed in the context of its likely sampling error.

The empirical likelihood–based method (Einmahl and McKeague 2003) and the density-based empirical likelihood ratio test (Vexler et al. 2014e) possess the good property of a stable power and are suggested for use in the considered cases and the real data examples. The approaches based on the empirical likelihood technique, that is, the empirical likelihood–based method and the density-based empirical likelihood ratio test, avoid specifying a specific dependence structure. These empirical likelihood–based approaches and data-driven tests work very efficiently and are fast in the detection of linear, nonlinear, and random effects forms of dependence structures. Note that the data-driven rank test was developed given that data distributions satisfy a special assumption. In the case of the coexistence of additive and multiplicative random effects, the dependence is mostly difficult to recognize compared to other random effects formulations. We introduce a new and efficient dependence measure, AUK, based on the ROC curve concept. We present theoretical properties and applications of AUK. Furthermore, the graphical method of heat maps can be efficiently used in order to visually compare powers and various tests, providing clustering of methods.

10.8 Supplement

1. Fieller et al. (1957) investigated three measures of rank correlation, including Spearman's coefficient r_S, Kendall's coefficient r_K, and the Fisher–Yates coefficient (Fisher and Yates 1938), with the aid of the data, the sampling distributions, and relationships in the case where the basic variables, which have been ranked, follow bivariate normal distributions. The authors examined some known results on the distribution theory of r_S and r_K, for example, results of Kendall (1948) and Moran (1950). It was noted that for independent random rankings, the complete distributions of r_S and r_K have been obtained for small n by combinatorial enumeration and adequate approximations have been evolved for larger n, while in the case of correlated rankings, it is necessary to specify the nature of the dependence. The authors proposed a simple solution to deal with correlated rankings arising from the class of population models, for example, rankings generated by sampling from a bivariate normal parent (can be extended to a wider class of parental distributions) with correlation ρ. It was shown that if n is not too large the z-transforms, $z_S = \tanh^{-1} r_S = \dfrac{1}{2} \log_e \dfrac{1+r_S}{1-r_S}, z_K = \tanh^{-1} r_K$, are approximately normally distributed with variances nearly independent of ρ. It was shown that if the rankings are generated by one of a wide class of distributions of paired variables, then the z-transforms of the rank correlation measures z_S, z_K are normally distributed with variances dependent only on the sample size. This result makes it possible to make approximate comparisons of the rank coefficients r_S and z_K, for example, comparisons of their power in detecting differences in population ρ values.

2. Certain tests of independence by use of various simple functionals of the sample distribution function (d.f.) may possess superior power properties compared to other tests of independence, for example, tests based on $T_n(r) = S_n(r) - \prod_{j=1}^{m} S_{nj}(r_j)$, where $S_n(x)$ is n^{-1} times the number of X_i, all of whose components are less than or equal to the corresponding components of x. For example, the test based on $A_n = \sup |T_n(r)|$, a statistic constructed in the spirit of the Kolmogorov–Smirnov statistics, obviously has such properties. Motivated by this observation, Blum et al. (1961) derived the characteristic functions of the limiting d.f.'s of a class of test criteria of independence and tabled the corresponding d.f. in the bivariate case, where the test is equivalent to the one originally proposed by Hoeffding (1948). The authors also investigated the computational problems that arise in the inversion of characteristic functions, as well as techniques for computing the statistics and approximating the tail probabilities.

3. Bhuchongkul (1964) proposed a class of rank tests for the independence of two random variables X, Y on the basis of a random bivariate sample, (X_1, Y_1),

(X_2, Y_2), ..., (X_N, Y_N). Let $Z_{N,r_i} = 1$ $(Z'_{N,r_i} = 1)$ when $X_i(Y_i)$ is the r_ith(s_ith) smallest of the $X's(Y's)$ and $Z_{N,r_i} = 0$ $(Z'_{N,r_i} = 0)$ otherwise, and $E_{N,r_i}(E'_{N,s_i})$ be the expected value of the r_ith(s_ith) standard normal order statistic from a sample of size N. Then normal score test statistics have the form $T_N = N^{-1} \sum_{i=1}^{N} E_{N,r_i} E'_{N,s_i} Z_{N,r_i} Z'_{N,s_i}$ and

belong to the class of statistics considered by Fisher and Yates (1949), Terry (1952), and Hoeffding (1994). When $E_{N,r_i} = r_i$ and $E_{N,s_i} = s_i$, the resulting test statistic is equivalent to the Spearman rank correlation statistic. The author showed that the normal score test is the locally most powerful rank test, and asymptotically as efficient as the parametric correlation coefficient.

4. Bell and Doksum (1967) focused on characterizing the family of all distribution-free tests of independence, and those subfamilies that are optimal for specified alternative classes. It was shown that each distribution-free statistic is a function of a Pitman (or permutation) statistic and that the rank statistics are those whose distributions depend appropriately on the maximal invariant (Lehmann 1959). For parametric alternatives, the most powerful (Lehmann and Stein 1949) and the locally most powerful tests were shown to be Pitman tests based on the likelihood, while the corresponding optimal rank tests are analogous to those in the two-sample case (Capon 1961), and are closely related to those of Bhuchongkul (1964). The authors demonstrated that the normal score test is minimax for one reasonable nonparametric class of alternatives, while minimax for the other class is an unexpected statistic. The authors also extended the ideas of monotone tests developed by Chapman (1958) and others and derived analogous results for minimum power.

5. Bhattacharyya et al. (1970) presented exact one-sided rejection regions and Type I error control for the normal score test based on third-quadrant layer ranks. Given a random sample of (X_1,Y_1), (X_2,Y_2),..., (X_n,Y_n), the third-quadrant layer rank (Woodworth 1966) of Z_j, is defined as the number of points $(X_i - X_j, Y_i - Y_j)$, $1 \le i \le n$, that lie in the closed third quadrant (Woodworth 1966). The normal score layer rank test proposed was shown to be asymptotically locally most powerful for positive dependence in the bivariate normal distribution. The authors also proposed a simplified ad hoc version of the normal score test analogously to Kendall's τ-statistic and tabulated its rejection regions. The good performance of proposed tests was confirmed via Monte Carlo evaluation of power from two different types of bivariate distributions, both of which have positive correlation coefficients.

6. Schweizer and Wolff (1981) demonstrated that the copula of a pair of random variables X, Y is invariant under almost surely strictly increasing transformations of X and Y, and that any property of the joint distribution function of X and Y that is invariant under such transformations is solely a function of their copula. The authors proposed several natural nonparametric measures of dependence for pairs of random variables based on copulas and showed that these measures possess many pleasant properties when evaluated according to a reasonable modification of Renyi's set of criteria (Rényi 1959).

7. Jupp and Spurr (1985) proposed two families of invariant tests for independence of random variables on compact Riemannian manifolds, based on Gine's Sobolev norms, which are obtained by mapping the manifolds into Hilbert spaces. The authors applied this approach to uniform scores to obtain a class of distribution-free tests in the bivariate circular case. It was suggested to employ randomization

tests for general compact manifolds and distribution-free tests based on uniform scores for the bivariate circular case. The tests were illustrated with a study in the directions of magnetization of rock before and after heat treatment.

8. Schriever (1987) introduced a partial ordering for positive-dependent bivariate distributions, called "more associated," which expresses the strength of positive dependence. The ordering "more associated" can easily be generalized to the multivariate. The ordering makes precise an intuitive notion of one bivariate distribution being more positive dependent than another. The author showed that tests of independence based on rank statistics such as Spearman's rho, Kendall's tau, Fisher–Yates normal score statistic, van der Waerden's statistic, and the quadrant statistic are more powerful under increasing positive dependence. These measures of positive dependence were demonstrated to be able to preserve the ordering stochastically in samples when the ordering "more associated" is present between two underlying distributions (with continuous marginals).

9. Kimeldorf and Sampson (1989) developed a structure for studying concepts of positive dependence and explored the relationships between and among three sets of positive dependence concepts: positive dependence orderings, positive dependence properties (such as positive quadrant dependence and total positivity of order 2), and measures of positive association (such as Spearman's ρ_S and Kendall's τ). With regards to dependence properties and measures of association, Kimeldorf and Sampson claimed that "it is often unclear exactly what dependence (property) a specific measure of positive association is attempting to describe." As a partial response, Nelsen (1992) presented that as both a population parameter and a sample statistic, Spearman's ρ_S is a measure of average positive (and negative) quadrant dependence, while Kendall's τ is a measure of average total positivity (and reverse regularity) of order 2.

10. In order to develop families of bivariate distributions to model nonnormal variations, Genest and Rivest (1993) provided statistical inference procedures for a wide class of bivariate distributions that are generated by so-called Archimedean copulas. A bivariate distribution function $H(x, y)$ with marginals $F(x)$ and $G(y)$ is said to be generated by an Archimedean copula if it can be expressed in the form $H(x, y) = \phi^{-1}[\phi\{F(x)\} + \phi\{G(y)\}]$ for some convex, decreasing function ϕ defined on $(0,1]$ in such a way that $\phi(1) = 0$. Archimedean copulas encompass many well-known systems of bivariate distributions, including those of the Gumbel, Clayton, Frank, Hougaard, and frailty models. Providing a suitable representation of the dependence structure between two variates X and Y in the light of a random sample $(X_1, Y_1), \ldots, (X_n, Y_n)$, Genest and Rivest (1993) examined the problem of selecting an Archimedean copula and proposed a method-of-moments estimation technique based on Kendall's tau. The methods were illustrated by a uranium exploration data set (Cook and Johnson 1981).

11. Blest (1999) extended the use of Kendall's measure τ as an extent of disarray of permuted data, from the cases based on originally ordered data to the cases where a limited number of the original set are selected and reordered. A choice (and ordering) of a subset may be of interest in various ways, for example, in the case where a team is to be selected from a group of possible members presented in a particular order and where the psychological constructs of "recency" and "primacy" may come into play so that the order of selection is not independent of the order of presentation of the data. Consider the case where only

m ($m \in \{2, 3, 4, ..., n - 3, n - 2\}$) of the original n items are chosen and ranked. The author presented a new set of integer sequences representing the frequency of permutations of $m \leq n - 1$ chosen items requiring a given number of transpositions for each integer $n \geq 4$. For large n and m, it was shown that the distribution of relative frequencies follows a normal distribution for sufficiently large m, effectively for $m \geq 10$.

12. Wilcox (2001) discussed the use of testing the hypothesis that the correlation between two variables is zero using a standard Student's t-test in order to detect an association and the marginal τ-distributions. The author noted two practical problems with this strategy. One is that even though the hypothesis of a zero correlation is true, the probability of rejecting could be 1 for large sample sizes in the cases where the correlation between two random variables is 0, while Student's τ-test is not even asymptotically correct. The same practical problems arise when standard methods based on a linear regression model and the least-squares estimators are applied. The other problem is that Student's t-test can miss nonlinear associations. Motivated by these practical problems, especially the latter problem, the author suggested an approach that avoids both of the difficulties by testing $H_0 : E(Y|X) = E(Y)$. This method may have less power than Student's t-test in some situations due in part to the t-test's use of an incorrect estimate of the standard error. It was shown that the Cramer–von Mises form of the test statistic is generally better than the Kolmogorov–Smirnov form based on simulations.

13. Fisher and Switzer (2001) suggested dealing with specific forms of association by visualization since graphs have the potential to assess a far richer class of bivariate dependence structures than any collection of tests. The authors described the use of a combination of chi-plots and the usual scatterplot to provide a practical tool for manifesting dependence structures. The chi-plot depends on the data only through the values of their ranks and supplements a scatterplot of the data by providing a graph that has characteristic patterns depending on whether the variates (a) are independent, (b) have some degree of monotone relationship (i.e., nonzero grade correlation), or (c) have a more complex dependence structure. The authors illustrated some of the wide variety of forms of dependence that a single chi-plot can highlight and presented a catalog of the typical behavior of the chi-plot in the presence of more complex forms of dependence. The authors illustrated the methods via three examples: (a) a set of 88 measurements of the relationship between the equivalence ratio and a measure of the richness of the air–ethanol mix (Simonoff 1996), (b) a set of 28 measurements of the size of the annual spawning stock of salmon compared with corresponding production of new catchable-sized fish in the Skeena River (Simonoff 1996), and (c) an application to multivariate data.

14. Ding and Wang (2004) presented a nonparametric procedure for testing marginal independence between two failure time variables given only bivariate current status data. The procedure can be regarded as a generalization of the Mantel–Haenszel test. The authors demonstrated that bivariate current status data can be naturally represented by 2×2 tables formed at observed monitoring times. The asymptotic properties of the test were derived and the finite sample performance was investigated based on simulations. The authors illustrated the method by analyzing data from a community-based study of cardiovascular epidemiology in Taiwan.

15. Two random variables are positive quadrant dependent (PQD) when the probability that they are simultaneously large (or small) is at least as great as it would be if they were independent (Lehmann 1966). Scaillet (2005) considered a consistent test of PQD, which is similar to a Kolmogorov–Smirnov test, of the complete set of restrictions that relate to the copula representation of positive quadrant dependence. Inference of the test was made and justified relying on a simulation-based multiplier method and a bootstrap method. The finite sample behavior of both methods was studied based on Monte Carlo experiments. The methods were illustrated with American insurance claim data and a study of the presence of positive quadrant dependence in life expectancies at birth of males and females across countries.

16. Taskinen et al. (2005) proposed new multivariate extensions of Kendall's tau and Spearman's rho statistics for multivariate nonparametric tests of independence. Two different approaches were discussed. One approach employs interdirection proportions to estimate the cosines of angles between centered observation vectors and between differences of observation vectors. The other approach uses covariances between affine-equivariant multivariate signs and ranks. The tests have advantages over the quadrant test extensions in that they do not require centering (i.e., subtracting a location estimator) and generally have better power properties than the quadrant test extensions. When each vector is elliptically symmetric, the test statistics arising from these two approaches appear to be asymptotically equivalent. For data in common dimensions, the spatial sign versions are easy to compute, and they provide intuitive, practical, robust alternatives to multivariate normal theory methods. The authors developed asymptotic theory to approximate the finite sample null distributions and calculate limiting Pitman efficiencies. Small sample null permutation distributions were presented. The tests were compared with the classical Wilks test via a simple simulation study, and the theory was illustrated by a study of the effect of an aerobic conditioning program on cholesterol levels (McNaughton and Davies 1987).

17. Rukhin and Osmoukhina (2005) focused on comparisons of two different algorithms based on their similarity scores for face recognition. The authors explored the possibility of using nonparametric dependence characteristics to evaluate biometric systems or algorithms and investigated the extensions of classical rank correlation coefficients to the case when only a given number of top matches is used. Noticing that difficulties may arise with these coefficients in capturing the total correlation, the author studied a version of a scan statistic that measures co-occurrence of rankings for two arbitrary algorithms. The exact covariance structure of the statistic was presented for a pair of independent algorithms. Classical results on linear rank statistics were to derive the asymptotic normality of the test statistic in general. The concept of copula was shown to be useful for the study of nonparametric dependence characteristics. In particular, it was demonstrated that the random scores of considered recognition methods can be modeled by a two-parameter family of copulas exhibiting strong tail dependence. The results were applied to an example from a face recognition technology program (Phillips et al. 2000), in which four recognition algorithms each produced rankings from a gallery.

18. Bolboaca and Jäntschi (2006) studied a sample of 67 pyrimidine derivatives with inhibitory activity on *Escherichia coli* dihydrofolate reductase (DHFR) by the use of molecular descriptor families on structure–activity relationships. The use of

Pearson, Spearman, Kendall, and gamma correlation coefficients in the analysis of structure–activity relationships of biologic active compounds was studied and presented.

19. Many joint distributions may exhibit weak dependence. In this case, the sample value of Spearman's rho could be about 50% larger than the sample value of Kendall's tau. Fredricks and Nelsen (2007) employed the theory of copulas to investigate the relationship between Spearman's rho and Kendall's tau for pairs of continuous random variables. The authors showed that under mild regularity conditions, the limit of the ratio of Spearman's rho to Kendall's tau is 3/2 as the joint distribution of the random variables approaches that of two independent random variables. Sufficient conditions were presented for determining the direction of the inequality between three times tau and twice rho when the underlying joint distribution is absolutely continuous. In particular, the authors provided an elegant analytical proof of a result due to Capéraà and Genest (see Fredricks and Nelsen [2007] for the reference), namely, that $\rho \geq \tau \geq 0$ whenever one of X or Y is simultaneously left-tail decreasing and right-tail increasing in the other variable. Fredricks and Nelsen (2007) noted that Daniels' inequality (see Fredricks and Nelsen [2007] for the reference) amounts to saying that if C is an arbitrary copula with partial derivatives $C_1(u, v) = \partial C(u, v)/\partial u$ and $C_2(u, v) = \partial C(u, v)/\partial v$, then $\left| \int_{[0,1]^2} \{u - C_2(u,v)\}\{v - C_1(u,v)\} \, du \, dv \right| \leq \frac{1}{12}$. Fredricks and Nelsen presented refined bounds $\tau - (1 - \tau^2) \leq 3\tau - 2\rho \leq \tau + (1 - \tau^2)$, independently found by Daniels as well as Durbin and Stuart (see Fredricks and Nelsen [2007] for the reference). In this context, we note that Genest and Nešlehová (2009) presented a simple analytical proof related to the Daniels' inequality.

20. Schmid and Schmidt (2007) considered the nonparametric estimation of multivariate population versions of Spearman's rho via the empirical copula. The estimators were shown to be asymptotically normally distributed using empirical process under rather weak assumptions concerning the copula. The asymptotic variances were derived for some copulas of simple structure, which are determined by the copula and its partial derivatives. The obtained formulas were shown to be suitable for explicit computations if the copula possesses a simple structure. Otherwise, a bootstrap algorithm can be employed to obtain the asymptotic variances.

21. Zhang (2008) proposed a class of quotient correlations that can be used as an alternative to Pearson's correlation, and a class of rank-based quotient correlations that can be used as an alternative to Spearman's rank correlation. The newly proposed quotient correlation coefficients can measure nonlinear dependence where the regular correlation coefficient is generally not applicable and are more intuitive and flexible in cases where the tail behavior of data is important. A test for independence was developed based on the quotient correlation concept, in which the test statistic was shown to follow a limiting gamma distribution and therefore a gamma statistic, unlike most test statistics, which are either normal or χ^2 asymptotically. When testing nonlinear dependence, even in cases where the Fisher's Z-transformation test may fail to reach a correct conclusion, the test statistic based on the quotient correlations possesses high power. The quotient correlation can also easily and intuitively be adjusted to values at tails that generate two new gamma statistics: the tail quotient correlation and the tail independence

test statistics. The authors employed both simulated data and a real data analysis of Internet traffic to illustrate the advantages of using these new concepts. The methods were illustrated with a study of testing tail (in)dependence of the joint behavior of large values of three Internet traffic variables: size of response, time duration of response, and throughput (rate = size/time), which are in the context of HTTP (web browsing) responses.

22. Székely and Rizzo (2009) proposed new approaches to measuring multivariate dependence and testing the joint independence of random vectors in arbitrary dimension, including distance correlation as well as distance and Brownian covariance with respect to a stochastic process. Distance covariance and distance correlation are analogous to product–moment covariance and correlation, but generalize and extend these classical bivariate measures of dependence. The distance covariance statistic is defined as the square root of $V_n^2 = n^{-2} \sum_{k,l=1}^{n} A_{kl} B_{kl}$, where A_{kl} and B_{kl} are simple linear functions of the pairwise distances between sample elements. Distance correlation, a standardized version of distance covariance, is zero if and only if the random vectors are independent. It was shown that population distance covariance coincides with the covariance with respect to Brownian motion; thus, both can be called Brownian distance covariance. In the bivariate case, Brownian covariance is the natural extension of product–moment covariance, since Pearson product–moment covariance is obtained by replacing the Brownian motion in the definition with identity. Note that while uncorrelatedness can sometimes replace independence, uncorrelatedness is too weak to imply a central limit theorem even for strongly stationary summands. Therefore, Brownian covariance and correlation can be recommended compared to the classical Pearson covariance and correlation.

23. Gretton and Györfi (2010) developed three simple and explicit procedures for testing the independence of two multidimensional random variables. The first two procedures partition the underlying space and evaluate the test statistics, including generalizations of the L_1 divergence measure and log-likelihood, on the resulting discrete empirical measures. The third test statistic was defined as a kernel-based independence measure. Distribution-free strong consistent tests, meaning that both on H_0 and its complement the tests make almost no error after a random sample size based on large deviation bounds, were derived. Asymptotically α-level tests were obtained from the limiting distribution of the test statistics. For the latter tests, the Type I error converges to a fixed nonzero value, and the Type II error drops to zero, for increasing sample size. All tests reject the null hypothesis of independence if the test statistics become large. The performance of the tests was evaluated experimentally on benchmark data proposed by Gretton et al. (2008).

24. Nazarov and Stepanova (2009) considered a multivariate version of Spearman's rho for testing independence and derived the asymptotic efficiency under a general distribution model specified by the dependence function. The multivariate version of Spearman's rho was compared with other multivariate Spearman-type test statistics in terms of asymptotic efficiency. Conditions for Pitman optimality of the test were established.

25. Quessy (2012) proposed new tests for the hypothesis of bivariate extreme-value dependence and investigated test statistics that are continuous functionals of

either Kendall's process or its version with estimated parameters. The procedures considered were based on linear combinations of moments and on Cramer–von Mises distances. A suitably adapted version of the multiplier central limit theorem for Kendall's process enables the computation of asymptotically valid p-values. The author considered a generalization of the moment-based methodology of Ghoudi et al. and Ben Ghorbal et al. (see Quessy [2012] for the references) to higher-order moments of T. The author developed tests based on the distribution function of T, rather than only some of its moments. The power of the tests was evaluated for small, moderate, and large sample sizes, as well as asymptotically, under local alternatives. An illustration with a real data set was presented.

26. Zheng et al. (2012) examined the applicability of Pearson's correlation as a measure of explained variance. The authors noted that one of its limitations is that asymmetry in explained variance has not been accounted for. Aiming to develop broad applicable correlation measures, the authors studied a pair of generalized measures of correlation (GMC) that deals with asymmetries in explained variances, and linear or nonlinear relations between random variables. The authors presented scenarios under which the paired measures are identical, and they become a symmetric correlation measure that is the same as the squared Pearson's correlation coefficient. The efficiency of the test statistics was illustrated in simulation examples. In real-data analysis, the authors presented an important application of GMC in explained variances and market movements among three important economic and financial monetary indicators.

27. Birnbaum (2012) developed tests of independence and stationarity in choice data collected with small samples, based on the approach of Smith and Batchelder (2008). The technique was intended to distinguish cases where a person is systematically changing "true" preferences (from one group of trials to another) from cases in which a person is following a random preference mixture model with independently and identically distributed sampling in each trial. Preference reversals were counted between all pairs of repetitions. The variance of these preference reversals between all pairs of repetitions was then calculated. The distribution of this statistic was simulated by a Monte Carlo procedure in which the data are randomly permuted and the statistic was obtained in each simulated sample. A second test was obtained based on the computation of the correlation between the mean number of preference reversals and the difference between replicates, which was also simulated by Monte Carlo. The author illustrated the method using the data of Regenwetter et al. (2011), where 8 of 18 subjects showed significant deviations from the independence assumptions by one or both of these tests.

28. Xu et al. (2013) conducted a comparative analysis of Spearman's rho and Kendall's tau with respect to samples drawn from bivariate normal and contaminated normal populations. The authors suggested by theoretical and simulation results that contrary to the opinion of equivalence between Spearman's rho and Kendall's tau in some literature, the behaviors of Spearman's rho and Kendall's tau are strikingly different in the aspects of bias effect, variance, mean squared error, and asymptotic relative efficiency. The new findings provided deeper insights into the two most widely used rank-based correlation coefficients, as well as a guidance for choosing which one to use under the circumstances where Pearson's product–moment correlation coefficient fails to apply.

29. When the goal is the quantification of a relationship between two variables, not simply the establishment of its existence, Reimherr and Nicolae (2013) presented a framework for selecting and developing measures of dependence. The authors started with only a few nonrestrictive guidelines focused on existence, range, and interpretability, which provide a very open and flexible framework. For quantification, the most crucial is the notion of interpretability, whose foundation can be found in the work of Goodman and Kruskal (1979), and whose importance can be seen in the popularity of tools such as R^2 in linear regression. While Goodman and Kruskal developed measures with probabilistic interpretations, the authors demonstrated how more general measures of information can be used to achieve the same goal. To that end, the authors presented a strategy for building dependence measures that is designed to allow practitioners to tailor measures to their needs, and it was demonstrated how many well-known measures fit in with the framework. The authors illustrated the guide in the selection and development of a dependence measure with two real data examples, including a study exploring U.S. income and education and a study examining measures of dependence for functional data of geomagnetic storms.

11

Goodness-of-Fit Tests (Tests for Normality)

11.1 Introduction

Many statistical procedures are, strictly speaking, only appropriate when the corresponding parametric assumptions that are made regarding data distributions are sufficiently accurate. If the data distribution under the null hypothesis is completely known, then testing for goodness of fit is equivalent to testing for uniformity. For example, when we observe independent and identically distributed (i.i.d.) data points $X_1, \ldots, X_n$ with $F(u) = \Pr(X_1 \le u)$, where the function $F(u)$ is completely defined and known under H_0, one can transform the observations as $F(X_1), \ldots, F(X_n)$ to test for H_0 that says $F(X_1), \ldots, F(X_n)$ are uniformly [0, 1] distributed. In general, testing distributional assumptions for normality and uniformity is widely employed. Tests focused on these two distributions have been one of the major areas of continuing statistical research both theoretically and practically. Thus, tests for goodness of fit, especially tests for normality, have a very important role in statistical inference applied to clinical experiments. Testing composite hypotheses of normality, i.e., H_0: the population is normally distributed, versus H_1: the population is not normally distributed, is well addressed in statistical literature (e.g., Vexler and Gurevich 2010b). Some well-known tests of fit are the Shapiro–Wilk test, the Kolmogorov–Smirnov test, and the Anderson–Darling test. Among these tests, the Shapiro–Wilk test is highly efficient (Razali and Wah 2011; Shapiro and Wilk 1965; Vexler and Gurevich 2010b). For more details regarding goodness-of-fit tests, we refer the reader to Huber-Carol et al. (2002), Vexler and Gurevich (2010b), Claeskens and Hjort (2004) and Vexler et al. (2011b).

11.2 Shapiro–Wilk Test for Normality

The Shapiro–Wilk test employs the null hypothesis principle to check whether a sample of i.i.d. observations $X_1, \ldots, X_n$ came from a normally distributed population. The test statistic has the form

$$W = \frac{\left(\sum_{i=1}^{n} a_i X_{(i)} \right)^2}{\sum_{i=1}^{n} (X_i - \bar{X})^2},$$

where $X_{(i)}$ is the ith order statistic, that is, the ith smallest number in the sample, and $\bar{X}$ is the sample mean; the constants a_i are given by

$$(a_1, \ldots, a_n) = \frac{m^T V^{-1}}{(m^T V^{-1} V^{-1} m)^{1/2}},$$

where $m = (m_1, \ldots, m_n)^T$ and $m_1, \ldots, m_n$ are the expected values of the order statistics of independent and identically distributed random variables sampled from the standard normal distribution, and V is the covariance matrix of those order statistics. For example, when the sample size is 10, we have $a_1 = 0.5739$, $a_2 = 0.3291$, $a_3 = 0.2141$, $a_4 = 0.1224$, and $a_5 = 0.0399$. The null hypothesis is rejected if W is below a pre-determined threshold. Note that the Shapiro–Wilk test does not depend on the distribution of data under the null hypothesis and the corresponding critical value can be calculated numerically using Monte Carlo techniques; see Chapter 16 for details.

It should be noted that tests for normality can be subject to low power, especially when the sample size is small. Thus, a Q–Q plot (see Chapter 3) is recommended for verification in addition to the test (Wilk and Gnanadesikan 1968).

Example 11.1: Testing for Normality Using the Shapiro-Wilk Test

The following program shows how to implement the Shapiro–Wilk test in practice. We use R to simulate $n = 100$ data points from $N(0,1)$, $Uniform(0,1)$, and $\exp(1)$ distributions and check the data for normality. The function `shapiro.test` yields the test statistic and the corresponding p-value, as seen below:

```
> n<-100
>
> # N(0,1)
> x<-rnorm(n,mean=0,sd=1)
> shapiro.test(x)

        shapiro-wilk normality test

data: x
w = 0.9876, p-value = 0.4825

> # Uniform(0,1)
> y<-runif(n,min=0,max=1)
> shapiro.test(y)

        shapiro-wilk normality test

data: y
w = 0.9545, p-value = 0.001674

> #exp(1)
> z<-rexp(n,rate=1)
> shapiro.test(z)

        shapiro-wilk normality test

data: z
w = 0.8113, p-value = 5.574e-10
```

For the data simulated from a $N(0,1)$ distribution, we fail to reject the null hypothesis at the 0.05 significance level with p-value = 0.4825, suggesting that there is not sufficient evidence to conclude the data are not from the normal distribution. For the data simulated from either the $Uniform(0,1)$ or $\exp(1)$ distributions, we reject the null hypothesis at the 0.05 significance level with p-values of 0.0017 and <0.0001, respectively, stating that there is sufficient evidence to conclude the data are not from the normal distributions.

11.3 Supplement

11.3.1 Tests for Normality

1. Kac et al. (1955) investigated testing whether the distribution function (d.f.) $G(x)$ of the observed independent variables $x_1, \ldots, x_n$ is a member of a given class, for example, a class of normal d.f.'s. The authors considered tests of normality based on $v_n = \delta(G_n^*(y), N(y \mid \bar{x}, s^2))$ and $w_n = \int (G_n^*(y), N(y \mid \bar{x}, s^2))^2 d_y N(y \mid \bar{x}, s^2))$, where $F(y)$ and $G(y)$ are any two d.f.'s, $G_n^*(y)$ is the empirical d.f. associated with $G(y)$, $\delta(F, G) = \sup_y |F(y) - G(y)|$, and $N(y|\mu, \sigma^2)$ is the normal d.f. with mean μ and variance σ^2. The asymptotic power of these tests was shown to be considerably greater than that of the optimum χ^2-test. For a certain Gaussian process $Z(t)$, $0 \le t \le 1$, it was shown that the sample functions of $Z(t)$ are continuous with probability 1, and that
$$\lim_{n \to \infty} \Pr\{nw_n < a\} = \Pr\{W < a\}, \text{ where } W = \int_0^1 [Z(t)]^2 dt.$$

2. In order to test a complete sample for normality, Shapiro and Wilk (1965) introduced a new statistical procedure in which the test statistic was obtained by dividing the square of an appropriate linear combination of the sample order statistics by the usual symmetric estimate of variance. The statistic is appropriate for a test of the composite hypothesis of normality since this ratio was shown to be both scale and origin invariant. The test procedure was illustrated with three examples: (a) a sample of weights in pounds of 11 men: 148, 154, 158, 160, 161, 162, 166, 170, 182, 195, and 236 (Snedecor 1946); (b) an extract of 200 random sampling numbers from the Kendall–Babington Smith Tracts for Computers No. 24 (Kendall 1948); and (c) an example of a confounded 2^5 factorial experiment on effects of five factors on yields of penicillin (Davies and Box 1956).

3. Stephens (1974) provided a practical guide to goodness-of-fit tests using statistics based on the empirical distribution function. The author examined five of the leading statistics and three important situations. The statistics considered include Durbin's D-test (1961), the Cramer–von Mises W^2-test (1928), the Kuiper U-tests (1960), Watson's U^2-test (1961), and the Anderson–Darling A test (1954). Three important situations considered include the cases where the hypothesized distribution $F(x)$ is completely specified and where $F(x)$ represents the normal or exponential distribution with one or more parameters to be estimated from the data. For each situation, empirical distribution function statistics can be easily calculated. The tests based on empirical distribution function require only one line of significance points and were shown to be competitive in terms of power.

4. Hegazy and Green (1975) classified existing tests of goodness of fit into four categories: (a) the likelihood ratio and Pearson tests, (b) tests based on the empirical distribution function, (c) tests based on sample moments, and (d) tests based on sample ordered statistics. The authors presented some new tests of the goodness of fit of the uniform and normal distributions (both with unknown parameters) using order statistic properties. The authors derived approximate distributions for some of these using formulas obtained for the first four moments and obtained critical values by simulation. Approximate relationships for the dependence of the critical values of the test criterion on the sample size so that the tabulation does not involve the sample size were presented.

The authors investigated powers of the tests under certain alternatives and revealed that some of them are some of the most powerful goodness-of-fit tests available for the related hypotheses.

5. The criteria of Shapiro and Wilk (1965) and Shapiro and Francia (1972) have the same form, differing only in the definition of the coefficients, where the computation of the Shapiro–Francia test is much simpler. Sarkadi (1975) proved that the Shapiro–Francia test of normality is consistent. More generally, the version of it that tests the hypothesis that the distribution belongs to a two-parameter family of distributions with location and scale parameters is consistent.

6. Pettitt and Stephens (1976) modified Cramer–von Mises-type statistics so that tests of goodness of fit could be made for the simple hypothesis with censored data. Pettitt (1976) developed asymptotic theory for the distribution of Cramer–von Mises statistics for testing the goodness of fit of censored samples when tests of fit were made with unknown parameters. Based on the derived limiting covariance function of the empirical process when estimators from censored samples were used, the asymptotic distributions of Cramer–von Mises statistics were derived when testing for normality, with the mean and variance unknown for single-sided and symmetric censoring. The authors presented asymptotic percentage points for the Cramer–von Mises statistic, the Anderson–Darling statistic, and the Watson statistic. By Monte Carlo methods, the author investigated the small sample distributions.

7. Spiegelhalter (1977) proposed a tractable location and scale-invariant test for normality against all symmetric alternatives. Focusing on symmetric alternatives with unknown location and scale, the test statistic was shown to closely approximate a combination of two traditional test statistics, and was shown to have a Bayesian interpretation. Based on a simulation study, it was shown that the test compares favorably with a number of existing tests. The author applied the test for normality to Darwin's data (Box and Tiao 2011), where the data were assumed to be drawn from an asymmetric population.

8. The Anderson–Darling goodness-of-fit statistic was shown to be a powerful omnibus test of normality when the mean and variance are unknown. Pettitt (1977) presented tables for calculating small sample percentage points of the statistic and the percentage points that were derived from smoothing empirical percentage points using the asymptotic percentage points. Based on these percentage points, a joint assessment of normality was made based on several independent samples using Fisher's method. The method was compared with the method based on the Shapiro–Wilk statistic in terms of empirical power, and it was shown that there is little difference between the methods based on the two different statistics.

9. Lin and Mudholkar (1980) demonstrated that the mean and the variance of a random sample are independently distributed if and only if the parent population is normal. This characterization was used as a basis for developing a test, termed the Z-test, for the composite hypothesis of normality against asymmetric alternatives. The null distribution of the Z-test statistic was for practical purposes satisfactorily approximated by a normal distribution for samples of size 5 up to 100. The author derived the large sample null distribution and the consistency of the test and showed that the Z-test has good power properties relative to some well-known competitors based on a Monte Carlo power study.

10. Shapiro and Wilk's (1965) *W*-statistic arguably provides the best omnibus test of normality, but is currently limited to sample sizes between 3 and 50. Royston (1982) extended *W* up to a sample size of 2000 and presented an approximate normalizing transformation suitable for computer implementation. The authors presented a novel application of using *W* to fit the three-parameter lognormal distribution.

11. Oja (1983) presented a family of statistics for testing normality that includes new tests for skewness, kurtosis, and bimodality alternatives. The tests were shown to be simple to use, and their power properties were demonstrated to be as good as those of the very similar U-statistics given by Oja (1981), that is,

$$T_1 = \left(\frac{n}{3}\right)^{-1} \sum \frac{X_{(k)} - X_{(j)}}{X_{(k)} - X_{(i)}}, \quad T_2 = \left(\frac{n}{4}\right)^{-1} \sum \frac{X_{(k)} - X_{(j)}}{X_{(l)} - X_{(i)}},$$

where $X_{(1)}, \ldots, X_{(n)}$ is an ordered sample from a distribution with an unknown cumulative distribution function, and the sums are respectively over $1 \le i < j < k \le n$ and $1 \le i < j < k < l \le n$.

12. Verrill and Johnson (1987) established the asymptotic equivalence of a class of statistics based on different choices of normal scores and concluded that the Shapiro–Francia, Filliben, Weisberg–Bingham, and de Wet–Venter versions of the statistic are asymptotically equivalent. It was shown that this asymptotic equivalence also holds for the Type I and Type II censored data cases.

13. Verrill and Johnson (1988) investigated the plausibility of the normal (or lognormal) model that is needed when the observations on strength or life length are right-censored in a wide variety of applications. The authors showed that the plotting procedure still applies if the observations are censored at a fixed-order statistic or a fixed time and investigated the corresponding distribution theory for some modified versions of the Shapiro–Wilk correlation statistic. Results from an empirical power study and large sample critical values were presented and compared with the Monte Carlo values.

14. Zhang and Wu (2005) proposed powerful omnibus tests of normality based on the likelihood ratio. It was shown that they outperform the best tests in the literature, including the Shapiro–Wilk and Anderson–Darling tests for normality in terms of power.

15. Dong and Giles (2007) derived the empirical likelihood ratio (ELR) (see Chapter 6) test for the problem of testing for normality and provided the sampling properties of the ELR test and four other commonly used tests. Using the Monte Carlo simulation technique, the power comparisons against a wide range of alternative distributions showed that the empirical likelihood ratio test is the most powerful of these tests in certain situations.

16. Coin (2008) introduced a new goodness-of-fit statistic test for normality based on a polynomial regression. Based on simulation studies, the authors made a comparison between the new procedure and some well-known tests. It was shown to be very effective in detecting nonnormality when the alternative distribution is symmetric.

17. Rahman and Govindarajulu (1997) modified Shapiro and Wilk's test for normality *W* such that it can be extended for all sample sizes. The critical values of the modified test statistic $\tilde{W}$ were given for sample sizes up to $n = 5000$. The empirical

moments showed that the null distribution of $\tilde{W}$ is skewed to the left and is consistent for all sample sizes. Empirical powers of $\tilde{W}$ were also comparable with those of W.

11.3.2 Tests for Normality Based on Characteristic Functions

1. Epps and Pulley (1983) proposed an omnibus test of normality, which uses a weighted integral of the squared modulus of the difference between the characteristic functions of the sample and of the normal distribution. It was shown that the test has high power against many alternative hypotheses.

2. In order to suggest a simple test of the composite hypothesis of normality against the alternative that the underlying distribution is long-tailed, Hall and Welsh (1983) presented a simple test for normality based on the behavior of the empirical characteristic function in the neighborhood of the origin. The test was shown to be very competitive with several well-known tests for normality, such as tests proposed by Shapiro and Wilk (1965) and the standardized fourth moment test.

3. Csorgo (1986) extended the univariate weak convergence theorem of Murota and Takeuchi (1981) for the Mahalanobis transform of the d-variate empirical characteristic function, $d \geq 1$. The author proposed a maximal deviation statistic for testing the composite hypothesis of d-variate normality. By using Fernique's inequality in conjunction with a combination of analytic, numerical analytic, and computer techniques, exact upper bounds for the asymptotic percentage points of the statistic were derived. The resulting conservative large sample test was shown to be consistent against every alternative with components having a finite variance. Based on Monte Carlo experiments, the performance of the test on some well-known data sets was evaluated. The performance of the test was illustrated on the well-known Norton's bank data of size 780 as given in Yule (1950, p. 205) and Fisher's *Iris* setosa data originally analyzed by Fisher (1936b).

11.3.3 Test for Normality Based on Sample Entropy

1. Vasicek (1976) introduced a test of the composite hypothesis of normality based on the property of the normal distribution that its entropy exceeds that of any other distribution with a density of the same variance. The test statistic was based on a class of estimators of entropy and was shown to be a consistent test of the null hypothesis for all alternatives without a singular continuous part. The power of the test was estimated against several alternatives. It was demonstrated that the test compares favorably with other tests for normality.

2. Vexler and Gurevich (2010b) introduced the density-based empirical likelihood methodology (see Chapter 6) for constructing powerful goodness-of-fit tests. The density-based empirical likelihood ratio test for normality was shown to be an extension of Vasicek's (1976) sample entropy-based test for normality.

3. Prescott (1976) examined the effect of outliers on a test of normality based on sample entropy using sensitivity contours. The contours were compared with those of the Shapiro–Wilk W-test, and it was shown that the entropy test is considerably less sensitive to outliers than the W-test. The test was illustrated with

an example of a confounded 2^5 experiment on effects of five factors on yields of penicillin described by Davies (1954).

4. Tusnady (1977) investigated sequences of tests with error $\exp(-nA)$ of the first type. It was shown that the error of the second type of such a sequence of tests is bounded by $\exp(-nB)$, where B is determined by the Kullback–Leibler information distance of the hypotheses tested. The author proposed using the information distance between the empirical measure and the null hypothesis on a finite partition of the sample space as a test statistic. The exact Bahadur slope of the proposed statistic was investigated. A sufficient condition was provided that ensures that this test has error of the second type about $\exp(-nB)$ with the best possible B. Tusnady (1977) discussed an asymptotic optimality of tests for normality based on sample entropy. Perhaps, the method of Tusnady (1977) can be applied to show an asymptotic optimality of density-based empirical likelihood ratio–type tests, since the distribution-free approximation to the most powerful test is used while constructing the nonparametric density-based likelihood ratio tests.

5. Arizono and Ohta (1989) provided a test of fit for normality based on Kullback–Leibler information. The test can be applied not only to the composite hypotheses, but also to the simple hypotheses.

6. Robinson (1991) employed the Kullback–Leibler information criterion as a basis for one-sided testing of nested hypotheses. The test statistic requires no distributional form, uses nonparametric density estimation, and a form of weighting was employed in order to obtain a normal null limiting distribution. The test was shown to be consistent against a class of alternatives. The tests were applied to testing the random walk hypothesis in several exchange-rate time series of varying lengths.

7. Park (1999) extended the theory of the sample entropy to the ordered sample. The author provided the sample entropy of order statistics, and presented one application of the sample entropy of order statistics as a test of normality versus skewness. The proposed test statistic was shown to possess comparable performance with other existing tests.

8. Mudholkar and Tian (2001) employed a superior normal generator to construct a corrected and extended tabulation for their test. It was shown that the same tables can be used for implementing the entropy test for the composite-inverse Gaussian hypothesis. The finding extended the known Gaussian and inverse Gaussian analogies. A Monte Carlo experiment was performed for the tabulation of the percentiles, and the empirical distributions of the two test statistics were compared. The author summarized some known similarities between the normal and inverse Gaussian distributions.

11.3.4 Tests for Multivariate Normality

1. Mardia (1968) obtained the exact power of a test U (Mardia 1967) for normal location alternatives. But the expression cannot be simplified even for small samples. The empirical power function of the U-test was obtained and compared with the power of Hotelling's T^2 by extending some efficiency measures and developing a new noncentral T^2 routine. It was shown that the efficiency of the U-test relative to Hotelling's T^2-test decreases with the sample size and lies between 79% and 93%.

For the bivariate case, the test was shown to be convenient and faster than the general noncentral routine developed by Bargmann and Ghosh (1964).

2. Wilk and Shapiro (1968) presented statistical methods for the joint assessment of the supposed normality of a collection of independent (small) samples, which may derive from populations having differing means and variances. The procedures were based on the use of the W-statistic (Shapiro and Wilk 1965) as a measure of departure from normality. The authors considered two modes of combination of a collection of W-statistics. These were proposed for use in conjunction with the probability plotting of the collection of these transforms. The authors demonstrated some summary empirical sampling results on the comparative sensitivities of these procedures, along with detailed consideration of several specific examples that illustrate the additional informative value of probability plotting. The proposed techniques were shown to have substantial data analysis value as adjuncts to other statistical methods.

3. Given data X_{ij}, $j = 1$ to n_i, $i = 1$ to g, in order to test whether the X_{ij}'s are normal with a common covariance matrix, Hawkins (1981) proposed using the quantities $V_{ij} = (X_{ij} - X_{i.})' S^{-1} (X_{ij} - X_{i.})$ as the test statistic, where $X_{i.}$ denote the mean of the ith group and S the pooled covariance matrix. The exact null distribution of V_{ij} was derived, and the Anderson–Darling statistic was proposed for testing whether the data fit this null distribution. The test was shown to be flexible, easily implemented, and have acceptable power. The method was illustrated with the data discussed in Aitchison et al. (1977).

4. Pierce and Kopecky (1979) showed that tests of normality appropriate for the identically distributed case are asymptotically valid when computed from residuals in regression situations. Based on numerical results via simulation, Pierce and Gray (1982) showed the adequacy of this result for sample sizes of 20 and 40. The Shapiro–Wilk and Anderson–Darling tests were found to be quite adequate for $n = 20$ in typical simple linear regression situations, and for $n = 40$ in certain multiple regression settings.

5. Quesenberry et al. (1983) provided transformations that are useful in studying the validity of the assumptions for a fixed-effects, one-way, normal errors, and analysis of variance model. The authors extended the techniques of Quesenberry et al. (1976) to the case where the variances of the parent distributions are assumed to be the same for all samples. The method can be used as a flexible tool in the model analysis of some rather complex data sets, for example, cases in which the samples are quite small, possibly as small as two, three, or four. The method was illustrated with a data set obtained as part of a large forage management study in which tall fescue was harvested at different heights throughout the growing season.

6. Bowman and Foster (1993) developed adaptive smoothing and density-based tests of multivariate normality, where the amount of smoothing applied varied according to local features of the underlying density. The authors investigated the difficulties of applying Taylor series arguments in this context and simple properties of the estimates by numerical integration and compared with the fixed kernel approach. The author derived optimal smoothing strategies based on the multivariate normal distribution and two tests of multivariate normality. One test for multivariate was based on the integrated squared error and the other test was based on entropy measures. The tests demonstrated good power properties.

7. Zhu et al. (1995) extended the test based on sample entropy proposed by Vasicek (1976) to the multivariate case with projection pursuit for searching for departure from the multivariate normal distribution. Tests for multinormality were based on density estimation, a number-theoretic method, projection pursuit techniques, and sample entropy. It was shown that the test may be recommended for practice due to its good powers under various alternatives.

8. Versluis (1996) compared 15 tests for bivariate normality with unknown parameters based on a Monte Carlo power analysis. Component-wise independent distributions with skewed, low-kurtosis, and high-kurtosis marginal distributions were considered as alternative hypotheses. Further, the family of bivariate gamma distributions was used to determine the effect of correlation as an alternative hypothesis. It was shown that the Shapiro–Wilk–Stephens test performs well for all alternative distributions analyzed. The Shapiro–Wilk–Stephens test exhibited good power against the lognormal and the family of bivariate gamma distributions, but showed poor power against independent uniform distributions. The test procedures were illustrated with a study of monofilament and multifilament yarn.

9. Darbellay and Vajda (2000) provided a series of analytical expressions for the entropy and mutual information of multivariate continuous probability distributions. It was noted that the entropy and mutual information were defined for all values of the distribution parameters for the distributions considered, but this was not always the case for the variances and the covariance, or even the means. The authors constructed several nonparametric estimators for the differential entropy and demonstrated the bias of these estimators on finite samples.

10. Plug-in estimates are wildly used to evaluate entropies of one-dimensional probability densities. The plug-in estimates first estimate a probability density and then compute its entropy. While plug-in estimates work well in low dimensions and for densities with known parametric form, the difficult problem of density estimation makes them impractical for small sample sizes in higher dimensions. Miller (2003) developed a new class of estimators for approximating the entropy of multidimensional probability densities based on the order statistics of a sample, by extending the classic plug-in estimators to multiple dimensions. Unlike plug-in estimators of entropy, Miller's estimators avoid the difficult intermediate step of density estimation. For fixed dimension, the estimators are polynomial in the sample size. The author showed that these consistent and rapidly converging estimators can result in effective and computationally efficient entropy estimators for multidimensional distributions.

11. Székely and Rizzo (2005) proposed a new class of rotation-invariant and consistent goodness-of-fit tests for multivariate distributions based on Euclidean distance between sample elements, which is applicable to any multivariate distribution with finite second moments. The method for testing multivariate normality was developed for when parameters are estimated. It was shown that the resulting test is affine invariant and consistent against all fixed alternatives. Based on a comparative Monte Carlo study, it was shown that the test is a powerful competitor to existing tests, and is very sensitive against heavy-tailed alternatives. Applications include one-sample goodness-of-fit tests for discrete or continuous multivariate distributions in arbitrary dimension.

12

Statistical Change-Point Analysis

The next day, the wind changes, meaning Mary must leave.

Mary Poppins (1964)*

12.1 Introduction

In health studies there may be a distributional shift, oftentimes in terms of a shift in location either due to random factors or due to some known factors at a fixed point in time that is either known or needs to be estimated. Change-point problems may be encountered in many disciplines, such as epidemiology, industrial processes, economics, biology, and geology. For example, biomarker measurements may be measured differently between two laboratories, and say a given research organization switches laboratories. Then there may be a shift in mean biomarker levels simply due to differences in sample processing. As another example, the speed limit on many expressways in the United States was increased from 55 miles per hour to 65 miles per hour in 1987. In order to investigate the effect of this increased speed limit on highway traveling, one may study the change in the traffic accident death rate after modification of the 55-mile per hour speed limit law. Problems closely related to the example above are called *change-point* problems in statistical literature. In this chapter, we outline the general aspects of change-point problems and the variety of methods to deal with change-point data analysis issues.

From the statistical viewpoint, suppose we have a random process that generates independent observations indexed by some nonrandom factor such as time or location. Since observations are obtained over varying values of the nonrandom factor, we suspect that there has been at least one change in the random process during the data collection period. A change point can be viewed as the location or time point such that the observations follow different distributions before and after that point. Multiple change points can be defined similarly. Statistical inference and predictions will be invalid if changes in the random process during the data collection period are not taken into account. In order to understand the consequences that a change point (or multiple change points) may have on a process and to harness potentially beneficial transitional information about the given point, we are generally interested in the following components:

1. Deciding if there is a change (or changes) in the sequence of observed random variables, which is often viewed as a hypothesis testing problem;
2. Estimating the number of changes and their corresponding locations if there has been at least one change in the process;
3. Investigating the type and importance of the changes that have occurred in the process.

---

* American musical fantasy film.

The statistical literature regarding the change-point problem is focused primarily on offline change-point detection or retrospective change-point analysis, where inference regarding the detection of a change occurs *retrospectively*, that is, after the data have already been collected. The example of traffic mortality rate illustrated above falls into this offline category. Various applications, for example, in the areas of biology, medicine, and economics, tend to generate offline change-point problems. For example, in genomics, detecting chromosomal DNA copy number changes or copy number variations in tumor cells can facilitate the development of medical diagnostic tools and personalized treatment regimens for cancer and other genetic diseases (e.g., Lucito et al. 2000). The offline change-point detection methods are also useful in studying the variation (over time) of share prices on the major stock exchanges.

In contrast to the offline change-point problem, the so-called online (sequential) change-point problem or an online surveillance change problem features methods in which a prospective analysis is performed *sequentially*. In this case, in order to detect a change as soon as possible, such that the consequences of such a change can be tackled effectively, the detection method is implemented after every new observation is collected; we refer the reader to Chapter 13 for general ideas regarding sequential data analysis, of which this is one type of such analysis. The online change-point problems are widely presented and studied in fields such as statistical quality control, public health surveillance, and signal processing (Mei 2006). For instance, in a continuous production process, the quality of the products is expected to remain stable. However, in practice, for some known or unknown reasons, the process may fail to produce products of equal quality. Therefore, one may be interested in investigating when the quality of a product starts to deteriorate. Under such circumstances, online change-point analysis can be used in the form of control charts to monitor output of industrial processes. Typically, control charts have a central line (the mean) and upper and lower lines representing control limits, which are usually set at three-sigma (standard deviations) detection limits from the mean. Any data points that fall outside these limits, or unusual patterns (determined by various run tests) on the control chart, suggest that systematic causes of variation are present. Under such circumstances, the process is said to be "out of control" and actions are taken to find and possibly eliminate the corresponding causes. A process is declared to be "in control" if all points charted lie randomly within the control limits. In order to illustrate the construction and operation of control charts, we consider the following two data examples.

Example 12.1: Control Charts

We consider a data example containing one-at-time measurements of a continuous process variable presented in Gavit et al. (2009). Figure 12.1 shows the *X*-chart or control chart for the data. Based on the *X*-chart shown in Figure 12.1, there is no evidence showing that the process is out of control.

Implementation of Figure 12.1 is shown in the following R code:

```
> # install.packages("qcc") # install it for the first time
> library(qcc)
> dat.raw <- c(10.9,9.7,8.6,9.3,9.2,10.4,9.6,10.0,8.8,11.0,10.3,9.3,
    11.1,9.9,8.9,10.2,10.6,12.2,10.7,11.2,10.9,11.2,11.5)
> dat <- qcc.groups(dat.raw, sample=1:length(dat.raw))
> obj <- qcc(dat, type="xbar.one",nsigmas = 3)
```

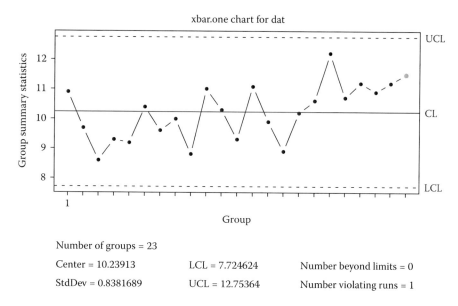

xbar.one chart for dat

FIGURE 12.1
X-chart for a data example containing one-at-time measurements of a continuous process variable presented in Gavit et al. (2009). The horizontal upper and lower dashed lines represent the upper and lower three-sigma control limits, respectively. The middle solid horizontal line is the mean.

Example 12.2

We consider another data example obtained from the inside diameter measurements of piston rings for an automotive engine produced by a forging process (Montgomery 1991). The inside diameter of the rings manufactured by the process is measured on 25 samples, each of size 5, for control phase I. Figure 12.2 presents the *X*-bar chart, a type of Shewhart control chart that is used to monitor the arithmetic means of successive samples of constant size, for this calibration data.

Implementation of Figure 12.2 is shown in the following R code:

```
> # install.packages("qcc") # install it for the first time
> library(qcc)
> data(pistonrings)
> diameter <- qcc.groups(pistonrings$diameter, pistonrings$sample)
>
> # Plot sample means to control the mean level of a continuous variable
> 'Phase I' <- diameter[1:25,]
> 'Phase II' <- diameter[26:40,]
> obj <- qcc('Phase I', type="xbar", newdata='Phase II', nsigmas = 3)
```

12.2 Common Change-Point Models

In this chapter, we concentrate on the offline (retrospective) change-point analysis problem and use the term *change point* throughout for simplicity. Before further discussion of change-point detection methods, the general change-point model must be rigorously defined and common change-point problems are introduced.

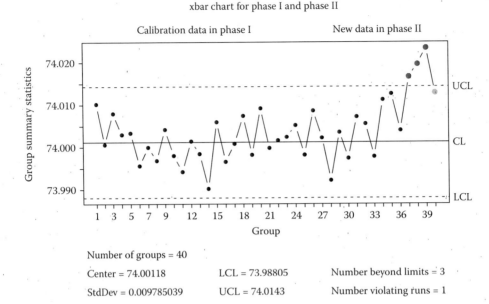

FIGURE 12.2
Shewhart chart (X-bar chart) for both calibration data and new data, where all the statistics and the control limits are solely based on the calibration data, that is, first 25 samples. The centerline (CL) is the horizontal solid line, the upper (UCL) and lower (LCL) control limits are the dashed lines, and the sample group statistics are drawn as points connected with lines.

Any properties of a random sequence are determined by its distribution, that is, by a probability measure in a certain functional space. Therefore, a change in any of the characteristics of a random process is generally a change in some characteristic of the distribution. In fact, a sequence with change points is linked with pieces of sequences with different distributions. In order to formulate the general change-point model, let $X_1, X_2, ...,$ X_n be a sequence of independent random vectors (variables) with probability distribution functions $F_1, F_2, ..., F_n$, respectively. The general change-point problem is to test the null hypothesis

$$H_0: F_1 = F_2 = ... = F_n$$

versus the alternative

$$H_1: F_1 = \cdots = F_{k_1-1} \neq F_{k_1} = \cdots = F_{k_2-1} \neq F_{k_2} = \cdots = F_{k_q-1} \neq F_{k_q} = \cdots = F_n,$$

where q is an unknown number of change points and $k_1, k_2, ..., k_q$ $(1 < k_1 < k_2 < ... < k_q < n)$ are the respective unknown change-point locations. Under the alternative hypothesis, the difference between distribution functions before and after the changes can be represented not only in the difference of their functional forms, but also in the difference between values of parameters involved in the distribution functions; for example, F_{k_1-1} and F_{k_1} could be normal distributions but with different means.

Statistical inference commonly involves two aspects: determining if any change point exists in the process and estimating the number and locations of change points.

The change-point problem can be categorized in terms of alternatives and model settings. When one change can be expected, that is, under $H_1 : F_1 = \cdots = F_{k_1-1} \neq F_{k_1} = \cdots = F_n$, we have the simple change-point model. When under the alternative we assume that there are q change points in the process, where $q > 1$ is an integer, we have a multiple-change-point model. In the case of multiple change points, when the number of change points is known, we can develop and employ testing procedures specific to change-point detection procedures. When the number of change points is unknown, for example, in the cases of climate change and stock price change, we can construct specific change-point detection procedures or employ the binary segmentation method extending any simple change-point method, for example, those discussed later in Section 12.3, to uncover all possible change points (Vostrikova 1981). A general description of the binary segmentation method can be summarized as follows:

Step 1: Choose and apply a simple change-point detection method to test for no change point versus a single change point. If we fail to reject the null hypothesis of no change point, then stop. If H_0 is rejected, then there is a change point. In this case, we estimate the change point and proceed to step 2.

Step 2: Based on the estimator of the change point, divide the random sample into two subsamples containing pre- and post-change-point observations, respectively. Test both subsamples for a change based on the simple change-point detection method chosen in step 1.

Step 3: Repeat the segmentation procedure until no further subsamples contain change points.

Step 4: The collection of change-point locations is found by steps 1–3, and accordingly, the total number of changes can be estimated.

Note that due to the iterative nature of the binary segmentation method described above, it may fail in some situations, for example, in the case of detecting a small segment of structural change that is among a large segments (Olshen et al. 2004).

Change-point detection problems can be considered using parametric approaches (Chen and Gupta 2011; Gurevich and Vexler 2005). However, in practice it may sometimes be difficult to assume pre-specified data distributions. When we have a possible change in the process, it is hard to verify the parametric assumptions, for example, applying a goodness-of-fit test. Moreover, if the assumptions are not met, the results are not robust without taking the change-point problem into consideration. Gurevich and Vexler (2010) presented extensive Monte Carlo simulations showing that a slight divergence from parametric assumptions leads to invalid statistical inference. Under such circumstances, one can consider nonparametric approaches (Ferger 1994; Gombay 2001; Gurevich 2006; Wolfe and Schechtman 1984; Zou et al. 2007) or semiparametric methods of change-point detection (Guan 2004, 2007; Guan and Zhao 2005).

In subsequent sections, we will present parametric, nonparametric, and semiparametric change-point detection methods in a variety of model settings, including the single change-point problem, the epidemic alternative, which is a special type of a multiple change-point problem, and change-point problems in regression models.

12.3 Simple Change-Point Model

There is a rich literature dealing with the simple change-point problem, that is, the case $q = 1$ (e.g., Chen and Gupta 2011; Chernoff and Zacks 1964; Gombay and Horvath 1994; Page 1954, 1955). It is usually assumed that if a change in the distribution did occur, then it is unique and the observations after the change all have the same distribution, which differs from the distribution of the observations before the change (e.g., Gombay and Horvath 1994; Page 1955). Let $X_1, X_2, ..., X_n$ be independent continuous random variables with fixed sample size n. In the formal context of hypotheses testing, we state the change-point detection problem as testing for

$$H_0: X_1, X_2, ..., X_n \sim F_0 \text{ versus } H_1: X_i \sim F_1, X_j \sim F_2, i = 1, ..., v - 1, j = v, ..., n,$$

where F_0, F_1, F_2 are distribution functions that correspond to density functions f_0, f_1, f_2. Note that the change point $v \in (1, n]$ should be an integer. The simple change-point model is termed a so-called *at most one change-point* (AMOC) model when $F_0 = F_1$. Following certain applied aspects of quality control studies, the literature assumes commonly that the function F_1 is equal to F_0 (e.g., Gombay and Horvath 1994; James et al. 1987).

12.3.1 Parametric Approaches

Efficient detection methods for the classical simple change-point problem include the cumulative sum and Shiryayev–Roberts approaches, both of which are known to have optimality properties when both pre-change and post-change distributions are known (Moustakides 1986; Pollak 1985; Yakir et al. 1999). When the post-change and pre-change distributions are partially or fully unknown, the cumulative sum and Shiryayev–Roberts methods are reasonably efficient procedures in the sequential statement of the problem (Gordon and Pollak 1997; Pollak 1987). These techniques can be well adapted to retrospective cases. Considering a general case when F_1 can be different from the null distribution F_0, in the parametric setting, we assume that the density functions f_0, f_1, and f_2 have known forms possibly with certain unknown parameters (Gombay and Horvath 1994; Gurevich 2007; James et al. 1987; Vexler 2006; Vexler and Gurevich 2009).

12.3.1.1 CUSUM-Based Techniques

When the parameter v is known, as defined above, and the density functions f_0, f_1, f_2 are assumed to be completely known, the likelihood ratio statistic Λ_v^n provides the most powerful test by virtue of the Neyman–Pearson lemma, where

$$\Lambda_k^n = \frac{\prod_{i=1}^{k-1} f_1(X_i) \prod_{i=k}^{n} f_2(X_i)}{\prod_{i=1}^{n} f_0(X_i)}.$$

We refer the reader to Chapter 4 for details regarding likelihood ratio tests.

When the parameter v is unknown, and if the density functions f_0, f_1, and f_2 are completely known, the maximum likelihood estimator

$$\hat{v} = \arg\max_{1 \leq k \leq n} \Lambda_k^n$$

of the parameter v can be applied. By plugging in the maximum likelihood estimator of the change-point location $\hat{v}$, we have

$$\Lambda_n = \Lambda_{\hat{v}} = \max_{1 \le k \le n} \Lambda_k^n,$$

which has the maximum likelihood ratio form. This corresponds to the well-known cumulative sum (CUSUM)–type test statistic (Gombay and Horvath 1994). The null hypothesis is rejected for large values of the CUSUM test statistic. Decision rules based on CUSUM-type statistics are well-accepted and very powerful parametric change-point detection schemes (e.g., Gurevich 2007; Gurevich and Vexler 2005; Lai 1995; Page 1955).

Remark 12.1

Under certain assumptions, one can show the estimator $\hat{v}$ is consistent (e.g., Borovkov 1999; Gurevich and Vexler 2005; Pollak and Tartakovsky 2007; Tartakovsky et al. 2009). However, it is reasonable to assume that estimation of a change point without testing its existence may be an erroneous procedure, since $\hat{v}$ provides a number even under H_0.

In the case that the density functions f_0, f_1, and f_2 have forms with unknown parameters, one needs to estimate the unknown parameters and then an approximated CUSUM-type test statistic can be defined. Gombay and Horvath (1994) considered the situation $f_0(x) = f(x; \theta_0)$, $f_1(x) = f(x; \theta_1)$, $f_2(x) = f(x; \theta_2)$, where the vector parameters $\theta_i \in \Theta \subseteq R^d$, $i = 0, 1, 2$, are unknown, $\theta_1 \ne \theta_2$. It is suggested to reject the null hypothesis for larger values of the log maximal likelihood ratio $Z_n = \max_{1 < k \le n} \left(2 \log(\Lambda_k^{*n}) \right)$, i.e., if $Z_n > C_1$ for a fixed test threshold $C_1 > 0$, where

$$\Lambda_k^{*n} = \frac{\sup_{\theta_1 \in \Theta} \prod_{i=1}^{k-1} f(X_i; \theta_1) \sup_{\theta_2 \in \Theta} \prod_{i=k}^n f(X_i; \theta_2)}{\sup_{\theta_0 \in \Theta} \prod_{i=1}^n f(X_i; \theta_0)}.$$

In order to control the Type I error rate of CUSUM-type tests, evaluation of the null distribution of the corresponding CUSUM test statistics is commonly required. Toward this end, a simulation study or complex asymptotic propositions ($n \to \infty$) can be employed to approximate the Type I error rate of CUSUM-type tests. For the asymptotic null distribution of the approximated CUSUM-type test statistic defined above and the rate of convergence of this approximation, we refer the reader to Gombay and Horvath (1994, 1996). Note that likelihood ratio–type tests have high power (e.g., Lai 1995) and evaluation of the significance level may be a major issue. Vexler and Wu (2009) demonstrated that an inflated Type I error rate can be expected in tests based on the CUSUM statistic. Therefore, the idea of a nonasymptotic optimality of the retrospective CUSUM test is problematic. The change-point literature concludes, generally speaking, that there are no uniformly most powerful tests in the context of the retrospective change-point problem (James et al. 1987).

Example 12.3

We give an application of the CUSUM test procedure to search a change point in a subset of high-density lipoprotein (HDL) cholesterol data. The study sample consists of 50 measurements of HDL, which are assumed to be normally distributed. It is assumed that the first series of observations (an unknown number) are measurements from individuals with myocardial infarction (diseased), and the subsequent series of observations are measurements from controls (healthy). Figure 12.3 presents the scatterplot of the study sample. We would like to test for a possible mean and variance change. To be specific, let $X_1, X_2, \ldots, X_n$ be a sequence of independent normal random variables with parameters $(\mu_1, \sigma_1^2), (\mu_2, \sigma_2^2), \ldots, (\mu_n, \sigma_n^2)$ respectively ($n = 50$). We are interested in testing the null hypothesis,

$$H_0: \mu_1 = \mu_2 = \ldots = \mu_n = \mu \text{ and } \sigma_1^2 = \sigma_2^2 = \cdots = \sigma_n^2 = \sigma^2,$$

versus the alternative,

$$H_1: \mu_1 = \ldots = \mu_{v-1} \neq \mu_v = \ldots = \mu_n \text{ and } \sigma_1^2 = \cdots = \sigma_{v-1}^2 \neq \sigma_v^2 = \cdots = \sigma_n^2,$$

where the parameters μ, σ^2, and $v \in (1, n]$ are unknown.

Under the null hypothesis from above, the log-likelihood function is

$$\log L_0\left(\mu, \sigma^2\right) = -\frac{n}{2}\log(2\pi) - \frac{n}{2}\log(\sigma^2) - \frac{1}{2\sigma^2}\sum_{i=1}^{n}(X_i - \mu)^2.$$

Define $\hat{\mu}_{k, m} = \sum_{i=k}^{m} X_i \big/ (m - k + 1)$ and $\hat{\sigma}_{k, m}^2 = \sum_{i=k}^{m} \left(X_i - \hat{\mu}_{k, m}\right)^2 \big/ (m - k + 1)$. Then under the null hypothesis, the maximum likelihood estimators of μ and σ^2 can be easily found to be $\hat{\mu}_{1, n}$ and $\hat{\sigma}_{1, n}^2$, respectively. Therefore, the maximum likelihood under H_0 is

$$\log L_0\left(\hat{\mu}_{1, n}, \hat{\sigma}_{1, n}^2\right) = -\frac{n}{2}\log(2\pi) - \frac{n}{2}\log\left(\hat{\sigma}_{1, n}^2\right) - \frac{n}{2}$$

Under the alternative hypothesis with the change point at k, the maximum likelihood is

$$\log L_1\left(\hat{\mu}_{1, k-1}, \hat{\sigma}_{1, k-1}^2, \hat{\mu}_{k, n}, \hat{\sigma}_{k, n}^2\right) = -\frac{n}{2}\log(2\pi) - \frac{v-1}{2}\log\left(\hat{\sigma}_{1, k-1}^2\right) - \frac{n-v+1}{2}\log\left(\hat{\sigma}_{k, n}^2\right) - \frac{n}{2}.$$

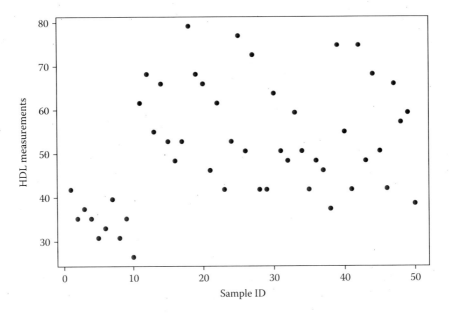

FIGURE 12.3
Scatterplot of the study sample of HDL measurements.

Therefore, the log-maximal likelihood ratio is $Z_n = \max_{2<k\leq n-1}\left(2\log(\Lambda_k^{*n})\right)$, where the statistic

$$2\log\left(\Lambda_k^{*n}\right) = n\log\left(\hat{\sigma}_{1,n}^2\right) - (k-1)\log\left(\hat{\sigma}_{1,k-1}^2\right) - (n-k+1)\log\left(\hat{\sigma}_{k,n}^2\right).$$

We reject the null hypothesis if $Z_n > C_1$ for a fixed test threshold $C_1 > 0$. The test threshold C_1 can be found according to the asymptotic distribution of Z_n. Under H_0, the asymptotic distribution of Z_n satisfies

$$\lim_{n\to\infty}\Pr\left\{a_nZ_n^{1/2} - b_n \leq t\right\} = \exp(-2\exp(-t)), \quad -\infty < t < \infty,$$

where $a_n = (2\log\log n)^{1/2}$ and $b_n = 2\log\log n + \log\log\log n$. The result is shown in Chen and Gupta (2011). Note that under H_0, based on the fact that the maximum likelihood estimator of σ^2 follows a scaled chi-square distribution, for example, $n\hat{\sigma}^2/\sigma^2 \sim \chi_{n-1}^2$, we have as $n \to \infty$,

$$Z_n = \max_{2<k\leq n-1}\left\{n\log\left(\hat{\sigma}_{1,n}^2/\sigma^2\right) - (k-1)\log\left(\hat{\sigma}_{1,k-1}^2/\sigma^2\right) - (n-k+1)\log\left(\hat{\sigma}_{k,n}^2/\sigma^2\right)\right\}$$

$$\sim \max_{2<k\leq n-1}\left\{n\log\left(\chi_{n-1}^2/n\right) - (k-1)\log\left(\chi_{k-2}^2/(k-1)\right) - (n-k+1)\log\left(\chi_{n-k}^2/(n-k+1)\right)\right\},$$

where χ_j^2 denotes the chi-square distributed random variable with j degrees of freedom; for more details, we refer the reader to Chen and Gupta (2011). Based on this property, the test threshold C_1 can be obtained by means of a classical Monte Carlo (MC) simulation technique; for details, we refer the reader to Chapter 16.

The following R code inputs the study sample and implements the CUSUM testing procedure based on the asymptotic distribution of Z_n:

```
> X<-c(41.8,35.2,37.4,35.2,30.8,33.0,39.6,30.8,35.2,26.4,61.6,68.2,55.0,
  66.0,52.8,48.4,52.8,79.2,68.2,66.0,46.2,61.6,41.8,52.8,77.0,50.6,72.6,
  41.8,41.8,63.8,50.6,48.4,59.4,50.6,41.8,48.4,46.2,37.4,74.8,55.0,41.8,
  74.8,48.4,68.2,50.6,42.0,66.0,57.2,59.4,38.6)
> n<-length(X)
>
> plot(1:n,X,pch=16,xlab="Sample ID",ylab="HDL Measurements") #
  scatterplot
>
> alpha=0.05
> MC=10000
>
> # CUSUM: critical distribution based on asymptotic distribution
  (normal)
> get.cv.CUSUM.asym.N<-function(n,alpha){
+ a.n<-(2*log(log(n)))^(1/2)
+ b.n<-2*log(log(n))+log(log(log(n)))
+ cv.CUSUM<-((b.n-log(-(log(1-alpha))/2))/a.n)^2
+ }
>
> get.LR<-function(x,v){
+ # MLE of mu and sigma2 under H_0
+ mu0<-mean(x)
+ var0<-mean((x-mu0)^2)
+
+ # MLE under H_1
+ x1.v<-x[1:(v-1)]
+ mu1<-mean(x1.v)
```

```
+ var1.v<-mean((x1.v-mu1)^2)
+
+ x2.v<-x[v:n]
+ mu2<-mean(x2.v)
+ var2.v<-mean((x2.v-mu2)^2)
+
+ # 2log(LR)
+ return(n*log(var0)-(v-1)*log(var1.v)-(n-v+1)*log(var2.v))
+ }
>
> get.max.LR<-function(x){
+ n<-length(x)
+ tmp<-sapply(3:(n-1),function(v) get.LR(x,v))
+ max(tmp[!is.infinite(tmp)])
+
+ }
>
> cv.asym.N<-get.cv.CUSUM.asym.N(n,alpha)
> cv.asym.N
[1] 16.46402
>
> # test stat
> test.stat<-get.max.LR(X)
> test.stat
[1] 35.44201
>
> # decision rule based on C1 obtained from the asymptotic distribution
> if (test.stat>cv.asym.N) print("Reject H_0") else {print("Fail to
  reject H_0")}
[1] "Reject H_0"
```

In this case, we have $Z_n > C_1$ at the 0.05 significance level. Therefore, we reject the null hypothesis and conclude that there is a change in mean and/or variance.

12.3.1.2 Shiryayev–Roberts Statistic-Based Techniques

In previous subsections, we considered the case where the change-point location is known or estimated, which leads to the CUSUM scheme. Applying the Bayesian concept (see Chapter 7), we can simply integrate the unknown change point with respect to the prior information regarding a point where the change is occurring. In this change-point problem, the integration will correspond to simple summation. Thus, based on the Neyman–Pearson lemma, one can construct the following test statistic

$$R_n = \sum_{k=1}^{n} \Lambda_k^n.$$

This approach is well addressed in the change-point literature as the Shiryayev–Roberts (SR) scheme (Vexler 2006; Vexler and Gurevich 2009; Vexler and Wu 2009). The SR approach is well-accepted for developing optimal procedures in the field of sequential change-point detections (see, e.g., Krieger et al. 2003; Pollak 1985; Pollak and Tartakovsky 2007; Tartakovsky et al. 2009). In the retrospective setting, when the density functions f_0, f_1, and f_2 are completely known, the SR test statistic has the form R_n presented above. The null hypothesis is rejected if

$$R_n > C_2,$$

for a fixed test threshold $C_2 > 0$. This retrospective change-point detection policy based on the SR statistic is nonasymptotically optimal in the sense of average most powerful (via $v = 1, \ldots, n$); see Vexler and Wu (2009), Gurevich and Vexler (2010), and Tsai et al. (2013) for more details.

Example 12.4

In order to show the implementation of the parametric change-point method described above, we consider testing for a change point in a sequence of exponential random variables with unknown parameters. Let $X_1, X_2, \ldots, X_n$ be a sequence of independent exponentially distributed random variables. We are interested in testing the null hypothesis:

$$H_0 : X_1, X_2, \ldots, X_n \overset{i.i.d.}{\sim} f(x) = \exp(-x)$$

versus the alternative

$$H_1 : X_1, X_2, \ldots, X_{v-1} \overset{i.i.d.}{\sim} f(x; \lambda_1) = \lambda_1 \exp(-\lambda_1 x), \ X_v, X_{v+1}, \ldots, X_n \overset{i.i.d.}{\sim} f(x; \lambda_2) = \lambda_2 \exp(-\lambda_2 x),$$

where the parameters $\lambda_1, \lambda_2 > 0$, and $v \in (1, n]$ are unknown.

Under the null hypothesis, the likelihood function is

$$L_0 = \Pi_{i=1}^n f(X_i) = \exp\left(-\sum_{i=1}^n X_i \right).$$

Under the alternative hypothesis with the change point at k, the maximum likelihood under H_1 is

$$\sup_{\theta_1 \in \Theta} \Pi_{i=1}^{k-1} f(X_i; \theta_1) \sup_{\theta_2 \in \Theta} \Pi_{i=k}^n f(X_i; \theta_2)$$

$$= \left((k-1) \Big/ \sum_{i=1}^{k-1} X_i \right)^{k-1} \exp\left(-(k-1) \right) \left((n-k+1) \Big/ \sum_{i=k}^n X_i \right)^{n-k+1} \exp\left(-(n-k+1) \right).$$

Therefore, the maximum likelihood ratio test statistic is

$$\Lambda_k^{*n} = \frac{\left((k-1) \Big/ \sum_{i=1}^{k-1} X_i \right)^{k-1} \left((n-k+1) \Big/ \sum_{i=k}^n X_i \right)^{n-k+1} \exp(-n)}{\exp\left(-\sum_{i=1}^n X_i \right)}.$$

Based on the CUSUM-type test statistic $Z_n = \max_{1 < k \le n} \left(2 \log(\Lambda_k^{*n}) \right)$, following Gombay and Horvath (1994), we can reject the null hypothesis if $Z_n > C_1$ for a fixed test threshold $C_1 > 0$. Based on the SR-type test statistic, we can reject the null hypothesis if $\sum_{v=2}^n \Lambda_v^{*n} > C_2$. The critical values C_1 and C_2 can be found by Monte Carlo (MC) evaluations; for details, we refer the reader to Haccou and Meelis (1988) and Chapter 16.

Below we present simulation results comparing the CUSUM approach and the SR approach in terms of power. Toward this end, we simulated data sets of sizes $n = 30, 50,$ and 200 with a variety of change points v. The underlying distribution of the first $v - 1$ observations is the exponential distribution with parameter $\lambda_1 = 1$, and the remaining observations are from the exponential distribution with parameter λ_2, where $|\lambda_1 - \lambda_2| =$ 1.6, 1.8, and 2. At the 0.05 significance level, the critical values for CUSUM test statistics and SR test statistics are found via the MC technique, and the corresponding powers are presented in Table 12.1. It can be noted that in the scenarios considered, the SR test is more powerful than the CUSUM test. For both methods, when the change point v is around $n/2$, a larger power can be expected, but this property is reversed if the change point v is close to the edges, that is, when $v \approx n$ or $v \approx 1$.

TABLE 12.1

Monte Carlo Power Comparisons between the CUSUM Approach and the SR Approach Based on Exponentially Distributed Data Sets of Sizes $n = 30, 50,$ and 200

n	Change Point v	Method	$\|\lambda_1 - \lambda_2\| = 1.6$	$\|\lambda_1 - \lambda_2\| = 1.8$	$\|\lambda_1 - \lambda_2\| = 2.0$
30	5	CUSUM	0.086	0.120	0.141
		SR	0.092	0.118	0.159
	10	CUSUM	0.117	0.174	0.219
		SR	0.153	0.216	0.281
	15	CUSUM	0.144	0.181	0.274
		SR	0.156	0.224	0.316
	25	CUSUM	0.095	0.128	0.146
		SR	0.099	0.130	0.160
50	5	CUSUM	0.086	0.115	0.147
		SR	0.092	0.130	0.160
	15	CUSUM	0.180	0.263	0.367
		SR	0.220	0.316	0.456
	25	CUSUM	0.211	0.327	0.430
		SR	0.264	0.383	0.526
	35	CUSUM	0.189	0.252	0.350
		SR	0.212	0.298	0.426
	45	CUSUM	0.088	0.113	0.148
		SR	0.093	0.122	0.130
200	5	CUSUM	0.078	0.112	0.146
		SR	0.078	0.098	0.137
	25	CUSUM	0.358	0.546	0.692
		SR	0.403	0.578	0.736
	50	CUSUM	0.596	0.801	0.928
		SR	0.659	0.860	0.951
	100	CUSUM	0.735	0.907	0.980
		SR	0.808	0.954	0.990
	150	CUSUM	0.545	0.788	0.915
		SR	0.625	0.839	0.944
	175	CUSUM	0.289	0.463	0.639
		SR	0.318	0.494	0.657
	180	CUSUM	0.238	0.379	0.534
		SR	0.248	0.388	0.533

Note: The differences between the pre-change parameter and the post-change parameter are considered to be 1.6, 1.8, and 2.

The following R code implements the simulation procedure:

```
> ###### Compare CUSUM and SR based on exponential distributed observations
> # CUSUM: obtain the statistic Z(x1,...xn, v.true;lambda0,lambda1)
> CUSUM<-function(lambda.pre=1,lambda.post=1.5,n,v.true){
+ X<-c(rexp(v.true-1,lambda.pre),rexp(n-v.true+1,lambda.post))
+ n<-length(X)
+ LR.ks<-sapply(2:n,function(v){
+ beta<-sum(X[1:(v-1)])/sum(X)
+ r<-(v-1)/n
+ 2*n*(-r*log(beta/r)-(1-r)*log((1-beta)/(1-r)))
+ })
+ Zn<-max(LR.ks) # maximal likelihood ratio
+ }
>
> # SR: obtain the statistic R(x1,...xn, v.true;lambda0,lambda1)
> SR<-function(lambda.pre=1,lambda.post=1.5,n=100,v.true=50){
+ X<-c(rexp(v.true-1,lambda.pre),rexp(n-v.true+1,lambda.post))
+ LR.ks<-sapply(2:n,function(v){
+ beta<-sum(X[1:(v-1)])/sum(X)
+ r<-(v-1)/n
+ exp(n*(-r*log(beta/r)-(1-r)*log((1-beta)/(1-r))))
+ })
+ sum(LR.ks)
+ }
>
> # set up parameter for simulations
> alpha<-0.05 # significance level
> MC<-10000
> lambda0<-1
> n.seq<-c(30,50,200)
> lambda1.seq<-lambda0+seq(0.6,1,by=0.2)
> methods<-c("CUSUM","SR")
>
> out<-nm<-c()
> for (n in n.seq){
+ if (n==30) v.seq<-c(5,10,15,25)
+ if (n==50) v.seq<-c(5,15,25,35,45)
+ if (n==200) v.seq<-c(5,25,50,100,150,175,180)
+ for (v.true in v.seq){
+ tmp<-c()
+ for (lambda1 in lambda1.seq){
+ ############ CUSUM ############
+ # critical value based on asymptotic distribution
+ #cv.CUSUM.asym<-get.cv.CUSUM.asym(n,alpha)
+
+ # critical value based on Monte Carlo Simulation
+ CUSUM.all.H0<-replicate(MC,CUSUM(lambda.pre=lambda0,lambda.
  post=lambda0,n,v.true))
+ cv.CUSUM.MC<-quantile(CUSUM.all.H0,1-alpha)
+
+ # power
+ CUSUM.all.H1<-replicate(MC,CUSUM(lambda.pre=lambda0,lambda.
  post=lambda1,n,v.true))
+ #power.CUSUM.asym<-mean(CUSUM.all.H1>cv.CUSUM.asym)
+ power.CUSUM.MC<-mean(CUSUM.all.H1>cv.CUSUM.MC)
+
+ ############ SR ############
+ # critical value based on Monte Carlo Simulation
+ SR.all.H0<-replicate(MC, SR(lambda.pre=lambda0,lambda.
  post=lambda0,n,v.true))
```

```
+  cv.SR<-quantile(SR.all.H0,1-alpha)
+
+  # power
+  SR.all.H1<-replicate(MC, SR(lambda.pre=lambda0,lambda.
   post=lambda1,n,v.true))
+  power.SR.MC<-mean(SR.all.H1>cv.SR)
+
+  powers<-c(power.CUSUM.MC,power.SR.MC)
+  tmp<-cbind(tmp,sprintf("%4.3f", powers))
+  }
+  tmp<-cbind(c(v.true,""),methods,tmp)
+  colnames(tmp)<-c("v","Methods",paste0("lambda=",lambda1.seq))
+  out<-rbind(out,tmp)
+  }
+
+  nm<-c(nm,paste0("n=",n),rep("",length(v.seq)*2-1))
+
+  }
>  rownames(out)<-nm
>  out # print the powers shown in Table 12.1.
```

Detecting a change point occurring in other data distributions, for example, a gamma distribution, can follow in a similar manner. For a survey of methods, we refer the reader to Section 12.6. The simple change-point problem can be considered in the regression model, for example, in the model of logistic regression (Gurevich and Vexler 2005). For more details regarding the change-point detection in regression models, we refer the reader to Sections 12.5 and 12.6.

12.3.2 Nonparametric Approaches

When little information is available regarding the statistical data structure before and after a given change point, nonparametric detection methods can be employed for arbitrary changes in distribution. When the AMOC model is stated nonparametrically, there is no universally most powerful methodology (e.g., as the parametric likelihood methods described in Section 12.3.1). In this case, many nonparametric test statistics for change-point detection are based on signs, ranks, or U-statistics (e.g., Csörgö and Horváth 1997; Gombay 2001; Gurevich 2006; Horváth and Shao 1996). In particular, when the type of change point is known in advance, such as a change in location, mean, or variance, more powerful tests are available, which take into account the type of change (Hawkins and Deng 2010). In this section, we describe nonparametric detection methods for change in location with AMOC and general U-statistics-based approaches that can be applied in the AMOC model.

12.3.2.1 Change in Location

The majority of work in the change-point literature focuses on the shift in the location parameter (Hawkins and Zamba 2005). The basic AMOC problem was first considered by Page (1954, 1955) in the special case of $F_0(x) = F_1(x)$ and $F_2(x) = F_0(x - \Delta)$ for the setting of continuous inspection schemes, where Δ is an unknown location parameter. It is of interest to test the null hypothesis of no change H_0: $\Delta = 0$ against either one- or two-sided alternatives. Let θ_0 be the initial mean of the process (i.e., the mean of X_1). Define $S_0 = 0$ and the partial sums $S_k = \sum_{j=1}^{k} V_j$, $k = 1, \ldots, n$, where

$$V_j = \begin{cases} a & \text{if } X_j \geq \theta_0, \\ -b & \text{if } X_j < \theta_0. \end{cases}$$

The constants $a > 0$, $b > 0$, possibly dependent on F_0, are chosen so that $F_{\theta_0}(v_j) = 0$, $j = 1, \ldots, n$.

Assuming that the initial mean of the process θ_0 is known a priori, Page (1954, 1955) proposed rejecting H_0: $\Delta = 0$ in favor of the alternative of one change $\Delta > 0$ for large values of T, where

$$T = \max_{1 \le k \le n}\left\{ S_k - \min_{1 \le j < k}(S_j) \right\}.$$

Note that if θ_0 is the median, then we can choose $a = b$ and it holds that $E_{\theta_0}(V_j) = 0$. In particular, when $a = b = 1$, the V_j's are simply the signs associated with the $(X_j - \theta_0)$'s, where zero is identified with a positive sign. The resulting change-point detection method is nonparametric distribution-free over the class of continuous variables.

When initial level θ_0 is unknown, Bhattacharyya and Johnson (1968) formulated the change-point model in terms of stochastically increasing variables and proposed rejecting H_0: $\Delta = 0$ in favor of H_1: $\Delta > 0$ for large values of

$$J = \sum_{i=1}^{n} L_i E\left[-f_0'(V^{(R_i)})/f_0(V^{(R_i)}) \right],$$

where $L_i = \sum_{t=1}^{i} I_t$ are cumulative weights with $I_1 = 0$, $\mathbf{R} = (R_1, \ldots, R_n)$ is the vector of ranks of $X_1, \ldots, X_n$, and $V^{(1)} < \ldots < V^{(n)}$ are the order statistics for a random sample of size n from continuous population with distribution function F_0 and density function f_0. Therefore, the Bhattacharyya–Johnson statistic, J, has the general appearance of an optimal linear rank statistic. Note that from a Bayesian point of view, the weight I_t can be interpreted as the prior probability that X_t is the initial shifted variable. For instance, with uniform weights $I_t \equiv (n - 1)^{-1}$, $t = 2, \ldots, n$, which correspond to an uninformative prior, we have $L_i = \sum_{t=1}^{i} I_t = (i - 1)/(n - 1)$. In this case, the statistic J is equivalent to

$$J' = \sum_{i=1}^{n} (i-1)E\left[-f_0'\left(V^{(R_i)}\right)/f_0\left(V^{(R_i)}\right) \right].$$

Let $M = \mathrm{median}_{1 \le j \le n}(X_j)$. Consider two special cases of the general statistic J with uniform weights, J_1 and J_2, which are similar to linear rank statistics with median scores and Wilcoxon scores, respectively, where

$$J_1 = \sum_{i=1}^{n} (i-1)I\{X_i - M \ge 0\}, \quad J_2 = \sum_{i=1}^{n}\sum_{j=1}^{n} (i-1)I\{X_i - X_j \ge 0\},$$

and $I\{\cdot\}$ is the indicator function. Let $M_{k,n-k}$ be the number of observations among the last $(n - k)$ that exceed the median of all n observations, that is,

$$M_{k,n-k} = \sum_{i=k+1}^{n} I\{X_i - M \ge 0\}.$$

The statistic $M_{k,n-k}$ is simply a two-sample median statistic applied to the total of n observations viewed as an initial sample of k observations and a second sample of $n - k$ observations. Similarly, the statistic

$$U_{k,n-k} = \sum_{i=k+1}^{n} \sum_{j=1}^{k} I\{X_i - X_j \geq 0\}$$

is just a two-sample Mann–Whitney statistic applied to the same breakdown of the data into two subsamples of sizes n and $n - k$. Accordingly, J_1 and J_2 can be written as

$$J_1 = \sum_{k=1}^{n-1} M_{k,n-k} \text{ and } J_2 = \sum_{k=1}^{n-1} U_{k,n-k}.$$

In analogy to parametric likelihood ratio procedures for one-sided alternatives in the case where both the initial level θ_0 and variance σ^2 are unknown, Sen and Srivastava (1975) proposed two additional nonparametric tests. They suggested rejecting H_0: $\Delta = 0$ in favor of one-sided alternative H_1: $\Delta > 0$ for large values of

$$D_1 = \max_{1 \leq k \leq n-1} \left\{ \frac{M_{k,n-k} - E_0(M_{k,n-k})}{\left[\mathrm{var}_0(M_{k,n-k}) \right]^{1/2}} \right\},$$

$$D_2 = \max_{1 \leq k \leq n-1} \left\{ \frac{U_{k,n-k} - E_0(U_{k,n-k})}{\left[\mathrm{var}_0(U_{k,n-k}) \right]^{1/2}} \right\} = \max_{1 \leq k \leq n-1} \left\{ \frac{U_{k,n-k} - (k(n-k))/2}{\left[k(n-k)(n+1)/12 \right]^{1/2}} \right\},$$

where $E_0(M_{k,n-k})$ and $\mathrm{var}_0(M_{k,n-k})$ are the null mean and variance of the statistic $M_{k,n-k}$, respectively.

In a structure similar to the statistic D_2, but with different weightings assigned to the difference terms $U_{k,n-k} - [k(n - k)/2]$ that lead to the maximums, Pettitt (1979) proposed rejecting H_0: $\Delta = 0$ in favor of the one-sided alternative H_0: $\Delta > 0$ for large values of

$$K_1 = \min_{1 \leq k \leq n-1} \left\{ \sum_{i=1}^{k} \sum_{j=k+1}^{n} Q_{ij} \right\},$$

where

$$Q_{ij} = \mathrm{sign}(X_i - X_j) = \begin{cases} 1 & \text{if } X_i > X_j, \\ 0 & \text{if } X_i = X_j, \\ -1 & \text{if } X_i < X_j. \end{cases}$$

Note that the statistic K_1 can be rewritten as

$$K_1 = \max_{1 \leq k \leq n-1} \left\{ -\sum_{i=1}^{k} \sum_{j=k+1}^{n} Q_{ij} \right\} = 2 \max_{1 \leq k \leq n-1} \left\{ U_{k,n-k} - (k(n-k))/2 \right\}.$$

It is clear that the statistic K_1 employs equal weightings, while the statistic D_2 weights these differences by $[\mathrm{var}_0 \, (U_{k, n-k})]^{-1/2}$.

In the same vein, Pettitt (1979) proposed rejecting $H_0: \Delta = 0$ in favor of the two-sided alternative $H_1: \Delta \neq 0$ for large values of

$$K_2 = \max_{1 \leq k \leq n-1} \left| \sum_{i=1}^{k} \sum_{j=k+1}^{n} Q_{ij} \right| = 2 \max_{1 \leq k \leq n-1} \left\{ \left| U_{k,n-k} - \frac{k(n-k)}{2} \right| \right\}.$$

Schechtman and Wolfe (1988) studied the two-sided analogue of K_2 based on the unequal weightings as the one employed in the one-sided statistic D_2. They suggest rejecting H_0: $\Delta = 0$ in favor of H_0: $\Delta \neq 0$ for the large values of

$$D_3 = \max_{1 \leq k \leq n-1} \left\{ \frac{|U_{k, n-k} - (k(n-k))/2|}{\left[k(n-k)(n+1)/12 \right]^{1/2}} \right\}.$$

Schechtman and Wolfe (1988) studied the relative merits of these two weighting schemes. Pettitt (1979) and Sen (1978) derived some of the asymptotic properties of the change-point procedures based on K_1 and K_2. The large sample properties of the tests associated with D_2 and D_3 are discussed in Sen (1978) and Schechtman and Wolfe (1988).

12.3.2.2 U-Statistics-Based Approaches

Consider the AMOC model in a general case where $F_0(x) = F_1(x) = F(x)$ and $F_2(x) = G(x)$, $G(x) \neq F(x)$ for some x. Let $X_1, X_2, \ldots, X_n$ be a sequence of independent random variables. It is of interest to test the null hypothesis

$$H_0: X_1, X_2, \ldots, X_n \sim F$$

against the alternative

$$H_1: X_i \sim F, \, X_j \sim G, \; i = 1, \ldots, \tau, \; j = \tau + 1, \ldots, n,$$

where the distribution functions F, G and the change point τ (which is equivalent to $v - 1$ described in Section 3.1) are unknown. Let the change point $\tau = [n\lambda]$ for some $\lambda \in (0, 1)$, where $[x]$ denotes the largest integer not larger than x.

Consider comparing the first τ observations to the last $(n - \tau)$ observations via a bivariate function $h(u, v)$, which is termed the kernel function in the theory of U-statistics. Kernels of U-statistics can be symmetric, that is,

$$h(x,y) = h(y,x), \; -\infty < x,y < \infty,$$

or antisymmetric, that is,

$$h(x,y) = -h(y,x), \; -\infty < x,y < \infty.$$

Kernels of U-statistics can be categorized as nondegenerate or degenerate. Let

$$\tilde{h}_1(t) = Eh(X_1, t) = \int h(u,t) \, dF(u),$$

and

$$\tilde{h}_2(t) = Eh(X_{\tau+1}, t) = \int h(u, t) dG(u).$$

If $\mathrm{var}\!\left(\tilde{h}_1(X_1)\right) > 0$, we have a nondegenerate kernel, whereas if $\mathrm{var}\!\left(\tilde{h}_1(X_1)\right) = 0$, then we have a degenerate kernel. Define a U-statistic of degree 2 with kernel $h(x, y)$ as

$$\binom{n}{2}^{-1} \sum_{1 \le i < j \le n} h(X_i, X_j).$$

The generalized U-statistic

$$U_k = \sum_{i=1}^{k} \sum_{j=k+1}^{n} h(X_i, X_j),$$

is well suited for two-sample and change-point problems. For a general review of U-statistics, we refer the reader to Lee (1990) and Serfling (2009).

Under the null hypothesis of no change, different types of kernels lead to U-statistics with completely different large sample behaviors; see Csörgö and Horváth (1997) for the results. However, under the alternative H_1, if

$$\mathrm{var}\!\left(\tilde{h}_1(X_{\tau+1})\right) > 0 \text{ or } \mathrm{var}\!\left(\tilde{h}_2(X_1)\right) > 0,$$

then a unified treatment is available for all possible types of kernels, symmetric, antisymmetric, degenerate, and nondegenerate. Let $\theta_1 = Eh(X_1, X_2)$ and $\theta_{12} = Eh(X_1, X_{\tau+1})$. Gombay (2001) proposed using the test statistic $\max_{1 \le k \le n} Z_k$, a functional of

$$Z_k = U_k - k(n - k)\theta_1,$$

and let the estimator of $\tau = \tau(n)$ be

$$\hat{\tau} = \hat{\tau}(n) = \min\left\{ j : Z_j = \max_{1 \le k \le n} Z_k \right\}.$$

Under certain regularity conditions, it is shown that under H_1,

$$|\tau(n) - \hat{\tau}(n)| = O_p(1),$$

and as $n \to \infty$, the test statistic is asymptotically normally distributed,

$$\frac{\max\limits_{1 \le k \le n} Z_k - \tau(n - \tau)(\theta_{12} - \theta_1)}{n^{3/2}(D_1^2 \lambda(1 - \lambda)^2 + D_2^2 \lambda^2(1 - \lambda))^{1/2}} \xrightarrow{d} N(0, 1),$$

where

$$D_1^2 = \int \left(\int h(u, v) dG(v) \right)^2 dF(u) - \theta_{12}^2 = \text{var}\left(\tilde{h}_2(X_1) \right),$$

$$D_2^2 = \int \left(\int h(u, v) dF(v) \right)^2 dG(u) - \theta_{12}^2 = \text{var}\left(\tilde{h}_1(X_{\tau+1}) \right).$$

In other words, the asymptotic distribution of the test statistic $\max_{1 \le k \le n} Z_k$ is the same as that of Z_τ, the test statistic we would use if τ were known.

Note that the conditions to be held depend on types of kernels. Consider symmetric kernels that are commonly employed. The following conditions are required to hold for degenerate symmetric kernels:

1. $Eh^2(X_1, X_2) < \infty$, $Eh^2(X_{\tau+1}, X_{\tau+2}) < \infty$, $Eh^2(X_1, X_{\tau+1}) < \infty$, and $Eh(X_1, X_{\tau+1}) h(X_1, X_{\tau+2}) < \infty$ to guarantee all integrals are finite
2. $\theta_{12} \ne \theta_2$ for consistency of the estimator of $\tau = \tau(n)$
3. $\lambda(\theta_{12} - \theta_1) - (1 - \lambda)(\theta_2 - \theta_1) > 0$ as a sufficient condition for asymptotic normality of the statistic $\max_{1 \le k \le n} Z_k$

    For nondegenerate symmetric kernels, in addition to conditions 1–3, one more technical condition is assumed:

4. $E\left\{ \tilde{h}_1^2(X_1) \log\log \left(|\tilde{h}_1(X_1)| + 1 \right) \right\} < \infty, E\left\{ \tilde{h}_2^2(X_{\tau+1}) \log\log \left(|\tilde{h}_2(X_{\tau+1})| + 1 \right) \right\} < \infty$

For more details and conditions regarding antisymmetric kernels, we refer to Csörgö and Horváth (1997).

In the applications of U-statistics, typical choices of kernels are $h(x,y) = (x-y)^2/2$ (the sample variance), $h(x,y) = |x-y|$ (Gini's mean difference), and $h(x,y) = \text{sign}(x+y)$ (Wilcoxon's one-sample statistic). A variety of kernels can be employed to detect a change point in the AMOC model, where the choice of the kernel depends on the type of change point of interest. We illustrate some common scenarios in the following examples.

Example 12.5

We may use the symmetric kernel $h(x,y) = (x-y)^2/2$ to test for a change in the variance of independent observations. The kernel is usually nondegenerate. But when $(\text{var}(X_1))^2 = E(X_1 - EX_1)^4$, it is degenerate (Serfling 2009). In this case, $\theta_1 = \text{var}(X_1)$, $\theta_2 = \text{var}(X_{\tau+1})$, and $\theta_{12} = \left(EX_1^2 - 2(EX_1)(EX_{\tau+1}) + EX_{\tau+1}^2 \right)/2$. The terms in asymptotic variance are

$$D_1^2 = \frac{1}{4} EX_1^4 + \left(EX_1^2 \right)(EX_{\tau+1})^2 + \frac{1}{4}\left(EX_{\tau+1}^2 \right)^2 - \left(EX_1^3 \right)(EX_{\tau+1})$$

$$+ \frac{1}{2}\left(EX_1^2 \right)\left(EX_{\tau+1}^2 \right) - (EX_1)(EX_{\tau+1})\left(EX_{\tau+1}^2 \right) - \theta_{12}^2,$$

$$D_2^2 = \frac{1}{4} EX_{\tau+1}^4 + \left(EX_{\tau+1}^2 \right)(EX_1)^2 + \frac{1}{4}\left(EX_1^2 \right)^2 - \left(EX_{\tau+1}^3 \right)(EX_1)$$

$$+ \frac{1}{2}\left(EX_1^2 \right)\left(EX_{\tau+1}^2 \right) - (EX_{\tau+1})(EX_1)\left(EX_1^2 \right) - \theta_{12}^2.$$

Example 12.6

Assume a distribution F is symmetric about 0; we then may use the symmetric kernel $h(x,y) = (x+y)/2$, which gives the Walsh average, to test for a change to a distribution G that is not symmetric about 0. In this case, $\theta_1 = E((X_1+X_2)/2) = 0$, $\theta_2 = E((X_{\tau+1}+X_{\tau+2})/2) = EX_{\tau+1}, \theta_{12} = 2\theta_2$, and the conditions above hold when $\theta_2 > 0$ and $\lambda > 2/3$. The terms in asymptotic variance are $D_1^2 = \text{var}(X_1)/4$ and $D_2^2 = \text{var}(X_{\tau+1})/4$.

Example 12.7

In order to test for a change in location of continuous random variable, one may use the antisymmetric kernel function $h(x,y) = \text{sign}(x-y)$. In this case, $\theta_1 = \theta_2 = 0$, and we assume that $\theta_{12} = 2\Pr(X_{\tau+1} \le X_1) - 1 > 0$. The terms in asymptotic variance are $D_1^2 = 4\,\text{var}(G(X_1))$ and $D_2^2 = 4\,\text{var}(F(X_{\tau+1}))$.

12.3.2.3 Empirical Likelihood–Based Approach

Einmahl and McKeague (2003) proposed an empirical likelihood–based test (see Chapter 6) for changes in distribution based on retrospectively collected data. The approach is to localize the empirical likelihood using a suitable time variable implicit in the null hypothesis and then form an integral of the log-likelihood ratio statistic.

Let $X_1, \ldots, X_n$ be independent, and assume that for some $\tau \in \{2, \ldots, n\}$ and some continuous distribution functions F, G,

$$X_1, \ldots, X_{v-1} \sim F \text{ and } X_v, \ldots, X_n \sim G,$$

with v, F, and G are unknown. In order to test the null hypothesis of no change point, $H_0: F = G$, we define the local likelihood ratio test statistic

$$R(t,x) = \frac{\sup\left\{L(\tilde{F},\tilde{G},v) : \tilde{F}(x) = \tilde{G}(x), v = [nt = +1]\right\}}{\sup\left\{L(\tilde{F},\tilde{G},v) : [nt] + 1\right\}},$$

for $1/n \le t < 1$ and $x \in R$, with

$$L\left(\tilde{F},\tilde{G},v\right) = \prod_{i=1}^{v-1}\left(\tilde{F}(X_i) - \tilde{F}(X_i-)\right)\prod_{i=v}^{n}\left(\tilde{G}(X_i) - \tilde{G}(X_i-)\right).$$

Set $n_1 = [nt]$, $n_2 = n-[nt]$, and let F_{1n} and F_{2n} be the empirical distribution functions of the first n_1 observations and last n_2 observations, respectively. Let F_n be the empirical distribution function of the full sample, so $F_n(x) = (n_1 F_{1n}(x) + n_2 F_{2n}(x))/n$. Then

$$\log R(t,x) = n_1 F_{1n}(x)\log\frac{F_n(x)}{F_{1n}(x)} + n_1\left(1 - F_{1n}(x)\right)\log\frac{1 - F_n(x)}{1 - F_{1n}(x)}$$

$$+ n_2 F_{2n}(x)\log\frac{F_n(x)}{F_{2n}(x)} + n_2\left(1 - F_{2n}(x)\right)\log\frac{1 - F_n(x)}{1 - F_{2n}(x)},$$

where $0 \log(a/0) = 0$. Consider the test statistic

$$T_n = -2 \int_{1/n}^1 \int_{-\infty}^\infty \log R(t, x) \, dF_n(t, x) \, dt = -\frac{2}{n} \sum_{i=1}^n \int_{1/n}^1 \log R(t, X_i) \, dt.$$

Clearly, T_n is distribution-free. Let W_0 be a four-sided tied-down Wiener process on $[0,1]^2$ defined by

$$W_0(t,y) = W(t,y) - tW(1,y) - yW(t,1) + tyW(1,1),$$

where W is a standard bivariate Wiener process. Let F and G be continuous. Then, under H_0, the limit distribution of T_n is

$$T_n \xrightarrow{D} \int_0^1 \int_0^1 \frac{W_0^2(t, y)}{t(1-t)y(1-y)} \, dy \, dt.$$

The empirical likelihood–based statistic is shown through simulations to have greater power than corresponding Cramer–von Mises type statistics. We refer the reader to Einmahl and McKeague (2003) for more details regarding the simulation results.

12.3.2.4 Density-Based Empirical Likelihood Approaches

Vexler and Gurevich (2010a) provided a general method for constructing distribution-free change-point detection schemes that have approximate likelihood structures. It is of interest to test the null hypothesis

$$H_0: X_1, X_2, \ldots, X_n \sim F_0,$$

against the alternative

$$H_1: X_1, X_2, \ldots, X_{v-1} \sim F_1, X_v, X_{v+1}, \ldots, X_n \sim F_2,$$

where $X_1, X_2, \ldots, X_n$ are independent observations, and F_0, F_1, F_2 are distribution functions with corresponding density functions $f_0, f_1,$ and f_2. Assume that density functions $f_0, f_1,$ and f_2 are completely unknown and the change point $v \in [2,n]$. When we consider the hypothesis test nonparametrically, we would like to obtain test statistics having distribution functions that do not depend on the nonasymptotic Type I error of the test statistics.

In view of the maximum empirical likelihood (EL) methodology, we write the parametric likelihood function $L_f^{(1,k)}$ in the form of

$$L_f^{(1,k)} = \prod_{i=1}^k f(X_i) = \prod_{i=1}^k f(X_{(i)}) = \prod_{i=1}^k f_i,$$

where f is a density function of independent observations $X_1, \ldots, X_k, f_i = f(X_{(i)})$, and $X_{(1)} \le X_{(2)} \le \ldots \le X_{(k)}$ are the order statistics based on $X_1, \ldots, X_k$. Derive the maximum EL estimates of

f_i, $i = 1, \ldots, k$ that maximize $L_f^{(1,k)}$ and satisfy an empirical constraint; we define $X_{(j)} = X_{(1)}$ if $j \leq 1$ and $X_{(j)} = X_{(k)}$ if $j \geq k$. We have

$$\Lambda_k^n = \frac{\prod_{i=1}^{k-1} f_1(X_i) \prod_{i=k}^{n} f_2(X_i)}{\prod_{i=1}^{n} f_0(X_i)} = \prod_{i=1}^{k-1} \frac{f_1(Z_i)}{f_0(Z_i)} \prod_{j=k}^{n} \frac{f_2(Y_j)}{f_0(Y_j)} = \prod_{i=1}^{k-1} \frac{f_1(Z_{(i)})}{f_0(Z_{(i)})} \prod_{j=1}^{n-k+1} \frac{f_2(Y_{(j)})}{f_0(Y_{(j)})},$$

where $Z_{(1)} \leq Z_{(2)} \leq \ldots \leq Z_{(k-1)}$ and $Y_{(1)} \leq Y_{(2)} \leq \ldots \leq Y_{(n-k+1)}$ are the order statistics based on the observations $Z_1 = X_1, Z_2 = X_2, \ldots, Z_{k-1} = X_{k-1}$ and $Y_1 = X_k, Y_2 = X_{k+1}, \ldots, Y_{n-k+1} = X_n$, respectively. Denote

$$\prod_{i=1}^{k-1} f_1(Z_{(i)}) = \prod_{i=1}^{k-1} g_i, \quad g_i = f_1(Z_{(i)}).$$

Note that we have

$$\frac{1}{2m} \sum_{j=1}^{k-1} \int_{Z_{(j-m)}}^{Z_{(j+m)}} f_1(x) dx = \frac{1}{2m} \sum_{j=1}^{k-1} \int_{Z_{(j-m)}}^{Z_{(j+m)}} \frac{f_1(x)}{f_0(x)} f_0(x) dx \doteq \frac{1}{2m} \sum_{j=1}^{k-1} \frac{g_j}{f_0(Z_{(j)})} \int_{Z_{(j-m)}}^{Z_{(j+m)}} dF_0(x) \leq 1,$$

where $Z_{(i)} = Z_{(1)}$ if $i \leq 1$ and $Z_{(i)} = Z_{(k-1)}$ if $i \geq k - 1$. The equation $\int f_1 = 1$ constrains values of g_i, $i = 1, \ldots, k - 1$. Therefore, the empirical condition on g_i, $i = 1, \ldots, k - 1$ is

$$\tilde{S}_m \leq 1, \tilde{S}_m = \frac{1}{2m} \sum_{i=1}^{k-1} \frac{g_i}{f_0(Z_{(i)})} \left(F_{0n}(Z_{(i+m)}) - F_{0n}(Z_{(i-m)}) \right),$$

where $F_{0n}(x) = n^{-1} \sum_{i=1}^{n} I(X_i \leq x)$ is the empirical distribution function that estimates $F_0(x)$. The values of $g_1, \ldots, g_{k-1} = \arg\max_{g_1, \ldots, g_{k-1}} \left\{ \prod_{i=1}^{k-1} g_i : \text{satisfying the empirical conditions} \right\}$ are

$$g_i = \frac{2m f_0(Z_{(i)})}{(k-1)(F_{0n}(Z_{(i+m)}) - F_{0n}(Z_{(i-m)}))},$$

Thus, the density-based approximation of $\prod_{i=1}^{k-1} g_i$ is

$$\max_{1 \leq m \leq (k-1)^{1-\delta}} \left(\prod_{i=1}^{k-1} \frac{2m f_0(Z_{(i)})}{(k-1)(F_{0n}(Z_{(i+m)}) - F_{0n}(Z_{(i-m)}))} \right).$$

Hence, the ratio $\prod_{i=1}^{k-1} f_1(Z_{(i)})/f_0(Z_{(i)})$ in Λ_k^n defined above is approximated by the density-based EL ratio

$$\max_{1 \le m \le (k-1)^{1-\delta}} \left(\prod_{i=1}^{k-1} \frac{2mf_0(Z_{(i)})}{(k-1)(F_{0n}(Z_{(i+m)}) - F_{0n}(Z_{(i-m)}))} \frac{1}{f_0(Z_{(i)})} \right)$$

$$= \max_{1 \le m \le (k-1)^{1-\delta}} \left(\prod_{i=1}^{k-1} \frac{2m}{(k-1)(F_{0n}(Z_{(i+M)}) - F_{0n}(Z_{(i-m)}))} \right).$$

Similarly, we obtain that the nonparametric approximation of the ratio $\prod_{j=1}^{n-k+1} f_2(Y_{(j)})/f_0(Y_{(j)})$ by Λ_k^n defined above has the form

$$\min_{1 \le r \le (n-k+1)^{1-\delta}} \left(\prod_{j=1}^{n-k+1} \frac{2r}{(n-k+1)(F_{0n}(Y_{(j+r)}) - F_{0n}(Y_{(j-r)}))} \right),$$

where $Y_{(j)} = Y_{(1)}$ if $j \le 1$ and $Y_{(j)} = Y_{(n-k+1)}$ if $j \ge n - k + 1$. Then, we can construct nonparametric approximation of the likelihood ratio in the form

$$\tilde{\Lambda}_k^n = \min_{1 \le m \le (k-1)^{1-\delta}} \left(\prod_{i=1}^{k-1} \frac{2m}{(k-1)(F_{0n}(Z_{(i+m)}) - F_{0n}(Z_{(i-m)}))} \right)$$

$$\times \min_{1 \le r \le (n-k+1)^{1-\delta}} \left(\prod_{j=1}^{n-k+1} \frac{2r}{(n-k+1)(F_{0n}(Y_{(j+r)}) - F_{0n}(Y_{(j-r)}))} \right),$$

with $\delta \in (0,1)$. Based on this, two nonparametric tests can be proposed as nonparametric forms of the CUSUM and SR procedures that reject H_0 if

1. $\log\left(\tilde{\Delta}_n\right) = \log\left(\max_{2 \le k \le n} \tilde{\Delta}_k^n\right) > C,$

2. $\log\left(\tilde{R}_n\right) = \log\left(\sum_{k=2}^{n} \tilde{\Lambda}_k^n\right) > H,$

for fixed test thresholds $C, H > 0$. Similar to Canner (1975), we will arbitrarily define $F_{0n}(x) - F_{0n}(y) = 1/n$ if $F_{0n}(x) = F_{0n}(y)$. Since $I(X > Y) = I(F_0(X) > F_0(Y))$, we have

$$\Pr_{H_0}\left\{\log\left(\tilde{\Delta}_n\right) > C\right\} = \Pr_{X_1, \dots, X_m \sim UNIF(0,1)}\left\{\log\left(\tilde{\Delta}_n\right) > C\right\},$$

$$\Pr_{H_0}\left\{\log\left(\tilde{R}_n\right) > H\right\} = \Pr_{X_1, \dots, X_m \sim UNIF(0,1)}\left\{\log\left(\tilde{R}_n\right) > H\right\}.$$

Therefore, the Type I error rates of the test procedures defined in (1) and (2) above can be calculated exactly, for all sample sizes n and $0 < \delta < 1$; for more details regarding the Monte Carlo technique to obtain critical values, we refer the reader to Chapter 16.

A large area of change-point research has concentrated on various aspects for the simple change-point problems. For a survey of other nonparametric detection methods, we refer the reader to the supplemental materials (Section 12.6).

12.3.3 Semiparametric Approaches

Guan (2004) considered a semiparametric change-point model and focused on the estimation of and testing for a change point to a biased sample. We present the detailed work of Guan (2004) in the subsequent sections.

Using the empirical likelihood method (Owen 1988; Qin and Lawless 1994; Zhang 1997), auxiliary information regarding the relationship between the two population distributions can be employed efficiently. Let $x_1, \ldots, x_n$ be independent vectors in $\mathbf{R}^d$. We would like to test between the following hypotheses:

H_0: $x_1, \ldots, x_n$ is a random sample from a population with distribution function F.

H_1: For some $n^{-1} \leq \theta_n < 1$, $x_1, \ldots, x_{n\theta_n}$ is a random sample from F and $x_{n\theta_n+1}, \ldots, x_n$ is a random sample from a weighted G, where

$$G(y) = \frac{1}{w} \int_{-\infty}^{y} w(x, \beta)\, dF(x), w(\cdot, \cdot) > 0,$$

in which $w = \int_{-\infty}^{\infty} w(s, \beta)\, dF(s) < \infty$ is the normalizing constant and the weight function $w(x, \beta)$ is of known form, but may depend on an unknown parameter $\beta \in R^d$. It is assumed that $w(x, \beta)$ is positive and differentiable with respect to β. If $\beta \neq 0$, $w(x, \beta) \neq 1$ and $w(x, 0) = 1$ for all x. Here θ_n is an unknown parameter taking a value from $\Theta_n = \{k/n : k = 1, \ldots, n\}$, and it is assumed that $\theta_n \to \theta_0 \in (0,1)$ as $n \to \infty$.

In this semiparametric model, the distributions F and G are treated in a nonparametric fashion with the exception that the ratio of the density or probability functions has a known parametric form. We focus on the change from F to the weighted G. Although most of the technical results of this section are given for a general weight $w(x, \beta)$, the most important model in practice is the semiparametric exponential model, with weight $w(x, \beta) = \exp\{\beta^T \tau(x)\}$. In this case, the log ratio of the two density or probability functions, say, f and g, is of the form

$$\log \frac{g(x)}{f(x)} = \alpha + \beta^T \tau(x),$$

where $\alpha = -\log w$. Typically, we use $\tau(x) = x$, or $\tau(x)$ is chosen to contain second- or higher-order powers of x. These choices correspond to the first-, second-, or higher-order approximation of $\log\{g(x)/f(x)\}$. When it can be assumed that both f and g belong to a parametric exponential family, then the model of the log ratio of the two density or probability functions is an exact parametric expression, and we also have other choices for $\tau(x)$, such as $\tau(x) = \log x$. This exponential model can be used to detect a possible change in $E\{\tau(X)\}$.

Let $x_1,\dots,x_{n\theta_n}$ and $x_{n\theta_n+1},\dots,x_n$ be independent and identically distributed (i.i.d.) observations from population F and a weighted population G as specified in H_1, respectively. The likelihood L of the data is

$$L = \prod_{i=1}^{n} p_i \prod_{j=n\theta_n+1}^{n} w(x_j) \left\{ \sum_{i=1}^{n} p_i w(w_i) \right\}^{-n(1-\theta_n)},$$

where $p_i = dF(x_i)$ ($i = 1, \dots, n$). For each fixed $\theta_n \in \Theta_n \cap (0,1)$, let $l(\theta_n, w, \beta)$ be the maximum value of $\log L + n\log n$ with respect to $p_i (i = 1, \dots, n)$ subject to the constraints

$$\sum_{i=1}^{n} p_i w(x_i) = w, \quad \sum_{i=1}^{n} p_i = 1 \left(p_i \geq 0, i = 1, \dots, n \right).$$

As in Qin (1993) and Vardi (1982), the Lagrange multiplier method leads to

$$l(\theta_n, w, \beta) = -\sum_{i=1}^{n} \log\left\{ \theta_n w + 1(1 - \theta_n)w(x_i, \beta) \right\} + \sum_{i=n\theta_n+1}^{n} \log\left\{ w(x_i, \beta) \right\} + n\theta_n \log w.$$

Therefore, the score functions are

$$\psi_1(\theta_n, w, \beta) = \frac{\partial l(\theta_n, w, \beta)}{\partial w} = \frac{\theta_n(1 - \theta_n)}{w} \sum_{i=1}^{n} \frac{w(x_i, \beta) - w}{(1 - \theta_n)w(x_i, \beta) + \theta_n w},$$

$$\psi_2(\theta_n, w, \beta) = \frac{\partial l(\theta_n, w, \beta)}{\partial w} = \sum_{i=n\theta_n+1}^{n} \frac{w'_\beta(x_i, \beta)}{w(x_i, \beta)} \sum_{i=1}^{n} \frac{(1, 0)w'_\beta(x_i, \beta)}{(1 - \theta_n)w(x_i, \beta) + \theta_n w},$$

where $w'_\beta(x, \beta) = \partial w(x, \beta)/\partial \beta$. Let $\left(\hat{w}, \hat{\beta}^T \right) = \left(\hat{w}(\theta_n), \hat{\beta}^T(\theta_n) \right)$ be the solution to

$$\psi_1(\theta_n, w, \beta) = 0, \psi_2(\theta_n, w, \beta) = 0.$$

Consequently,

$$\hat{p}_i = \frac{1}{n} \frac{\hat{w}}{(1 - \theta_n)w(x_i, \hat{\beta}) + \theta_n \hat{w}}, i = 1, \dots, n.$$

And the profile log-likelihood function of the unknown change point θ_n is given by

$$l(\theta_n) = -\sum_{i=1}^{n\theta_n} \log\left\{ (1 - \theta_n)\frac{w(x_i, \hat{\beta})}{\hat{w}} + \theta_n \right\} - \sum_{i=n\theta_n+1}^{n} \log\left\{ 1 - \theta_n + \theta_n \frac{\hat{w}}{w(x_i, \hat{\beta})} \right\},$$

with $l(0) = l(1) = 0$. The estimator $\hat{\theta}_n$ can be defined as

$$\hat{\theta}_n = \min\left[\arg\max\{l(\theta_n) : \theta_n \in \Theta_n\}\right].$$

A significantly large value of the empirical log-likelihood ratio statistic

$$S_n = 2l\left(\hat{\theta}_n\right) = 2\max_{\theta_n} l(\theta_n)$$

will lead to rejection of H_0 in favor of H_1. Define $\Lambda_0 = \Lambda_n = 0$ and, for $k = 1, \ldots, n-1$, $n\Lambda_k = l(k/n)$ so that $S_n = 2\max_{0 \le k \le n}\{n\Lambda_k\}$. For $k = 1, \ldots, n-1$, write $\hat{w}_k = \hat{w}(k/n)$ and $\hat{\beta}_k = \hat{\beta}(k/n)$, the maximum semiparametric likelihood estimators of w and β, respectively, when $\theta_n = (k/n)$. Under H_0, it can be derived that

$$\lim_{n \to \infty} \Pr\{C(\log n)Z_n \le t + D_d(\log n)\} = \exp\left(-2e^{-t}\right),$$

for all t, where $Z_n = S_n^{1/2}$, $C(x) = (2\log x)^{1/2}$, $D_d(x) = 2\log x + \frac{1}{2}d\log\log x - \log\Gamma\left(\frac{1}{2}d\right)$, and $\Gamma(t)$ is a gamma function.

The testing procedure based on the statistic S_n is asymptotically equivalent to the nonparametric test statistic based on the tied-down partial sum (Csörgö and Horváth 1997); see Guan (2004) for details. Note that the nonparametric test proposed by Csörgö and Horváth (1997) is equivalent to the parametric maximum likelihood ratio test when samples are drawn from normal distributions with unknown constant variance. When samples are from normal distributions, the semiparametric model proposed by Guan (2004) is a little less powerful than the nonparametric test proposed by Csörgö and Horváth (1997), but otherwise the semiparametric test is more powerful than the nonparametric test.

12.4 Epidemic Change Point Problems

In health-related studies, investigators often encounter epidemic problems. The epidemic problem is a special multiple change points problem of great practical interest. Let $X_1, X_2, \ldots, X_n$ be independent continuous random variables from the distributions $F_1, F_2, \ldots, F_n$, respectively. The epidemic problem is defined by testing the null hypothesis of no change in distribution,

$$H_0: F_1 = F_2 = \ldots = F_n = F$$

versus the alternative hypothesis,

H_1: there are integers $1 \le k < m \le n$ such that

$$F_1 = \ldots = F_k = F^{(1)} \ne F_{k+1} \ldots = F_m = F^{(2)} \ne F_{m+1} = \ldots = F_n = F^{(3)},$$

where F and $F^{(i)}$, $i = 1, 2, 3$, are unknown.

The essence of this epidemic alternative (sometimes called the square-wave alternative) is that the distribution in question is assumed to have changed after k, and then is restored to the original state after m, where the epidemic occurred between k and m (see, e.g., Guan 2004; Levin and Kline 1985; Ramanayake and Gupta 2003; Yao 1993b). Vexler (2006) considered the hypothesis testing of change points in the context of regression models with the epidemic change as a special case; for details, refer to Section 12.5.2.

The epidemic problem has many practical applications in many fields, such as medical studies. For instance, certain flu may break out at a time point, and the mortality rate may start to increase at that breakout time, endure that change for a certain period, and then be restored to the original mortality rate after the flu dies out.

12.4.1 Parametric Approaches

12.4.1.1 Simple Case of the Problem

If the distributions $F_1, F_2, \ldots, F_n$ of continuous random variables $X_1, X_2, \ldots, X_n$ belong to a common parametric family $F(\cdot, \theta)$, where $\theta \in \mathbf{R}^d$, then the epidemic problem is defined by testing the null hypothesis of no change in the population parameters θ_i, $i = 1, \ldots, n$,

$$H_0: \theta_1 = \theta_2 = \ldots = \theta_n = \theta$$

versus the alternative hypothesis,

$$H_1: \text{there are integers } 1 \leq k < m \leq n \text{ such that}$$

$$\theta_1 = \ldots = \theta_k = \alpha_1 \neq \theta_{k+1} \ldots = \theta_m = \beta \neq \theta_{m+1} = \ldots = \theta_n = \alpha_2,$$

where the nuisance parameters θ, α_1, α_2, and β are unknown.

For simplicity and ease of exposition, we consider the normally distributed data and a particular case of the alternative where $\alpha_1 = \alpha_2 = \theta$ and $\beta = \theta + \delta$ with the one-sided alternative, where we assume that the sign of δ is known, say $\delta > 0$. A typical normally distributed data pattern with epidemic change is illustrated in Figure 12.4, where observations are simulated from normal distributions $N(\theta, 1)$ with $\theta = 1$, $\delta = 3$, $k = 30$, $m = 60$, and $n = 90$. The following R code implements the simulation procedure:

```
> theta<-1
> delta<-3
> k<-30
> m<-60
> n<-90
> X<-c(rnorm(k,theta,1),rnorm(m-k,theta+delta,1),rnorm(n-m,theta,1))
> plot(1:n,X,pch=16,xlab="ID")
```

Yao (1993b) studied a variety of tests to detect an epidemic alternative in the mean value of a sequence of independent normal variables, including Levin and Kline's statistic, the semilikelihood ratio, the likelihood ratio, the scorelike statistic, and the recursive residual statistic. We present the detailed work of Yao (1993a, 1993b) in subsequent sections.

Assume that X_i, $i = 1, \ldots, n$, are normally distributed with mean θ_i and variance 1. Let $S_j = \sum_{i=1}^{j} X_i$, Pr_0 denote the probability measure under the null hypothesis H_0, and

$$\omega(x) = 2x^{-2} \exp\left\{-2\sum_{n=1}^{\infty} n^{-1}\Phi\left(-n^{1/2} x/2\right)\right\}, x > 0,$$

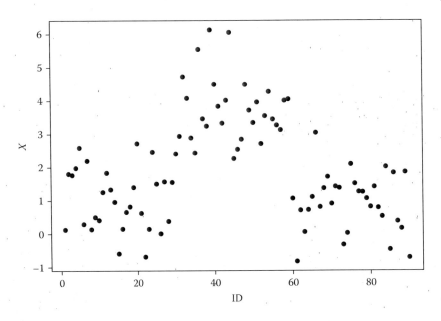

FIGURE 12.4
Scatterplot of a simulated sequence of observations from normal distributions $N(\theta, 1)$ with $\theta = 1$, $\delta = 3$, $k = 30$, $m = 60$, and $n = 90$.

where Φ denotes the standard normal distribution functions. The special function $\omega(x)$ is involved in some large-deviation approximations to the significance levels. For numerical purposes, it is often sufficient to use the approximation for small x (Siegmund 1985, Section 10.4), where

$$\omega(x) = \exp\{-0.583x\} + o(x^2).$$

12.4.1.1.1 Levin and Kline's Statistic

When θ and δ are known, the log-likelihood ratio statistic for testing H_0 against H_1 is proportional to

$$\max_{1 \le i < j \le n} \left\{ S_j - j\theta - (S_i - i\theta) - (j - i)\delta/2 \right\}.$$

However, in many practical situations, it is very unlikely that θ and δ would be known. Levin and Kline (1985) suggested using this statistic by replacing θ with its maximum likelihood estimator under H_0, namely, $\hat{\theta} = S_n/n$, and δ taken as the smallest increment in means, which is considered important to detect, say δ_0, to obtain

$$Z_1 = \max_{1 \le i < j \le n} Z_1(i, j) = \max_{1 \le i < j \le n} \left\{ S_j - S_i - (j - i)S_n/n - (j - i)\delta_0/2 \right\}.$$

Suppose that b and n tend to infinity in such a way that $b/n = \zeta$ is a fixed positive constant. Then under the null hypothesis, as $n \to \infty$, the asymptotic relation of Z_1 follows:

$$\Pr_0(Z_1 \ge b) \sim (2w(2\zeta + \delta_0/2))^2 \{2n(2\zeta + \delta_0/2)(\zeta + \delta_0/2)\} \exp\{-2n\zeta(\zeta + \delta_0/2)\}.$$

For technical details, we refer to Theorem 2 of Hogan and Siegmund (1986).

12.4.1.1.2 Semilikelihood Ratio Statistic

Inspired by Levin and Kline (1985), Siegmund (1986) considered the likelihood ratio when δ and μ are unknown. This statistic is in the form

$$Z_2 = \max_{1 \le i < j \le n} Z_2(i,j) = \max_{1 \le i < i \le n} \left\{ S_j - S_i - (j-i)S_n/n - \tfrac{1}{2}\delta_0(j-i)\big(1 - (j-i)/n\big) \right\}.$$

Siegmund (1986) developed an asymptotic approximation for its significance level under the same assumptions of the asymptotic relation of Z_1, where

$$\mathrm{Pr}_0(Z_2 \ge b) \sim \begin{cases} \dfrac{1}{4}w^2(\delta_0)n\delta_0^2\left(\dfrac{1}{4} - 2\zeta/\delta_0\right)^{-1/2}\exp(-n\delta_0\zeta), & \text{if } \delta_0 > 8\zeta, \\[2ex] 4w^2\big(\delta_0/2 + 4\zeta\big)n(\zeta + \delta_0/8)^{5/2}\,(\zeta - \delta_0/8)^{-\frac{1}{2}}\exp\big\{-2n(\zeta + \delta_0/8)^2\big\}, & \text{if } 0 \le \delta_0 < 8\zeta. \end{cases}$$

It seems that Z_1 is easier to study than Z_2. However, when the duration of the epidemic state $m - k$ is close to n, intuitively Z_1 would not perform as well as Z_2.

12.4.1.1.3 Likelihood Ratio Statistic

For θ and δ, both unknown but $\delta > 0$, the square root of a slightly generalized log-likelihood ratio statistic can be proposed as

$$Z_3 = \max_{n_0 \le i < j \le n_1} Z_3(i,j) = \max_{n_0 \le i < j \le n_1} \left\{ \frac{(S_j - S_i - (j-i)S_n/n)}{\big((j-i)(1-(j-i)/n)\big)^{1/2}} \right\},$$

for some $1 \le n_0 < n_1 < n$. Here the generalization is taken by maximizing $Z_3(i,j)$ over $n_0 \le i < j \le n_1$ instead of over $1 \le i < j \le n$, as suggested by Siegmund (1985, 1986). Assuming that $b = n^{1/2}$, $n_0 = nt_0$, and $n_1 = nt_1$, with $0 < t_0 < t_1 < 1$ and $c > 0$ fixed, then as $n \to \infty$,

$$\mathrm{Pr}_0(Z_3 \ge b) \sim \frac{1}{4}b^3 \varphi(b) \int_{t_0}^{t_1} \frac{1}{(1-t)t^2}\left(w\left[c/\{t(1-t)\}^{\frac{1}{2}}\right]\right)^2 dt,$$

where φ denotes the standard normal density function. This large-deviation approximation provides quite good approximation even for moderate sample size n (Yao 1993a, 1993b). For more details and some stochastic simulations regarding the large-deviation approximations for the significance level of Z_3, we refer to Siegmund (1988) and Yao (1993a, 1993b).

In the case where the observations $X_1, X_2, \ldots, X_n$, have an unknown constant variance σ^2, the likelihood ratio statistic for testing the epidemic change can be taken as $Z_3/\hat{\sigma}^2$, where $\hat{\sigma}^2$ is the maximum likelihood estimator of σ^2 under the null hypothesis (Yao 1993a, 1993b).

12.4.1.1.4 Score-Type Statistic

Without the maximization, Z_3 is the normalized difference between the mean of $X_{i+1}, \ldots, X_j$ and the overall mean; that is, it is somehow the standard two-sample test statistic for testing that the mean of $X_{i+1}, \ldots, X_j$ is the greatest. In the case of two-sample testing, the problem is invariant under common shifts in location of all observations, so one might restrict consideration to invariant procedures, that is, those that depend on X's only through the maximal invariants $Y_j = X_j - X_1$ ($j = 2, ..., n$). By the Neyman–Pearson lemma, the likelihood ratio based on $Y_2, ..., Y_n$, is the most powerful invariant test for testing the null hypothesis H_0 against H_1 with fixed (k,m) and δ, which gives the test statistic

$$Z_\delta = \delta\left(S_m - S_k - \frac{m-k}{n} S_n \right) - \frac{1}{2}(m-k)\left(1 - \frac{m-k}{n} \right)\delta^2.$$

However, in practice, usually δ is unknown. By differentiating Z_δ with respect to δ and setting $\delta = 0$, we obtain the invariant efficient score statistic $S_m - S_k - (m-k)S_m/n$, which leads to the locally most powerful invariant test in the sense that it maximizes the slope of the power function at $\delta = 0$ (Cox and Hinkley 1974). Maximizing this score function over $k < m$ suggests a score-type statistic for testing the epidemic change

$$Z_4 = \max_{1 \le i < j \le n} Z_4(i, j) = \max_{1 \le i < j \le n} \left\{ S_j - S_i - (j-i)S_n/n \right\}.$$

Note that when $j = n$, Z_4 is equivalent to Pettitt's method, which was designed for testing one change-point hypothesis (James et al. 1987; Pettitt 1979). On the other hand, if we let $\delta_0 = 0$ in Z_1, then the test statistic Z_1 equals Z_4, which manifests that Z_4 can be viewed as a special case of the Levin and Kline statistic when we aim to detect any change in means, even though the increment is very small. As a consequence, the special case of the large-deviation approximation to Z_1 with $\delta_0 = 0$ provides as asymptotic approximation for the tail probability of the statistic Z_4.

Obviously, the statistic Z_4 is in a simpler form than all of Z_1, Z_2, and Z_3. When δ_0 is small, the statistics Z_2 and Z_4 perform similarly. However, the behavior of Z_3 is very different. Note that intuitively, the primary contribution to the power of Z_3 comes from the probability that the process $S_j - S_i - (j - i) S_n/n$ exceeds the boundary of $b[(j - i) \{1 - (j - i)/n\}]^{1/2}$, denoted by b_{Z_3}, for some (i, j) in a neighborhood of $(i, j) = (k, m)$. Suppose that the rejection region of Z_4 is

$$\left[\max_{1 \le i < j \le n} \left\{ S_j - S_i - (j-i)S_n/n \right\} \ge b_1 \right].$$

In order that the two tests based on Z_3 and Z_4 have the same significance level, b_1 must be less than b_{Z_3} in a neighborhood of $j - i = n/2$. Hence, we expect that Z_4 has greater power than Z_3 when $m - k$ is near $n/2$ because in this case, the process is more likely to go above b_1 than above b_{Z_3}. The converse is true when $m - k$ is near 0 or n. Introduction of n_0 and n_1 in Z_3 gives the statistician the flexibility to trade some power to detect changes with $m - k < n_0$ and $m - k > n_1$ for an increase in power to detect changes with $m - k$ near $n/2$.

12.4.1.1.5 Recursive Residual Statistic

Inspired by an ad hoc so-called recursive test statistic (for more details, we refer to Section 12.4), which was proposed initially by Brown et al. (1975) for testing a change point in a linear model, Yao (1993a, 1993b) considered the standardized residual r_j of X_j from the mean value of the first $j - 1$ random variables, where

$$r_j = \left\{ (j-1)/j \right\}^{1/2} \left(X_j - \bar{X}_{j-1} \right), \, j = 2, ..., n,$$

and

$$\overline{X}_{j-1} = (X_1 + \ldots + X_{j-1})/(j-1).$$

It can be easily shown that under H_0, the recursive residuals r_j, $j = 2, \ldots, n$, are independent standard normal variables. Let the cumulative sum of the standardized residual be $\tilde{S}_j = \sum_{i=2}^{j} r_i$, and define a test statistic

$$Z_5 = \max_{n_0 \leq j-i < n} Z_5(i, j) = \max_{n_0 \leq j-i < n} \left\{ \left(\tilde{S}_j - \tilde{S}_i \right) \middle/ (j-i)^{1/2} \right\}.$$

Assume $b \to \infty$, $n \to \infty$, and $n_0 \to \infty$ in such a way that for some $c > 0$ and $t_0 \in (0, 1)$, $b = cn^{1/2}$, $n_0 = t_0 n$. Yao (1993a, 1993b) presented that as $n \to \infty$, we have the following results:

1. For each $\zeta_0 \in \left(t_0^{1/2} c, c \right)$,

$$\Pr_0 \left\{ Z_5 \geq b \,\middle|\, \tilde{S}_n = n\zeta_0 \right\} \sim (n/2) (c/\zeta_0)^3 \left(c^2 - \zeta_0^2 \right) \left\{ w \left(c^2/\zeta_0 \right) \right\}^2 \exp \left\{ -n \left(c^2 - \zeta_0^2 \right)/2 \right\};$$

2. $\Pr_0 \left\{ Z_5 \geq b \,\middle|\, \tilde{S}_n = bn^{1/2} \right\} \sim \left(b^3/2 \right) \varphi(b) \int_{bn^{-1/2}}^{bn_0^{-1/2}} x^{-1} \left(nx^2/b^2 - 1 \right) w^2(x) dx.$

For detailed proofs, we refer to the appendix of Yao (1993). Accordingly, the following approximation can be obtained:

$$\Pr_0 (Z_5 \geq b) \approx 1 - \varphi(b) + \left(b^3/2 \right) \varphi(b) \int_{bn^{-1/2}}^{bn_0^{-1/2}} x^{-1} \left(nx^2/b^2 - 1 \right) w^2(x) dx.$$

The approximation is demonstrated to be good even for moderate n when the probability is of the order 0.01–0.10 (Yao 1993a, 1993b).

12.4.1.1.6 Adaption to Two-Sided Alternative Hypothesis

For the two-sided alternative hypothesis, that is, not to restrict $\delta > 0$ in the H_1, we can replace the statistic $Z_p(i, j)$, $p = 3, 4, 5$, by its corresponding absolute value. Take the likelihood ratio statistic Z_3, for example, in which case we can use $|S_j - S_i - (j - i) S_n/n|$ for the two-sided alternative hypothesis in place of $S_j - S_i - (j - i) S_n/n$. Yao (1989, 1993a, 1993b) presented that asymptotically, the significance levels are twice the corresponding levels for a one-sided alternative hypothesis, if we make such a replacement in the likelihood ratio statistic, score-type statistic, and recursive residual statistic.

12.4.1.1.7 Asymptotic Distributions under the Alternative Hypothesis

Assume that the hypothesis H_1 holds with fixed (k,m) and $\delta > 0$. Then the probability measure under the alternative hypothesis at the fixed change points (k,m) and the drift δ with $1 < k < m < n$ and $\delta > 0$ can be denoted by $\Pr_{\gamma\delta}$, with $\gamma = m - k$ since all probabilities depend asymptotically on (k, m) only through γ. By integrating approximations to conditional boundary-crossing probabilities and employing Cramer's approximation for the probability of ruin of a risk process (Siegmund 1985, Chapter 8), Yao (1993a, 1993b) developed numerically feasible approximations to the powers of Z_p, $p = 1, \ldots, 4$. Define the following constants that are involved in the approximation:

$$\gamma_0 = \gamma/n; \; u_1 = u_4 = b/\gamma, \; u_2 = b/\gamma + \delta_0\gamma_0/2, \; u_3 = \{\gamma(1 - \gamma_0)\}^{-1/2} b/2;$$

$$v_1 = b/(n - \gamma) + \delta_0/(2(1 - \gamma_0)), \; v_2 = b/(n - \gamma) + \delta_0/(1 - \gamma_0)/2, \; v_3 = u_3, \; v_4 = b/(n - \gamma);$$

$$\lambda_1 = \delta\{\gamma_0(1 - \gamma_0)\}^{1/2} - \{\gamma(n - \gamma)\}^{-1/2} b - (n - \gamma)^{-1/2} \delta_0\gamma^{1/2}/2,$$

$$\lambda_2 = (\delta - \delta_0/2)\{\gamma_0(1 - \gamma_0)\}^{1/2} - \{\gamma(n - \gamma)\}^{-1/2} b,$$

$$\lambda_3 = \delta\{\gamma_0(1 - \gamma_0)\}^{1/2} - n^{-1/2} b, \; \lambda_4 = \delta\{\gamma_0(1 - \gamma_0)\}^{1/2} - \{\gamma(n - \gamma)\}^{-1/2} b.$$

If $\gamma_0 \in (0, 1)$ is fixed, then as $n \to \infty$ with $|u_p - v_p| < \delta$, $p = 1, \ldots, 4$, we have

$$\mathrm{Pr}_{\gamma, \delta}(Z_p \geq b) \approx \Phi\left(n^{1/2}\lambda_p\right) + \frac{\phi\left(n^{1/2}\lambda_p\right)}{\{\gamma(1 - \gamma_0)\}^{1/2}} \times \begin{cases} H(u_p, v_p) \text{ if } u_p \neq v_p, \\ H(u_p) \text{ if } u_p = v_p, \end{cases}$$

where

$$H(x, y) = 2\left\{w(2x)w(2y)\right\}^2 \frac{x + y}{(\delta + x + y)^2} + 2x\left\{\frac{w(2x)}{\delta + x - y}\right\}^2 + 2y\left\{\frac{w(2y)}{\delta - x + y}\right\}^2$$

$$+ \left\{w(2x)w(2y)\right\}^2 \frac{1 + 2y^{-1} x/w(2y) + 2x^{-1} y/w(2x)}{\delta + x + y}$$

$$- \left\{w(2x)\right\}^2 \frac{2w(2y)(x + y)/y + 2(x - y)^{-1}w(2y) y/w(2x) - 1}{\delta + x - y}$$

$$- \left\{w(2y)\right\}^2 \frac{2w(2x)(x + y)/x + 2(y - x)^{-1}w(2x) y/w(2y) - 1}{\delta - x + y}$$

for $x \neq y$, and

$$H(x) = w^2(2x)\left\{\frac{4xw^2(2x)}{(\delta + 2x)^2} + \frac{w^2(2x) + 4w(2x)}{\delta + 2x} + \frac{8x}{\delta^2} + \frac{4[1 - 2w(2x)]}{\delta}\right\}.$$

This approximation to the powers of Z_p, $p = 1, \ldots, 4$, at the fixed change points (k, m), $1 < k < m < n$, and the drift $\delta > 0$, although not as accurate as the approximations of the probability measure under the null hypothesis H_0, is sufficient for use in practice without fear of being misled. For more details, we refer to Yao (1993a, 1993b).

Remark 12.2

In the approach above, it is suggested that one choose a test statistic subjectively, based on the length of epidemic durations that are considered most likely. For example, if $m - k$ is around $n/2$, a suitable choice would be the score-type statistic Z_4. Otherwise, one would choose the modified likelihood ratio test based on Z_3 with $n_0 > 1$ and $n_1 < n$. In general, the modified likelihood ratio test based on Z_3 is perhaps slightly preferred because it performs better than the others when $m - k$ is near 0 or n, where all tests are weak.

12.4.1.1.8 Estimators of the Change Points
Consider the estimators of the change point in the mean value of a sequence of independent normal variables in the case of epidemic alternatives. Let $S_j^* = \sum_{i=1}^{j} (X_i - \bar{X}_n)$, $j = 1, \ldots, n$, where $\bar{X}_n = n^{-1} \sum_{i=1}^{n} X_i$. The estimator of the change point related to the maximum likelihood is defined as follows:

$$(\hat{k}, \hat{m}) = \underset{1 \le i < j \le n, n\varepsilon \le j - i \le n(1-\varepsilon)}{\arg \max} \left\{ \sqrt{n \, | S_j^* - S_i^* | / \{(j - i)(n - j + i)\}} \right\}$$

where $0 < \varepsilon < 1/2$. Hušková (1995) developed the asymptotic properties of estimators of the change points for local changes ($\delta = \delta_n \to 0$) and presented the consistency and the limit distribution of the estimators of the change points in this situation. For the case of estimators of the change points in a sequence of dependent observations, we refer to Brodsky and Darkhovsky (1993).

The detection of the epidemic problem based on other data distributions, such as the exponential distribution, can follow in a similar manner; for more details, we refer the reader to Ramanayake and Gupta (2003), Chen and Gupta (2011), and the supplement (Section 12.6).

12.4.1.2 General Case of the Problem

Let $X_1, X_2, \ldots, X_n$ be independent continuous random variables from the density functions $g_1, g_2, \ldots, g_n$, respectively. We are interested in testing a general case of epidemic changes for the null hypothesis,

$$H_0: g_i = f_0 \text{ for all } i = 1, \ldots, n$$

versus the alternative hypothesis,

$$H_1 : g_1 = \ldots = g_{v_1-1} = f_1; \, g_{v_1} = \ldots = g_{v_2-1} = f_2; \, g_{v_2} = \ldots = g_n = f_3,$$

v_1, v_2 are unknown change points, $2 \le v_1 < v_2 \le n$. The density functions $f_0, f_1, f_2,$ and f_3 are not necessarily known. By virtue of the general principle of the Neyman–Pearson fundamental lemma, Tsai et al. (2013) proposed the adjusted Shiryayev–Roberts statistic

$$\frac{1}{n} R_n^{(2)} = \frac{1}{n} \sum_{k_1=1}^{n} \sum_{k_2=k_1}^{n} \frac{\prod_{i=1}^{k_1-1} f_1(X_i) \prod_{j=k_1}^{k_2-1} f_2(X_j) \prod_{l=k_2}^{n} f_3(X_l)}{\prod_{i=1}^{n} f_0(X_i)}.$$

The decision-making rule is to reject H_0 if

$$\frac{1}{n} R_n^{(2)} > C_\alpha,$$

where C_α is a test threshold at the significance level of α.

This Shiryayev–Roberts statistic is the average most powerful test statistic, that is,

$$\frac{1}{n}\sum_{k_1=1}^{n}\sum_{k_2=k_1'}^{n}\Pr_{k_1,k_2}\left\{\frac{1}{n}R_n^{(2)}>C_\alpha\right\}\geq\frac{1}{n}\sum_{k_1=1}^{n}\sum_{k_2=k_1}^{n}\Pr_{k_1,k_2}\left\{\delta\text{ rejects }H_0\right\},$$

for any decision rule $\delta\in[0,1]$ with fixed $\Pr_{H_0}\{\delta\text{ rejects }H_0\}=\alpha$ and based on the observations $X_1,\ldots,X_n$, where $\Pr_{k_1,k_2}$ denote probability conditional on $v_1=k_1$ and $v_2=k_2$. The proof is shown in the appendix.

When forms of the density functions $f_0, f_1, f_2,$ and f_3 depend on unknown parameters, one can apply either the mixture approach or the estimation approach described below:

1. In the *mixture approach*, a class of likelihood ratio test statistics is constructed via the Bayesian methodology (see, e.g., Vexler and Gurevich 2011). Let $f_s(u)=f(u;\theta_s)$, $s=0,\ldots,3$, where θ_0 is an unknown parameter and the vector of unknown parameters $(\theta_1,\theta_2,\theta_3)$ has a known prior $\pi(\theta_1,\theta_2,\theta_3)$. Then the mixture Shiryayev–Roberts statistics takes the form of

$$\frac{1}{n}R_n^{(3)}=\frac{1}{n}\sum_{k_1=1}^{n}\sum_{k_2=1}^{n}\iiint\frac{\prod_{i=1}^{k_1-1}f_1(X_i;\theta_1)\prod_{j=k_1}^{k_2-1}f_2(X_j;\theta_2)\prod_{l=k_2}^{n}f_3(X_l;\theta_3)}{\prod_{i=1}^{n}f_0(X_i;\hat{\theta}_0)}\,d\pi(\theta_1,\theta_2,\theta_3),$$

where $\hat{\theta}_0=\arg\max_\theta\prod_{i=1}^{n}f_0(X_i;\theta)$ is the maximum likelihood estimator, under the null hypothesis, of θ_0 based on the observations $X_1,\ldots,X_n$. The appropriate test rejects H_0 if

$$\frac{1}{n}R_n^{(3)}>C_\alpha,$$

where C_α is a test threshold at the significance level of α. Under such a scenario, in a class of any detection rules $\delta\in[0,1]$ with the density functions $f_s(u)=f(u;\theta_s)$, $s=0,\ldots,3$, this test is the average integrated most powerful test with respect to a prior $\pi(\theta_1,\theta_2,\theta_3)$ for a fixed estimate of the significance level $\hat{\alpha}=\int\delta(x_1,x_2,\ldots,x_n)f_0(x_1,x_2,\ldots,x_n;\hat{\theta}_0)\prod_{i=1}^{n}dx_i$, that is,

$$\frac{1}{n}\sum_{k_1=1}^{n}\sum_{k_2=k_1}^{n}\iiint\Pr_{k_1,k_2}\left\{\frac{1}{n}R_n^{(3)}>C_{\hat{\alpha}}\right\}d\pi(\theta_1,\theta_2,\theta_3)-C_{\hat{\alpha}}\Pr_{H_0}\left\{\frac{1}{n}R_n^{(3)}>C_{\hat{\alpha}}\right\}$$

$$\geq\frac{1}{n}\sum_{k_1=1}^{n}\sum_{k_2=k_1}^{n}\iiint\Pr_{k_1,k_2}\left\{\delta\text{ rejects }H_0\right\}d\pi(\theta_1,\theta_2,\theta_3)-C_{\hat{\alpha}}\Pr_{H_0}\left\{\delta\text{ rejects }H_0\right\}.$$

2. In the *estimation approach,* a class of likelihood ratio test statistics is constructed via the maximum likelihood estimation of the parameters. Let $f_s(u) = f(u; \theta_s)$, $s = 0, \ldots, 3$. Then the proposed modified Shiryayev–Roberts statistic has the form of

$$\frac{1}{n} R_n^{(4)} = \frac{1}{n} \sum_{k_1=1}^{n} \sum_{k_2=k_1}^{n} \frac{\sup_{\theta_1 \in \Theta} \prod_{i=1}^{k_1-1} f_1(X_i; \theta_1) \sup_{\theta_2 \in \Theta} \prod_{j=k_1}^{k_2-1} f_2(X_j; \theta_2) \sup_{\theta_3 \in \Theta} \prod_{l=k_2}^{n} f_3(X_l; \theta_3)}{\sup_{\theta_0 \in \Theta} \prod_{i=1}^{n} f_0(X_i; \theta_0)}.$$

The appropriate test rejects H_0 if

$$\frac{1}{n} R_n^{(4)} > C_\alpha,$$

where C_α is a test threshold at the significance level of α.

Example 12.8

Let $f_s(x) = f_{N(\mu_s, \theta_s^2)}(x)$, $s = 0, 1, 2, 3$, where θ_s^2, $s = 0, 1, 2, 3$, are fixed known parameters, and μ_0 is an unknown parameter. We assume that the priors for the parameters μ_j, $j = 1, 2, 3$, under the alternative hypothesis, are normal densities, that is, $\mu_j \sim N\left(\lambda_j, \phi_j^2\right)$, $j = 1, 2, 3$. Then the mixture Shiryayev–Roberts statistic is

$$\frac{1}{n} R_n^{(3)} = \frac{1}{n} \frac{\sum_{k_1=1}^{n} \sum_{k_2=k_1}^{n} \left(\frac{\sigma_1^2}{(k_1-1)} + \phi_1^2\right)^{\frac{(k_1-1)}{2}} \left(\frac{\sigma_2^2}{(k_2-1)} + \phi_2^2\right)^{\frac{-(k_2-1)}{2}} \left(\frac{\sigma_3^2}{(n-k_2-1)} + \phi_3^2\right)^{\frac{-(n-k_2+1)}{2}} \exp\left\{-\frac{A_{k_1,k_2}}{2}\right\}}{(\sigma_0)^{-n} \exp\left\{-\sum_{i=1}^{n}(X_i - \bar{X}_0)^2 / 2\sigma_0^2\right\}},$$

where

$$A_{k_1, k_2} = \frac{(\bar{X}_1 - \lambda_1)^2}{(\sigma_1^2/(k_1-1) + \phi_1^2)} + \frac{(\bar{X}_2 - \lambda_2)^2}{(\sigma_2^2/(k_2-k_1) + \phi_2^2)} + \frac{(\bar{X}_3 - \lambda_3)^2}{(\sigma_3^2/(n-k_2+1) + \phi_3^2)},$$

and

$$\bar{X}_0 = \sum_{i=1}^{n} X_i / n$$

$$\bar{X}_1 = \sum_{i=1}^{k_1-1} X_i/(k_1-1), \quad \bar{X}_2 = \sum_{i=k_1}^{k_2-1} X_i/(k_2-k_1), \quad \bar{X}_3 = \sum_{i=k_2}^{n} X_i/(n-k_2+1).$$

Example 12.9

Assume $f_s(x) = f_{N(\mu_s, \theta_s^2)}(x), s = 0, 1, 2, 3,$ where expectations μ_s and variances $\sigma_s^2, s = 0, 1, 2, 3,$ are unknown. Then, the statistic defined in the estimation approach has the form

$$\frac{1}{n} R_n^{(4)} = \frac{1}{n} \sum_{k_1=1}^{n} \sum_{k_2=k_1}^{n} \frac{\hat{\sigma}_0^{n/2}}{\hat{\sigma}_1^{(k_1-1)/2} \hat{\sigma}_2^{(k_2-k_1)/2} \hat{\sigma}_3^{(n-k_2+1)/2}},$$

where

$$\hat{\sigma}_0 = \frac{\sum_{i=1}^{n}(X_i - \hat{\mu}_0)^2}{n}, \hat{\mu}_0 = \frac{\sum_{i=1}^{n} X_i}{n}; \hat{\sigma}_1 = \frac{\sum_{i=1}^{k_1-1}(X_i - \hat{\mu}_1)^2}{k_1 - 1}, \hat{\mu}_1 = \frac{\sum_{i=1}^{k_1-1} X_i}{k_1 - 1},$$

$$\hat{\sigma}_2 = \frac{\sum_{i=k_1}^{k_2-1}(X_j - \hat{\mu}_2)^2}{k_2 - k_1}, \hat{\mu}_2 = \frac{\sum_{i=k_1}^{k_2-1} X_j}{k_2 - k_1}, \hat{\sigma}_3 = \frac{\sum_{\ell=k_2}^{n}(X_\ell)^2}{n - k_2 + 1}, \hat{\mu}_3 = \frac{\sum_{\ell=k_2}^{n}(X_\ell)^2}{n - k_2 + 1}.$$

The epidemic problem can also be considered in a linear regression model. For example, Vexler (2006) proposed and examined a class of generalized maximum likelihood asymptotic power one retrospective tests based on martingale-structured Shiryayev–Roberts statistics for detection of epidemic changes of a linear regression model. Guaranteed non-asymptotic upper bounds for the significance levels of the considered tests are presented. For more details regarding the problems in regression models, we refer the reader to Section 12.5 and the supplemental material (Section 12.6).

12.4.2 Nonparametric Approaches

Based on the empirical likelihood methodology (see Chapter 6 for details), Ning et al. (2012) developed a nonparametric method to detect epidemic change points without the constraint of the data distributions.

Let $X_1, X_2, \ldots, X_n$ be a sequence of independent random variables from a common parametric family $F(\cdot, \theta)$, where $\theta \in \mathbf{R}^d$. Consider the problem with the epidemic alternative stated in Section 12.4, where θ denotes the population mean; that is, we want to test the null hypothesis of no change in the mean versus the epidemic change in the mean. Denote $\theta^* = \theta + \delta$. Then the null hypothesis of no change is equivalent to the hypothesis $\theta^* = \theta$ or $\delta = 0$. For a fixed (k, m), the empirical log-likelihood function is

$$l(\theta, \theta^* \mid k, m) = \sum_i \log u_i + \sum_j \log v_j,$$

where $i = 1, \ldots, k, m + 1, \ldots, n, j = k + 1, \ldots, m, u_i = \Pr(X = x_i), v_j = \Pr(X = x_j),$ and X is a random variable. With the constraints $\sum_i u_i = \sum_j v_j = 1,$ $l(k, m)$ reaches the maximum value at $u_i = (n - m + k)^{-1}$ and $v_j = (m - k)^{-1}$ by the Lagrange multiplier method. Therefore, the empirical log-likelihood ratio function is

$$\log ELR\left(\theta, \theta^* \mid k, m\right) = \sum_i \log((n - m + k)u_i) + \sum_j \log((m - k)v_j).$$

Then, the profile empirical likelihood ratio function for given θ and θ^* has the form

$$EL\left(\theta, \theta^* \mid k, m\right) = \sup\left\{\log ELR\left(\theta, \theta^* \mid k, m\right): \sum_i u_i = \sum_j v_j = 1, \sum_i u_i x_i = \theta, \sum_j v_j x_j = \theta^*\right\},$$

where $u_i \geq 0$ and $v_j \geq 0$. In order to test the null hypothesis $\theta^* = \theta$, the test statistic is defined as

$$Z_{n, k, m} = -2\sup_\theta\left\{EL(\theta, \theta^* \mid k, m)\right\}$$

$$= -2\sup_\theta\left\{\sum_i \log((n - m + k)u_i) + \sum_j \log((m - k)v_j)\right\}.$$

In the practical case where the change points k, m are unknown, Ning et al. (2012) suggested the trimmed maximally selected empirical likelihood ratio statistic as

$$Z_n = \max_{k_0 < k < m < n - k_1} \{Z_{n, k, m}\}.$$

The values of k_0 and k_1 can be chosen arbitrarily, as Lombard (1987) suggested. Ning et al. (2012) employed $k_0 = k_1 = 2[\log n]$ and presented the asymptotic null distribution of Z_n under mild conditions. Suppose that $E_F \|X\|^3 < \infty$, and $E_F(XX')$ is positive definite. Under H_0, we have

$$\Pr(A(\log(t(n)))(Z_n)^{1/2} \leq x + D_r(\log(t(n))) \to \exp(-e^{-x})$$

as $n \to \infty$ for all x, where

$$A(x) = (2\log x)^{1/2},$$

$$D_d(x) = 2\log x + (d/2)\log\log x - \log\Gamma(d/2),$$

$$t(n) = \frac{n^2 + (2[\log n])^2 - 2n[\log n]}{(2[\log n])^2},$$

and d is the dimension of the parameter space. The test is also proved to be consistent. The empirical likelihood ratio test is robust to the data distribution and behaves reasonably well in terms of power performance. However, this test may not detect the change points close to 1 or n since the empirical estimators may not exist due to the properties of the empirical likelihood method. For more details regarding the proofs and discussions, we refer to Ning et al. (2012).

12.4.3 Semiparametric Approaches

Guan (2007) considered the tests of change points with epidemic alternatives (e.g., Levin and Kline 1985; Yao 1993a, 1993b; see Section 12.4.1 for details) and constructed empirical likelihood ratio–based semiparametric tests of change points with epidemic alternatives. We present the detailed work of Guan (2007) in the subsequent sections.

Let $X_1, \ldots, X_n$ be independent vectors in $\mathbf{R}^p$. Let F be any distribution and G a weighted distribution defined as

$$G(y) = w^{-1} \int_{-\infty}^{y} w(x, \beta) \, dF(x),$$

where $w = \int_{-\infty}^{\infty} w(x, \beta) \, dF(x) < \infty$ and $w(x, \beta) > 0$ is a known weight function, but may depend on a vector of unknown parameters $\beta \in \mathbf{R}^d$. Define $X_k^m = \{X_{k+1}, \ldots, X_m\}$ and $\Theta_n = \{(k/n, m/n): 1 \le k \le m \le n\}$. We will consider the null hypothesis

$$H_0 : X_0^n \sim F,$$

versus the alternative

$$H_1 : X_0^k \cup X_m^n \sim F, X_k^m \sim G \text{ for some } (k_n, \mu_n) \in \Theta_n, k_n = nk_n, m_n = n\mu_n.$$

The most important special case is the semiparametric exponential model with weight function $w(x, \beta) = \exp\{\beta^T H(x)\}$, where $H(x) = [h_1(x), \ldots, h_d(x)]^T$ is a vector of measurable functions. This exponential model contains many important families of distributions, such as the exponential family and the "partially exponential" family.

The goal is to make inference on $\theta_n = (k_n, \mu_n)$ using the empirical likelihood techniques of Owen (1988, 1990) (see Chapter 6 for details). Note that when $0 = k_n < \mu_n < 1$ or $0 < k_n < \mu_n = 1$, this model reduces to a semiparametric model with AMOC. In this case, the empirical likelihood ratio test has been shown to be more powerful and sensitive than the non-parametric test based on cumulative sums (Guan 2004). If the change points are known, the above model is a semiparametric two-sample model. We consider the case when the change points are unknown in the following subsections.

Define the proportion of the epidemic state by $\pi_n = d(\theta_n) = \mu_n - k_n$. The likelihood based on the observed data $x_1, \ldots, x_n$ is

$$L = \prod_{i=1}^{n} p_i \prod_{j=nk_n+1}^{n\mu_n} w(x_j, \beta) \left\{ \sum_{i=1}^{n} p_i w(x_i, \beta) \right\}^{-n\pi_n},$$

where $p_i = dF(x_i)$, $i = 1, \ldots, n$. For each fixed $\theta_n = (k_n, \mu_n)$ with $0 \le k_n \le \mu_n \le 1$ and (w, β), let $l(\theta_n, w, \beta)$ be the maximum value of $\log L + n \log n$ with respect to p_i, subject to constraints $\sum_{i=1}^{n} p_i w(x, \beta) = w$, $\sum_{i=1}^{n} p_i = 1$, $p_i \ge 0$, $i = 1, \ldots, n$. Using the Lagrange multiplier method, we can easily obtain

$$l(\theta_n, w, \beta) = -\sum_{i=1}^{n} \log\{(1 - \pi_n)w + \pi_n w(x_i, \beta)\} + \sum_{i=nk_n+1}^{n\mu_n} \log\{w(x_i, \beta)\} + n(1 - \pi_n)\log w.$$

For each θ_n, let $\left(\hat{w}, \hat{\beta}\right) = \left\{\hat{w}(\theta_n), \hat{\beta}(\theta_n)\right\}$ be a solution to

$$\psi_1(\theta_n, w, \beta) = \frac{\pi_n(1-\pi_n)}{w} \sum_{i=1}^{n} \frac{w(x_i, \beta) - w}{(1-\pi_n)w + \pi_n w(x_i, \beta)} = 0,$$

$$\psi_2(\theta_n, w, \beta) = \sum_{i=nk_n+1}^{n\mu_n} \frac{w'_\beta(x_i, \beta)}{w(x_i, \beta)} - \sum_{i=1}^{n} \frac{\pi_n w'_\beta(x_i, \beta)}{(1-\pi_n)w + \pi_n w(x_i, \beta)} = 0,$$

where $w'_\beta(x, \beta) = \partial w(x, \beta)/\partial\beta$. The profile likelihood of θ_n is $l(\theta_n) = l\left\{\theta_n, \hat{w}(\theta_n), \hat{\beta}(\theta_n)\right\}$, with $l(\theta_n) = l(0, 1)$ 0 for $0 \le k_n = \mu_n \le 1$. The maximum likelihood change-point estimates $\hat{\theta}_n = \left(\hat{k}_n, \hat{\mu}_n\right)$ can be obtained as

$$\hat{\theta}_n = \arg\max\left\{l(\theta_n); 0 \le k_n \le \mu_n \le 1\right\}.$$

Let $\Lambda_{k_n, m_n} = l(\theta_n)/n$, $S_n = 2 \max_{0 \le k_n < m_n \le n}\{n\Lambda_{k_n, m_n}\}$, where $k_n = nk_n$ and $m_n = n\mu_n$. Then the weighted likelihood ratio process is defined as $Z_n(s, t)$ if $0 \le s \le t \le 1$ or $Z_n(t, s)$ if $0 \le t < s \le 1$, where

$$Z_n(s, t) = 2n|t - s|(1 - |t - s|)\,\Lambda_{[sn], [tn]}.$$

We can obtain test statistics $V_{n,d}$ and $W_{n,d}$ as functionals of $Z_n(s, t)$, where

$$V_{n,d} = \int_0^1\int_0^1 Z_n(s, t)\,ds\,dt = 4n \sum_{1 \le k < m < n} a_{km}\Lambda_{k,m} \text{ with } a_{ij} = \frac{6(j-i)(n-j+i)-1}{6n^4},$$

$$W_{n,d} = \sup_{0 \le s \le t \le 1} Z_n(s, t).$$

With some mild conditions, under H_0 for each n, there exist independent Brownian bridges $B_n^{(1)}, \ldots, B_n^{(d)}$ on $[0, 1]$ such that

$$\sup_{0 \le s, t \le 1}\left| Z_n(s, t) - \sum_{1 \le i \le d}\left\{B_n^{(i)}(s) - B_n^{(i)}(t)\right\}^2 \right| = o_p(1).$$

Note that the conditions are quite general. For example, all the conditions are met for exponential model. For detailed conditions and proofs, we refer to Guan (2007). This result demonstrates that the approximate null distribution of the weighted likelihood ratio process $Z_n(s, t)$ is the same as that in the parametric case (see Theorem 1.7.3 of Csörgő and Horváth 1997). Based on this result, the weak convergence of some test statistics that are functionals of Z_n can be obtained. For example,

$$V_{n,d} \xrightarrow{d} V_d = \sum_{i=1}^{d}\int_0^1\int_0^1 |B^{(i)}(t) - B^{(i)}(s)|^2\,ds\,dt,$$

$$W_{n,d} \xrightarrow{d} \sup_{0 \le s \le t \le 1}\sum_{i=1}^{d} |B^{(i)}(t) - B^{(i)}(s)|^2.$$

Here V_d can be written as $V_d = \sum_{i=1}^{d} V^{(i)}$, where $V^{(1)}, \ldots, V^{(d)}$ are i.i.d. random variables and

$$\Pr\{V_1 \geq v\} = \Pr\{V^{(1)} \geq v\} = 2\sum_{j=1}^{\infty}(-1)^{j+1}e^{-\pi^2 j^2 v}, \quad v > 0.$$

When $d = 1$, the limiting distribution of $W_{n,1}$ is the same as that of the Kuiper statistic. Therefore, for $x > 0$,

$$\lim_{n \to \infty} \Pr\{W_{n,1} \geq x\} = 2\sum_{k=1}^{\infty}(4k^2 x - 1)e^{-2k^2 x}.$$

A table of this limiting distribution can be found in Shorack and Wellner (2009, p. 144).

Remark 12.3

It is assumed that under H_1 as $n \to \infty$, $k_n \to k_0$ and $\mu_n \to \mu_0$, $0 < k_0 < \mu_0 < 1$. Under the alternative H_1, the maximum likelihood estimates $\hat{\theta}_n = (\hat{k}_n, \hat{\mu}_n)$ of the change points $\theta_n = (k_n, \mu_n)$ are asymptotically unique and consistent. When we use the model with $w(x, \beta) = \exp(\beta x)$, the proposed test has the same limiting null distribution as the nonparametric test of epidemic change in the mean value, which was proposed by Lombard (1987).

12.5 Problems in Regression Models

Regression analysis is applied in many disciplines, including clinical trials and medical studies. In practice, ignoring changes in the data structure may lead to a poorly fitting regression model, which in turn may lead to incorrect inference. The statistical literature has several research studies of the problems associated with regression models.

Kim (1994) considered a test for a change point in linear regression by using the likelihood ratio statistic when the alternative specifies that only the intercept changes and when the alternative permits the intercept and the slope to change. In contrast, one may consider problems of segmented regression with two segments separated by a *breakpoint* (also called broken line [stick] regression, piecewise regression, join-point regression, or two or more phases regression when there are two or more segments), where one constrains the regression function to be continuous at the change point. Segmented linear regression can be useful to quantify an abrupt change of the response function given a varying influential factor. The breakpoint can be interpreted as a *critical, safe,* or *threshold* value beyond or below which (un)desired effects occur. The breakpoint can be important in decision making. A motivating example for segmented linear regression is dose–response curves, where there is a more or less sudden change in the rate at which response varies with dose. In epidemiologic studies, segmented regression models often occur as threshold models (Küchenhoff and Ulm 1997), where it is assumed that the exposure has no influence on the response up to possibly unknown thresholds (also termed threshold limiting values).

In this chapter, we present the problem for the simple linear regression model (Kim 1994; Kim and Siegmund 1989), as well as for segmented regression models (Vexler 2006).

12.5.1 Linear Regression

Given explanatory variables $x_1, \ldots, x_m$, suppose that observations y_i ($i = 1, \ldots, m$) are independent and normally distributed with common variance σ^2. For some j, the change point, the expectation of y_i equals $\alpha_0 + \beta_0 x_i$ if $i \leq j$ and equals $\alpha_1 + \beta_1 x_i$ if $i > j$. Kim and Siegmund (1989) considered the likelihood ratio tests of the hypothesis of no change, $H_0: \beta_0 = \beta_1$ and $\alpha_0 = \alpha_1$, against one of the alternatives, $H_1: \beta_0 = \beta_1 = \beta$ and there exists a j ($1 \leq j < m$) such that $\alpha_0 \neq \alpha_1$, or H_2: there exists a j ($1 \leq j < m$) such that $\beta_0 \neq \beta_1$ or $\alpha_0 \neq \alpha_1$. A secondary consideration is when H_1 holds, to obtain confidence regions for j and jointly for j, $\alpha_0 - \alpha_1$, and β. Since problems similar to these have been widely discussed in a variety of formulations with a variety of applications in mind, we begin with a brief review and motivation for our formulation. The following notation will be used:

$$\bar{y}_i = i^{-1} \sum_{k=1}^{i} y_k, \bar{y}_i^* = (m-i)^{-1} \sum_{k=i+1}^{m} y_k,$$

$$Q_{yyi} = \sum_{k=1}^{i} (y_k - \bar{y}_i)^2, Q_{yyi}^* = \sum_{k=i+1}^{m} (y_k - \bar{y}_i^*)^2, Q_{xyi} = \sum_{k=1}^{i} (x_k - \bar{x}_i)(y_k - \bar{y}_i),$$

$$\hat{\beta} = Q_{xym}/Q_{xxm}, \hat{\alpha}_i = \bar{y}_i - \hat{\beta}\bar{x}, \hat{\alpha}_i^* = \bar{y}_i^* - \hat{\beta}\bar{x}_i^*, \hat{\alpha}^2 = m^{-1}(Q_{yym} - Q_{xym}^2/Q_{xxm}).$$

A tedious calculation shows that the likelihood ratio test of H_0 against H_1, generalized slightly as suggested by James et al. (1987), rejects H_0 for large values of

$$\max_{m_0 \leq i \leq m_1} |U_m(i)|/\hat{\sigma},$$

where

$$U_m(i) = \left(\frac{i}{1-1/m}\right)^{1/2} \left(\frac{\bar{y}_i - \bar{y}_m - \hat{\beta}(\bar{x}_i - \bar{x}_m)}{[1 - i(\bar{x}_i - \bar{x}_m)^2/\{Q_{xxm}(1-i/m)\}]^{1/2}}\right)$$

$$= (\hat{\alpha}_i - \hat{\alpha}_i^*)\left[\frac{i(1-i/m)}{1 - i(\bar{x}_i - \bar{x}_m)^2/\{Q_{xxm}(1-i/m)\}}\right]^{1/2}.$$

Under H_0, we have $y_i = \alpha + \beta x_i + \varepsilon_i$ ($i = 1, \ldots, m$), where the ε_i are independent $N(0, \sigma^2)$. Suppose $x_i = f(i/m)$ and let g be defined as

$$g(t) = \left\{\int_0^1 f(u)\,du - t^{-1}\int_0^t f(u)\,du\right\} \Bigg/ \left\{(1-t)\left(\int_0^1 f^2(u)\,du - \left(\int_0^1 f(u)\,du\right)^2\right)^{1/2}\right\},$$

and let

$$\mu(t) = 1/[2t(1-t)\{1-g^2(t)t(1-t)\}].$$

Assume $b, m \to \infty$ such that for some $0 < c < 1$ and $0 \leq t_0 < t_1 \leq 1$,

$$b/\sqrt{m} \to c, \, m_i \sim mt_i \, (i = 0,1).$$

Then for U_m defined above, the probability $p_1 = \Pr\left\{ \max_{m_0 \leq i \leq m_1} \hat{\sigma}^{-1} |U_m(i)| \geq b \right\}$ satisfies

$$p_1 \sim (2/\pi)^{1/2} b(1 - b^2/m)^{1/2(m-5)} \int_{t_0}^{t_1} \mu(t) v\left[\{2c^2\mu(t)/(1-c^2)\}^{1/2} \right] dt,$$

where

$$v(x) = 2x^{-2} \exp\left\{ -2 \sum_{n=1}^{\infty} n^{-1} \Phi\left(-\tfrac{1}{2} x\sqrt{n} \right) \right\}, \, x > 0,$$

and Φ denotes the standard normal distribution function. For numerical purposes, it often suffices to use the small x approximation (Siegmund 1985, Chapter 10), which leads to the approximation $v(x) \approx \exp(-\rho x)$, where ρ is a numerical constant approximately equal to 0.583.

12.5.2 Segmented Linear Regression

Let the observed sample be $\{Y_i, x_{1i}, x_{2i}\}_{i=1}^n$. Without loss of generality and for the sake of clarity of exposition, we assume that x_{1i} and x_{2i} are scalar values. Let

$$Y_i = (\beta_{00} + \beta_{01}x_{1i} + \varepsilon_{0i}) \, I\{i < v\} + (\beta_{10} + \beta_{11}x_{1i} + \beta_{12}x_{2i} + \varepsilon_{1i}) \, I\{v \leq i < y\}$$

$$+ (\beta_{00} + \beta_{01}x_{1i} + \varepsilon_{0i}) \, I \, \{i \geq y\}, \, v < y, \, v < y, \, i = 1, \ldots, n$$

denote the segmented linear regression model, where β_{km}, $m = 0, \ldots, k+1, k = 0, 1$ are regression parameters, x_{1i}, x_{2i} are fixed predictors, $I\{\cdot\}$ is the indicator function, v, y are the change points, and $\varepsilon_{0i}, \varepsilon_{1i}$ are independent random disturbance terms with $g_0(u, \theta_0), g_1(u, \theta_1)$ densities (θ_0 and θ_1 are parameters), respectively. The model corresponds to a situation where up to an unknown change point $v > 0$, the observations satisfy the linear regression model with parameters β_{00}, β_{01}. Beyond that (if $v \leq n$), an epidemic state runs from time v through $y - 1$, after which (if $y < n$) the normal state is restored.

Vexler (2006) considered the hypothesis testing where

$$H_0: v > n \text{ versus } H_1: 1 \leq v \leq n; v, y: 0 < v < y \text{ are unknown}$$

Note that if $\beta_{12} = 0, \beta_{10} = \beta_{00} + \delta, \beta_{11} = \beta_{01} + \delta, \delta$ is a nuisance parameter and $\varepsilon_{0i}, \varepsilon_{1i}$ are normal distributed with zero expectation and variance σ^2, then we have the problem considered by Yao (1993a, 1993b); if $\beta_{01} = \beta_{11} = \beta_{12} = 0, \beta_{10} = \beta_{00} + \delta, \theta_0 = \theta_1$, and $g_0 = g_1$, then we have the problem analyzed by Hušková (1995); if $y > n$, then it is a standard problem of regression models (e.g., Gurevich and Vexler 2005; Julious 2001). For other investigations of such problems, see, for example, Račkauskas and Suquet (2006). We present the method by Vexler (2006) in the following subsections, considering a simple case where β_{00}, β_{01}, θ_0, β_{10}, β_{11}, β_{12}, θ_1 are known and a general case where β_{00}, β_{01}, θ_0, β_{10}, β_{11}, β_{12}, θ_1 are unknown.

12.5.2.1 Simple Case of the Problem

We consider the segmented linear regression model where β_{00}, β_{01}, θ_0, β_{10}, β_{11}, β_{12}, θ_1 are known. Let $\Pr_0$ denote the probability measure under H_0 and P_{km} denote the probability measure under H_1 with $v = k$, $y = m$ Likewise, let E_0 and E_{km} denote expectation under P_0 and P_{km}, respectively. Denote the likelihood ratio

$$\Lambda_{km} = \prod_{i=k}^{m} \frac{g_1(Y_i - \beta_{10} - \beta_{11}x_{1i} - \beta_{12}x_{2i}, \theta_1)}{g_0(Y_i - \beta_{00} - \beta_{01}x_{1i}, \theta_0)}$$

The standard test statistics for the hypothesis test stated above are some modifications of CUSUM statistics, for instance, $\max_1 \leq m \leq n$, $\max_1 \leq k \leq m \Lambda_{km}$ (e.g., Yao 1993a, 1993b). In sequential analysis of solving problems, there are methods related to substitution of maximum of likelihood ratios by the Shiryayev–Roberts statistics. Hence, that leads us to the Shiryayev–Roberts detection policy aimed at obtaining guaranteed characteristics of procedures (e.g., Pollak 1987). In this situation, the statistical decision-making rule is to reject H_0 if and only if

$$\frac{1}{n} \max_{1 \leq m \leq n} R_m > c,$$

where $R_m = \sum_{k=1}^{m} \Lambda_{km}$, and the threshold $C > 0$. The significance level α of the test satisfies

$$\alpha = \Pr_0 \left\{ \max_{1 \leq m \leq n} R_m > nC \right\} \leq 1/C.$$

12.5.2.2 General Case of the Problem

This section considers the segmented linear regression model where β_{00}, β_{01}, θ_0, β_{10}, β_{11}, β_{12}, θ_1 are unknown. Denote

$$\Lambda_{km}^{(2)} = \prod_{i=k}^{m} \frac{g_1\left(Y_i - \hat{\beta}_{10}^{(k,i-1)} - \hat{\beta}_{11}^{(k,i-1)}x_{1i} - \hat{\beta}_{12}^{(k,i-1)}x_{2i}, \hat{\theta}_1^{(k,i-1)}\right)}{g_0\left(Y_i - \tilde{\beta}_{00}^{(k,m)} - \tilde{\beta}_{01}^{(k,m)}x_{1i}, \tilde{\theta}_0^{(k,m)}\right)},$$

where $\left\{\hat{\beta}_{10}^{(1,m)}, \hat{\beta}_{11}^{(1,m)}, \hat{\beta}_{12}^{(1,m)}, \hat{\theta}_1^{(1,m)}\right\}$ are some (any) estimators of $\{\beta_{01}, \beta_{11}, \beta_{12}, \theta_1\}$ based on $\{Y_l, \ldots, Y_m\}$ with $\left\{\hat{\beta}_{10}^{(l,l-1)}, \hat{\beta}_{11}^{(l,l-1)}, \hat{\beta}_{12}^{(l,l-1)}, \hat{\theta}_1^{(l,l-1)}\right\} = \{0,0,0,1\}$, and $\left\{\tilde{\beta}_{00}^{(k,m)}, \tilde{\beta}_{01}^{(k,m)}, \tilde{\theta}_0^{(k,m)}\right\}$ are maximum likelihood estimators of $\{\beta_{00}, \beta_{01}, \theta_0\}$ in the σ-algebra generated by $\{Y_k, \ldots, Y_m\}$

$$\left\{\tilde{\beta}_{00}^{(k,m)}, \tilde{\beta}_{01}^{(k,m)}, \tilde{\theta}_0^{(k,m)}\right\} = \arg \max_{\beta_{00}^*, \beta_{01}^*, \theta_0^*} \prod_{i=k}^{m} g_0\left(Y_i - \beta_{00}^* - \beta_{01}^* x_{1i}, \theta_0^*\right).$$

The same idea appears in Gurevich and Vexler (2005) in a different context. By definition of maximum likelihood estimators, we obtain the inequality

$$\prod_{i=k}^{m} g_0\left(Y_i - \tilde{\beta}_{00}^{(k,m)} - \tilde{\beta}_{01}^{(k,m)} x_{1i}, \tilde{\theta}^{(k,m)}\right) \geq \prod_{i=k}^{m} g_0(Y_i - \beta_{00} - \beta_{01} x_{1i}, \theta_0)$$

and use it to consider the significant level of a test. In this situation, the statistical decision-making rule is to reject H_0 if and only if

$$\frac{1}{n} \max_{1 \leq m \leq n} R_m^{(2)} > C,$$

where $R_m^{(2)} = \sum_{k=1}^{m} \Lambda_{km}^{(2)}$, and threshold $C > 0$. The significance level $\alpha^{(2)}$ of the test satisfies

$$\alpha^{(2)} = \Pr_0 \left\{ \max_{1 \leq m \leq n} R_m^{(2)} > nC \right\} \leq 1/C.$$

12.6 Supplement

12.6.1 Simple Change Point

12.6.1.1 Parametric Methods

1. Quandt (1960) explored several approaches for testing the hypothesis that no switch has occurred in the true values of the parameters of a linear regression system. The distribution of the relevant likelihood ratio λ is analyzed on the basis of the empirical distribution resulting from some sampling experiments. The hypothesis that $-2\log \lambda$ has a χ^2-distribution with the appropriate degrees of freedom is rejected and an empirical table of percentage points is obtained.

   A sequence of independent random variables $X_1, X_2, \ldots, X_N$ is said to have a change point at n if $X_1, X_2, \ldots, X_n$ have a common distribution $F(x)$ and $X_{n+1}, \ldots, X_N$ have a common distribution G, $G \neq F$. Consider the problem of testing the null hypothesis of no change against the alternative of a change $G < F$ at an unknown change point n. Praagman (1988) compared two classes of statistics based on two-sample linear rank statistics (max and sum type) in terms of their Bahadur efficiency. Assuming that a distribution of observations x is defined by a real parameter θ and that it is of interest to test H_0: $\theta = \theta_0$ versus H_1: $\theta \neq \theta_0$, Bahadur asymptotic relative efficiency of two sequences of statistics $\{V_n\}$ and $\{T_n\}$ is the ratio of the corresponding Bahadur exact slopes, where the Bahadur exact slope of a test statistic T_n is defined by $-\lim_{n \to \infty} 2n^{-1} \log\left(\Pr_\theta(T_n \geq T_n(\mathbf{x}))\right)$. It is shown that for every sequence of sum-type statistics, a sequence of max-type statistics can be constructed with at least the same Bahadur slope at all possible alternatives. Special attention is paid to alternatives close to the null hypothesis.

2. Hirotsu (1997) derived exact null and alternative distributions of the two-way maximally selected χ^2 for interaction between the ordered rows and columns for each of the normal and Poisson models, respectively. This method is one of the multiple comparison procedures for ordered parameters and is useful for defining a block interaction or a two-way change-point model as a simple alternative to the two-way additive model. The construction of a confidence region for the two-way change point is then described.

3. Borovkov (1999) proposed asymptotically optimal procedures in the classical problem, which are established under the assumption that the change point, being an unknown parameter, increases in an unbounded fashion.

4. Let $\beta_n(t)$ denote the weighted (smooth) bootstrap process (see Chapter 17 for details) of an empirical process. Horváth et al. (2000) showed that the order of the best Gaussian approximation for $\beta_n(t)$ is $n^{-1/2}\log n$ and constructed a sequence of approximating Brownian bridges achieving this rate. The authors also obtained an approximation for $\beta_n(t)$ using a suitably chosen Kiefer process. The result is applied to detect a possible change in the distribution of independent observations.

5. Change-point problems arise when different subsequences of a data series follow different statistical distributions, commonly of the same functional form but having different parameters. Hawkins (2001) developed an exact approach for finding maximum likelihood estimates of the change points and within-segment parameters when the functional form is within the general exponential family. The algorithm, a dynamic program, has an execution time, which is linear in the number of segments and quadratic in the number of potential change points. The details are worked out for the normal, gamma, Poisson, and binomial distributions.

6. Desmond et al. (2002) applied analysis on a herpes zoster pain data set. The analysis of pain severity data was complicated by the nonlinear rate of resolution. Using two clinical trial data sets as the bases for analyses, the rates of baseline pain resolution were computed across each of three phases and compared for age, severity of pain at onset, and number of lesions at baseline. The model of Desmond et al. verified three phases of zoster pain—acute, subacute, and chronic—and delineated the impact of treatment and other factors on the phase-specific rates of pain cessation.

7. Vexler (2008) adapted the Shiryayev–Roberts approach to detect various types of changes in distributions of non-i.i.d. observations. By utilizing the martingale properties of the Shiryayev–Roberts statistic, this technique provides distribution-free, nonasymptotic upper bounds for the significance levels of asymptotic power one tests for change points with epidemic alternatives. Since optimal Shiryayev–Roberts sequential procedures are well investigated, the proposed methodology yields a simple approach for obtaining analytical results related to retrospective testing. In the case when distributions of data are known up to parameters, an adaptive estimation was presented that is more efficient than a well-accepted non-anticipating estimation described in the literature. The adaptive procedure can also be used in the context of sequential detection.

8. Vexler et al. (2009b) considered a specific classification problem in the context of detection. The authors presented generalized classical maximum likelihood tests for homogeneity of the observed sample in a simple form that avoids the complex direct estimation of unknown parameters. A martingale approach was proposed for transformation of test statistics. For sequential and retrospective testing

problems, the authors proposed the adapted Shiryayev–Roberts statistics in order to obtain simple tests with asymptotic power one. An important application of the developed methods is in the analysis of exposure's measurements subject to limits of detection in occupational medicine.

9. Vexler and Wu (2009) presented and examined an approach to nonsequential detections based on the Shiryayev–Roberts scheme. The authors showed that retrospective detection policies based on Shiryayev–Roberts statistics are nonasymptotically optimal in the context of most powerful testing.

10. Gurevich and Vexler (2010) reviewed recent retrospective parametric and distribution-free generalized detection policies, attending to different contexts of optimality and robustness of the procedures, as well as proposed new relevant procedures. The authors conducted a broad Monte Carlo study to compare various parametric and nonparametric tests, also investigating the sensitivity of the detection policies with respect to assumptions required for correct executions of the procedures. An example based on real biomarker measurements was provided to judge our conclusions.

11. Habibi (2011) applied the CUSUM method to transformed observations and showed this method works better than the usual CUSUM procedure, which uses the original data. Two main transformations are the null distribution function and score function. Test statistics were presented with their limiting null distributions.

12. In accordance with a given risk function of hypothesis testing, investigators commonly try to derive an optimal property of a test. Vexler and Gurevich (2011) demonstrated that criteria for which a given test is optimal can be declared by the structure of this test, and hence almost any reasonable test is optimal. In order to establish this conclusion, the principal idea of the fundamental Neyman–Pearson lemma is applied to interpret the goodness of tests, as well as retrospective and sequential detections are considered in the context of the proposed technique. Aside from that, the authors evaluated a specific classification problem that corresponds to measurement error effects in occupational medicine.

12.6.1.2 Nonparametric Methods

1. Horváth and Shao (1996) presented that the maximally selected standardized U-statistic converges in distribution to an infinite sum of weighted chi-square random variables in the degenerate case and applied the result to the detection of possible changes in the distribution of a sequence observation.

2. Dumbgen (1991) considered a sequence $X_1, X_2, ..., X_n$ of independent random variables, where $X_1, X_2, ..., X_{n\theta}$ have distribution P and $X_{n\theta+1}, X_{n\theta+2}, ..., X_n$ have distribution Q. The change point $\theta \in (0,1)$ is an unknown parameter to be estimated, and P and Q are two unknown probability distributions. The nonparametric estimators of Darkhovskh (1976) and Carlstein (1988) are embedded in a more general framework, where random seminorms are applied to empirical measures for making inference about θ. Darkhovskh's and Carlstein's results about consistency are improved, and the limiting distributions of some particular estimators are derived in various models. The author further proposed asymptotically valid confidence regions for the change point θ by inverting bootstrap tests. This method was illustrated with Nile data.

3. The critical values for various tests based on U-statistics to detect a possible change are obtained through permutations (see Chapter 17 for details) of the observations. Horváth and Hušková (2005) obtained the same approximations for the permutated U-statistics under the no-change null hypothesis as well as under the exactly one-change alternative. The results are used to show that the simulated critical values are asymptotically valid under the null hypothesis, and the tests reject with the probability tending to 1 under the alternative.

4. Zou et al. (2007) proposed a nonparametric method based on the empirical likelihood (see Chapter 6 for details) to detect the change point from a sequence of independent random variables. The empirical likelihood ratio test statistic is proved to have the same limit null distribution as that with classical parametric likelihood. Under some mild conditions, the maximum empirical likelihood estimator of change point is also shown to be consistent. The simulation results demonstrate the sensitivity and robustness of the proposed approach.

5. Ning (2012) discussed a model with the mean being constant up to some unknown point, increasing linearly to another unknown point, and then dropping back to the original level. A nonparametric method based on the empirical likelihood test was proposed to detect and estimate the locations of change points. Under some mild conditions, the asymptotic null distribution of an empirical likelihood ratio test statistic is shown to have the extreme distribution. The consistency of the test was also proved. Simulations of the powers of the test indicate that it performs well under different assumptions of the data distribution. The test was applied to the aircraft arrival time data set and the Stanford heart transplant data set.

12.6.2 Multiple Change Points

12.6.2.1 Parametric Methods

1. Csörgő and Horváth (1997) reviewed and described a variety of methods to deal with problems. The authors presented the limit theorem of various techniques and illustrated the applicability of the main results via discussing a number of data sets using different methods.

2. Braun et al. (2000) considered situations where a step function with a variable number of steps provides an adequate model for a regression relationship, while the variance of the observations depends on their mean. This model provides for discontinuous jumps at change points and for constant means and error variances in between change points. The basic statistical problem consists of identification of the number of change points, their locations, and the levels that the function assumes in between. The authors embedded this problem into a quasi-likelihood formulation and employed the minimum deviance criterion to fit the model; for the choice of the number of change points, the authors discussed a modified Schwarz criterion. A dynamic programming algorithm makes the segmentation feasible for sequences of moderate length. The performance of the segmentation method is demonstrated in an application to the segmentation of the bacteriophage λ sequence.

3. Consider a sequence of independent exponential random variables that is susceptible to a change in the means. Ramanayake and Gupta (2003) proposed testing whether the means have been subjected to an epidemic change after an unknown

point, for an unknown duration in the sequence. The likelihood ratio statistic and a likelihood ratio–type statistic are derived. The distribution theories and related properties of the test statistics are discussed. Percentage points and powers of the tests are tabulated for selected values of the parameters. The powers of these two tests are then compared to the two statistics proposed by Aly and Bouzar (1992). The tests are applied to find epidemic changes in the set of Stanford heart transplant data and air traffic arrival data. Define $S_j = \sum_{i=1}^{j} X_i$. Then the equivalent test statistic is $T_0 = \sum_{m=1}^{n-1} \sum_{k=1}^{m-1} (S_m - S_k)/\theta = \sum_{m=1}^{n-1} (n-i)(i-1)X_i/\theta$. In most practical situations, it is highly unlikely that θ would be known. The authors suggested replacing θ with $\bar{X} = n^{-1} \sum_{i=1}^{n} X_i$, the maximum likelihood estimator of θ under H_0. For convenience, the authors recommended the statistic

$$T = \sum_{i=1}^{n-1} (n-1)(i-1)X_i \bigg/ \left(M \sum_{i=1}^{n} X_i \right),$$

where $M = 2n^{-1} \sum_{i=1}^{n-1} (n-i)(i-1) = (n-1)(n-2)/3$. Define $T_1 = (T-0.5)/\sqrt{\operatorname{var}(T)}$ to be the standardized statistic corresponding to statistic T. Then by the Lyapunov central limit theorem and Slutky's theorem, under H_0, the statistic T_1 follows an asymptotic normal distribution. Employing a three-term Edgeworth expansion for the distribution function of statistic T_1 (e.g., see Gombay 1994), the critical values of T_0 for moderate sample sizes can be calculated as

$$F_{T_1}(x) = \Phi(x) - \left\{ \frac{\sqrt{\beta_1(T)}}{6}(x^2-1) + \frac{1}{24}(\beta_2(T_1)-3)(x^3-3x) + \frac{1}{72}\beta_1(T_1)(x^5-10x^3+15x) \right\} \varphi(x),$$

where $\Phi(x)$ and $\varphi(x)$ are the distribution function and the density function of a standard normal random variable, respectively.

4. Ganocy (2003) developed estimators for the change points in two ways, which in the two-dimensional case is equivalent to edge reconstruction in images. One is based on the likelihood approach. Two procedures are established using maximum likelihood estimation. The first, an unconstrained procedure, is derived without assuming continuity at the location of the change points, while the second, a constrained estimation method, imposes a continuity restriction at these locations. Additionally, the continuity-restricted model is extended to allow for the middle segment to be a quadratic function instead of a straight line. A model selection procedure is derived to test for the significance of the quadratic component. Algorithms are produced to solve for the unknown parameters. Second, a Bayesian approach is used to estimate the unknown change point and variance (or precision) parameters. In addition to developing standard Bayesian methodology for maximizing a posterior (MAP), a new Bayesian-type algorithm, maximization–maximization–posterior (MMP), is proposed. Under both the likelihood and Bayesian approaches, the algorithms can be accelerated by choosing good starting values using knowledge of the approximate location of the change points, which can be obtained visually from a preliminary plot of the data. The author studied the performance of the two approaches by simulation and analysis. From the performance characteristics, the different algorithms were compared.

5. In order to detect epidemic change in the mean of a sample of size n, Alfredas and Charles (2004) introduced new test statistics UI and DI based on weighted increments of partial sums. The authors obtained their limit distributions under the null hypothesis of no change in the mean. Under the alternative hypothesis, our statistics can detect very short epidemics of length $\log^{\gamma} n$, $\gamma > 1$. Using self-normalization and adaptiveness to modify UI and DI allows us to prove the same results under very relaxed moment assumptions. Trimmed versions of UI and DI are also studied.

6. Many long instrumental climate records are available and might provide useful information in climate research. These series are usually affected by artificial shifts, due to changes in the conditions of measurement and various kinds of spurious data. A comparison with surrounding weather stations by means of a suitable two-factor model allows us to check the reliability of the series. Caussinus and Mestre (2004) employed an adapted penalized log-likelihood procedure to detect an unknown number of breaks and outliers. An example concerning temperature series from France confirmed that a systematic comparison of the series together is valuable and allows us to correct the data even when no reliable series can be taken as a reference.

7. Chen and Gupta (2011) presented different models, including gamma and exponential models, rarely examined thus far in the literature. Extensive examples throughout the text emphasize key concepts and different methodologies used, namely, the likelihood ratio criterion and the Bayesian and information criterion approaches. New examples of analysis in modern molecular biology and other fields, such as finance and air traffic control, are added.

8. Killick and Eckley (2011) developed the package to provide users with a choice of multiple search methods to use in conjunction with a given method, and in particular provide an implementation of the recently proposed PELT algorithm. The authors described the search methods that are implemented in the package, as well as some of the available test statistics, while highlighting their application with simulated and practical examples. Particular emphasis was placed on the PELT algorithm and how results differ from the binary segmentation approach.

12.6.2.2 Nonparametric Methods

1. Brodsky and Darkhovsky (1993) present a summary of results in a variety of nonparametric detection methods, which have been developed for practical applications and computer programs. Some of them were realized in the VERDIA program package of nonparametric change-point detection, which is included in the MESOSAUR package for statistical analysis.

2. James and Matteson (2013) designed the *ecp* package to perform multiple analysis while making as few assumptions as possible. While many other methods are applicable only for univariate data, this R package is suitable for both univariate and multivariate observations. Hierarchical estimation can be based on either a divisive or agglomerative algorithm. Divisive estimation sequentially identifies change points via a bisection algorithm. The agglomerative algorithm estimates locations by determining an optimal segmentation. Both approaches are able to detect *any* type of distributional change within the data. This provides an advantage over many existing algorithms that are only able to detect changes within the marginal distributions

12.6.3 Problems in Regression Models

12.6.3.1 *Linear Regression*

1. Kim and Cai (1993) examined the robustness of the likelihood ratio tests for a change point in simple linear regression. The authors first summarized the normal theory of Kim and Siegmund (1989), where the likelihood ratio test was considered for no change in the regression coefficients versus the alternatives with a change in the intercept alone and with a change in the intercept and slope. The authors then discussed the robustness of these tests. Using the convergence theory of stochastic processes, we show that the test statistics converge to the same limiting distributions regardless of the underlying distribution. The authors performed simulations to assess the distributional insensitivity of the test statistics to a Weibull, a lognormal, and a contaminated normal distribution in two different cases: fixed and random independent variables. Numerical examples illustrated that the test has a correct size and retains its power when the distribution is nonnormal. The effects of the independent variable's configuration with the aid of a numerical example were studied.

2. Kim (1994) considered a problem of detecting a change point in a linear model and discussed analytic properties of the likelihood ratio statistic and studied its asymptotic behavior. An approximation for the significance level of the test is provided, assuming values of the independent variables are effectively random. The author also discussed the power and the robustness of the likelihood ratio test.

3. Andrews et al. (1996) determined a class of finite sample optimal tests for the existence of a change point at an unknown time in a normal linear multiple regression model with known variance. Optimal tests for multiple change points were also derived. It was shown that the results cover some models of cointegration. Power comparisons of several tests were provided based on simulations.

4. Spokoiny (1998) proposed a method of adaptive estimation of a regression function that is near optimal in the classical sense of the mean integrated error and is shown to be very sensitive to discontinuities or change points of the underlying function or its derivatives. For example, in the case of a jump of a regression function, beyond the intervals of length (in order) $n^{-1}\log n$ around change points, the quality of estimation is essentially the same as if locations of jumps were known. The method is fully adaptive and no assumptions are imposed on the design, number, and size of jumps. The results were formulated in a nonasymptotic way and can be applied for an arbitrary sample size.

5. Julious (2001) introduced the two-line model when the location of the change point is known, with an F-test to detect a change in the regression coefficient. The situation when the change point is unknown was then introduced and an algorithm proposed for parameter estimation. It was demonstrated that when the location of the change point is not known, the F-test does not conform to its expected parametric distribution. Nonparametric bootstrap methods were proposed as a way of overcoming the problems encountered. A physiology example was illustrated where the regression change represents the change from aerobic to anaerobic energy production.

6. Pastor-Barriuso et al. (2003) introduced transition methods for logistic regression models in which the dose–response relationship follows two different straight lines, which may intersect or may present a jump at an unknown change point.

In these models, the logit includes a differentiable transition function that provides parametric control of the sharpness of the transition at the change point, allowing for abrupt changes or more gradual transitions between the two different linear trends, as well as for estimation of the location of the change point. Linear–linear logistic models are particular cases of the proposed transition models. The authors present a modified iteratively reweighted least-squares algorithm to estimate model parameters, and we provide inference procedures, including a test for the existence of the change point. These transition models are explored in a simulation study, and they are used to evaluate the existence of a change point in the association between plasma glucose after an oral glucose tolerance test and mortality using data from the mortality follow-up of the second national health and nutrition examination survey.

7. Liu et al. (2008) proposed a nonparametric method based on the empirical likelihood to detect the change point in the coefficient of linear regression models. The empirical likelihood ratio test statistic is proved to have the same asymptotic null distribution as that with classical parametric likelihood. Under some mild conditions, the maximum empirical likelihood estimator is also shown to be consistent. The simulation results showed the sensitivity and robustness of the proposed approach. The method was applied to some real data sets to illustrate the effectiveness.

8. The product partition model (PPM) is a powerful tool for clustering and analysis, mainly because it considers the number of blocks or segments as a random variable. Loschi et al. (2010) applied the PPM to identify multiple change points in linear regression models, extending some previous works. In addition, the authors provided a predictive justification for the within-block linear model. This way of modeling provides a non–ad hoc procedure for treating piecewise regression models. The authors also modified the original algorithm proposed by Barry and Hartigan (1993) in order to obtain samples from the product distribution posteriors of the parameters in the regression model, say in the contiguous-block case. Consequently, posterior summaries (including the posterior means or product estimates) can be obtained in the usual way. The product estimates were obtained considering both the proposed and Barry and Hartigan's algorithms, which are compared to least-squares estimates for the piecewise regression models. Some financial data sets were analyzed to illustrate the use of the proposed methodology.

9. Chen et al. (2011) considered two problems concerning locating change points in a linear regression model. One involves jump discontinuities (change points) in a regression model, and the other involves regression lines connected at unknown points. The authors compared four methods for estimating single or multiple change points in a regression model, when both the error variance and regression coefficients change simultaneously at the unknown points: Bayesian, Julious, grid search, and segmented methods. The proposed methods were evaluated via a simulation study and compared via some standard measures of estimation bias and precision. Finally, the methods were illustrated and compared using three real data sets. The simulation and empirical results overall favor both the segmented and Bayesian methods of estimation, which simultaneously estimate the change point and the other model parameters, though only the Bayesian method is able to handle both continuous and discontinuous problems successfully. If it is known that regression lines are continuous, then the segmented method ranked first among methods.

12.6.3.2 Threshold Effects

1. Ulm (1991) presented a method for estimating and testing a threshold value in epidemiological studies within the framework of the logistic regression model, which is widely used in the analysis of the relationship between some explanatory variables and a dependent dichotomous outcome. In most available programs for this and also for other models, the concept of a threshold is disregarded. The method for assessing a threshold consists of an estimation procedure using the maximum likelihood technique and a test procedure based on the likelihood ratio statistic, following under the null hypothesis (no threshold) a quasi-one-sided χ^2-distribution with one degree of freedom. The use of this distribution is supported by a simulation study. The method is applied to data from an epidemiological study of the relationship between occupational dust exposure and chronic bronchitic reactions. The results are confirmed by bootstrap resampling.

2. Küchenhoff and Ulm (1997) reviewed several statistical methods for assessing threshold limiting values in occupational epidemiology. The authors summarized the statistical properties of those methods and briefly compared them from a theoretical point of view and in more detail with respect to their behavior in a concrete data analysis. The techniques are applied to a study concerning the relationship between dust concentration at the working place and chronic bronchitis (CBR), where a special interest was to determine a threshold limiting value for the total inhalable dust with respect to developing chronic bronchitis.

3. Küchenhoff and Carroll (1997) considered the estimation of parameters in a particular segmented generalized linear model with additive measurement error in predictors, with a focus on linear and logistic regression. The authors showed that in threshold regression, the functional and structural methods differ substantially in their performance. In one of their simulations, approximately consistent functional estimates can be as much as 25 times more variable than the maximum likelihood estimate for a properly specified parametric model. Structural (parametric) modeling ought not to be a neglected tool in measurement error models. An example involving dust concentration and bronchitis in a mechanical engineering plant in Munich was used to illustrate the results.

4. Bender (1999) proposed a method for quantitative risk assessment in epidemiological studies investigating threshold effects. The simple logistic regression model is used to describe the association between a binary response variable and a continuous risk factor. By defining acceptable levels for the absolute risk and the risk gradient, the corresponding benchmark values of the risk factor can be calculated by means of nonlinear functions of the logistic regression coefficients. Standard errors and confidence intervals of the benchmark values are derived by means of the multivariate delta method. This approach is compared with the threshold model of Ulm (1991) for assessing threshold values in epidemiological studies.

5. Gössl and Kuechenhoff (2001) discussed Bayesian estimation of a logistic regression model with an unknown threshold limiting value (TLV). In these models, it is assumed that there is no effect of a covariate on the response under a certain unknown TLV. The estimation of these models in a Bayesian context by Markov chain Monte Carlo (MCMC) methods is considered with a focus on the TLV. The authors extended the model by accounting for measurement error in the covariate. The Bayesian solution is compared with the likelihood solution proposed

by Küchenhoff and Carroll (1997) using a data set concerning the relationship between dust concentration in the working place and the occurrence of chronic bronchitis.

6. Gurevich and Vexler (2005) considered generalized maximum likelihood asymptotic power one tests that aim to detect a change point in logistic regression when the alternative specifies that a change occurred in parameters of the model. A guaranteed nonasymptotic upper bound for the significance level of each of the tests is presented. For cases in which the test supports the conclusion that there was a change point, the authors proposed a maximum likelihood estimator of that point and present results regarding the asymptotic properties of the estimator. An important field of application of this approach is occupational medicine, where for a lot of chemical compounds and other agents, so-called threshold limit values (TLVs) are specified. The authors demonstrated applications of the test and the maximum likelihood estimation of the change point using an actual problem that was encountered with real data.

7. Lee and Seo (2008) proposed a semiparametric estimation method of a threshold binary response model, where the parameters for a regression function are finite-dimensional, while allowing for heteroscedasticity of unknown form. In particular, the authors considered Manski's (1975, 1985) maximum score estimator. The model is irregular because of a change point due to an unknown threshold in a covariate. This irregularity coupled with the discontinuity of the objective function of the maximum score estimator complicates the analysis of the asymptotic behavior of the estimator. Sufficient conditions for the identification of parameters are given and the consistency of the estimator is obtained. It is shown that the estimator of the threshold parameter, γ_0, is n^{-1} consistent, and the estimator of the remaining regression parameters, θ_0, is $n^{-1/3}$ consistent. Furthermore, the authors obtained the asymptotic distribution of the estimator. It turns out that both estimators $\hat{\gamma}$ and $\hat{\theta}$ are oracle efficient in that $n(\hat{\gamma}_n - \gamma_0)$ and $n^{1/3}(\hat{\theta}_n - \theta_0)$ converge weakly to the distributions to which they would converge weakly if the other parameters were known.

8. Lee et al. (2011) developed a general method for testing threshold effects in regression models, using sup–likelihood ratio (LR)–type statistics. While the standard approach in the literature for obtaining the asymptotic null distribution of the sup-LR-type test statistic requires that there exist a certain quadratic approximation to the objective function, the method proposed here can be used to establish the asymptotic null distribution, even when the usual quadratic approximation is intractable. The authors illustrated the usefulness of our approach in the examples of the maximum score estimation, maximum likelihood estimation, quantile regression, and maximum rank correlation estimation. The authors established consistency and local power properties of the test and presented some simulation results and also an empirical application to tipping in racial segregation.

12.6.3.3 Segmented Regression

1. Küchenhoff (1996) considered the problem of estimating the unknown breakpoints in segmented generalized linear models. Exact algorithms for calculating maximum likelihood estimators were derived for different types of models. After discussing the case of a general linear model (GLM) with a single covariate having

one breakpoint, a new algorithm was presented for when further covariates are included in the model. The essential idea of this approach was then used for the case of more than one breakpoint. As a further extension, an algorithm for the situation of two regressors each having a breakpoint was proposed. These techniques were applied for analyzing the data of the Munich rental table. It can be seen that these algorithms are easy to handle without too much computational effort. The algorithms are available as GAUSS programs.

2. Pastor and Guallar (1998) presented a two-segmented logistic regression model, in which the linear term associated with a continuous exposure in standard logistic regression is replaced by a two-segmented polynomial function with unknown change point, which is also estimated. A modified, iteratively reweighted least-squares algorithm was presented to obtain parameter estimates and confidence intervals, and the performance of this model is explored through simulation. Finally, a two-segmented logistic regression model was applied to a case-control study of the association of alcohol intake with the risk of myocardial infarction and compared with alternative analyses. The ability of two-segmented logistic regression to estimate and provide inferences for the location of change points and for the magnitude of other parameters of effect makes this model a useful complement to other methods of dose–response analysis in epidemiologic studies.

3. Wu et al. (2001) developed a test based on isotonic regression for monotonic trends in short-range dependent sequences and applied it to Argentina rainfall data and global warming data. This test provided another perspective for problems. The isotonic test was shown to be more powerful than some existing tests for trend.

4. Staudenmayer and Spiegelman (2002) considered the problem of segmented regression in the presence of covariate measurement error (see Chapter 15) in main study and validation study designs. A closed and interpretable form for the full likelihood was derived. Employing the likelihood results, the bias of the estimated change point was computed in the case when the measurement error is ignored. The authors found the direction of the bias in the estimated change point to be determined by the design distribution of the observed covariates, and the bias can be in either direction. The method was illustrated with data from a nutritional study that investigates the relation between dietary folate and blood serum homocysteine levels and found that the analysis that ignores covariate measurement error would have indicated a much higher minimum daily dietary folate intake requirement than is obtained in the analysis that takes covariate measurement error into account.

5. Muggeo (2003) considered fitting piecewise terms in regression models where one or more breakpoints are true parameters of the model. For estimation, a simple linearization technique is called for, taking advantage of the linear formulation of the problem. As a result, the method is suitable for any regression model with linear predictor, and so current software can be used; threshold modeling as a function of explanatory variables is also allowed. Differences between the other procedures available are shown and relative merits discussed. In order to make useful comparisons, the following two routinely used data sets in segmented regression analysis were presented to illustrate the method: (a) Stanford heart transplant data, which consist of survival of patients on the waiting list for the Stanford heart transplant program begun in October 1967, along with subject-specific covariates, including age, sex, and several prognosis factors; and

(b) chronic bronchitis and dust concentration data. Muggeo (2008) developed an R package *segmented* to fit regression models with broken-line relationships, aiming to estimate linear and generalized linear models (and virtually any regression model) having one or more segmented relationships in the linear predictor. The package includes testing and estimating functions and methods to print, summarize, and plot the results. Estimates of the slopes and of the possibly multiple breakpoints are provided.

6. Auh and Sampson (2006) proposed an isotonic logistic discrimination procedure that generalizes linear logistic discrimination by allowing linear boundaries to be more flexibly shaped as monotone functions of the discriminant variables. Under each of three familiar sampling schemes for obtaining a training data set, namely, prospective, mixture, and retrospective, the authors provided the corresponding likelihood-based inference. This method was theoretically compared with monotone discrimination procedures. A cancer study was used to illustrate the applicability of the method.

7. Regression splines in linear mixed models for longitudinal analysis of continuous variables offer the analyst additional flexibility in the formulation of descriptive analyses, exploratory analyses, and hypothesis-driven confirmatory analyses. Edwards et al. (2006) proposed a method for fitting piecewise polynomial regression splines with varying polynomial orders in the fixed effects or random effects of the linear mixed model. The polynomial segments are explicitly constrained by side conditions for continuity and some smoothness at the points where they join. By reparameterizing this explicitly constrained linear mixed model, an implicitly constrained linear mixed model is constructed that simplifies implementation of fixed-knot regression splines. The proposed approach is relatively simple, handles splines in one variable or multiple variables, and can be easily programmed using existing commercial software such as SAS or S-Plus. The method is illustrated with an analysis of longitudinal viral load data from a study of subjects with acute HIV-1 infection and an analysis of 24-hour ambulatory blood pressure profiles.

8. Czajkowski et al. (2008) considered a general model for anomaly detection in a longitudinal cohort mortality pattern based on logistic join-point regression with unknown join points. The authors discussed backward and forward sequential procedures for selecting both the locations and the number of join points. Estimation of the model parameters and selection algorithms was illustrated with longitudinal data on cancer mortality in a cohort of chemical workers.

12.6.3.4 Structural Change

1. Chu et al. (1995) investigated tests for structural change based on moving sums (MOSUM) of recursive and least-squares residuals. The authors obtained and tabulated the asymptotic critical values of the MOSUM test with recursive residuals and showed that the asymptotic critical values of the MOSUM test with least-squares residuals can easily be obtained from already existing tables for the moving-estimates test. The authors also showed that these MOSUM tests are consistent and have nontrivial local power against a general class of alternatives. The simulations further indicate that the proposed MOSUM tests can complement other tests when there is a single structural change and have power advantage when there are certain double structural changes.

2. Zeileis et al. (2001) developed the R package *strucchange* for testing for structural change in linear regression, which reviews tests for structural change in linear regression models from the generalized fluctuation test framework, as well as from the *F*-test (Chow test) framework. Since Zeileis et al. (2001), various extensions have been added to the package, in particular related to breakpoint estimation (also known as dating, discussed in Zeileis et al. [2003]) and to structural change tests in other parametric models (Zeileis 2006). A more unifying view of the underlying theory is presented in Zeileis (2005) and Zeileis et al. (2010). Here, we focus on the linear regression model and introduce a unified approach for implementing tests from the fluctuation test and *F*-test framework for this model, illustrating how this approach has been realized in *strucchange*. Enhancing the standard significance test approach, the package contains methods to fit, plot, and test empirical fluctuation processes (like CUSUM, MOSUM, and estimate-based processes) and to compute, plot, and test sequences of *F*-statistics with the sup*F*, ave*F*, and exp*F* tests. Thus, it makes powerful tools available to display information about structural changes in regression relationships and to assess their significance. Furthermore, it describes how incoming data can be monitored.

3. Bai and Perron (2003) presented a comprehensive discussion of computational aspects of multiple structural change models along with several empirical examples. Using the R statistical software package, Zeileis and Kleiber (2005) reported on the results of a replication study. The authors verified most of their findings; however, some confidence intervals associated with breakpoints cannot be reproduced. These confidence intervals require computation of the quantiles of a nonstandard distribution, the distribution of the argmax functional of a certain stochastic process. Interestingly, the difficulties appear to be due to numerical problems in GAUSS, the software package used by Bai and Perron.

12.6.3.5 Change Points on Phylogenetic Trees

Assume that we observe n sequences at each of m sites and assume that they have evolved from an ancestral sequence that forms the root of a binary tree of known topology and branch lengths, but the sequence states at internal nodes are unknown. The topology of the tree and branch lengths are the same for all sites, but the parameters of the evolutionary model can vary over sites. Persing et al. (2014) considered a piecewise constant model for these parameters, with an unknown number of change points and hence a transdimensional parameter space over which we seek to perform Bayesian inference. The authors proposed two novel ideas to deal with the computational challenges of such inference. First, the authors approximated the model based on the time machine principle: the top nodes of the binary tree (near the root) are replaced by an approximation of the true distribution; as more nodes are removed from the top of the tree, the cost of computing the likelihood is reduced linearly in n. The approach introduced a bias. Second, the authors developed a particle marginal Metropolis–Hastings (PMMH) algorithm that employs a sequential Monte Carlo (SMC) sampler and can use the first idea. The time machine PMMH algorithm copes well with one of the bottlenecks of standard computational algorithms: the transdimensional nature of the posterior distribution. The algorithm was implemented on simulated and real data examples, and the authors empirically demonstrated its potential to outperform competing methods based on approximate Bayesian computation (ABC) techniques.

12.6.3.6 Statistical Quality Control Schemes

1. Bakir (2004) proposed a distribution-free (or nonparametric) statistical quality control chart for monitoring a process center. The proposed chart is of the Shewhart type and is based on the signed ranks of grouped observations. The exact false alarm rate and the in-control average run length of the proposed chart were computed by using the null distribution of the well-known Wilcoxon signed-rank statistic. The out-of-control run lengths were computed exactly for normal underlying distributions and by simulation for uniform, double exponential, and Cauchy shift alternatives. Efficiency studies showed that the proposed chart is more efficient than the traditional Shewhart X-bar chart under heavy-tailed distributions (the double exponential and the Cauchy), but is less efficient under light-tailed distributions (the uniform and the normal).

2. Zou et al. (2006) proposed a control chart based on the change point that is able to monitor linear profiles whose parameters are unknown but can be estimated from historical data. This chart can detect a shift in either the intercept, slope, or standard deviation. Simulation results showed that the proposed approach performs well across a range of possible shifts, and that it can be used during the start-up stages of a process. Simple diagnostic aids were given to estimate the location of the change and determine which of the parameters has changed.

3. Harel et al. (2008) adapted and developed methodology in quality control to monitor data collection in epidemiologic studies. There are no procedures currently used by epidemiologists to evaluate quality control during the actual process of data collection; methods are implemented only after the data have been collected. The authors focused on procedures that can be used during data collection: instrument calibration and population sampling. For the first, the authors proposed methods utilizing Shewhart control charts and Westgard stopping rules. For evaluating population sampling, methods utilizing regression analysis were presented. A motivating example was provided to highlight the utility of these methods. The proposed methodology may help investigators to identify data quality problems that can be corrected while data are still being collected, and also to identify biases in data collection that might be adjusted later.

4. Exponential CUSUM charts are used in monitoring the occurrence rate of rare events because the interarrival times of events for homogeneous Poisson processes are independent and identically distributed exponential random variables. In these applications, it is assumed that the exponential parameter, that is, the mean, is known or has been accurately estimated. However, in practice, the in-control mean is typically unknown and must be estimated to construct the limits for the exponential CUSUM chart. Zhang et al. (2014) investigated the effect of parameter estimation on the run-length properties of one-sided lower exponential CUSUM charts. In addition, analyzing conditional performance measures shows that the effect of estimation error can be significant, affecting both the in-control average run length and the quick detection of process deterioration. The authors provided recommendations regarding phase I sample sizes. This sample size must be quite large for the in-control chart performance to be close to that for the known parameter case. Finally, an industrial example was illustrated to highlight the practical implications of estimation error and to offer advice to practitioners when constructing or analyzing a phase I sample.

12.7 Appendix

Proof that the adjusted Shiryayev–Roberts statistic is the average most powerful (Section 12.4.1.2).
Based on the inequality $(A - B)(I\{A \geq B\}) \geq 0$, with $A = R_n^{(2)}/n$ and $B = C_\alpha$, we can write

$$\left(\frac{1}{n}R_n^{(2)} - C_\alpha\right)\left(I\left\{\frac{1}{n}R_n^{(2)} \geq C_\alpha\right\} - \delta\right) \geq 0.$$

Deriving the H_0 expectation from both the sides of the inequality above, we have

$$\frac{1}{n}E_{H_0}\left(R_n^{(2)}I\left(\frac{1}{n}R_n^{(2)} > C_\alpha\right)\right) - C_\alpha E_{H_0}\left(I\left(\frac{1}{n}R_n^{(2)} > C_\alpha\right)\right) \geq \frac{1}{n}E_{H_0}\left(R_n^{(2)}\delta\right) - C_\alpha E_{H_0}(\delta).$$

We have

$$E_{H_0}\left(R_n^{(2)}\delta\right) = \sum_{k_1=1}^{n}\sum_{k_2=k_1}^{n}E_{H_0}\left\{\frac{\prod_{i=1}^{k_1-1}f_1(X_i)\prod_{j=k_1}^{k_2-1}f_2(X_j)\prod_{l=k_2}^{n}f_3(X_l)}{\prod_{i=1}^{n}f_0(X_i)}\delta(X_1,\ldots,X_n)\right\}$$

$$= \sum_{k_1=1}^{n}\sum_{k_2=k_1}^{n}\int\cdots\int\frac{\prod_{i=1}^{k_1-1}f_1(X_i)\prod_{j=k_1}^{k_2-1}f_2(X_j)\prod_{l=k_2}^{n}f_3(X_l)}{\prod_{i=1}^{n}f_0(X_i)}\delta(X_1,\ldots,X_n)\prod_{i=1}^{n}f_0(X_i)\prod_{i=1}^{n}dX_i$$

$$= \sum_{k_1=1}^{n}\sum_{k_2=k_1}^{n}\int\cdots\int\prod_{i=1}^{k_1-1}f_1(X_i)\prod_{j=k_1}^{k_2-1}f_2(X_j)\prod_{l=k_2}^{n}f_3(X_l)\delta(X_1,\ldots,X_n)\prod_{i=1}^{n}dX_i$$

$$= \sum_{k_1=1}^{n}\sum_{k_2=k_1}^{n}\Pr_{k_1,k_2}\{\delta=1\} = \sum_{k_1=1}^{n}\sum_{k_2=k_1}^{n}\Pr_{k_1,k_2}\{\delta \text{ rejects } H_0\}.$$

Since the rule $\{\delta$ based on $X_1, \ldots, X_n$ rejects $H_0\}$ includes also $\left\{\frac{1}{n}R_n^{(2)} > C_\alpha\right\}$, the proof is complete.

13

A Brief Review of Sequential Testing Methods

> In most randomized clinical trials, patient entry is sequential so that the results become available sequentially. Both medical ethics and the natural curiosity of investigators require an ongoing assessment of the accumulating data to see if a treatment difference is sufficient to stop the trial.
>
> **Pocock (1977)**

13.1 Introduction

The focus of this book is on testing procedures based on observed data, from either a retrospectively or prospectively designed study. Retrospective studies are generally derived from already existing databases or combining existing pieces of data, for example, using electronic health records to examine risk or protection factors in relation to a clinical outcome, where the outcome may have already occurred prior to the start of the analysis. The investigator collects data from past records, with no or minimal patient follow-up, as is the case with a prospective study. Many valuable studies, such as the first major case-control study published by Lane-Claypon (1926), investigating risk factors for breast cancer, were retrospective investigations. Prospective studies may be analyzed similar to retrospective studies, or they may have a sequential element to them, which we will describe below; that is, data may be analyzed continuously or in stages during the course of study.

In retrospective studies it is common to have sources of error due to confounding and various biases, such as selection bias, misclassification, or information bias. In addition, the inferential decision procedures for retrospective studies are based on complete data sets, where the sample size is fixed in advance and can oftentimes be quite large. It is possible in these settings to have underpowered or overpowered designs. For example, medical claims data may lead to an overpowered design, that is, a study that will detect small differences from the null hypothesis that may not be scientifically interesting. Consequently, retrospective studies may induce unnecessarily high financial or human cost or statistically significant results that are not necessarily meaningful. Armitage (1991) stated,

> The classical theory of experimental design deals predominantly with experiments of predetermined size, presumably because the pioneers of the subject, particularly R.A. Fisher, worked in agricultural research, where the outcome of a field trial is not available until long after the experiment has been designed and started.

In fact, in an experiment in which data accumulate steadily over a period of time, it is natural to monitor results as they occur, with a view toward taking action, such as certain modification or early termination of the study. For example, a disease prevention trial or an epidemiological cohort study of occupational exposure may run on a timescale of tens of years. It is not uncommon for phase III cancer clinical trials, where the primary objective is final confirmation of safety and efficacy, with a survival endpoint to run 10 years.

From a logistical and cost-effectiveness point of view, it is natural to employ sequential testing approaches. Sequential analysis will be performed as "a method allowing hypothesis tests to be conducted on a number of occasions as data accumulate through the course of a trial. A trial monitored in this way is usually called a sequential trial" (Everitt and Palmer 2010). In fully sequential approaches, statistical tests are conducted after the collection of every observation. In group-sequential testing, tests are conducted after batches of data are observed. Both approaches allow one to draw conclusions during the data collection and possibly reach a final conclusion at a much earlier stage, as is the case in classical hypothesis testing. In classical retrospective hypothesis testing the sample size is fixed at the beginning of the experiment and the data collection is conducted without considering the data or the analysis, whereas the sample size in a sequential analysis is a random variable.

The sequential analysis methodology possesses many advantages, including economic savings in sample size, time, and cost. It also has advantages in terms of ethical considerations and monitoring; for example, a clinical trial might be stopped early if a new treatment is more efficacious than originally assumed. Sequential analysis methods have different operating characteristics compared to fixed sample size tests; for example, different methods for obtaining unbiased estimates of effects are needed. Given the potential cost savings and the interesting theoretical properties of sequential tests, many variations have become well established and thoroughly investigated. There are formal guidelines for using sequential tests in many research areas (DeGroot 2005; Dmitrienko et al. 2005). For example, in terms of government-regulated trials in the United States, there are formal published requirements pertaining to interim analyses and the reporting of the corresponding statistical results. It is stated in a Food and Drug Administration (1988) guideline that

> the process of examining and analyzing data accumulating in a clinical trial, either formally or informally, can introduce bias. Therefore all interim analyses, formal or informal, by any study participant, sponsor staff member, or data monitoring group should be described in full even if treatment groups were not identified. The need for statistical adjustment because of such analyses should be addressed. Minutes of meetings of the data monitoring group may be useful (and may be requested by the review division).

Armitage (1975, 1991) argued that ethical considerations demand a trial be stopped as soon as possible when there is clear evidence of the preference for one or more treatments over the standard of care or placebo, which logically leads to the use of a sequential trial. In his publications cited above, Armitage described a number of sequential testing methods and their application to trials comparing two alternative treatments.

Sequential methods are well suited for use in clinical trials with short-term outcomes, for example, a 1-month follow-up value. When dealing with human subjects, regular examinations of accumulating results and early termination of the study are ethically desirable (Armitage 1975). Sequential methods touch much of modern statistical practice, and hence we cannot possibly include all relevant theory and examples. In this chapter, we outline several of the more well-applied sequential testing procedures, including two-stage designs, the sequential probability ratio test, group-sequential tests, and adaptive sequential designs.

Note that the scheme of sequential testing may result in very complicated estimation issues in the postsequential analyses of the data. Investigators should be careful in applying standard estimation techniques to data obtained via a sequential data collection procedure. For example, estimation of sample mean and variance of the data can be very problematic in terms of obtaining unbiased estimates (Liu and Hall 1999; Martinsek 1981).

13.2 Two-Stage Designs

The rudiments of sequential analysis can be traced to the works of Huyghens, Bernoulli, DeMoivre, and Laplace on the gambler's ruin problem (Lai 2001). The formal application of sequential procedures started in the late 1920s in the area of statistical quality control in manufacturing production. The early two-stage designs, which can be extended to multistage designs, were proposed for industrial acceptance sampling of a production lot where the decision was that the lot met specification or the lot was defective. In a two-stage acceptance sampling plan, there are six parameters: the sample sizes for each stage (n_1 and n_2), acceptance numbers (c_1 and c_2), and rejection numbers (d_1 and d_2), where $d_1 > c_1 + 1$ and $d_2 = c_2 + 1$. To implement the plan, one first takes an initial sample of n_1 items, and if this contains c_1 defective items or fewer, the lot is accepted, but if d_1 defective items or more are found, the lot is rejected. Otherwise, the decision is deferred until a second sample of size n_2 is inspected. The lot is then accepted if the total cumulative number of defective items is less than or equal to c_2 and rejected if this number is greater than or equal to d_2; see Dodge and Romig (1929) for more details. The two-stage sequential testing idea can be generalized to a multistage sampling plan where up to K stages are permitted (see Bartky [1943] for details). This approach was subsequently developed by Freeman et al. (1948) to form the basis of the U.S. military standards for acceptance sampling.

A similar problem arises in the early stages of drug screening and in phase II clinical trials, where the primary objective is to determine whether a new drug or regimen has a minimal level of therapeutic efficacy, that is, sufficient biological activity against the disease under study, to warrant more extensive development. Such trials are often conducted in a multi-institution setting where designs of more than two stages are difficult to manage. Simon (1989) proposed an optimal two-stage design, which has the goal to "minimize the expected sample size if the new drug or regimen has low activity subject to constraints upon the size of the Type I error rate (α) and the Type II error rate (β)." These types of interim stopping rules are often termed a futility analysis; we discuss futility analysis in detail in Section 13.7.

Simon's two-stage designs are based on testing for the true response probability p that $H_0: p \leq p_0$ versus $H_1: p \geq p_1$ for some desirable target level p_0 and p_1. Each Simon's two-stage design is indexed by four numbers, n_1, n_2, r_1, and r, where n_1 and n_2 denote the numbers of patients studied in the first and second stages, and r_1 and r denote the stopping boundaries in the first and second stages, respectively. Let the total sample size be $n = n_1 + n_2$. The study is terminated at the end of the first stage, and the drug is rejected for further investigation if r_1 or fewer responses out of n_1 participants are observed; otherwise, the study proceeds to the second stage, with a total sample size n, and the drug is rejected for further development if r or fewer responses are observed at the end of the second stage, that is, at the end of the study. A Type I error occurs when there are more than r_1 responses at the end of the first stage and more than r responses at the end of the study when $p \leq p_0$. A Type II error occurs if there are r_1 or fewer responses in the first stage or there are r or fewer responses at the end of the study when $p \geq p_1$. The values of n_1, n_2, r_1, and r are found for fixed values of p_0, p_1, α (the Type I error rate), and β (the Type II error rate), and are determined as follows.

The decision of whether to terminate after the first or the second stage is based on the number of responses observed. The number of responses X, given a true response rate p and a sample size m, follows a binomial distribution, that is, $\Pr(X = x) = b(x; p, m)$ and $\Pr(X \leq x) = B(x; p, m)$, where b and B denote the binomial probability mass function and the binomial cumulative distribution function, respectively. Therefore, the total sample size is random. The probability of early termination and the expected sample size depend on the true probability of response p. By using exact binomial probabilities, the probability of early termination after the first stage, denoted as $\mathrm{PET}(p)$, has the form $B(r_1; p, n_2)$, and the expected sample size based on a true response probability p for this design can be defined as $E(N|p) = n_1 + (1-\mathrm{PET}(p))n_2$. The probability of rejecting a drug with a true response probability p, denoted as $\bar{R}(p)$, is

$$\bar{R}(p) = B(r_1; p, n_2) + \sum_{x=r_1+1}^{\min\{n_1, r\}} b(x; p, n_1) B(r - x; p, n_2).$$

For pre-specified values of the parameters p_0, p_1, α, and β, if the null hypothesis is true, then we require that the probability that the drug should be accepted for further study in other clinical trials should be less than α, that is, concluding that the drug is sufficiently promising. We also require that the probability of rejecting the drug for further study should be less than β under the alternative. That is, an acceptable design is one that satisfies the error probability constraints $\bar{R}(p_0) \geq 1 - \alpha$ and $\bar{R}(p_1) \geq 1 - \beta$. Let Ω be the set of all such designs. A grid search is used to go through every combination of n_1, n_2, r_1, and r, with an upper limit for the total sample size n, usually between 0.85 and 1.5 times the sample size for a single stage design (Lin and Shih 2004). The optimal design under H_0 is the one in Ω that has the smallest expected sample size $E(N|p_0)$. For more details, we refer the reader to Simon (1989). Extensions of this design for testing both efficacy and futility after the first set of subjects has enrolled are well developed (e.g., see Kepner and Chang 2003).

13.3 Sequential Probability Ratio Test

The modern theory of sequential analysis originates from the research of Barnard (1946) and Wald (1947). In particular, the method of the sequential probability ratio test (SPRT) has been the predominant influence of the subsequent developments in the area. Inspired by the Neyman–Pearson lemma (Neyman and Pearson 1933), Wald (1947) proposed the SPRT, which provides a method of constructing an efficient sequential statistical test.

Let X_1, X_2, ... be a sequence of random variables with joint probability density function $f(x_1, ..., x_n)$ for $n = 1, 2, ...$. Consider a basic form for testing a simple null hypothesis $H_0: f = f_0$ against a simple alternative hypothesis $H_1: f = f_1$, where f_0 and f_1 are known. Recall that the likelihood ratio has the form

$$L_n = \frac{f_1(X_1, ..., X_n)}{f_0(X_1, ..., X_n)}.$$

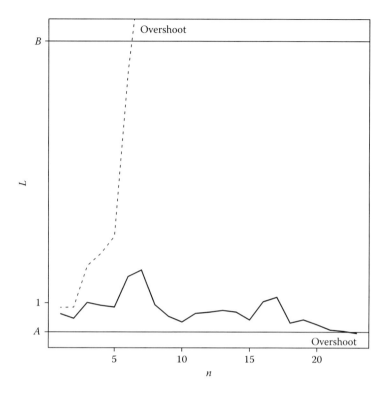

FIGURE 13.1

Sampling process via SPRT; the solid line shows the case where the sampling process stops when $L_N \leq A$ and that leads to the decision not to reject H_0, and the dashed line represents the case where the sampling process stops when $L_N \geq B$ and we decide to reject H_0. The shown overshoots have the values of $L_N - A$ or $L_N - B$, respectively.

The goal of the SPRT is to inform a decision as to which hypothesis is more likely as soon as possible relative to the desired Type I and Type II error rates. To accomplish this goal, observations are collected sequentially one at a time; when a new observation has been made, a decision rule has to be made among the following options: (1) not to reject the null hypothesis and stop sampling, (2) reject the null hypothesis and stop sampling, or (3) collect another observation as a piece of information and repeat 1 and 2. Toward this end, we specify boundaries for the decision process given as $0 < A < 1 < B < \infty$, and sample $X_1, X_2, \ldots$ sequentially until the random time N, where $N = N_{A,B} = \inf\{n \geq 1: L_n \notin (A,B)\}$. In other words, we stop sampling at time N and decide not to reject H_0 if $L_N \leq A$ or decide to reject H_0 if $L_N \geq B$; see Figure 13.1 for illustration. The determination of A and B is given below.

Graphically, we plot the likelihood value as a function of the sample size and examine the time series process as to whether it crossed either the A or B boundary. The R code for producing the plot is

```
> # For any pre-specified A and B (0<A<1<B). For example, A=.11, B=0.
> A=.11
> B=9
> muX0<-0 # A simple example where X~i.i.d. N(0,1) under H0
> muX1<-0.5 # A simple example where X~i.i.d. N(0.5,1) under H1
> L<-1
> n<-0
> L.seq.A<-c()
```

```
> while(L>A & L<B){
+     x<-rnorm(1,muX0,1)
+     L<-L*exp((muX1-muX0)*x+(muX0^2-muX1^2)/2)  #dnorm(x,muX1,1)/
          dnorm(x,muX0,1)
+     L.seq.A<-c(L.seq.A,L)
+     n<-n+1
+ }
>
> L<-1
> n<-0
> L.seq.B<-c()
> while(L>A & L<B){
+     x<-rnorm(1,muX1,1)
+     L<-L*exp((muX1-muX0)*x+(muX0^2-muX1^2)/2)
+     L.seq.B<-c(L.seq.B,L)
+     n<-n+1
+ }
> # to plot
> par(mar=c(4,4,2,2))
> plot(L.seq.A,type="l",lty=1,ylim=c(0,9.3),yaxt="n",xlab="n",ylab="L")
> lines(L.seq.B,type="l",lty=2)
> abline(h=c(A,B))
> axis(2,c(A,1,B),label=c("A","1","B"),las=2)
```

13.3.1 SPRT Stopping Boundaries

The constants A and B are chosen so that the Type I and Type II error probabilities are approximately equal (bounded appropriately) to the pre-specified values α and β, respectively, and formally defined as

$$\alpha = \Pr_{H_0}(L_N \geq B) \leq B^{-1}(1-\beta) \text{ and } \beta = \Pr_{H_1}(L_N \leq A) \leq A(1-\alpha).$$

The proof of these probability relationships is provided in the appendix. Note that the inequality accounts for values of the likelihood that "overshoots" the boundaries A and B (e.g., see Figure 13.1). Treating the above inequalities as approximate equalities and solving for α and β leads to the useful error rate approximations

$$\alpha \approx \frac{1-A}{B-A} \text{ and } \beta \approx \frac{A(B-1)}{B-A};$$

or equivalently, solving for A and B leads to practical (bounded above) approximations of the boundaries

$$A \approx \frac{\beta}{1-\alpha} \text{ and } B \approx \frac{1-\beta}{\alpha},$$

when the overshoots are not taking into account.

13.3.2 Wald Approximation to the Average Sample Number

The expected stopping time $E(N)$ is often called the average sample number (ASN). Being able to calculate the ASN is practically relevant in terms of the logistics of planning a given study. To study the ASN and the asymptotic properties of the stopping time N, we consider the following reformulation and make an additional assumption that the observations x_i are independent and identically distributed (i.i.d.). Therefore, the log-likelihood ratio $\log L_n$ is a sum of i.i.d. random variables $Z_i = \log[f_1(X_i)/f_0(X_i)]$, that is, $\log L_n = \sum_{i=1}^{n} Z_i = S_n$ (define $\log L_n$ as S_n for simplicity). Then the stopping time can be rewritten as $N = N_{c_1, c_2} = \inf\{n \geq 1 : S_n \leq -c_1 \text{ or } S_n \geq c_2\}$, where $c_1 = -\log A$ and $c_2 = \log B$ are positive. Denote $\mu_{Zi} = E_i(Z_1) = \int \{\log[f_1(x)/f_0(x)]\} f_i(x) dx$ and $\sigma_{Zi}^2 = E_i(Z_1 - \mu_{Zi})^2$, under the simple hypothesis H_i, $i = 0, 1$. By Wald's fundamental identity (Wald 1947), the Wald approximation to the expected sample size can be expressed in the forms

$$E_0 N \cong \begin{cases} \mu_{Z0}^{-1} \left\{ \alpha \log\left(\dfrac{1-\beta}{\alpha}\right) + (1-\alpha) \log\left(\dfrac{\beta}{1-\alpha}\right) \right\}, & \text{if } \mu_{Z0} \neq 0, \\[2mm] \sigma_{Z0}^{-2} \log\left(\dfrac{\beta}{1-\alpha}\right) \log\left(\dfrac{\alpha}{1-\beta}\right), & \text{if } \mu_{Z0} = 0, \end{cases}$$

and

$$E_1 N \cong \begin{cases} \mu_{Z1}^{-1} \left\{ (1-\beta) \log\left(\dfrac{1-\beta}{\alpha}\right) + \beta \log\left(\dfrac{\beta}{1-\alpha}\right) \right\}, & \text{if } \mu_{Z1} \neq 0. \\[2mm] \sigma_{Z1}^{-2} \log\left(\dfrac{\beta}{1-\alpha}\right) \log\left(\dfrac{\alpha}{1-\beta}\right), & \text{if } \mu_{Z1} = 0. \end{cases}$$

Note that the Wald approximation to $E(N)$ underestimates the true ASN. The accuracy of the Wald approximation to $E(N)$ is mostly determined by the amount that S_N will tend to overshoot $-c_1$ or c_2. If this overshoot tends to be small, the approximations will be quite good; otherwise, the approximation can be poor (Berger 1985).

13.3.3 Asymptotic Properties of the Stopping Time N

Define $c = \min(c_1, c_2)$ and suppose that $E(Z_1) = \mu \neq 0$, where c_1 and c_2 are defined above. Based on the central limit theorem result shown by Siegmund (1968), it is easy to check that for $\mu > 0$,

$$(c_2/\mu)^{-1/2}[N - (c_2/\mu)] \xrightarrow{d} N(0, \sigma^2/\mu^2) \text{ as } c \to \infty,$$

Similarly, if $\mu < 0$, then $(c_1/|\mu|)^{-1/2}[N - (c_1/|\mu|)] \xrightarrow{d} N(0, \sigma^2/\mu^2)$ as $c \to \infty$. See Martinsek (1981) for more detail. Additionally, Martinsek (1981) presented the following result:

Theorem 13.1

Let $Z_1, Z_2, \ldots$ be i.i.d. with $E(Z_1) = \mu \neq 0$, $\text{var}(Z_1) = \sigma^2 \in (0, \infty)$, and assume $E|Z_1|^p < \infty$, where $p \geq 2$. Then

1. If $\mu > 0$ and $c_2 = o(c_1)$ as $c \to \infty$, then $\{c_2^{-p/2}|N - (c_2/\mu)|^p : c \geq 1\}$ is uniformly integrable, and hence $E|N - (c_2/\mu)|^r \sim (c_2/\mu)^{r/2}(\sigma/\mu)^r E|N(0,1)|^r$ as $c \to \infty$, for $0 < r \leq p$.

2. If $\mu < 0$ and $c_1 = o(c_2)$ as $c \to \infty$, then $\{c_1^{-p/2}|N - (c_1/\mu)||^p : c \geq 1\}$ is uniformly integrable, and hence $E|N - (c_1/|\mu|)|^r \sim (c_1/|\mu|)^{r/2}(\sigma/|\mu|)^r E|N(0,1)|^r$ as $c \to \infty$, for $0 < r \leq p$.

When $p = 2$, the asymptotic behavior of var(N) is shown in the following corollary (Martinsek 1981):

Corollary 13.1

Let $Z_1, Z_2, \ldots$ be i.i.d. with $E(Z_1) = \mu \neq 0$, var(Z_1) = $\sigma^2 \in (0, \infty)$. Then

1. If $\mu > 0$ and $c_2 = o(c_1)$ as $c \to \infty$, then var(N) $\sim c_2 \sigma^2/\mu^3$ as $c \to \infty$.
2. If $\mu > 0$ and $c_2 = o(c_1)$ as $c \to \infty$, then var(N) $\sim c_1 \sigma^2/|\mu|^3$ as $c \to \infty$.

Consider the one-parameter case where $f_0 = f(x; \theta_0)$ and $f_1 = f(x; \theta_1)$. Ghosh (1969) derived the asymptotic behavior of the expectation and variance of the stopping time N in the cases of several sample distributions (normal, binomial, exponential, and Poisson) as $\Delta = \theta_1 - \theta_0 \to 0$. Ghosh's approximation is good for small values of Δ, and the approximation given in Corollary 13.1 is good for larger values of Δ. Based on Corollary 13.1 and Theorem 2.1 of Berk (1973), it can be derived that

$$\text{var}_{\theta_0}(N)/E_{\theta_0}^2(N) \cong (4c_1\theta_0^2/(2\theta_0^2)^3)/(c_1^2/2\theta_0^2)^2) = 2/c_1,$$

which is in fact constant for fixed c_1 and c_2 as Δ varies. This computation implies that the constant of proportionality should be close to $2/c_1$ if c is large. Martinsek (1981) presented in Table 2 the actual observed rations calculated from Cox and Roseberry (1966), along with values of $2/c_1$. For more details, see, for example, Martinsek (1981).

Example 13.1: Sequential Probability Ratio Test about a Single Mean

As a typical example of the SPRT, we consider the situation where $X \sim N(\mu, \sigma^2)$, $\sigma^2 = 1$, and it is desired to test $H_0: \mu = \mu_0$ versus $H_1: \mu = \mu_1$ with $\alpha = 0.05$ and $\beta = 0.2$, where $\mu_0 = -1/2$ and $\mu_1 = 1/2$. For the purpose of the comparison of the required sample size, in addition to the SPRT, we also considered the nonsequential LRT (i.e., fixed sample size test). Define $\bar{X}_n = n^{-1}\sum_{i=1}^{n} X_i$. It is clear that the likelihood ratio is

$$L_n = \exp\left(n(\mu_1 - \mu_0)\bar{X}_n + n(\mu_0^2 - \mu_1^2)/2\right),$$

and

$$\alpha = \Pr(L > C_\alpha | H_0) = \Pr(\bar{X}_n > \log(C_\alpha)/(n(\mu_1 - \mu_0)) + (\mu_1 + \mu_0)/2 | H_0),$$

$$\beta = \Pr(L > C_\alpha | H_1) = \Pr(\bar{X}_n > \log(C_\alpha)/(n(\mu_1 - \mu_0)) + (\mu_1 + \mu_0)/2 | H_1).$$

Therefore, one can easily obtain that $\log(C_\alpha)/(n(\mu_1 - \mu_0)) + (\mu_1 + \mu_0)/2 = \Phi_{(\mu_0, \sigma^2/n)}^{-1}(1 - \alpha)$, where $\Phi_{(\mu_0, \sigma^2/n)}^{-1}(1 - \alpha)$ denotes the $(1-\alpha)$th quantile of a normal distribution with a mean of μ_0 and a variance of σ^2/n. As a consequence, $\beta = \Pr(\bar{X}_n > \Phi_{(\mu_0, \sigma^2/n)}^{-1}(1 - \alpha) | H_1)$, and hence the fixed sample size in the nonsequential LRT test can be obtained by solving

$\Phi^{-1}_{(\mu_1,\sigma^2/n)}(1-\beta) = \Phi^{-1}_{(\mu_0,\sigma^2/n)}(1-\alpha)$. In this example, assuming $\alpha = 0.05$ and $\beta = 0.2$, the non-sequential LRT test requires a sample size ≥ 6.1826 (6.1826 corresponds to how much sample information is required to achieve the desired error probabilities). Here we use the `uniroot` function in R to obtain the sample size. The R code to obtain the results is shown below:

```
> ## set up parameters
> alpha <- 0.05 # the significance level
> beta <- 0.2 # power=1-beta=0.8
> muX0 <- -1/2
> muX1 <- 1/2
>
> ### Likelihood ratio test
> # power as a function of the number of observations n
> get.power <- function(n){
+    right.part <- qnorm(alpha,mean=muX0,sd=1/sqrt(n),lower=FALSE)
+    pnorm(right.part,mean=muX1,sd=1/sqrt(n),lower=FALSE)
+ }
> power <- 1-beta
> n.LR <- uniroot(function(n) get.power(n)-power, c(0, 10000))$root
> n.LR
[1] 6.182566
```

For the sequential test, it can be easily obtained that the stopping boundaries of the SPRT are $A = 4/19$ and $B = 16$ based on $\alpha = 0.05$ and $\beta = 0.2$. Note first by simple calculation that $\mu_{zi} = \mu_i$ and $\sigma^2_{Zi} = 1$, $i = 0,1$, and thus the Wald approximations to the ASN are 2.6832 and 3.8129 under H_0 and H_1, respectively. The ASNs obtained via the Monte Carlo simulations (we refer the reader to Chapter 16 for more details related to Monte Carlo studies) are 4.1963 and 5.6990 under the null and alternative hypotheses, respectively. This proves that the Wald approximations are indeed underestimates of the ASN (however, considerably smaller than the sample size required in the nonsequential LRT test). The R code to obtain the results is shown below:

```
> ##### the function to get the ASN via Monte Carlo simulations ######
> # case: "H0" for the null hypothesis; "H1" or "Ha" for the alternative
> # alpha: the type I error rate, i.e., presumed significance level
> # beta: the type II error rate, where the power is 1-beta
> # muX0: the mean specified under the null hypothesis
> # muX1: the mean specified under the alternative hypothesis
> # MC: the number of Monte Carlo repetitions
>
> get.n<-function(case="H0",alpha=0.05,beta=0.2,muX0=-1/2,muX1=1/2,
    MC=5000){
+    if (missing(alpha)|missing(beta)) stop("missing alpha value or beta
       value")
+    if (missing(muX0)|missing(muX1)) stop("missing mean value under H_0
       or H_1") else {
+       if (case=="H0") mu<-muX0 else if (case=="H1"|case=="Ha") mu<-muX1
          else stop("wrong specification of case")
+    }
+    if (!missing(alpha) & !missing(beta) & !missing(muX0) &
       !missing(muX1) & case%in%c("H0","H1","Ha")){
+       if (missing(MC)) MC<-5000
+       A<-beta/(1-alpha)
+       B<-(1-beta)/alpha
+       n.seq<-c()
+       for (i in 1:MC){
+          L<-1
+          n<-0
```

```
+           while(L>A & L<B){
+               x<-rnorm(1,mu,1)
+               L<-L*exp(-(2*(muX0-muX1)*x+muX1^2-muX0^2)/2)
+               n<-n+1
+           }
+           n.seq[i]<-n
+       }
+       return(n.seq)
+   }
+ }
>
> ## SPRT under H_0
> n.seq.0<-get.n(case="H0",alpha=0.05,beta=0.2,
      muX0=-1/2,muX1=1/2,MC=50000)
> mean(n.seq.0)
[1]  4.1963
> var(n.seq.0)
[1]  11.2889
>
> ## SPRT under H_1
> n.seq.1<-get.n(case="H1",alpha=0.05,beta=0.2,
      muX0=-1/2,muX1=1/2,MC=50000)
> mean(n.seq.1)
[1]  5.6990
> var(n.seq.1)
[1]  13.5441
```

The SPRT is very simple to apply in practice, and this procedure typically leads to lower sample sizes on average than fixed sample size tests given fixed α and β.

For this example, the asymptotic ASNs calculated based on Theorem 13.1 (Martinsek 1981) under H_0 and H_1 are 3.1163 and 5.5452, respectively. The result is closer to the ASN obtained via the Monte Carlo simulations than the Wald approximation to the ASN. The asymptotic var(N) values calculated based on Corollary 13.1 (Martinsek 1981) under H_0 and H_1 are 12.4652 and 22.1807, respectively, whereas those obtained via the Monte Carlo simulations are 11.2889 and 13.5441, respectively.

In conclusion, there are a variety of fully sequential tests. The SPRT is theoretically optimal in the sense that it attains the smallest possible expected sample size before a decision is made compared to all sequential tests that do not have larger error probabilities than the SPRT (Wald and Wolfowitz 1948). However, it should be noted that the expected sample size based on the SPRT can be large when the parameter to be tested is not equal to the value specified under the null or alternative hypothesis. In addition, the SPRT is an open scheme with an unbounded sample size; as a consequence, the distribution of sample size can be skewed with a large variance; for more detail, we refer the reader to Martinsek (1981) and Jennison and Turnbull (2010).

13.4 Group-Sequential Tests

In practice, especially in the context of clinical trials, it is convenient to analyze the data after collecting groups of observations, as opposed to a fully sequential test in which the collection of a single observation at a time and continuous data monitoring can be a serious practical burden.

The introduction of group-sequential tests has led to a wide use of sequential methods and has achieved the most efficient gains compared with fully sequential tests. The group-sequential designs and corresponding methods of analysis are particularly useful in clinical trials, where it is standard practice that monitoring committees meet at regular intervals to assess the progress of a study and add formal interim analyses of the primary patient response. Group-sequential tests address the ethical and efficiency concerns in clinical trials. Group-sequential tests can be conducted conveniently with most of the benefits of fully sequential tests in terms of lower expected sample sizes and shorter average study lengths (Jennison and Turnbull 2010).

In this section, we introduce the general idea of group-sequential tests. In group-sequential designs, subjects are allocated in up to K groups of an equal group size m, according to a constrained randomization scheme, which ensures m subjects receive each treatment in every group and the accumulating data are analyzed after each group of $2m$ responses. The experiment can stop early to reject the null hypothesis if the observed difference is sufficiently large. For each $k = 1, \ldots, K$, assume that S_k is the test statistic computed from the first k groups of observations, C_k is the corresponding threshold, and the decision rule is to reject H_0 when $S_k > C_k$; then the test terminates if H_0 is rejected, that is, $S_k > C_k$. If the test continues to the Kth analysis and $S_K > C_K$, it stops at that point and H_0 is accepted.

The problem in which many authors are interested in the field of sequential analysis is the calculation of the sequence of critical values, $\{C_1, \ldots, C_K\}$, to give an overall Type I error rate. Various different types of group-sequential tests give rise to different sequences. In choosing the appropriate number of groups K and the group size m, there may be external influences, such as a predetermined cost or length of trial to fix mK or a natural interval between analyses to fix m. However, it is useful to evaluate the statistical power constraint by the possible designs under consideration. Note that when significance tests at a fixed level are repeated at stages during the accumulation of data, the probability of obtaining a significant result rises above the nominal significance level in the case that the null hypothesis is true. Therefore, repeated significance testing of the accumulated data is applied after each group is evaluated, with critical boundaries adjusted for multiple testing (see Chapter 14 for details). For more details, we refer the reader to, for example, Jennison and Turnbull (2010).

As a specific example, consider a clinical trial with two treatments, A and B, where the response variable for each patient to treatment A or B is normally distributed with known variance, σ^2, and unknown mean, μ_A or μ_B, respectively. The group-sequential procedure for testing $H_0: \mu_A = \mu_B$ versus $H_1: \mu_A \neq \mu_B$ is specified by the maximum number of stages, K, the number of patients, m, to be accrued on A and B at each stage (assume equal sample sizes for each stage and for A and B), and decision boundaries $a_1, \ldots, a_K$. The sequential procedure is as follows: upon completion of each stage k of sampling ($1 \leq k \leq K$), compute the test statistic

$$S_k = \sqrt{m} \sum_{i=1}^{k} (\bar{X}_{Ai} - \bar{X}_{Bi})/(\sqrt{2}\sigma),$$

where $\bar{X}_{Ai}$ and $\bar{X}_{Bi}$ denote the sample mean to treatments A and B at the ith stage of m patients, respectively. If $|S_k| < a_k$ and $k < K$, continue to stage $k + 1$; if $|S_k| \geq a_k$ and $k = K$, stop sampling. Let M denote the stopping stage. The null hypothesis is accepted if $|S_M| < a_M$ or rejected if $|S_M| \geq a_M$. Note that $S_1, S_2 - S_1, \ldots, S_k - S_{k-1}$ are independent and identically distributed normal random variables with mean $\mu = \sqrt{n}\,(\mu_A - \mu_B)/(\sqrt{2}\sigma)$ and variance 1. Pocock (1977) proposed the boundaries $a_k = ak^{1/2}$, $k = 1, 2, \ldots, K$, where constant a satisfies

$$\alpha = 1 - \Pr(|S_1| < a, \ |S_2| < a2^{1/2}, \ \ldots, \ |S_k| < ak^{1/2} | \mu = 0).$$

This group-sequential design can sometimes be statistically superior to standard sequential designs. And the results based on a normal response can be easily adapted to other types of response data. For more details and discussion regarding other types of response data, we refer the reader to Pocock (1977).

The assumption of equal numbers of observations in each group can be relaxed, and then more flexible methods for handling unequal and unpredictable group sizes can be developed (Jennison and Turnbull 2010). The mathematical results of (group) sequential analysis are straightforward. Certain risks of error will be achieved and corresponding inferences will be valid if the stopping rules are followed rigorously. However, major issues involved in the practical implementation of (group) sequential clinical trial designs are whether stopping rules should be followed rigorously and, if not, what degree of flexibility is appropriate (Whitehead 1999).

13.5 Adaptive Sequential Designs

In recent years, there has been a great deal of interest in the work of adaptive sequential designs, an alternative and somewhat dissimilar methodology to the sequential approaches described above. Adaptive designs allow the modification of the design and the sample size after a portion of the data has been collected. This can be done using sequentially observed and estimated treatment effects at interim analyses to modify the maximal statistical information to be collected or by reexamining the variance assumptions about the original design based on estimates.

For each $k = 1, \ldots, K$, assume that S_k is the test statistic computed from the first k groups of observations. Essentially, the technique of the adaptive design is based on the assumption of multivariate normality for $S_1, \ldots, S_k$ and was first described by Bauer and Kohne (1994). The authors focused on a two-stage design and assumed that the data from each stage are independent of those from the previous stage. We outline the basic idea with a simple two-arm parallel clinical trial as follows: Suppose that it is desired to test the null hypothesis H_0: $\theta = 0$, where θ represents the treatment difference between the experimental and control groups. Based on the data obtained from each of the two stages, two p-values, p_1 and p_2, can be obtained. Using Fisher's combination method, Bauer and Kohne (1994) showed that $-2\log(p_1 p_2)$ follows a chi-square distribution on four degrees of freedom under the null hypothesis, giving the ability to combine the data from the two stages in a single test. The approach only assumes the independence of data from the two stages, leading to great flexibility in the design and analysis of trials without inflating the Type I error rate. The adaption methodology can be extended to trials with greater numbers of stages. The adaptations can be based on unblinded data collected in a trial, as well as external information. In addition, the adaptation rules need not be specified in advance.

Note that the adaptive design approach makes use of a test statistic, which is not a sufficient statistic for the treatment difference, resulting in a lack of power for the test. However, the enhanced flexibility of the adaptive design makes it extremely attractive and important.

13.6 Futility Analysis

We described Simon's two-stage designs in Section 13.2, which provide a simple futility rule for an early stop in clinical trials. The term *futility* refers to the inability to achieve its objectives in a clinical trial. Futility analyses involve the decision-making process to terminate a trial prior to completion conditional on the data accumulated so far when the interim results suggest that it is unlikely to achieve statistical significance. It can save resources that could be used on more promising research. One can combine the sequential testing concept with futility analysis.

Stochastic curtailment is one approach to futility analysis. It refers to a decision to terminate the trial based on an assessment of the conditional power, where conditional power is the probability that the final result will be statistically significant conditional on the data observed thus far and a specific assumption about the pattern of the data to be observed in the remainder of the study. Common assumptions include the original design effect, or the effect estimated from the current data, or under the null hypothesis. While a conditional power computation could be used as the basis for terminating a trial when a positive effect emerges, a group-sequential procedure is usually employed for such decisions. A conditional power assessment is usually used to assess the futility of continuing a trial when there is little evidence of a beneficial effect. In some studies, such monitoring for conditional power is done in an ad hoc manner, whereas in others, a futility stopping criterion is specified.

There are other approaches proposed to assess futility, such as group-sequential methods described in Section 13.4, predictive power, and predictive probability. For more details, we refer the reader to, for example, Snapinn et al. (2006).

13.7 Postsequential Analysis

In the previous sections, we discussed advantages of sequential procedures for statistical tests. However, in the framework of sequential experiments, once data have been collected, the hypothesis testing paradigm may no longer be the most useful one for the following statistical analysis; see, for example, the discussion in Cutler et al. (1966). In practice, medical studies usually require a more complete analysis rather than the simple accept or reject decision of a hypothesis test. Once a sequential procedure is executed, generally speaking, we will meet disadvantages of postsequential analysis. The problem is that all simple sequential approaches based on retrospectively collected data should be completely modified when data are collected via sequential schemes. Moreover, analyzing the data arising from sequential experiments commonly requires very complicated adjustments.

The probability properties of the statistics obtained in a trial that is stopped early at only n samples are different from those attained in a similar trial that is run for a predetermined number of trials, even if they end up collecting the same number of samples. Because the sampling procedure stops randomly during a sequential study, classical methods related to the fixed sample size test do not work for the sequential designs. If these issues are not accounted for in the interpretation of the sequential trial, the results of analysis of data collected via sequential procedures will be biased. For example, assuming N is a stopping time based on sequentially obtained i.i.d. observations $X_1, X_2, \ldots, X_n$, $\sum_{i=1}^{N} X_i \Big/ N$ may not be an unbiased estimator of $E(X_1)$, that is, $E\left(\sum_{i=1}^{N} X_i \Big/ N\right) \neq E(X_1)$. Piantadosi (2005) argued that the estimate of a treatment effect will be biased when a trial is terminated at an early stage. The earlier the decision, the larger the bias. Whitehead (1986) also investigated the bias of maximum likelihood estimates calculated at the end of a sequential procedure. Liu and Hall (1999) showed that in a group-sequential test about the drift θ of a Brownian motion $X(t)$ stopped at time T, the sufficient statistic $S = (T, X(T))$ is not complete for θ. In addition, there exist infinitely many unbiased estimators of θ, and none has uniformly minimum variance.

Furthermore, most sequential analyses involve parametric approaches, especially in the group-sequential designs. In contrast with the analysis of data obtained retrospectively, the parametric assumptions are posed before data points are observed. Even if we have strong reasons to assume parametric forms of the data distribution, it will be extremely hard, for example, to test for the goodness of fit of data distributions after the execution of sequential procedures. In this case, perhaps, for example, the known Shapiro–Wilk test for normality will not be exact, and its critical value will depend on the underlying data distribution.

Therefore, it is important that proper methodology is followed in order to avoid invalid conclusions based on sequential data. For more information about the analysis following a sequential test, we refer the reader to Liu and Hall (1999), as well as Jennison and Turnbull (2010).

13.8 Supplement

1. Pitman (1949) derived a method to construct and compare nonsequential tests based on asymptotically normal statistics under the null hypothesis and the local alternatives. Lai (1978) extended Pitman's method to sequential testing. The author replaced the asymptotic normality assumption in Pitman's theory by its sequential analogue; that is, he used the weak convergence of normalized processes formed from these statistics under the null hypothesis and the local alternatives. The author developed uniform invariance principles for a large class of statistics, as well as uniform large-deviation theorems for the test statistics, under which the desired weak convergence assumption was proven to hold. As a result, the sequential tests under Lai's scheme have finite expected sample sizes under the null hypothesis and the local alternatives. The author illustrated the general method with the two-sample location problem. The asymptotic relative efficiencies of sequential tests agree with the corresponding Pitman efficiencies of their nonsequential analogues, the asymptotic relative efficiencies of the sequential Wilcoxon test, the sequential van der Waerden test, and the sequential normal score test relative to the two-sample sequential t-test.

2. Several authors considered nonparallel, curved boundaries for which the critical boundary values *A* and *B* depend on the cumulative sample size, thus ensuring an upper limit on the sample size. One simple modification discussed by Wald (1947) is to truncate the SPRT at a certain sample size; Aroian (1968) and Aroian and Robison (1969) showed how to compute the operating characteristic (the probability of accepting H_0 as a function of the parameter of interest) and the expected sample size curves for such plans using Aroian's direct numerical methods. The direct methods allow unlimited flexibility in the selection of test regions. Aroian (1968) illustrated the use of the direct method for obtaining the operating characteristic and ASN for truncated sequential tests with an example of the binomial distribution, investigating the probability of success in a single trial.

3. Given a test in a certain class of sequential tests, let α denote its (exact) level and $v < \infty$ its expected stopping time under the alternative. Then among all level α sequential tests whose expected stopping times under the alternative do not exceed v, the given test is locally most powerful. Berk (1975) discussed sequential tests that are locally most powerful for certain one-sided testing problems. For models in a one-parameter exponential family, each locally most powerful sequential test is shown to be a Wald SPRT for a family of paired (conjugate) simple hypotheses.

4. Armitage (1975) prescribed the use of traditional test statistics, such as the *t*-statistic or the chi-square statistic, for testing H_0 in the sequential approach. The progress of the trial was tracked in terms of the sample size. Nevertheless, nuisance parameters may cause problems, and consequently, the power and Type I error rate will be affected. To maintain the correct properties of a test, Whitehead and Jones (1979), as well as Jennison and Turnbull (2010), suggested monitoring trials in terms of information and not sample size. The suitable conversion from information to required sample size can then be implemented for various response types. Plotting directly against information helps guarantee power at a particular reference value of the treatment difference θ, regardless of the value of nuisance parameters.

5. The conduct of a sequential clinical trial is considered in two distinct stages, the planning of the trial and the analysis of the results. Whitehead and Jones (1979) considered the comparison of two treatments using sequential tests based on straight-line stopping boundaries. The authors presented existing theory and results in the sequential analysis only in the planning stage of the trial, which allows the calculation of significance levels and interval estimates at the analysis stage. The analysis of the data, including the terminal sample size as part of the data, was viewed as a separate process, involving the ordinary tools of nonsequential statistics.

6. In clinical experiments, practitioners often wish to design a clinical trial to stop as early as possible due to either better than anticipated efficacy or no apparent treatment effect (futility) following ethical and efficiency concerns. For data collected retrospectively, various authors proposed methods to stop in favor of the null hypothesis based on conditional power calculations for the end of the trial given the current data. Betensky (1997) modified and extended these methods from the traditional fixed sample size designs to sequential designs, including the O'Brien–Fleming test (O'Brien and Fleming 1979) and the repeated significance test (Armitage et al. 1969; Pocock 1977). Betensky derived boundaries for monitoring the test statistics to visualize the impact of the parameters on the operating

characteristics of the tests and the corresponding design of the tests. This method was applied to two clinical trials: one that concluded with no treatment difference (AIDS Clinical Trials Group Protocol 118) and one that stopped early for positive effect (Beta-Blocker Heart Attack Trial); for details, see Betensky (1997).

7. DeMets and Ware (1982) proposed a group-sequential method for the periodic analysis of accumulating data in clinical trials, which are essentially one-sided as in treatment–placebo studies. The proposed boundaries retain the early stopping properties of the procedure described by DeMets and Ware (1980), when treatment appears to be ineffective or harmful, but incorporate the more stringent requirements of the model proposed by O'Brien and Fleming (1979) for early rejection of the null hypothesis in favor of treatment.

8. Conditional power procedures allow for early stopping in favor of the null hypothesis if the probability of rejecting the null at the planned end of the trial given the current data and a value of the parameter of interest is below some threshold level. Gordon Lan et al. (1982) demonstrated a stochastic curtailment procedure that calculates the conditional power under the alternative hypothesis. Alternatively, predictive power procedures incorporate information from the observed data by averaging the conditional power over the posterior distribution of the parameter. For complex problems in which explicit evaluation of conditional power is not possible, Betensky (1998) proposed solving the problem of projecting the outcome of a trial by considering the current data as a missing data problem. Accordingly, using the multiple imputation method, it eliminates the need for explicit calculation of conditional power.

9. Tsiatis et al. (1984) computed a confidence interval for the mean μ based on an intuitive sample space ordering that depends on (a) the boundary crossed ($S_k \leq -a_k$ or $S_k \geq a_k$), (b) the stopping stage M, and (c) the value of S_M. This confidence interval has exact coverage probabilities for the mean of a normal distribution following a group-sequential test. However, concern arises from the possibility that this ordering of the sample space may not be reasonable in many cases. In addition, the 90% confidence intervals proposed by Tsiatis et al. (1984) sometimes do not cover the sample average, a situation difficult to explain.

10. Irle (1984) considered the problem of sequentially testing two simple hypotheses for a stochastic process. Let α and β be the error probabilities of the SPRT and a competing test has error probabilities $\alpha' \leq \alpha$ and $\beta' \leq \beta$. For an SPRT that stops on its boundaries, the author proved $E_0 g(D_\tau) \geq E_0 g(D_{\tau'})$ for any convex function g satisfying some minor requirement, provided $\Pr_1(\tau' < \infty) = 1$ for the competing test, where $\Pr_0$ and $\Pr_1$ are arbitrary distributions, and D_τ and $D_{\tau'}$ are the terminal likelihood ratios under the SPRT and the competitor. An analogous statement holds for expectation under $\Pr_1$.

11. Bayesian inference (see Chapter 7 for details) is unaffected by data-dependent stopping rules in a formal sense. However, violations of prior assumptions and data-dependent stopping rules are concerns. Rosenbaum and Rubin (1984) noted the fact that the violations of prior assumptions may have more severe consequences in repeated practice with the use of data-dependent rules. The authors showed that when using a flat prior, when in fact the correct prior is normal with positive prior precision p, the coverage probabilities are less tightly concentrated around the desired 0.95 region with the use of data-dependent stopping rules, and the effect becomes stronger when p increases.

12. In experiments designed for sequential analyses, it may not be necessary to use distributional results that are valid for fixed designs in order to make repeated sampling inference. Sometimes the sequential nature of design can be ignored from an asymptotic point of view. Ford et al. (1985) presented alternative approaches and made inference for stochastic processes and missing data problems. The author presented a few simple illustrative examples, including the following: (a) a first-order autoregression; (b) a simple linear regression through the origin with two observations y_1 and y_2, where $y_1 \sim N(\theta, 1)$ and $y_2 \sim N(c_1\theta, 1)$ if $y_1 > a$; otherwise, $y_2 \sim N(c_2\theta, 1)$; and (c) a two-parameter regression.

13. Jennison (1987) derived a parametric family of group-sequential tests, which minimize the expected sample size among all group-sequential tests, and can be implemented when group sizes are unequal and unpredictable. The tests can achieve the expected error rates in a wide range of situations and are efficient when compared with other tests based on the same group sizes at the same error rates.

14. Based on the likelihood ratio test, Chang (1989) developed the confidence interval estimation for μ under H_0: $\mu = \mu_0$ versus H_1: $\mu \neq \mu_0$, following a group-sequential test in a clinical trial with two treatments. The likelihood ratio test statistic is

$$T(\mu_0, M, S_M) = \exp((S_M/M - \mu_0)^2 M/2),$$

which is equivalent to $T_1(\mu_0, M, S_M) = \sqrt{M} \, |S_M/M - \mu_0|$. Confidence intervals produced by this method have accurate nominal coverage probability and a shorter average length than that proposed by Tsiatis et al. (1984).

15. Edelman (1989) proposed a sequential t-test based on a simple function of the nonsequential Student t-statistic. The martingale property that this function holds, that is, the conditional expectation of a future increment on previous observations is zero, facilitates calculation of error probabilities and expected sample sizes. This test behaves in a manner similar to that of the locally most powerful test for the mean of a normal distribution with known variance against the one-sided alternative, and might be viewed as its logical analogue when the variance is unknown.

16. Lin (1991) addressed sequential testing in randomized clinical trials with multiple endpoints, where patients may be subject to random loss to follow-up and the endpoints of interest may be time-to-event variables or other quantitative measurements. The author proposed a test statistic in terms of a weighted sum of the linear rank statistics with respect to the marginal distributions of the multiple endpoints, where the weights maximize asymptotic power against certain local alternatives. Based on the asymptotic joint distribution of the test statistics, stopping boundaries can be derived. This approach preserves the Type I error rate and stops quicker than sequential procedures based on single endpoints. The method was illustrated with an example taken from an AIDS clinical trial evaluating therapies in the treatment of patients with human immunodeficiency virus, where the major clinical events of interest in AIDS trials are opportunistic infections and deaths.

17. For the comparison of responses in two groups of subjects, with either continuous or discrete repeated measurements, Lee and DeMets (1992) proposed a group-sequential procedure based on linear rank statistics and obtained the asymptotic

normality of the sequentially computed linear rank statistics, as well as the corresponding group-sequential boundaries. This method can be applied to test the equality of two changes and rates of change, as well as the equality of two means of the responses.

18. The SPRT and related procedures are concerned primarily with the problem of selecting one of two competing hypotheses. For the multihypothesis problem, Baum and Veeravalli (1994) have developed a procedure that generalizes the SPRT, which they term the MSPRT. The authors provided bounds on error probabilities and asymptotic expressions for the stopping time and error probabilities. Under Bayesian assumptions (we refer the reader to Chapter 7 for more details), it is argued that the MSPRT approximates the much more complicated optimal test when error probabilities are small and expected stopping times are large. Compared with Bayesian fixed sample size tests, the MSPRT requires two to three times fewer samples on average. The use of MSPRT was illustrated with two examples involving Gaussian densities, where the first is for sequential detection of a signal with one of M amplitudes, and the second is for sequential detection of one of M orthogonal signals.

19. Pampallona and Tsiatis (1994) considered a class of boundaries for group-sequential clinical trials that allow for early stopping when small treatment differences are observed. They are based on the one-parameter family of boundaries introduced by Wang and Tsiatis (1987) and can be derived exactly for any choice of Type I and Type II error probabilities. The authors provide tables of relevant parameters to help in the design of group-sequential tests. The proposed procedures can be easily applied to both one- and two-sided hypothesis testing.

20. Bakeman and Quera (1995) proposed the log-linear analysis, which can be thought of as a multidimensional extension of chi-square tests (Bakeman and Robinson 2013), as a promising coherent analytic view for sequential phenomena. Bakeman (1997) considered log-linear techniques in sequential analysis that simplify matters and integrate lag-sequential analysis with an established and well-supported statistical tradition. The author depicted several advantages of a log-linear approach to sequential problems, including its ability to deal routinely with the structural zeros created when consecutive codes cannot repeat and its integration of sequential methods into an established and well-supported statistical tradition. Bakeman (1997) introduced descriptions related to how to conceptualize, preprocess, and analyze sequential data, providing fundamental concepts and relevant practical tools and techniques for the analysis of sequential data.

21. Proschan and Hunsberger (1995), Fisher (1998), and Müller and Schäfer (2001) proposed related schemes in the possibilities in adaptive sequential designs to include dropping or adding treatment arms, changing the primary endpoint, changing the patient population, and even changing objectives, for example, switching from noninferiority to superiority. Müller and Schäfer (2001) illustrated their method with a clinical trial evaluating the effect of deep brain stimulation on motor function (part III of the Unified Parkinson's Disease Rating Scale [UPDRS III]) and quality of life (Parkinson's Disease Questionnaire with 39 items [PDQ-39]) in patients suffering from Parkinson's disease.

22. Scharfstein et al. (1997) presented that the time-sequential joint distributions of many statistics used to analyze group-sequential time-to-event data and

longitudinal data are multivariate normal with an independent increments covariance structure. The authors developed an information-based design and a monitoring procedure that can be applied to any type of model in any type of group-sequential study in the case that a unique parameter of interest can be tested efficiently. The procedure was illustrated with a phase III clinical trial, where the primary objective is final confirmation of safety and efficacy (AIDS Clinical Trial Group Protocol 019 [ACTG 019]), in which 1338 adults with asymptomatic human immunodeficiency virus (HIV) infection who had CD4+ cell counts of fewer than $500/mm^3$ were randomized to receive one of three treatment protocols: placebo (428 subjects); zidovudine, 500 mg/day (453); or zidovudine, 1500 mg/day (457).

23. Lai (1997) gave a brief survey and a unified treatment of a variety of optimal stopping problems in sequential testing theory by introducing a general class of loss functions and prior distributions. This unified treatment results in relatively simple sequential tests based on generalized likelihood ratio statistics or mixture likelihood ratio statistics in the context of a one-parameter exponential family. As a simple example, the author considered the case where $X_1, X_2, \ldots$ are i.i.d. $N(\theta, 1)$ random variables and the problem of testing H_0: $\theta < 0$ versus H_1: $\theta > 0$.

24. Volodin and Novikov (1998) considered a sequential Wald test for discrimination of two simple hypotheses $\theta = \theta_1$ and $\theta = \theta_2$ to distinguish composite hypotheses $\theta < \theta_0$ and $\theta > \theta_0$, where the parameters θ_1, θ_2 as well as the boundaries A and B are chosen in such a way that d-posteriori probabilities of errors do not exceed the given restrictions β_0 and β_1. The authors studied the asymptotic behavior of boundaries A and B, as well as the average observation time, as $\beta = \max\{\beta_0, \beta_1\} \to 0$, and compared asymptotically $E_\theta v$ with the least given number of observations necessary for discrimination of composite hypotheses with the same restrictions β_0, β_1 on d-posteriori probabilities of errors. It was shown that the minimum (in a neighborhood of the point $\theta = \theta_0$) gain of the average observation time makes up 25%. Consequently, sequential tests within the bounds of a d-posteriori approach give a gain in sample size for every value of a parameter tested.

25. Posch and Bauer (2000) investigated sample size reassessment for adaptive two-stage designs, modifying the sample size of the second stage based on the predicted power of the trial at the end of the first stage. The authors demonstrated that stopping rules allowing for the early acceptance of the null hypothesis that are optimal with respect to the ASN may lead to a great decrease of the overall power if the sample size is a priori underestimated. This issue can be dealt with by choosing designs with low probabilities of early acceptance or by midtrial adaptations of the early acceptance boundary using the variability observed in the first stage. This modified approach preserves the power and is negligibly anticonservative.

26. Many randomized clinical trials apply a group-sequential monitoring procedure for assessing treatment efficacy during the course of the trial. For a group-sequential trial in which the null hypothesis is ultimately rejected, the nominal p-value generally overstates the statistical significance of the result and some adjustment is required. Several orderings of the sample space, such as stagewise ordering, maximum likelihood estimator ordering, likelihood ratio ordering, and score test ordering, have been proposed for performing this adjustment. Cook (2002) compared the aforementioned four methods and concluded that the sample space induced by the observed z-score ordering has the most desirable operating

characteristics with respect to the extent of the strength of evidence against the null hypothesis implied by the data.

27. Freidlin and Korn (2002) discussed futility monitoring of randomized clinical trials and investigated several concerns associated with aggressive monitoring for lack of activity in studies comparing experimental and control treatment arms: (a) stopping for futility when the experimental arm is doing better than the control arm, (b) conditional power not being low at the time of stopping, (c) potential loss of power to detect clinically interesting differences that are smaller than the design alternative, and (d) sensitivity of the power to the departure from the proportional hazards assumption. The authors suggested that aggressive futility rules do not generally reduce power (relative to less aggressive rules) under incorrect design assumptions, such as overstatement of the target treatment effect or mild violations of the proportional hazards assumption. On the other hand, aggressive monitoring rules may result in an early termination for futility when the experimental arm is doing better than the control arm (in some cases nontrivially better, especially when trials are designed for unrealistically large effects). Therefore, aggressive monitoring rules may fail to provide sufficiently convincing evidence to influence clinical practice or establish a standard of treatment.

28. The adaptive design does not use the classical test statistics for some types of sample size reassessments, and the adaptive test may reject the null hypothesis while the classical one-sample test does not. To avoid such inconsistencies, Posch et al. (2003) characterized sample size reassessment rules based on conditional power arguments using either the observed or the prefixed effect size. Although these reassessment rules may tend to lead to a large ASN for small actual effects, more favorable properties can be obtained due to the application of a maximal bound for the second-stage sample size. Additionally, the authors explored the extension of flexibility to the number of stages. In the first interim analysis, a second interim analysis is only planned if the chance to achieve a decision there is high. This leads to a reduction in the average number of interim analyses performed, without paying a noticeable price in terms of the ASN.

29. Van Der Tweel and Van Noord (2003) investigated disadvantages of the conditional power approach and proposed (group) sequential continuation of the trial or study as a less arbitrary strategy. The authors reanalyzed the Lupus Nephritis Collaborative Study (LNCS) data (Lachin and Lan 1992) and the Atherosclerosis Study in Communities (ASC) data (Hunsberger et al. 1994) to illustrate the advantages of a sequential approach. It is concluded that (group) sequential analyses have several advantages over the conditional power approach. To save valuable resources for more promising hypotheses, more studies should consider a sequential design and analysis to enable early stopping when enough evidence has accumulated to conclude a lack of the expected effect.

30. Tsiatis and Mehta (2003) pointed out that the adaptive designs are inefficient in terms of the power and the sample size and can be improved uniformly using standard group-sequential tests based on the sequentially computed likelihood ratio test statistic. The authors illustrated their arguments with a clinical trial comparing a new treatment to placebo, in which up to n pairs of patients were recruited into the trial and one member of the pair was randomized to receive treatment and the other placebo.

31. Whitehead and Matsushita (2003) introduced a simple futility design that allows a comparative clinical trial to be stopped due to lack of effect at any of a series of planned interim analyses. Stopping due to apparent benefit is not permitted. The design is for use when any positive claim should be based on the maximum sample size, for example, to allow subgroup analyses or the evaluation of safety or secondary efficacy responses. Any frequentist analysis can be performed that is valid for the type of design employed. Its advantages and disadvantages relative to the use of stochastic curtailment are presented and discussed.

32. Lawson (2004) explored futility from an ethical perspective and assessed its relevance to the goals of medicine in general. As a tool for making clinical decisions, futility avoids the balance between the benefits and harms of specific treatments and ignores the fundamental issue of the goals of medicine. There is a lack of coherence in descriptions of futility, which may conflict with the concept of patient autonomy. The subjectivity character suggests that futility is of little use when used alone to consider how patients should be treated.

33. Lai and Shih (2004) proposed a class of flexible and efficient group-sequential designs for one-sided and two-sided tests of the natural parameter θ of an exponential family $f_\theta(x) = \exp(\theta x - \psi(\theta))$. The designs can achieve asymptotic efficiency by adapting to the information about the unknown parameters during the course of the trial, under pre-specified constraints on the maximum sample size and Type I error probability. Such flexible designs avoid the need for sample size reestimation for fixed sample size trials and obviate the difficulties due to information time (at which the total number of patients accrued reaches some pre-specified level) versus calendar time that arise in more complex settings, for example, time-sequential clinical trials comparing the failure times of two treatments. As an illustrative example, the authors considered Table 2 of Eales and Jennison (1992), where the number of groups $K = 5$ and the Type I error probability and the Type II error probability are both 0.05; see Eales and Jennison (1992) more details.

34. The error probabilities of Wald's SPRT, the weight function SPRTs, and subsequent invariant SPRTs have simple closed-form approximations because the stopped likelihood ratio statistics in these tests have simple two-point distributions if excess over the boundary is ignored, and Wald's likelihood ratio identity expresses these probabilities as expectations of the stopped likelihood ratio statistics. Lai (2004) gave a review of how likelihood ratio identities have been applied to analyze much more complicated sequential testing and change-point detection, and addressed an open problem concerning the asymptotic optimality of sequential generalized likelihood ratio procedures.

35. In an experiment, flexible designs allow large modifications of a design. A standard flexible method combines a weighted test with the modifications of the sample size in response to interim data or external information, which guarantees the Type I error level. However, in this case, the basic inference principles are violated. For example, with independent $N(\mu, 1)$ observations, the test rejects the null hypothesis of $\mu \leq 0$, while the average of the observations is negative. Burman and Sonesson (2006) provided several possible modifications of the flexible design methodology with a focus on alternative hypothesis tests. The authors concluded that flexible design is not valid in its most general form with the corresponding weighted test.

36. Methods for unplanned design change are defined in terms of nonsufficient statistics to keep the Type I error rate. However, their efficiency and the credibility of conclusions reached are doubtful. Jennison and Turnbull (2006) evaluated schemes for adaptive redesigned clinical trials, extending the theoretical results proposed by Tsiatis and Mehta (2003) that use sufficient statistics. By numerical computation of optimal tests, the authors assessed the benefits of pre-planned adaptive designs, including sequentially planned sequential tests proposed by Schmitz et al. (1993). The authors concluded that the flexibility of unplanned adaptive designs comes at the cost of efficiency and recommended that the power requirement should be determined carefully at the start of the study.

37. Snapinn et al. (2006) described and compared several widely used approaches to assess futility, including stochastic curtailment, predictive power, predictive probability, and group-sequential methods. The authors discussed issues associated with futility analyses, such as ethical considerations, whether or not Type I error can or should be reclaimed, one-sided versus two-sided futility rules, and the impact of futility analyses on power.

38. Todd (2007) reviewed and examined the recent theoretical developments and subsequent uptake of sequential methodology in clinical studies from the perspective of the contributions made to all four phases into which clinical trials are traditionally classified. The author reviewed and highlighted major statistical advancements and their applications, emphasizing the phase III clinical trials, where the vast majority of research focuses on work.

39. The group-sequential stopping rule is usually used in a clinical trial as the monitoring criteria to deal with the ethical and efficiency matters intrinsic in testing a new therapeutic or preventive treatment or agent. According to various criteria, stopping rules have been proposed in both statistical aspects (e.g., the frequentist Type I error rate, Bayesian posterior probabilities, and a stochastic curtailment) and scientific perspectives (e.g., estimates of treatment effect). However, it is easy to show that a stopping rule according to one of these criteria induces one based on all other criteria. Therefore, the criteria specified initially are relatively unimportant if the operating characteristics of stopping rules are fully inspected. Emerson et al. (2007) reviewed and evaluated the frequentist operating characteristics of a particular stopping rule so that the constraints imposed by various disciplines specified by the collaborators are satisfied by the selected clinical trial design.

40. Thall et al. (2007) presented the results of a clinical trial that makes use of sequential randomization, a novel trial design that allows the investigator to study adaptive treatment strategies. During this trial, prostate cancer patients who were found to be responding poorly to their initially assigned regimen were randomly reassigned to one of the remaining candidate regimens. Different from conventional trials that are based on a single randomization, sequential randomization designs allow the investigator to study adaptive treatment strategies that adjust a patient's treatment in response to the observed course of the illness.

41. Bembom and van der Laan (2007) reviewed several statistical methods available for analyses of sequential randomization trials. The authors focused on two different approaches for estimating the success rates of different adaptive treatment strategies of interest. By emphasizing the intuitive appeal and simple implementation of these methods, sequential randomization trials are shown to provide a rich

source of information that is made readily accessible through current analytical approaches.

42. The comparison of the accuracy of two diagnostic tests based on the receiver operating characteristic (ROC) curve methodology (see Chapter 8 for details) is typically conducted using fixed sample designs. However, human experimentation argues for periodic monitoring and interim analyses to address the ethics and efficiency issues in the medical study. In the context of comparative ROC studies, Tang et al. (2008) proposed a nonparametric group-sequential design plan, adapting a nonparametric family of weighted area under the ROC curve statistics (Wieand et al. 1989) and a group-sequential sampling plan. In addition, the authors introduced a semiparametric sequential method based on proportional hazards models. Through simulation studies, the nonparametric approach was shown to be robust to model misspecification and has great finite sample performance, compared with the alternative semiparametric and parametric analyses.

43. For a large phase III study, when many candidate regimens are possible but with limited resources, the multiarmed randomized selection trial is a useful strategy to remove inferior treatments from further consideration. In the case of a relatively quickly ascertained endpoint, for example, an imaging-based lesion volume change in acute stroke patients, frequent interim monitoring of the trial is ethically and practically appealing to clinicians. In the context of multiarmed clinical trials where the objective is to select a treatment with clinically significant improvement over the control group, or to declare futility if no such treatment exists, Cheung (2008) proposed a class of sequential selection boundaries. The proposed boundaries are easy to implement in a blinded fashion and can be applied on a flexible monitoring schedule in terms of calendar time. Design calibration with respect to pre-specified levels of confidence is simple and can be accomplished when the response rate of the control group is known only up to an interval. Compared to an optimal two-stage design, the proposed method was demonstrated to have a smaller sample size on average, especially when there is in fact a superior treatment to the control group. The method was illustrated with a phase II (where the primary objective is to establish the efficacy of the drug) selection trial in acute stroke patients using MRI response as the primary endpoint, where a two-stage design given in Table 2 of Fisher et al. (2006) was adopted.

44. In a sequential clinical trial where the stopping rule depends on the primary endpoint, the inference on secondary endpoints is problematic with possible substantial bias. Commonly used bias correction approaches estimate the bias by means of joint asymptotic normality of the statistics associated with the primary and secondary endpoints, assuming bivariate normal outcomes. Lai et al. (2009) proposed a method that uses resampling and a novel ordering scheme in the sample space of sequential statistics observed up to a stopping time. This approach provides accurate inference in complex clinical trials, for example, time-sequential trials with survival endpoints and covariates. The authors illustrated their method in the case of bivariate normal outcomes, nonnormal bivariate outcomes, Cox model with two covariates, and median survival.

45. The nested case-control design is a comparatively new kind of observational study, where cases and controls are observed longitudinally by sampling all cases whenever they occur, but controls at time points randomly scheduled or prefixed for

operational convenience. The nested case-control design is efficient in terms of cost and duration, especially in the case of a rare disease or the assessment of exposure levels is difficult. In the context of the nested case-control design, Park and Chang (2010) proposed a method of simultaneous sequential sampling on both subjects and replicates and studied both (group) sequential testing and estimation methods so that the study can be stopped as soon as the stopping rule is fulfilled. Different from the classical approaches used in longitudinal studies, the proposed sampling scheme is more efficient and more flexible. In order to accommodate the new sampling scheme, the authors defined a new σ-field, which contains mixtures of independent and correlated observations. Based on the martingale theories, the authors proved the asymptotic optimality of sequential estimation and verified that the independent increment structure is retained so that the group-sequential method is applicable. The author illustrated the method with real data on children's diarrhea, where controls are collected at prefixed time points. This study "assess the role of Enterotoxigenic *Escherichia coli* (ETEC) in children's diarrhea performed by the United States Naval Medical Research Unit Number Three conducted in two villages in the Abu Homos district of Beheira Governorate, Egypt (Clemens et al. 2004; Park and Kim 2004). From February 1995 to February 1998, 375 children were visited twice a week until 36 months of age. At these twice-weekly visits, information was collected on diarrheal symptoms for each day since the last visit. If any diarrheal symptoms were reported, rectal swabs were collected to identify diarrhea severity, from which only cases, not controls, were defined if diarrhea was confirmed. In addition, at every eighth-week visit rectal swabs were collected regardless of diarrheal symptoms. The collected rectal swabs were evaluated to define diarrhea status and to identify the existence of ETEC. The final number of diarrhea cases was 2201 and the number of controls was 2028 with the numbers of cases and controls with ETEC infection 610 and 380, respectively. Even though our major interest lies in assessing the causal association of ETEC with incidence of diarrhea symptoms, there are some confounding effects to incorporate into analysis in practice. In this study, two models with and without confounding variables have been compared. Confounding variables considered to adjust for the ETEC effect are seasonality and age" (see Park and Chang [2010] for more details).

46. In a survival analysis or time-to-event setting, statistical information, and hence efficiency, is most closely related to the observed number of events, while trial costs depend on the number of patients accrued. Due to the need to consider both the number of patients accrued and the calendar time of follow-up necessary to observe the desired number of events, an adaptive design is appealing since it offers the possibility that early trends in the estimated treatment effect may suggest a modification of the number of subjects that need to be accrued. Emerson et al. (2011) investigated and compared the trade-offs between efficiency (as measured by average number of observed events required), power, and cost (a function of the number of subjects accrued and length of observation) for standard group-sequential methods and an adaptive design that allows for early termination of accrual. The authors found that when certain trial design parameters are constrained, an adaptive approach to terminating subject accrual may improve the cost efficiency of a group-sequential clinical trial investigating time-to-event endpoints. However, when the spectrum of group-sequential designs considered is broadened, the advantage of the adaptive designs is less clear.

47. Although generally meta-analyses are regarded as retrospective activities, they are increasingly being applied to provide the latest evidence on specific research topics. In the meta-analysis, the possibility of false positive findings due to repeated significance tests should be considered. Higgins et al. (2011) discussed the use of sequential methods in meta-analyses that include random effects to account for heterogeneity across studies. The authors recommended using an approximate semi-Bayes approach to update evidence on the among-study variance, with an informative prior distribution based on findings from previous meta-analyses. Through simulation studies, the method was shown to have Type I and Type II error rates close to the nominal level. The method was illustrated with an example in the treatment of bleeding peptic ulcers, where the data are obtained from 23 trials that compare endoscopic hemostasis with a control treatment for the treatment of bleeding peptic ulcers, and the outcome of interest is post-treatment bleeding and the treatment effect recorded here is the log-odds ratio of no bleeding; see Sacks et al. (1990) for more details about the data.

48. Yi et al. (2012) proposed a hybridization of the conditional and predictive power methods, along with a novel resampling method, to assess futility in sequential trials with time-to-event outcomes. The proposed approach to futility assessment applies to sequential clinical trials with interim analyses planned at either fixed calendar times or fixed number of events. In addition, it does not resort to asymptotics and applies to general test statistics of either single or multiple dimensions.

49. There has been extensive commentary on the Type I error rate control and efficiency considerations in the adaptive clinical trial methodology. Levin et al. (2014) evaluated the reliability and precision of different inferential procedures in the presence of an adaptive design with pre-specified rules for modifying the sampling plan. The authors extended group-sequential orderings of the outcome space based on the stopping stage, likelihood ratio statistic, and sample mean to the adaptive setting in order to compute median-unbiased point estimates, exact confidence intervals, and p-values uniformly distributed under the null hypothesis. The likelihood ratio ordering is found to average shorter confidence intervals and produce higher probabilities of p-values below important thresholds than alternative approaches. The bias-adjusted mean demonstrates the lowest mean squared error among candidate point estimates. In order to quantify the cost of failing to plan ahead in settings where adaptations could realistically be pre-specified at the design stage, the authors compared the performance of the conditional error-based approach, which is the only method to accommodate unplanned adaptations and other methods. The authors concluded the cost to be meaningful across all designs and treatment effects that were considered, and to be substantial for designs frequently proposed in the literature.

50. Kirk and Fay (2014) reviewed sequential designs, including group-sequential and two-stage designs, for testing or estimating a single binary parameter. The authors introduced ideas common to many sequential designs, which can be explained without explicitly using stochastic processes. The authors provided an R package *binseqtest* with procedures that exactly bound the Type I error rate of tests while maintaining proper coverage of confidence intervals. Moreover, the authors reviewed some practical adaptations of the sequential design and demonstrated relevant issues, including the following: (a) the modification of the design if no assessment was made at one of the planned sequential stopping times, (b) the

estimation of the parameter if the study needs to be stopped early, (c) the allowable reasons for stopping early, and (d) the validity of inferences when the study is stopped for crossing the boundary, but later information is collected about responses of subjects that had enrolled before the decision to stop but had not responded by that time.

13.9 Appendix: Determination of Sample Sizes Based on the Errors' Control of SPRT

We have

$$\alpha = \Pr_{H_0}(L_N \geq B) = \sum_{n=1}^{\infty} \Pr_{H_0}(L_n \geq B, N = n)$$

$$= \sum_{n=1}^{\infty} E_{H_0} I(L_n \geq B, N = n) = \sum_{n=1}^{\infty} \int I(L_n \geq B, N = n) f_0(x_1, \ldots, x_n) dx_1 \ldots dx_n$$

$$= \sum_{n=1}^{\infty} \int I(L_n \geq B, N = n) \frac{f_0(x_1, \ldots, x_n)}{f_1(x_1, \ldots, x_n)} dx_1 \ldots dx_n$$

$$= \sum_{n=1}^{\infty} \int I(L_n \geq B, N = n) \frac{f_1(x_1, \ldots, x_n)}{L_n} dx_1 \ldots dx_n$$

$$\leq B^{-1} \sum_{n=1}^{\infty} \int I(L_n \geq B, N = n) f_1(x_1, \ldots, x_n) dx_1 \ldots dx_n = B^{-1} \sum_{n=1}^{\infty} E_{H_1} I(L_n \geq B, N = n)$$

$$= B^{-1} \Pr_{H_1}(L_N \geq B) = B^{-1}(1 - \beta).$$

Similarly, it can be derived that $\beta = \Pr_{H_1}(L_N \leq A) \leq A \Pr_{H_0}(L_N \leq A) = A(1 - \alpha)$.

14

A Brief Review of Multiple Testing Problems in Clinical Experiments

14.1 Introduction

Multiplicity issues are generally encountered in preclinical and clinical trials with multiple comparisons, tests for multiple endpoints, and multiple objectives. In preclinical applications, the objectives may correspond to testing across multiple genetic markers. In clinical settings, the objectives can be defined, for example, in terms of multiple dose levels, endpoints, or subgroup analyses. The types of multiplicity problems that arise in clinical trials depend on how these trials are designed for assessing clinically meaningful benefits of the treatments under investigation. That any given trial may collect data on multiple endpoints at different time points on patients randomized to test and control groups at different dose levels leads to potential myriad statistical tests. In addition, some trials may incorporate multiple interim analyses (e.g., see Chapter 13) during the course of the trial and change some design features adaptively based on the results of interim analyses. This creates additional layers of multiplicity problems. Some trials may also be multiregional, for which treatment benefit evaluations may require addressing regional differences, for example, differences in clinical practice, patient ethnicity, and other clinical and biological factors. These trials may pose challenging design and multiplicity problems when, in the absence of consistency of treatment effects, evidence of treatment benefits may be sought for specific regions or subpopulations. In general, the most common sources of multiplicity in clinical trials include the following:

1. Multiple dose–control comparisons in dose-finding studies to evaluate the efficacy and safety properties of a treatment compared with a control or between dose levels.

2. Multiple criteria for assessing the efficacy profile of a treatment, for example, both a safety and an efficacy endpoint or multiple efficacy endpoints. These criteria assist in the evaluation of multiple dimensions of the treatment effect, and the overall outcome can be declared positive if (a) one or more criteria are met, (b) all criteria are met, or (c) some composite criterion is met, depending on the trial's objectives.

3. Multiple secondary analyses, for example, analysis of secondary endpoints or subgroup effects that are typically evaluated after the trial's primary objective is met.

When multiple hypotheses are tested without adjusting the per comparison significance level, it will lead to an inflated Type I error rate across all tests. This is oftentimes referred to as the family-wise error rate, described in detail below. For example, if two independent tests are tested at a significance level of 0.05, then using basic probability, we can calculate the chance of at least one false positive result under both null hypotheses being true as 0.0975, that is, roughly double. If 10 tests are tested at 0.05, then the chance of a false positive across the 10 tests is 0.40 given all 10 null hypotheses are true.

Similarly, the concept of the Type II error rate needs to be extended from the univariate case to the multiple hypotheses testing case. A trial can fail due to poor planning or disregarding multiplicity issues with respect to multiple endpoints and multiple comparisons (Dmitrienko et al. 2010). For example, Austin et al. (2006) illustrated how multiple hypotheses testing can produce associations with no clinical plausibility with a study of all 10,674,945 residents of Ontario aged between 18 and 100 years in 2000. In this study, residents were randomly assigned to equally sized derivation and validation cohorts and classified according to their astrological sign. The authors tested 24 associations in the independent validation cohort and found that residents born under Leo had a significant higher probability of gastrointestinal hemorrhage, while Sagittarians had a significant higher probability of humerus fracture than all other signs combined. However, after adjusting the significance level to account for multiple comparisons, none of the identified associations remained significant in either the derivation or validation cohort. The analyses suggest that the problem of multiplicity should be accounted for to avoid detecting implausible associations.

Therefore, it is important that clinical trials are designed to control the error rates at a pre-specified level through appropriate design and analysis strategies that are determined a priori. In this chapter, we present some useful definitions of error rates, the power evaluations in multiple testing problems, and simple Bonferroni procedures that counteract the problem of multiplicity.

14.2 Definitions of Error Rates

In order to choose an appropriate multiple testing method, it is critical to select the set of relevant hypotheses that reflect the objectives of a clinical study or preclinical experiment. These are oftentimes termed *primary* hypotheses. Overall, error rates are generally less controlled in more exploratory analyses in the same study and linked to so-called *secondary* hypotheses or discovery hypotheses, which then need to be validated with future experiments. This section introduces several error rate definitions that are commonly used in clinical trials. In addition, we provide definitions of error rates commonly employed in preclinical and biomarker studies, where additional logistical considerations, such as cost of an assay, are at play.

14.2.1 Family-Wise Error Rates

The concept of a Type I error rate, the probability of incorrectly rejecting null hypotheses, originates in the problem of testing a single hypothesis; see Chapter 1 for details. In the context of multiple hypotheses tests, the family-wise error rate (FWER) is defined as the probability of making one or more false positive decisions, or Type I errors, among all the hypotheses given all null hypotheses are true.

As an example, consider a dose-finding study with m doses tested versus placebo. Assume the primary endpoint is normally distributed, with larger values indicating a positive dose response. Let μ_0 be the mean response in the placebo arm and μ_i be the mean response in the ith dose group, $i = 1, \ldots, m$. Let δ be a nonnegative constant defining the clinically important difference. The testing problem, formulated in terms of the difference in the mean responses, is to test the hypothesis of treatment effect no greater than δ versus a one-sided alternative of treatment effect greater than δ, that is,

$$H_{0i}: \mu_i - \mu_0 \leq \delta \text{ versus } H_{1i}: \mu_i - \mu_0 > \delta, i = 1, \ldots, m.$$

The Type I error rate for the ith hypothesis is the probability of concluding that a clinically relevant treatment effect is present when the treatment difference is actually no greater than δ.

If each of the m hypotheses is tested separately at a pre-specified significance level α, for example, $\alpha = 0.05$, it can be shown that the proportion of incorrectly rejected hypotheses will not exceed α. This is known as the control of the comparison-wise error rate or per comparison error rate, where comparison-wise error rate refers to the probability of committing a Type I error on a single, pre-specified test. However, preserving the comparison-wise error rate for a single test is not the same concept as preserving the error rate for multiple tests under consideration.

When multiple independent tests are under consideration, the hypotheses of interest should be considered together as a family, and an incorrect decision may result from a single Type I error in this family. Accordingly, the FWER, that is, the probability of rejecting at least one true hypothesis erroneously, can be computed under the assumption that all m hypotheses are simultaneously true. This procedure controls the FWER in the *weak* sense, where the FWER control is guaranteed only when all null hypotheses are true (i.e., when the global null hypothesis is true).

In the context of clinical trials with multiple independent endpoints, the weak FWER control can be interpreted as the probability of concluding an effect on at least one endpoint when there is no effect on any endpoint, that is, the probability of falsely concluding an ineffective treatment has an effect. If clinical trial endpoints are highly correlated, for example, testing about both blood pressure and cholesterol level, then the FWER calculations are conservative in terms of a bound. Methods for estimating the overall FWER and adjusting the error rates in a date-driven sense are available via resampling (e.g., see Hutson 2004).

In general, the assumption that all hypotheses are simultaneously true may be restrictive in many clinical applications and is not appropriate when investigators are interested in making claims about specific outcomes. For example, in dose-finding clinical trials, the treatment difference may vary across the dose levels and investigators are generally interested in testing the drug effect at each particular dose in order to claim that this effect is significant. To achieve this goal, one needs to preserve the probability of erroneously finding a significant result for each dose regardless of the treatment effect size in other dose groups, that is, to control the probability of incorrectly rejecting any true hypothesis despite which and how many other hypotheses are true. This approach controls the FWER in the *strong* sense, where the FWER control is ensured for any configuration of true and nontrue null hypotheses (including the global null hypothesis). Let T be the index set of true null hypotheses. Mathematically, strong control of the FWER requires that

$$\sup \text{ FWER} = \max_{T} \sup_{\{\mu_i(T)\}} \text{Pr(Reject at least one } H_{0i}, i \in T) \leq \alpha,$$

where the supremum is taken over all μ_i satisfying $\mu_i - \mu_0 \leq \delta$ for $i \in T$ and $\mu_i - \mu_0 > \delta$ for $i \notin T$, and the maximum is taken over all index sets T. Regulators mandate strong control of the FWER for the primary objectives in all confirmatory clinical trials (Committee for Proprietary Medicinal Products 2002).

FWER control across multiple tests is a form of simultaneous inference, where all inferences in a family are jointly corrected up to a pre-specified error rate. This approach is reasonable when a few hypotheses are involved. For a description of some commonly used multiple testing FWER control methods in addition to the Bonferroni procedure described below, see Hutson (2013).

The Bonferroni procedure is a widely used single-step correction procedure to counteract the problem of multiple comparisons. It is considered the simplest and most conservative method for controlling the FWER. In the problem of testing m equally weighted and independent hypotheses, $H_1, \ldots, H_m$, let $p_1, \ldots, p_m$ be the corresponding p-values. Let I_0 be the subset of the (unknown) true null hypotheses with m_0 members. At a pre-specified significance level α, the Bonferroni procedure rejects H_i if $p_i \leq \alpha/m$. Following the (first-order) Bonferroni inequality, it can be derived that

$$FWER = \Pr\left\{\bigcup_{i \in I_0} (p_i \leq \alpha/m)\right\} \leq \sum_{i \in I_0} \Pr\left\{p_i \leq \alpha/m\right\} \leq m_0 \alpha/m \leq m\alpha/m = \alpha.$$

That is, the Bonferroni procedure controls the FWER for any joint distribution of the raw p-values.

Denote the multiplicity-adjusted p-values for multiple testing procedures by $\tilde{p}_1, \ldots, \tilde{p}_m$. In the case of equally weighted hypotheses, the adjusted p-value based on the Bonferroni procedure for the hypothesis H_i is $\tilde{p}_i = \min(1, mp_i)$, $i = 1, \ldots, m$. The hypothesis H_i is rejected if $\tilde{p}_i \leq \alpha$.

Example 14.1: p-Value Adjustments within Multiple Testing

As a simple example, we revisit the thiobarbituric acid reactive substances (TBARS) data described in Section 3.2, which consists of 542 measurements of TBARS with the sample mean and sample standard deviation of 1.3808 and 0.4166, respectively. We would like to obtain the Bonferroni adjusted p-values for the following two hypothesis tests: (1) the t-test for the population mean, H_{01}: the population mean of TBARS is 1.4 versus H_{11}: the population mean of TBARS is not 1.4, and (2) the Shapiro–Wilk test for normality, H_{02}: TBARS is normally distributed versus H_{12}: TBARS is not normally distributed.

The Bonferroni adjusted p-values can be simply conducted via the R command p.adjust. The following R code performs the Bonferroni adjustment for multiple comparisons based on the TBARS data:

```
> p.mu<-t.test(tbars,mu=1.4)$p.value # t test
> p.N<-shapiro.test(tbars)$p.value # Shapiro-Wilk test for normality
> p<-c(p.mu,p.N)
> p # unadjusted pvalues
[1] 2.834995e-01 1.003122e-22
> pval.adj<-p.adjust(p, method="bonferroni")
> pval.adj  # Bonferroni adjusted pvalues
[1] 5.669989e-01 2.006244e-22
```

The Bonferroni adjusted p-values for the t-test for the population mean and the Shapiro–Wilk test for normality are 0.567 and <0.001, respectively. Both are rejected at the $\alpha = 0.05$ level.

To define simultaneous confidence intervals based on Bonferroni-based procedures, consider a parametric multiple hypotheses testing of no treatment effect versus a one-sided alternative, that is,

$$H_{0i}: \theta_i \leq 0 \text{ versus } H_{1i}: \theta_i > 0, i = 1, \ldots, m,$$

where $\theta_1, \ldots, \theta_m$ are parameters of interest, for example, mean treatment differences or differences in proportions. Let $\hat{\theta}_i$ and s_i denote an estimate of θ_i and an estimate of the standard error of θ_i, $i = 1, \ldots, m$, respectively. Assume that $\hat{\theta}_i$ is normally distributed with mean θ_i and standard deviation σ_i. A one-sided $100(1-\alpha)\%$ Bonferroni-based confidence interval for $\theta_1, \ldots, \theta_m$ is given by $(\tilde{L}_i, \infty)$, $i = 1, \ldots, m$, where

$$\tilde{L}_i = \hat{\theta}_i - z_{\alpha/m} s_i,$$

and $z_{\alpha/m}$ denotes the $(1 - \alpha/m)$ quantile of the standard normal distribution.

Note that Bonferroni confidence intervals are conservative and the actual probability for the confidence interval is greater than $1 - \alpha$.

An extension of the method for setting up simultaneous confidence intervals for Bonferroni-based closed testing procedures proposed by Strassburger and Bretz (2008) can be used to define simultaneous confidence intervals for the fallback procedure. The lower limits of one-sided $100 (1 - \alpha)\%$ confidence intervals are derived as follows. First, for any nonempty index set $J \subseteq I$, let

$$\alpha_i(J) = \begin{cases} 0 & \text{if } i \notin J, \\ \alpha(i - \ell_i(J))/m & \text{if } i \in J, \end{cases}$$

where $\ell_i(J)$ is the largest index in J that is smaller than i if i is not the smallest index in J and $\ell_i(J) = 0$ if i is the smallest index in J. Similarly, for any nonempty index set $J \subseteq I$ and $i \notin J$, let

$$\alpha_i^*(J) = \frac{1}{m - |J|} \left(\alpha - \sum_{j \in J} \alpha_j(J) \right),$$

where $|J|$ is the number of elements in J. The lower limits are given by

$$\tilde{L}_i = \begin{cases} \min_{J \subseteq A} \max(0, \theta_i - z_{\alpha_i^*(J)} s_i) & \text{if } i \in R \text{ and } R \neq I, \\ \hat{\theta}_i - z_{\alpha_i(A)} s_i & \text{if } i \in A, \\ \max(0, \theta_i - z_{\alpha/m} s_i) & \text{if } R = I, \end{cases}$$

where A and R are the index sets of retained and rejected hypotheses, respectively. These lower limits take advantage of the fact that the fallback procedure is not α - exhaustive. Unlike the lower limits for the Holm and fixed-sequence procedures, the fallback-adjusted lower limits are not automatically set to 0 for parameters corresponding to rejected hypotheses of no treatment effect.

14.2.2 False Discovery Rate and False Discovery Proportion

In studies involving a large number of hypotheses, for example, microarray experiments, simultaneous inference may be impractical. Specifically, as the number of hypotheses m increases, the FWER control of multiple tests becomes conservative and may fail to detect significant results unless the treatment effect is overwhelmingly positive. In this case, selective inference approaches may be more appropriate, where any subgroup of hypotheses from the large-scale group can be viewed as a family. Selective inference can be performed by controlling the false discovery rate (FDR) criteria (Benjamini and Hochberg 1995).

The modern widespread use of the FDR stems from the development in technologies that allowed the collection and analysis of a large number of distinct variables in several individuals, for example, the expression level of each of 5000 different genes in 50 different persons. The FDR was motivated by biomarker studies where the goal was to determine a subset of biomarkers worthy of further investigation. For example, suppose out of our 5000 genes under consideration we want to develop a custom assay that costs much less to run around 100 of the most significant genes, and suppose we are willing to live with the fact that a proportion of these 100 genes are false discoveries. The proportion of those false discoveries can be controlled at a given rate around a defined error rate. Going forward with the smaller set of selected genes, one then would be more stringent and use the FWER as the testing criteria.

Toward this end, the false discovery proportion (FDP) (Korn et al. 2004) is defined as the proportion of false discoveries among all discoveries (rejected null hypotheses). That is,

$$FDP = \left(\frac{\text{Number of incorrectly rejected null hypotheses}}{\text{Number of rejected hypotheses}} \right),$$

if the number of rejected hypotheses is positive; FDP = 0, if no hypothesis is rejected. Then the FDR is defined as $E(FDP)$, that is, the expected proportion of incorrectly rejected null hypotheses among all rejected null hypotheses. The FDR is said to be controlled at the γ level if

$$FDR \leq \gamma.$$

FDR controlling seeks to reduce the expected proportion of false discoveries, as opposed to the probability of even one false discovery in the case of FWER controlling. The FDR controlling procedures exert a less stringent control over false discovery than the FWER procedures (such as the well-known Bonferroni correction). Control of the FDR at the α level does not imply control of the FWER at the α level. Therefore, FDR procedures have greater power at the cost of increased rates of Type I errors, that is, rejecting null hypotheses of no effect when they should be accepted.

Note that when FDR is controlled at the γ level, it does not imply that the FDP is less than or equal to γ with high probability. To guarantee this, one can specify a fraction β and an acceptable probability of exceedance α, and control that

$$\Pr(FDP > \beta) \leq \alpha.$$

It can be interpreted as follows: among those hypotheses that are rejected, the proportion of false discoveries may exceed β with probability no greater than α. The FDP control is suitable in many nonconfirmatory settings, for example, genetic or preclinical studies, where a certain proportion of errors is considered acceptable. The FDP control with $\beta = 0$ is equivalent to the FWER control. However, control of the FDP with $\beta > 0$ at the α level does not imply control of the FWER at the α level.

FDR or FDP error controlling procedures are generally used for biomarker discovery trials and are generally not suitable for confirmatory clinical trials. In fact, it is possible to manipulate the design of a clinical trial so that any desired conclusion can be almost surely inferred without inflating the FDR (Finner and Roters 2001).

14.3 Power Evaluation

The extension of statistical power, or Type II error rates, from the univariate case to the multiple hypotheses testing case is not as relatively straightforward as the case of the FWER control. There are several methods for evaluating the performance of a clinical trial in terms of power given multiple testing. A standard approach is to consider the probability of rejecting *at least one* false null hypothesis (disjunctive power). Following the notation described in Section 14.2, disjunctive power is defined as

$$\Pr(\text{Reject at least one } H_{0i}, i \notin T),$$

where the probability is evaluated for a given set of parameter values: $\mu_i > \mu_0 + \delta$ if $i \notin T$ and $\mu_i > \mu_0 + \delta$ if $i \in T$ if (Senn and Bretz 2007). Disjunctive power is recommended for use, for example, in studies involving multiple comparisons with a control or in studies with multiple endpoints, where it is suffcient to demonstrate the treatment effect on at least one endpoint. Alternatively, conjunctive power can be obtained as the probability of rejecting *all* false null hypotheses, that is,

$$\Pr(\text{Reject all } H_{0i}, i \notin T),$$

where probability is again evaluated given a set of parameter values as above. It is argued that conjunctive power should be used in studies such as fixed drug combination studies or studies in which the treatment effect must be established on two or more coprimary endpoints. For other existing power concepts, we refer to Maurer and Mellein (1988) and Westfall et al. (2011). Note that general software implementations of the approaches above are not readily available. Customized programming and the corresponding simulations need to be conducted in most cases.

In practice, the appropriate power methodologies should be balanced against other considerations in multiple testing and ultimately should be chosen according to the study objectives; see Hommel and Bretz (2008) for details.

14.4 Remarks

In any analysis involving testing or estimation of multiple parameters, it is important to clarify the research questions to discern whether multiple inference procedures will be needed (Rothman et al. 2008). Multiple inference procedures will be needed if and only if joint hypotheses are of interest. It should be noted that conventional approaches to multiple inference questions, for example, Bonferroni adjustments, may not be the optimal choice due to their conservative nature (Greenland 1993). More modern procedures, such as hierarchical (empirical Bayes) modeling (Kass and Steffey 1989), will provide improved performance over some classical approaches.

14.5 Supplement

1. Bretz et al. (2010) described the common underlying theory of multiple comparison procedures through numerous examples, including the Bonferroni method and Simes's test. The book also depicts applications of parametric multiple comparisons in standard linear models and general parametric models, Dunnett's test, Tukey's all-pairwise comparison method, and general methods for multiple contrast tests for standard regression models, mixed-effects models, and parametric survival models. There is a detailed discussion and analysis regarding many multiple testing techniques, of which many examples are implemented in R.

2. In order to compare multiple outcomes commonly encountered in biomedical research, Huang et al. (2005) improved O'Brien's (1984) rank-sum tests via replacing the ad hoc variance by the asymptotic variance of the test statistics. When the differences between the two comparison groups in each outcome variable have the same direction (sign), that is, all positive or all negative, the improved tests control the Type I error rate at the desired level and increase power. When the signs of the differences vary, for example, some positive and some negative, the improved tests may lose power. Alternatively, Liu et al. (2010) proposed a so-called rank-max test statistic, which takes the maximum of the individual rank-sum statistics. The rank-max test statistic controls the Type I error rate and maintains satisfactory power regardless of the direction (sign) of the differences. The rank-max test has higher power than other tests in a certain alternative parameter space of interest. When applied to compare heart rates from a clinical trial to evaluate the effect of a procedure to remove the cardioprotective solution HTK (Domhof and Langer 2002), the popular Bonferroni correction, Huang et al.'s improved tests failed to show important significant differences, while the rank-max test yielded satisfactory results.

15

Some Statistical Procedures for Biomarker Measurements Subject to Instrumental Limitations

15.1 Introduction

In clinical trials involving measurements of biomarkers, the values supplied are typically estimates and hence subject to measurement errors (MEs). MEs may arise from assay or instrument inaccuracies, biological variations, or errors in questionnaire-based self-report data. For instance, it is well known that systolic blood pressure (SBP) is measured with errors mainly due to strong daily and seasonal variations relative to determining a normal or abnormal value. In this case, Carroll et al. (1984) suggested that approximately one-third of the observed variability is due to MEs. In such a circumstance, it makes sense to hypothesize an unbiased additive error model, assuming we observe the true value plus an error in each measurement. Subsequently, measurements may be subject to limits of detection (LODs) where values of biospecimens below certain detection thresholds are undetectable, leading to limitations of the information one can utilize in the analysis. Ignoring the presence of ME effects in the corresponding data can result in biased estimates and invalid statistical inferences. For example, in a study of polychlorinated biphenyl (PCB) congeners as potential indicators of endometriosis, a gynecological disease, Perkins et al. (2011) pointed out that the biomarker PCB 153 is unobservable below 0.2 ng/g serum due to the sensitivity of the measurement process. The authors proved that in the case of disregarding LOD problems in the data, PCB 153 might be discarded as potentially lacking the discriminatory ability for endometriosis.

To deal with additive ME issues, several approaches have been suggested, including study design methods based on repeated measurements, as well as statistical techniques that utilize Bayesian methodology (see Chapter 7 for details). We introduce the repeated measurements design first, where multiple measurements are assumed to be taken on the same experimental subjects at different times or under different conditions. The repeated measurements design provides the following merits: relatively small number of assumptions required on distributions of biomarker values, the feasibility of parameter identifiability that yields the ME effect-adjusted statistical inferences, and so forth (Fuller 2009). However, the repeated measurements design can lead to the following critical issues. One is that measurement processes based on bioassays can be relatively expensive, time-consuming, dangerous, or even unfeasible. To illustrate, the cost of the F2-isoprostane assay, an important biomarker for oxidative stress, was about $130 in a BioCycle study conducted to assess the reproducibility of F2-isoprostane (Malinovsky et al. 2012). It makes the reproducibility assessment an expensive proposition that cannot easily be repeated in practice. An additional example can be found in Faraggi et al. (2003). The authors focused on the interleukin 6 biomarker of inflammation that has been suggested to present a potential discriminatory ability for a myocardial infarction disease. However, since the cost of a single assay was $74, examination of its usefulness has been hindered. In addition to the issue of the potential high cost, the repeated measurements mostly provide information regarding ME distributions. This information can be considered a nuisance and is not directly related to parameters of interest in general. Another problem of the repeated measurements design is that investigators may not have enough observations to achieve the desired power or efficiency in statistical inferences when the number of replicates or individual biospecimens available is restricted (Vexler et al. 2012b).

Due to the limitations of the repeated measurements design mentioned above, one may consider tackling additive ME problems from the Bayesian perspective as an alternative and well-developed approach. Bayesian methods (e.g., Carroll et al. 2012; Schmid and Rosner 1993) allow one to efficiently incorporate prior knowledge regarding ME distributions with information extracted from data. However, the high computational cost, along with the possible nonrobustness of inferences due to model misspecification, prior selections, and distributional assumptions of data, complicates applications of Bayesian methods in several situations in practice (e.g., Kass 1993).

Another sort of ME mechanism can be caused by LOD issues. Statistical estimation and inferences based on LOD-affected data are often further complicated by the inability of laboratory methods or machinery to detect biomarker levels below some detection limits (e.g., Gupta 1952; Schisterman et al. 2011; Vexler et al. 2011c). Ignoring the LOD problem in data results in a loss of information and may lead to significant bias in the relevant statistical analysis. As a concrete example, we consider the following case related to a receiver operating characteristic (ROC) curve. The ROC curve is a well-known statistical tool in evaluation of biomarkers' abilities to discriminate healthy and diseased populations (e.g., Pepe 2003). In the context of the ROC curve applications, Perkins et al. (2007, 2009) showed that ignoring the LOD effects leads to an underestimation of the areas under the ROC curves (AUCs). To cope with the LOD problems, different techniques are suggested. Note that nonparametric approaches can be very nonrobust since a part of the data is unobserved numerically when data are subject to LOD effects. The Bayesian method, as one of the possible approaches to deal with LOD issues, may suffer from the high computational cost and the nonrobustness of inferences due to model misspecification and subjective prior selections. In this case, when LOD issues are in effect, parameter assumptions on data distributions are complicated to test. In the context of statistical techniques used to solve LOD issues, the modern statistical literature also introduces the single imputation method (e.g., Schisterman et al. 2006) and the multiple imputation method (e.g., Rubin and Schenker 1986). The single imputation method suggests substituting each missing value by a single parameter. In this case, optimal or appropriate values of this parameter can be defined corresponding to aims of relevant statistical problems (e.g., Schisterman et al. 2006). Though it is simple to implement and easy to understand, the single imputation process does not reflect the uncertainty of data. Alternatively, the multiple imputation method creates multiple data sets with different imputed values that are subsequently analyzed using multiple imputation combining rules (e.g., Rubin and Schenker 1986). However, this method is time-intensive and requires that missing observations satisfy different assumptions related to missing mechanisms and data distributions.

As we mentioned above, ME problems can be integrated with scenarios where assaying biomarkers can be expensive and labor-intensive in practice. Sometimes even the least expensive individual assays may be infeasible for analyzing large cohorts. As a result, it is advantageous to find cost-efficient strategies for sampling. The pooling strategy and random sampling are two different approaches commonly used by investigators to reduce overall costs of biological experiments (e.g., Schisterman et al. 2010, 2011; Vexler et al. 2006a, 2011a). The strategy of simple random sampling involves choosing and testing a random subset of available individual samples in accordance with a study budget. In this case, some individual biospecimens are ignored; however, no assumptions on data distributions should be assumed, and the estimation of operating characteristics of these individual biospecimens is straightforward.

The pooling design, on the other hand, involves randomly grouping and physically mixing individual biological samples. Assays are then performed on the smaller number of pooled samples. Thus, the pooling strategy reduces the number of measurements and then the overall cost of experiments without ignoring any individual biospecimens. For example, in the BioCycle study of F2-isoprostane mentioned above, the full design would cost $135,720, while the pooled designs with a similar efficiency of mean estimators would cost only $45,240 (Malinovsky et al. 2012). One can note that the pooling strategy has a great potential in operating with normal or gamma distributed data since the measurements of pooled observations are proven to be the averages of the individual measurements (e.g., Mumford et al. 2006; Vexler et al. 2006a, 2008b). The pooling approach is more efficient than random sampling when the mean is the only parameter of interest (Faraggi et al. 2003).

In the case of the LOD problems, the pooling design can be useful and efficient to reduce the number of unobserved measurements. This property of the pooling strategy can be utilized even if the cost of measurement processes is not a main concern (e.g., Mumford et al. 2006; Vexler et al. 2006a). However, applications of the pooling strategy may suffer from the following issues: (1) Information may be lost regarding distributions of individual measurements since these distribution functions are hard or even impossible to reconstruct based on pooled data in some situations (e.g., Schisterman et al. 2006; Vexler et al. 2010a). (2) The pooling design can be less efficient than the random sampling when the average is not close to be sufficient statistics, for example, in the case of lognormally distributed data (e.g., Mumford et al. 2006; Vexler et al. 2006a). (3) In the case of the LOD problems, the pooling design is not recommended when LOD affects more than 50% of the data (Mumford et al. 2006). (4) The efficiency of the pooling design is significantly dependent on data distribution (e.g., Mumford et al. 2006).

As a consequence of the benefits and drawbacks that the pooling design and random sampling possess, a natural idea is to consider a cost-efficient hybrid design involving a sample of both pooled and unpooled data in a reasonable proportion. It turns out that the hybrid design can be recommended for use when data are subject to additive MEs or LOD problems (e.g., Schisterman et al. 2010; Vexler et al. 2012b). In the presence of additive MEs, the hybrid design allows for the estimation of parameters related to distributions of MEs without repeated sampling when each measurement is informative (Vexler et al. 2012b). One can show that the hybrid design helps to reduce the number of LOD-affected observations (Schisterman et al. 2011).

In the following section, we formally address parametric and nonparametric methods based on classical approaches and the new hybrid design technique. In Section 15.3, we provide a Monte Carlo comparison of the methods considered above. A brief review of statistical literature related to the ME issues is presented in Section 15.4. In Section 15.5, we conclude this entry with remarks.

15.2 Methods

In this section, we present several methods for evaluating data subject to additive errors or errors caused by LOD problems.

15.2.1 Additive Errors

15.2.1.1 Repeated Measurements

In this section, we consider parametric and nonparametric inference based on data obtained following the repeated measurements design.

15.2.1.1.1 Parametric Likelihood Inference

Suppose that we repeatedly measure biospecimens observing scores $Z_{ij} = X_i + \varepsilon_{ij}$, where the true values of biomarker measurements X_i, $i = 1, \ldots, t$, are independent and identically distributed (i.i.d.), and ε_{ij}, $i = 1, \ldots, t, j = 1, \ldots, n_i$, are i.i.d. values of MEs. Here the subscript i denotes the ith individual, and j indicates the jth repeated measure. Define the total number of measures as $N = \sum_{i=1}^{t} n_i$. In this manner, it is assumed that there is an existence of a subset of t distinct bioassays, and each of them is measured n_i times repeatedly. For simplicity and without loss of generality, we assume that X_i and ε_{ij} are independent and normally distributed, that is, $X_i \sim N(\mu_x, \sigma_x^2)$ and $\varepsilon_{ij} \sim N(0, \sigma_m^2)$, where μ_x and σ_x^2 are the mean and variance of X_i, respectively, and 0 and σ_m^2 are the mean and variance of ε_{ij}, respectively. Accordingly, we have $Z_{ij} \sim N(\mu_x, \sigma_x^2 + \sigma_m^2)$. In this case, one can show that if $n_i = 1$, there are no unique solutions of estimation of σ_x^2 and σ_m^2. (This case can be titled as nonidentifiability since we can only estimate the sum, $\sigma_x^2 + \sigma_m^2$, but not the individual variances σ_x^2 and σ_m^2, e.g., Vexler et al. 2012b). Thus, we should assume $n_i > 1$. The observations Z in each group i are dependent because they are measured using the same bioarray. By the well-known techniques related to the maximum likelihood methodology, one can derive the maximum likelihood estimators (MLEs) of the parameters μ_x σ_x^2, and σ_m^2. That is, using the likelihood function,

$$L_R(Z \mid \mu_x, \sigma_x^2, \sigma_m^2) = \frac{\exp\left\{ -\left[(2\sigma_m^2)^{-1} \sum_i \sum_j (Z_{ij} - \mu_x)^2 - \sum_i \frac{n_i^2 \sigma_x^2 (\bar{Z}_{i\cdot} - \mu_x)^2}{2\sigma_m^2 (n_i \sigma_x^2 + \sigma_m^2)} \right] \right\}}{(2\pi)^{0.5N} \sigma_m^{2[0.5(N-t)]} \prod_i (n_i \sigma_x^2 + \sigma_m^2)^{0.5}},$$

where $\bar{Z}_{i\cdot} = n_i^{-1} \sum_{j=1}^{n_i} Z_{ij}$ (see Searle et al. 1992). If n_i s are assumed to be equal to n, the MLEs of μ_x, σ_m^2, and σ_x^2 are $\hat{\mu}_x = \bar{Z}.. = (nt)^{-1} \sum_{i=1}^{t} \sum_{j=1}^{n} Z_{ij}$, $\hat{\sigma}_m^2 = \sum_i \sum_j (Z_{ij} - \bar{Z}_{i\cdot})^2 / \{t(n-1)\}$, and $\hat{\sigma}_x^2 = \sum_i (\bar{Z}_{i\cdot} - \bar{Z}..)^2 / t - \sum_i \sum_j (Z_{ij} - \bar{Z}_{i\cdot})^2 / \{nt(n-1)\}$, respectively. For details about the properties of the MLEs, for example, asymptotic distributions of the estimators, see Searle et al. (1992) and Vexler et al. (2012b). It is clear that these properties derived using the standard maximum likelihood methodology provide a simple confidence interval estimation of the parameters, as well as can be used as basic ingredients for developing different statistical tests.

15.2.1.1.2 Nonparametric Likelihood Inference

In Section 15.2.1.1.1, we showed that the likelihood methodology can be easily applied to develop statistical procedures based on data subject to additive errors. In this section, we substitute the parametric likelihood by its nonparametric version to create distribution-free procedures based on data subject to additive errors. Toward this end, we propose employing the maximum likelihood concept. The empirical likelihood (EL) technique (we refer the reader to Chapter 6 for more details) has been extensively considered in both the theoretical and applied literature in the context of nonparametric approximations of the parametric likelihood (e.g., DiCiccio et al. 1989; Owen 1988, 1991, 2001; Vexler et al. 2009a, 2010c; Yu et al. 2010). We begin by outlining again the EL ratio method, and then we depict how to adapt the EL ratio technique based on data with repeated measures. Suppose i.i.d. data points $Y_1, \ldots, Y_n$ with $E|Y_1|^3 < \infty$ are observable. The problem of interest, for example, is to test the hypothesis H_0: $E(Y_1) = \mu_0$ versus H_1: $E(Y_1) \neq \mu_0$, where μ_0 is fixed and known. In this case, the EL function is defined as $L_n = \prod_{i=1}^{n} p_i$, where values of p_i should be found such that p_i will maximize L_n given the empirical constraints $\sum_{i=1}^{n} p_i = 1$, $\sum_{i=1}^{n} p_i Y_i = \mu_0$ and $0 < p_1, \ldots, p_n < 1$. These constraints correspond to an empirical version of $E(Y_1) = \mu_0$. This empirical likelihood function represents a nonparametric likelihood under H_0. Using the Lagrange method, one can show that the maximum EL function under H_0 has the form of

$$L(\mu_0) = \sup\left\{ \prod_{i=1}^{n} p_i : 0 < p_1, \ldots, p_n < 1, \sum_{i=1}^{n} p_i = 1, \sum_{i=1}^{n} p_i Y_i = \mu_0 \right\} = \prod_{i=1}^{n} \left[n\left\{1 + \lambda(Y_i - \mu_0)\right\}^{-1} \right],$$

where the Lagrange multiplier λ is a root of $\sum_{i=1}^{n} (Y_i - \mu_0) / \{1 + \lambda(Y_i - \mu_0)\} = 0$. Similarly, under the alternative hypothesis, the maximum EL function has the simple form of $L = \sup\left\{ \prod_{i=1}^{n} p_i : 0 < p_1, \ldots, p_n < 1, \sum_{i=1}^{n} p_i = 1 \right\} = \prod_{i=1}^{n} n^{-1} = n^{-n}$. As a consequence, the 2log EL ratio test statistic is $l(\mu_0) = 2[\log(L) - \log\{L(\mu_0)\}] = 2 \sum_{i=1}^{n} \log\{1 + \lambda(Y_i - \mu_0)\}$. The nonparametric version of Wilks's theorem shows that the $l(\mu_0)$ follows asymptotically a χ_1^2-distribution as $n \to \infty$ (e.g., Owen 1988, 2001). As mentioned in Section 15.2.1.1.1, the observations Z in each group i are dependent. Note that Z_{ij} is independent of Z_{kl} when $i \neq k$. Therefore, one can obtain an EL function for the block sample mean $\bar{Z}_i = n_i^{-1} \sum_{j=1}^{n_i} Z_{ij}$, $i = 1, \ldots, t$ $N = \sum_{i=1}^{t} n_i$, in a similar manner to the blockwise EL method given in Kitamura (1997). Then, the random variables become $\bar{Z}_1, \bar{Z}_2, \ldots \bar{Z}_t$, and the corresponding EL function for μ_x is defined as

$$L_R(\mu_x) = \sup\left\{ \prod_{i=1}^{t} p_i : 0 < p_1, \ldots, p_t < 1, \sum_{i=1}^{t} p_i = 1, \sum_{i=1}^{t} p_i \bar{Z}_i = \mu_x \right\} = \prod_{i=1}^{t} \left[t\left\{1 + \lambda(\bar{Z}_i - \mu_x)\right\} \right]^{-1},$$

where λ is a root of $\sum_{i=1}^{t} (\bar{Z}_i - \mu_x) / \left\{1 + \lambda(\bar{Z}_i - \mu_x)\right\} = 0$. In this case, the 2log EL ratio test statistic is $l_R(\mu_x) = 2 \sum_{i=1}^{t} \log\left\{1 + \lambda(\bar{Z}_i - \mu_x)\right\}$.

Assume $E|Z_{11}|^3 < \infty$. Then the 2log EL ratio, $l_R(\mu_x)$, is distributed as χ_1^2 when $\sum_{i=1}^{t} n_i^{-1} \to \infty$ as $t \to \infty$. The associated confidence interval estimator is then given by $CI_R = \{\mu_x : l_R(\mu_x) \leq C_{1-\alpha}\}$, where $C_{1-\alpha}$ is $100(1-\alpha)\%$ of a χ_1^2-distribution (for details, see Vexler et al. [2012b]).

15.2.1.2 Bayesian-Type Method

An alternative approach to address the additive ME problem is the Bayesian method. The Bayesian approach incorporates prior information of the distributions of the variance of the ME value, σ_m^2, with the likelihood function to correct ME bias. Assuming $X_i \sim N(\mu_x, \sigma_x^2)$ and $\varepsilon_{ij} \sim N(0, \sigma_m^2)$, the estimators of μ_x and σ_x^2 can be obtained by

$$(\hat{\mu}_x, \hat{\sigma}_x^2) = \max_{\mu_x, \sigma_x^2} \left\{ \int \left\{ 2\pi(\sigma_x^2 + \sigma_m^2) \right\}^{-n/2} \exp\left\{ -\frac{\sum_{i=1}^{n_i}(X_{i.} - \mu_x)^2}{2(\sigma_x^2 + \sigma_m^2)} \right\} \psi(\sigma_m^2) d\sigma_m^2 \right\},$$

where $\psi(\sigma_m^2)$ is the prior density function of σ_m^2. Possible prior distributions of σ_m^2 are, for example, chi-square distributions, Wishart distributions, gamma distributions, inverse gamma distributions, and inverse Gaussian distributions. In this case, uniform distributions can be used as noninformative priors. It turns out that the Bayesian estimators have relatively small variances even when prior distributions are noninformative. This approach is probably similar to the empirical Bayesian method (see Carlin and Louis [1997] for details), in which the parameters of priors are estimated by maximizing the marginal distributions.

15.2.1.3 Hybrid Pooled–Unpooled Design

15.2.1.3.1 Parametric Likelihood Inference

We briefly address the basic concept of the hybrid design. Let T be the number of individual biospecimens available and N be the total number of measurements that we can obtain due to the limited study budget, $N < T$. We obtain the pooling samples by randomly grouping individual samples into groups of size p. Let $Z_1^p, ..., Z_{n_p}^p$ present observations from pooled samples, and $Z_1, ..., Z_{n_{up}}$ denote the observations from unpooled samples. The ratio of pooled and unpooled samples is $\alpha/(1-\alpha)$, $\alpha \in [0,1]$. Namely, $T = \alpha Np + (1-\alpha)N$. Note that we can obtain pooled data by mixing p individual bioassays together, and we therefore divide the αNp bioassays into n_p groups, where $n_p = \alpha N$. We measure the grouped biospecimens as n_p single observations. In accordance with the pooling literature, we have $Z_i^p = p^{-1} \sum_{k=(i-1)p+1}^{ip} X_k + \varepsilon_{i1}$, $i = 1, ..., n_p = \alpha N$ (see, e.g., Faraggi et al. 2003; Liu and Schisterman 2003; Liu et al. 2004; Schisterman and Vexler 2008; Schisterman et al. 2006; Vexler et al. 2006a, 2008b, 2010a, 2011a). In this case, measurements of the unpooled samples based on $n_{up} = (1-\alpha)N$ independent individuals provide observations $Z_j = X_{pn_p+j} + \varepsilon_{j1}$, $j = 1, ..., n_{up} = (1-\alpha)N$. Since we assume that $X_i \sim N(\mu_x, \sigma_x^2)$ and $\varepsilon_{i1} \sim N(0, \sigma_m^2)$, $i = 1, ..., n_p$ we have $Z_i^p \sim N(\mu_x, \sigma_x^2/p + \sigma_m^2)$ and $Z_j \sim N(\mu_x, \sigma_x^2 + \sigma_m^2)$, $i = 1, ..., n_p$, $j = 1, ..., n_{up}$, $n_p + n_{up} = N$.

Thus, the likelihood function based on pooled–unpooled data takes the form of

$$L_H(Z \mid \mu_x, \sigma_x^2, \sigma_m^2) = (2\pi)^{-\frac{N}{2}} (\sigma_x^2 / p + \sigma_m^2)^{-\frac{n_p}{2}} (\sigma_x^2 + \sigma_m^2)^{-\frac{n_{up}}{2}}$$

$$\exp\left\{ -\sum_{i=1}^{n_p} \frac{(Z_i^p - \mu_x)^2}{2(\sigma_x^2 / p + \sigma_m^2)} - \sum_{j=1}^{n_{up}} \frac{(Z_j - \mu_x)^2}{2(\sigma_x^2 + \sigma_m^2)} \right\}.$$

Differentiating the log-likelihood function, $l_H = \log L_H$, with respect to μ_x, σ_x^2, and σ_m^2, respectively, to solve the ML equations $\{\partial l_H / \partial \mu_x = 0, \partial l_H / \partial \sigma_x^2 = 0, \text{ and } \partial l_H / \partial \sigma_m^2 = 0\}$, we obtain the MLEs of μ_x, σ_x^2, and σ_m^2 given by

$$\hat{\mu}_x = \frac{(\hat{\sigma}_x^2 + \hat{\sigma}_m^2) \sum_{i=1}^{n_p} Z_i^p + (\hat{\sigma}_x^2 / p + \hat{\sigma}_m^2) \sum_{j=1}^{n_{up}} Z_j}{n_{up}(\hat{\sigma}_x^2 / p + \hat{\sigma}_m^2) + n_p(\hat{\sigma}_x^2 + \hat{\sigma}_m^2)},$$

$$\hat{\sigma}_x^2 = \frac{p}{p-1}\left[\frac{\sum_{j=1}^{n_{up}}(Z_j - \hat{\mu}_x)^2}{n_{up}} - \frac{\sum_{i=1}^{n_p}(Z_i^p - \hat{\mu}_x)^2}{n_p} \right], \quad \hat{\sigma}_m^2 = \frac{\sum_{i=1}^{n_p}(Z_i^p - \hat{\mu}_x)^2}{n_p} - \frac{\hat{\sigma}_x^2}{p}.$$

Note that the estimator of μ_x has a structure that weighs estimations based on pooled and unpooled data in a manner similar to the Bayes posterior mean estimator based on normal–normal models (see Carlin and Louis 1997). For details related to the properties of the MLEs, see Vexler et al. (2012b) and Schisterman et al. (2010).

15.2.1.3.2 Nonparametric Likelihood Inference

Utilizing the EL methodology, Vexler et al. (2012b) constructed confidence interval estimators and test statistics based on pooled–unpooled data. Consider the situation described in Section 15.2.1.3.1. Assume we observe measurements under the null hypothesis H_0: $EZ_i^p = EZ_j = \mu_x$. In this case, the EL function for μ_x can be presented as

$$L_R(\mu_x) = \sup\left\{ \prod_{i=1}^{n_p} p_i \prod_{j=1}^{n_{up}} q_j : \right.$$

$$\left. 0 < p_1, \ldots, p_{n_p} < 1; 0 < q_1, \ldots, q_{n_{up}} < 1, \sum_{i=1}^{n_p} p_i = 1, \sum_{i=t}^{n_p} p_i Z_i^p = \mu_x; \sum_{j=1}^{n_{up}} q_j = 1, \sum_{j=1}^{n_{up}} q_j Z_j = \mu_x \right\}$$

$$= \prod_{i=1}^{n_p} \left[n_p \left\{ 1 + \lambda_1 \left(Z_i^p - \mu_x \right) \right\} \right]^{-1} \prod_{j=1}^{n_{up}} \left[n_{up} \left\{ 1 + \lambda_2 \left(Z_j - \mu_x \right) \right\} \right]^{-1},$$

where the Lagrange multipliers λ_1 and λ_2 are roots of the equations $\sum_{i=1}^{n_p} (Z_i^p - \mu_x) / \{1 + \lambda_1 (Z_i^p - \mu_x)\} = 0$ and $\sum_{j=1}^{n_{up}} (Z_j - \mu_x) / \{1 + \lambda_2 (Z_j - \mu_x)\} = 0$. Then, the $2\log$ EL ratio test statistic can be given in the form of

$$l_H(\mu_x) = 2\log\left\{ 1 + \lambda_1 (Z_i^p - \mu_x) \right\} + 2\sum_{j=1}^{n_{up}} \log\left\{ 1 + \lambda_2 (Z_j - \mu_x) \right\}.$$

If $E\,|\,Z_{11}\,|^3 < \infty$, then the 2log EL ratio, $l_H(\mu_x)$, is distributed as χ_2^2 when n_p, $n_{up} \to \infty$, under H_0 (Vexler et al. 2012b). The corresponding confidence interval estimator of μ_x is then given by $CI_H = \{\mu_x : l_H(\mu_x) \le H_{1-\alpha}\}$, where $H_{1-\alpha}$ is $100(1-\alpha)\%$ of a χ_2^2.

15.2.2 Limit of Detection

It is mentioned in Section 15.1 that in practice, measurements of biomarkers of interest may fall below a detection threshold d. For simplicity and clarity of explanation, we suppose that biomarker values are subject to an LOD and are only quantifiable above d (for situations related to multiple detection thresholds, see Vexler et al. [2011c]). Thus, we assume that for the ith subject, Z_i is observed instead of the true value of biomarker measurement X_i, whereby

$$Z_i = \begin{cases} X_i & ; X_i \ge d, \\ N/A & ; X_i < d. \end{cases}$$

15.2.2.1 Methods Based on the Maximum Likelihood Methodology

In the situation considered above, we assume true values of biomarker measurements $X \sim N(\mu_x, \sigma_x^2)$ and data are subject to the LOD. Assume k values are quantified and $n - k$ observations are censored below d. Putting the Z_i in an ascending order with N/A values leading, we have observations of biomarker values $Z_1^*, Z_2^*, \ldots, Z_n^*$. The logarithm of the likelihood function can be written as

$$\log L(Z^* \,|\, \mu_x, \sigma_x^2) = C - k \log \sigma_x - \sum_{i=n-k+1}^{n} \left(Z_i^* - \mu_x\right)^2 \big/ \left(2\sigma_x^2\right) + (n-k)\log \Phi(\eta),$$

where $\eta = (d - \mu_x)/\sigma_x$, C is a constant, $\Phi(\cdot)$ is the standard normal distribution function, and μ_x, σ_x^2 are parameters to be estimated. Let $\phi(\cdot)$ denote the standard normal density function. Differentiating the log-likelihood function with respect to μ_x and σ_x^2 yields the estimates in the form of

$$\hat{\sigma}_x = \left(d - \bar{Z}^*\right) \big/ \left(\eta + (n/k - 1)\phi(\eta)/\Phi(\eta)\right), \ \hat{\mu}_x = \bar{Z}^* + (\hat{\sigma}_x^2 - s_Z^2)/(d - \bar{Z}^*),$$

where

$$\bar{Z}^* = k^{-1} \sum_{i=n-k+1}^{n} Z_i^*, \ s_Z^2 = k^{-1} \sum_{i=n-k+1}^{n} \left(Z_i^* - \bar{Z}^*\right)^2.$$

These equations allow us to solve for $\hat{\sigma}_x$ numerically and, subsequently, $\hat{\mu}_x$ by substitution (e.g., Gupta 1952).

Similarly, consider the scenario where biomarker levels follow gamma distribution with shape parameter α and scale parameter β (e.g., Harter and Moore 1967). The log-likelihood equation is

$$\log L(Z \,|\, \alpha, \beta) = C - k\left[\log \Gamma(\alpha) + \log \beta\right] - (\alpha - 1)\sum_{i=n-k+1}^{n} \log\left(Z_i/\beta\right)$$

$$- \beta^{-1} \sum_{i=n-k+1}^{n} Z_i + (n-k)\log G(\eta),$$

where C is a constant, $\eta = d/\beta$, and $G(\eta) = \int_0^\eta (\Gamma(\alpha))^{-1} x^{\alpha-1} e^{-x} \, dx$. The MLEs for α and β can be obtained by maximizing the log-likelihood with respect to both parameters (for more details, see Perkins et al. [2007] and Harter and Moore [1967]).

15.2.2.2 Bayesian-Type Methods

In the LOD context, unobserved measurements of biomarkers below LOD can be treated via techniques developed for missing data problems. From the Bayesian perspective, these missing data can be considered unknown quantities. A posterior joint distribution of missing data and parameters of interest can be computed (e.g., Carlin and Louis 1997). Let Z_{obs} and Z_{mis} denote the observed data and missing data, respectively. Assume we are interested in the mean of biomarker measurements, μ_x, and the variance of biomarker measurements, σ_x^2. Incorporating prior information on missing data and the parameters of interest, one can show that the corresponding posterior distribution is proportional to

$$\phi\left(Z_{obs} \mid \mu_x, \sigma_x^2, Z_{mis}\right) \varphi\left(\mu_x, \sigma_x^2, Z_{mis}\right),$$

where $\varphi\left(\mu_x, \sigma_x^2, Z_{mis}\right)$ is the prior joint density of parameters of interest and the missing data, and $\phi\left(Z_{obs} \mid \mu_x, \sigma_x^2, Z_{mis}\right)$ is the density in the form of the likelihood of the observed data. Then we can estimate parameters of interest, as well as missing data, in the usual way using Markov chain Monte Carlo methods (e.g., Carlin and Louis 1997).

15.2.2.3 Single and Multiple Imputation Methods

The method of imputing data values is general and flexible for handling various missing data problems. Imputation methods are means or draws from a predictive distribution of the missing values. Thus, in the context of the problems discussed in this chapter, a method of creating a predictive distribution for the imputation based on the observed data is commonly required (e.g., Schisterman et al. 2006; Rubin and Schenker 1986).

We begin by outlining the single imputation method. Assume the observed continuous outcome, Y, satisfies the following linear regression model:

$$Y_i = \gamma + \eta X_i + \varepsilon_i, \, i = 1, \ldots, n,$$

with the exposure variable X_i and random noise ε_i, where $E(\varepsilon_i) = 0$, $var(\varepsilon_i) = \sigma_\varepsilon^2$, and $cov(X_i, \varepsilon_i) = 0$. When the LOD effect is present, we observe exposure measurements Z_i, $i = 1, \ldots, n$ instead of the unobserved true exposure values X_i, $i = 1, \ldots, n$. The formal definition of Z_i is mentioned at the beginning of Section 15.2.2. In order to estimate the linear regression coefficients above, one can use Z_i^a instead of unobserved X_i, where

$$Z_i^a = \begin{cases} X_i; & X_i \geq d, \\ a; & X_i < d. \end{cases}$$

Richardson and Ciampi (2003) demonstrated that to obtain asymptotically unbiased estimates of γ and η based on Y_i and Z_i^a, the value of a can be set up to be $E[X \mid X < d]$.

The application of this approach to practice requires investigators assuming to know how to calculate the conditional expectation $E[X|X < d]$, since no values of X_i below d are observed. Alternatively, Schisterman et al. (2006) showed that the simple solution $a = 0$ can provide the asymptotically normal unbiased least-squares estimators of the linear regression coefficients based on Y_i and Z_i^a without requirements of distributional assumptions. In these cases, assuming, for example, $\gamma = 0$, the unbiased estimator $\hat{\eta}_n$ has the form of

$$\hat{\eta}_n = \sum_{i=1}^n Y_i Z_i^a \bigg/ \sum_{i=1}^n \left(Z_i^a\right)^2.$$

For more details and more general cases, see Schisterman et al. (2006) and Nie et al. (2010).

In the example above, the single imputation method is applied to obtain the unbiased linear regression coefficient estimates via a replacement of the unobserved data by deriving special values for utilization. In a similar manner, the single imputation can be executed in various situations given aims of interest or risk functions. As an additional example, we refer to Perkins et al. (2007), where the single imputation method was applied to estimate ROC curves. The authors showed that without attending to the LOD problems, the estimated ROC curves are very biased.

Note that the single imputation method substitutes each missing observation only once. Due to imprecision caused by the estimated distribution of the variables, the single imputation method commonly results in an underestimation of the standard errors or results in p-values that are too small when statistical tests are based on data subject to the LOD problem (Rubin and Schenker 1986). This issue can be solved by creating multiple data sets that replace the missing data. Each imputation is based on a random draw from an estimated underlying conditional distribution. For example, in the considerations mentioned at the beginning of this section, one can use $Z_i^{\xi_i}$ instead of Z_i^a, where ξ_i is generated from the distribution function $G(u) = \Pr(X_1 < u | X_1 < d)$. Subsequently, results from individual data sets are averaged using multiple imputation combining rules.

As a concrete example, we assume $X \sim N(\mu_x, \sigma_x^2)$ and is subject to the LOD problem. We create K (typically K is from 5 to 10) new data sets $D_1, \ldots, D_K$, based on the original data X by replacing missing values with values generated from the underlying distribution. Let θ denote the vector of parameters of interest. In this example, $\theta = \mu_x$ or $\theta = \sigma_x^2$. And then $\hat{\theta}_i$ defines a vector of estimates based on the data set D_i, $i = 1, \ldots, K$. We average the results across all $\hat{\theta}_i$, $i = 1, \ldots, K$, by employing the following formulas:

$$\bar{\theta} = K^{-1} \sum_{i=1}^K \hat{\theta}_i, \quad \widehat{\text{var}}(\theta) = K^{-1} \sum_{i=1}^K \widehat{\text{var}}(\theta_i) + \left(1 + K^{-1}\right)(K-1)^{-1} \sum_{i=1}^K \left(\hat{\theta}_i - \bar{\theta}\right)^2,$$

which take into account both the within- and between-imputation variance (Rubin and Schenker 1986).

15.2.2.4 Hybrid Pooled–Unpooled Design

In this section, we describe a novel hybrid design that requires a consideration of assays on individual specimens and assays on pooled specimens when the measurement process is subject to the LOD problem. Refer to Section 15.2.1.3.1 for the notations of α, N, p, and T. Assume individual biomarker values are distributed as $X_i \sim N(\mu_x, \sigma_x^2)$. Thus, we obtain that pooled measurements are distributed as $X_i^{(p)} \sim N(\mu_x, \sigma_x^2 / p)$, where $X_i^{(p)} = p^{-1} \sum_{k=(i-1)p+1}^{ip} X_k$, $i = 1, \ldots, n_p = \alpha N$. Due to the LOD effect, we observe

$$Z_i^{(w)} = \begin{cases} X_i^{(w)} & ; X_i^{(w)} \geq d, \\ N/A & ; X_i^{(w)} < d, \end{cases}$$

where $w = 1, p$, $i = 1, \ldots, n_w$, and $X_i^{(1)}$ are the individual specimens.

In this case, the log-likelihood function based on $Z_i^{(w)}$, $w = 1, p$, say l_H, can be constructed. The maximum likelihood method can be used to estimate parameters μ_x and σ_x^2 (e.g., Gupta 1952). Toward this end, we solve the system of the equations $\{\partial l_H / \partial \mu_x = 0, \partial l_H / \partial \sigma_x^2 = 0\}$. Expressions for the solutions, the entries of the Fisher information matrix, related statistical inferences, and more general and complicated cases can be found in the supplementary materials of Schisterman et al. (2011).

15.3 Monte Carlo Experiments

To evaluate the performance of the reviewed methods, we applied the following simulation settings: $X_i \sim N(\mu_x = 1, \sigma_x^2 = 1)$, $i = 1, \ldots, N$, represent normally distributed exposure values; the total sample sizes $N = 100, 300$; normally distributed additive MEs $\varepsilon_{ij} \sim N(0, \sigma_m^2)$ with $\sigma_m^2 = 0.4, 1$, and the number of replicates $n = 2, 5, 10$ in the repeated measures sampling method; inverse gamma distributions, inverse Gaussian distributions, uniform distributions, and chi-square distributions as the prior distribution of MEs in the Bayesian method; the pooling group size $p = 2, 5, 10$ and the pooling proportion $\alpha = 0.5$ in the hybrid design. For each set of parameters, there were 10,000 Monte Carlo simulations. In this section, following the pooling literature, we assumed that the analysis of biomarkers was restricted to execute just N measurements and $T = 0.5N(p + 1)$ individual biospecimens are available, when the hybrid design was compared with the repeated measurements sampling method. For example, in the repeated measurements sampling method, the setting of $N = 100$ and $n = 2$ corresponds to 100 measurements from 50 individuals each measured twice. In the hybrid design, the setting of $N = 100$ and $p = 2$ corresponds to 100 measurements with $T = 150$ individual biospecimens available. It leads to a hybrid of $(1-\alpha) N = 50$ unpooled measurements and $\alpha N = 50$ pooled measurements with a pooling group size 2.

Table 15.1 shows the estimated parameters based on different design methods. For the repeated measurements data using the parametric likelihood method, the results show that as the replicates increase, the standard errors of the estimates of σ_m^2 decrease, indicating that the estimations of σ_m^2 appear to be better as the number of replicates increases. Apparently, the Monte Carlo standard errors of the estimators of μ_x and σ_x^2 increase when the number of replicates increases. Table 15.1 also shows that the Monte Carlo standard errors of the estimates for μ_x based on pooled–unpooled data are clearly less than those of the corresponding estimates utilizing repeated measurements, when $p \geq 2$ (respectively, $n \geq 2$). One observed advantage is that the estimation for σ_x^2 based on pooled–unpooled data is very accurate when the total number of measurements is fixed at the same level. Another advantage is that the standard errors of the estimates for the mean are much smaller than those based on repeated measurements.

TABLE 15.1

Monte Carlo Evaluations of the Maximum Likelihood Estimates Based on the Repeated Measurements and the Hybrid Design

Sample Size	Replicates n, Pooling Size p	Parameters $(\mu_x, \sigma_x^2, \sigma_m^2)$	Estimates			Standard Errors		
			$\hat{\mu}_x$	$\hat{\sigma}_x^2$	$\hat{\sigma}_m^2$	SE($\hat{\mu}_x$)	SE($\hat{\sigma}_x^2$)	SE($\hat{\sigma}_m^2$)
Repeated Measurements								
N = 100	n = 2	(1,1,0.4)	1.0021	0.9781	0.3997	0.1553	0.241	0.079
		(1,1,1.0)	1.0006	0.9688	0.9984	0.1726	0.3106	0.1994
	n = 5	(1,1,0.4)	0.9966	0.9462	0.399	0.2328	0.3305	0.0623
		(1,1,0.4)	1.0015	0.9362	0.9998	0.2442	0.3688	0.157
	n = 10	(1,1,1.0)	1.0026	0.8951	0.3999	0.3209	0.4346	0.0597
		(1,1,0.4)	1.0044	0.8917	0.9995	0.3299	0.469	0.1501
N = 300	n = 2	(1,1,0.4)	0.9987	0.9921	0.3999	0.0889	0.1405	0.0455
		(1,1,1.0)	1.0005	0.9883	0.9999	0.0995	0.1803	0.1162
	n = 5	(1,1,0.4)	0.9995	0.9797	0.3998	0.1356	0.195	0.0365
		(1,1,0.4)	0.999	0.9766	0.999	0.1409	0.2181	0.0906
	n = 10	(1,1,1.0)	0.9985	0.9682	0.3997	0.1864	0.2633	0.0344
		(1,1,0.4)	0.9985	0.966	1.0002	0.1914	0.2782	0.0861
Hybrid Design ($\alpha = 0.5$)								
N = 100	p = 2	(1,1,0.4)	1.0015	1.016	0.4365	0.1048	0.6712	0.4579
		(1,1,1.0)	1.0007	1.0754	1.0098	0.1327	1.0058	0.7275
	p = 5	(1,1,0.4)	0.9994	1.0045	0.3889	0.0924	0.3857	0.1662
		(1,1,0.4)	1.0008	1.0053	0.988	0.124	0.5932	0.3217
	p = 10	(1,1,1.0)	0.9993	1.0049	0.3918	0.0871	0.3341	0.1164
		(1,1,0.4)	0.9996	1.005	0.9836	0.1197	0.5082	0.2486
N = 300	p = 2	(1,1,0.4)	0.9999	0.9974	0.4066	0.0608	0.3868	0.2652
		(1,1,1.0)	1.0002	1.0069	0.9982	0.0758	0.5788	0.4179
	p = 5	(1,1,0.4)	0.9995	1.0013	0.3969	0.0534	0.2197	0.0954
		(1,1,0.4)	0.9993	1.0076	0.991	0.0711	0.3386	0.1819
	p = 10	(1,1,1.0)	0.9995	0.9995	0.3972	0.0497	0.1935	0.0671
		(1,1,0.4)	0.9992	1.0059	0.9922	0.0688	0.2928	0.1436

Table 15.2 shows the Monte Carlo properties of the estimators obtained via the Bayesian methods described in Section 15.2.1.2 in a variety of scenarios related to different choices of the prior distributions $\psi(\cdot)$ of MEs. The prior distributions were selected such that the mean of the prior distributions is very close to or very far from the true values of σ_m^2. Note that μ_x and σ_x^2 are parameters of interest, while σ_m^2 is a nuisance parameter. Table 15.2 demonstrates that the estimates of σ_x^2 depend on prior selections. For example, when the true σ_m^2 is set to be 1, the χ_1^2 prior distribution leads to very large Monte Carlo standard errors of the estimates. On the contrary, the uniform prior distributions give the minimum standard errors of the estimates compared to other choices of prior distributions. With uniform priors, the Bayesian method is comparable to the repeated measures designs, as well as the hybrid designs. In general, the Monte Carlo standard errors of the estimates of μ_x via the Bayesian methods are slightly bigger than those of estimates obtained via the hybrid designs, but still smaller than the estimates obtained via the repeated measurements designs in many scenarios.

TABLE 15.2

Monte Carlo Evaluations of the Maximum Likelihood Estimates Based on the Bayesian Methods

Sample Size	Prior Distribution	Parameters $(\mu_x, \sigma_x^2, \sigma_m^2)$	Estimates			Standard Errors		
			$\hat{\mu}_x$	$\hat{\sigma}_x^2$	$\hat{\sigma}_m^2$	$SE(\hat{\mu}_x)$	$SE(\hat{\sigma}_x^2)$	$SE(\hat{\sigma}_m^2)$
Bayesian Method								
N = 100	IGam(2.16,0.464)	(1,1,0.4)	0.9971	1.1615	0.2341	0.1203	0.2495	0.2118
	IGam(3,2)	(1,1,1.0)	0.9986	1.3855	0.6170	0.1396	0.4679	0.3849
	IGau(0.4,0.064)	(1,1,0.4)	1.0015	1.3656	0.0358	0.1178	0.4154	0.3642
	IGau(1,1)	(1,1,1.0)	0.9994	1.6316	0.3677	0.1424	0.6789	0.6361
	Unif(0,0.2)	(1,1,0.4)	0.9993	1.2910	0.1092	0.1181	0.3517	0.2909
	Unif(0,0.5)	(1,1,1.0)	0.9981	1.7160	0.2796	0.1424	0.7517	0.7269
	Unif(0.2,0.6)	(1,1,0.4)	0.9991	1.0046	0.3946	0.1174	0.1941	0.0072
	Unif(0.8,1.2)	(1,1,1.0)	0.9983	0.9932	1.0064	0.1428	0.2801	0.0103
	Unif(0.39,0.41)	(1,1,0.4)	1.0000	0.9855	0.4140	0.1177	0.1958	0.0141
	Unif(0.99,1.01)	(1,1,1.0)	0.9969	0.9810	1.0200	0.1406	0.2816	0.0202
	Chisq(0.4)	(1,1,0.4)	0.9997	1.3164	0.0781	0.1176	0.3679	0.3221
	Chisq(1)	(1,1,1.0)	0.9970	1.8119	0.1868	0.1414	0.8528	0.8135
	Chisq(0.3)	(1,1,0.4)	0.9997	1.3164	0.0781	0.1176	0.3679	0.3290
	Chisq(0.9)	(1,1,1.0)	0.9970	1.8119	0.1868	0.1414	0.8528	0.8292
N = 300	IGam(2.16,0.464)	(1,1,0.4)	1.0000	1.2027	0.2028	0.0690	0.2308	0.1972
	IGam(3,2)	(1,1,1.0)	1.0004	1.4445	0.5595	0.0819	0.4701	0.4406
	IGau(0.4,0.064)	(1,1,0.4)	0.9996	1.3572	0.0435	0.0678	0.3767	0.3608
	IGau(1,1)	(1,1,1.0)	0.9996	1.6545	0.3417	0.0817	0.6735	0.6585
	Unif(0,0.2)	(1,1,0.4)	0.9986	1.2999	0.0999	0.0684	0.3212	0.3001
	Unif(0,0.5)	(1,1,1.0)	1.0005	1.7579	0.2420	0.0816	0.7724	0.7586
	Unif(0.2,0.6)	(1,1,0.4)	0.9989	1.0152	0.3856	0.0686	0.1134	0.0145
	Unif(0.8,1.2)	(1,1,1.0)	1.0004	1.0078	0.9933	0.0805	0.1609	0.0069
	Unif(0.3967,0.4033)	(1,1,0.4)	0.9998	1.3533	0.0474	0.0683	0.3705	0.3526
	Unif(0.9967,1.0033)	(1,1,1.0)	1.0002	1.8859	0.1168	0.0812	0.8995	0.8833
	Chisq(0.4)	(1,1,0.4)	1.0002	1.3563	0.0429	0.0684	0.3733	0.3572
	Chisq(1)	(1,1,1.0)	0.9984	1.8978	0.1063	0.0813	0.9109	0.8937
	Chisq(0.3)	(1,1,0.4)	1.0000	1.2027	0.2028	0.0690	0.2308	0.1972
	Chisq(0.9)	(1,1,1.0)	1.0004	1.4445	0.5595	0.0819	0.4701	0.4406

Note: IGam(a,b) denotes the inverse gamma distribution with shape *a* and scale *b*; IGau(a,b) denotes the inverse Gaussian distribution with mean *a* and dispersion *b*; Unif(a,b) denotes the uniform distribution with minimum *a* and maximum *b*; Chisq(a) denotes the chi-square distribution with degrees of freedom *a*.

15.4 Concluding Remarks

In this chapter, we reviewed different methods to operate with data subject to various sorts of ME problems. When data are subject to additive errors, the methods based on repeated measurements designs and the hybrid pooled–unpooled technique, as well as Bayesian-type methods, have been proposed for properly modeling data with MEs. When the errors related to the LOD impact the data, the methods based on the maximum likelihood methodology, the Bayesian method, the single and multiple imputation techniques, and the scheme based on the hybrid pooled–unpooled design have been proposed as possible approaches to analyze the data. This chapter presented a limited number of Monte Carlo results to compare the efficiency and show the applicability of the considered methods. Based on the results in Section 15.3, we concluded that the novel hybrid pooled–unpooled design possesses very attractive properties of statistical procedures based on data subject to MEs. We also recommend using the Bayesian method to operate with ME-affected data. In general, one can conclude that instrumental limitations related to biostatistical studies should be taken into account to fix issues based on problematic biomarker measurements, by developing new statistical methods or modifying standard statistical methods.

15.5 Supplement

In this section, we briefly outline several recent publications regarding ME problems.

1. Consider the problem of the estimation of the distribution function, F_U, of a random variable U when observations from this distribution are contaminated by measurement error, that is, based on observations of random variables $Y = U + \varepsilon$, where ε represents measurement error. The estimation of F_U has been referred to as deconvolution, since the distribution of each Y_i is the convolution of the distributions of U_i and δ_i. Cordy and Thomas (1997) investigated the deconvolution of density by modeling the unknown distribution F_U as a mixture of a finite number of known distributions. The mixture model was shown to be able to approximate a wide range of distributions. The authors also demonstrated that this approach can be applied to estimation of a unimodal distribution. In both models, parameters were estimated and large sample confidence intervals were constructed based on the well-known likelihood theory. Based on simulation studies, the good performance of the estimators and the confidence interval procedures were confirmed. The authors illustrated their methods by an application of data from a dietary survey reported by Clayton (1992), where the ratio of polyunsaturated to saturated fat intake (P/S) was measured for 336 males in a 1-week full-weighted dietary survey, and the authors considered the measured values of P/S for the ith individual as normally distributed with mean equal to the true value, UM, of P/S and constant measurement error variance.

2. Failure in correcting a biomarker for measurement error may yield a lower perceived discriminating effectiveness, for example, a lower Youden index, which is a global measure of biomarker effectiveness, that is, the maximum difference between sensitivity (the probability of correctly classifying diseased individuals) and 1-specificity (the probability of incorrectly classifying health individuals); we refer the reader to Chapter 8 for more details regarding the concepts of sensitivity and specificity. Perkins and Schisterman (2005) provided an approach for estimating the Youden index and associated optimal cut point under normality assumptions in the presence of random normal measurement error, in the case of no available replications in the main study, and that measurement error is evaluated in an external reliability study. Confidence intervals for these corrected estimates were derived based on the delta method, and coverage probabilities were obtained via simulations over a variety of situations. Corrections for measurement errors may lead to biomarkers that were once naively considered ineffective becoming

useful diagnostic devices. The importance of the methods of correcting measurement errors was illustrated by a study of the biomarker thiobarbituric acid reactive substance (TBARS) that measures subproducts of lipid peroxidation and has been proposed as a discriminating measurement between cardiovascular disease cases and healthy controls (Schisterman 1999). It was demonstrated that incorporation of the correction for measurement errors leads to a 50% increase in diagnostic effectiveness at the optimal cut point.

3. In epidemiological studies, in addition to the cost limitation, many assays are affected by an LOD, depending on the instrument sensitivity. Mumford et al. (2006) investigated two common sampling strategies used to cut costs in the case that an LOD effect exists. The two sampling strategies considered are a random sample of the available samples and pooling biospecimens. These strategies were compared by examining the efficiency of the estimation of the area under the receiver operating characteristic curve (AUC) for normally distributed marker (we refer the reader to Chapter 8 for details). In the case where an LOD is in effect, the authors proposed a method to estimate AUC when dealing with data from pooled and unpooled samples. It was demonstrated that pooling is the most efficient cost-cutting strategy when the LOD affects less than 50% of the data. Nevertheless, use of the pooling design was not recommended when much more than 50% of the data is affected. The effect of pooling on ROC curve analysis with an LOD effect was illustrated by a real data example of individual cholesterol measurements on 80 volunteers (Faraggi et al. 2003).

4. In epidemiological studies of evaluation of the association between outcomes and exposures, measurements of exposures are often subject to measurement error. In this case, reliability studies are commonly employed to assess the reproducibility of the exposure's measures; that is, the consistency of the measurements of the exposure can be repeated on the same subject. In order to assess the measurement error problem, Liu et al. (2006) proposed sequential testing procedures for the planning and analysis of reliability studies. In the proposed multistage designs, repeated evaluation of reliability of the measurements is allowed. If at any early stage the data show substantial consistency in the measurements, then the evaluation process stops. Otherwise, it proceeds to the next stage until a conclusion with respect to the measurement error can be reached. The authors developed corresponding multistage methods for a number of two-stage designs and presented associated critical values. The authors also briefly reviewed the sample size and power calculation for one-stage reliability studies. Multistage designs were shown to be cost-effective compared to the traditional one-stage designs. A data example evaluating the reliability of biomarkers associated with oxidative stress was presented to illustrate the method of multistage evaluation of measurement error.

5. In the context of the estimation of the area under the receiver operating characteristic curve (AUC) (see Chapter 8 for details), Perkins et al. (2007) demonstrated that replacement values below the limit of detection provide guidance on the usefulness of these values in limited situations, even though they may result in a biased estimate of the AUC when properly accounted for. The authors demonstrated that maximum likelihood techniques lead to asymptotically unbiased estimators of the AUC under the assumptions of both normal and gamma distributions of biomarker levels. The authors also developed confidence intervals under normal and gamma distributional assumptions by applying the delta method, of which the

coverage probability was studied by simulation. The benefits of these methods to make inference for the AUC for a sample with a limit of detection were illustrated with an example using polychlorinated biphenyl levels to classify women with and without endometriosis.

6. Vexler et al. (2008b) considered incorporating additive measurement errors and pooling design into one stated problem, motivated by the fact that these two issues usually correspond to problems of reconstructing a summand's distribution of the biomarker by the distribution of the convoluted observations. The integrated approach allows for new fields of biospecimen evaluations, such as analysis of pooled data with measurement errors. Focused on the receiver operating characteristic (ROC) curve analysis (see Chapter 8 for details), the authors considered a wide family of distributions of biospecimens and biomarkers, mainly conditioned by the reconstructing problem. Maximum likelihood techniques, which are founded on characteristic functions, were proposed based on the following data: a biomarker with measurement error, pooled samples, and pooled samples with measurement error. A real data study of thiobarbituric acid reactive substance (TBARS), a biomarker that measures subproducts of lipid peroxidation, was used to illustrate the applicability of the methods to address issues such as whether pooling increases measurement errors and whether physical execution of pooled data leads to errors.

7. In order to examine parameter estimation for assays subject to a limit of detection, Schisterman and Vexler (2008) examined the effect of different sampling strategies of biospecimens for exposure assessment that cannot be detected below a detection threshold (DT). The authors compared the use of pooled samples with the use of a randomly selected sample from a cohort. It was demonstrated that a random sample strategy is less efficient than a pooling design under certain circumstances. In addition, in a context of a parametric estimation, the use of pooled data is preferable for certain values of the DT because pooling uses all available individual measurements and minimizes the amount of information lost below the DT. In order to capture the strengths of the different sampling strategies and overcome instrument limitations (i.e., DT), a hybrid design was proposed that applies pooled and unpooled biospecimens. The results were confirmed by several Monte Carlo simulations and a real study of evaluating cholesterol measurements censored below a detection threshold.

8. In order to compare the areas under correlated receiver operating characteristic (ROC) curves (see Chapter 8 for details) of diagnostic biomarkers whose measurements are subject to LOD, Vexler et al. (2008a) employed the likelihood ratio tests with operating characteristics that are easily obtained by the classical maximum likelihood methodology. The method was illustrated by an IQ study and a coronary heart disease study.

9. In the context of receiver operating characteristic (ROC) curves (see Chapter 8 for details), Perkins et al. (2009) proposed a method to correct ROC curves for measures subject to MEs and LOD simultaneously through replicate measures and the maximum likelihood methodology. Generalized ROC curve inference for a biomarker subject to a limit of detection and measurement error was developed. Simulation study was implemented to confirm the good performance of the method. The method was illustrated with a pre-eclampsia study of vascular endothelia growth factor.

10. When an independent variable is subject to an LOD, substitution methods are frequently used. Nie et al. (2010) investigated and compared the performance of substitution methods with that of a maximum likelihood method in a linear regression study for a left-censored independent variable X due to LOD. The following methods were considered and compared: (a) the deletion method, where unbiased estimates of parameters of interest can be obtained by simply discarding unobserved observations with $X_i \leq LOD_i$; (b) the commonly used substitution methods: replacing unobserved observations with $X_i \leq LOD_i$ by LOD_i, $LOD_i/2$, or $LOD_i/\sqrt{2}$; (c) the Schisterman, Vexler, Whitcomb, and Liu (SVWL) method (Schisterman et al. 2006), where LOD is assumed to be a constant; (d) the Richardson and Ciampi (RC) method (Richardson and Ciampi 2003), where LOD is assumed to be a constant and observations with $X_i \leq LOD$ are replaced by $E(X|X < LOD)$; and (e) the maximum likelihood (MLE) method, where parameter inference is estimated by the maximum likelihood method based on parametric distributional assumptions. The small sample performance was investigated based on a simulation study. The authors recommended the following. (a) If the exposure variable X approximately follows a normal distribution with unknown parameters or if X follows a known parametric distributional assumption other than a normal distribution with the likelihood changed to reflect this alternative distributional assumption, the MLE or RC method is suggested for use. (b) If the distribution of X cannot be assumed to be approximately normal, it is suggested to use the deletion method, which may be conservative.

11. In order to assess the relationship between exposure and disease outcome when an assay is subject to LOD, Albert et al. (2010) proposed a flexible class of regression models that incorporates multiple assay measurements and allows for continuous or binary outcomes. This proposed methodology is a structural model in which a parametric model is assumed for the true covariate values (compared with a functional model in which the true covariates are assumed fixed or are assumed random, with only minimal assumptions made about the distribution of the covariate). The methodology incorporated LODs in the assays and modeling of systematic differences between the multiple assays. Simulations were conducted to confirm the efficiency of the method under different designs. The method was illustrated by a study examining the relationship between polychlorinated biphenyl (PCB) environmental agents and the risk of endometriosis.

12. In order to estimate population distributions when some data are below a limit of detection, Gillespie et al. (2010) proposed employing the reverse Kaplan–Meier (KM) estimator to estimate population distributions. The authors facilitated broader use of the reverse KM estimator by describing its desirable properties and associated calculations. The method was illustrated with a dioxin exposure study of evaluating serum dioxin concentrations.

13. In order to assess potential associations between exposures to complex mixtures and health outcomes subject to limits of detection, Herring (2010) extended nonparametric Bayes shrinkage priors (see Chapter 7 for details) for model selection to investigations of complex mixtures by developing a formal hierarchical modeling framework to allow different degrees of shrinkage for main effects and interactions and to handle truncation of exposures at a limit of detection. The methods were illustrated with a study of endometriosis and exposure to environmental polychlorinated biphenyl congeners.

14. In the case where multiple biomarkers are available to evaluate the discrimination for the same outcome, levels of biomarkers can be combined to improve the discriminability. In the context of areas under the receiver operating characteristic (ROC) curve based on the best linear combination of biomarkers (see Chapter 8 for details), Perkins et al. (2011) developed asymptotically unbiased estimators via the maximum likelihood technique for two bivariate normally distributed biomarkers affected by LODs. Confidence intervals for the area under the curve were derived. Simulation study was conducted to evaluate the point estimation and confidence interval estimation with bias, root mean squared error, and coverage probability presented. The authors illustrated the method with a study of polychlorinated biphenyl (PCB) levels to classify women with and without endometriosis.

15. To compare populations based on longitudinal data subject to LOD, Vexler et al. (2011c) developed the maximum likelihood approach in conjunction with autoregressive modeling between successively measured observations by incorporating the limit of detection problem and the probability of dropout. Considering the characteristics of the longitudinal data in biomedical research, this approach allows practitioners to carry out powerful tests to detect a difference between study populations with respect to the growth rate and dropout rate. The method can be easily adapted for various different scenarios in terms of the number of groups to compare and a variety of growth trend patterns. The authors provided inferential properties for the proposed method based on well-developed theorems regarding the likelihood approach. A broad range of simulation studies was conducted to confirm the asymptotic results and good power properties. The method was illustrated with the following three data sets obtained from mouse tumor experiments: (a) a study evaluating the relationship between the loss of a gene (Thoc1) and mammary tumor progression (Kuang et al. 2004), (b) an animal tumor immunotherapy experiment (Koziol et al. 1981), and (c) a set of log-transformed data from a tumor xenograft model (Tan et al. 2002).

16. Consider the estimation of the regression of an outcome Y on a covariate X, where X is unobserved, but a variable W that measures X with error is observed. When calibration samples that measure pairs of values of X and W are available in the case that Y is measured (internal calibration) and not measured (external calibration), the following approaches for measurement error correction can be used: (a) the regression calibration method, which substitutes the unknown values of X by predictions from the regression of X on W estimated from the calibration sample, and (b) the imputation method: imputing the missing values of X given Y and W based on an imputation model and then using multiple imputation (MI) combining rules for inferences. Guo and Little (2011) investigated extensions of the regression calibration and MI methods that allow for heteroscedastic measurement error. Simulation studies were implemented to compare the regression calibration method with the MI method. It was shown that the MI method provides better inferences in the setting of covariates with heteroscedastic measurement error. A data set from the BioCycle study of evaluating the association between endogenous hormones and biomarkers of oxidative stress during the menstrual cycle was used to illustrate the method.

17. Zhang and Albert (2011) examined the problem of estimating the association of a binary outcome with a collection of covariates when an important exposure is subject to pooling. The author employed a regression calibration approach and

developed several methods, including plug-in methods that use a pooled measurement and other covariate information to predict the exposure level of an individual subject, and normality-based methods that make further adjustments by assuming normality of calibration error. Two ways were proposed within each class to perform the calibration (covariate augmentation and imputation). Simulation studies showed that these methods can effectively reduce the bias associated with the naive method by simply replacing all individual measurements in the pool by a pooled measurement. Specifically, the normality-based imputation method performs reasonably well in a variety of settings, even under skewed distributions of calibration errors. Data from the collaborative perinatal project were used to illustrate the methods.

18. Ma et al. (2011) investigated two types of pooling in lieu of a random sample, including the traditional random pooling and the "optimal" pooling method. The authors proposed the pooling method for regression analysis based on specimens ranked on the less expensive biomarker, where the more expensive assay is performed on the pool of relatively similar measurements. Monte Carlo simulation studies were conducted to confirm the considerable robustness and the optimality nature of the method, especially whenever expensive assays are involved. A coronary heart disease study of evaluation of interleukin 6 biomarker data was used to illustrate the method.

19. Based on cost-effectively sampled data, Vexler et al. (2011a) developed pooled data–based nonparametric inferences based on the empirical likelihood technique (see Chapter 6 for detail) to substitute for the traditional parametric-likelihood approach. The authors presented the associated true coverage, confidence interval estimation, and powerful tests based on data obtained after the cost-efficient designs. The pooled data–based nonparametric methodology was examined via a broad Monte Carlo study and a cholesterol study of MI disease.

20. Song (2011) developed empirical likelihood (see Chapter 6 for details) confidence intervals for the density function in the errors-in-variables model. It was demonstrated that the empirical likelihood–based confidence intervals have a theoretically accurate coverage rate for both ordinary and super smooth measurement errors. Simulation studies were conducted to compare the finite sample performances of the empirical likelihood confidence intervals and the z-type confidence intervals, which are constructed based on Fan's (1991) asymptotic normality theories.

21. Malinovsky et al. (2012) considered the problem of estimating the parameters of a Gaussian random effects model when the repeated outcome is subject to pooling in order to reduce the cost of performing multiple assays in longitudinal studies. Different pooling designs were considered for the efficient maximum likelihood estimation of variance components, focusing on the estimation of the intraclass correlation coefficient. Analytic and simulation study results confirmed the efficiencies of different pooling design strategies, as well as robustness of the designs to skewed distributions and unbalanced designs. The authors illustrated the design methodology of a longitudinal study of premenopausal women focusing on assessing the reproducibility of F2-isoprostane, a biomarker of oxidative stress, over the menstrual cycle.

22. Group testing is extensively used to reduce the cost of screening individuals for infectious diseases, and has since been expanded extensively to include more general statistical methodology when the data have to be gathered through grouping.

In the context of group testing for rare abnormalities, Delaigle and Hall (2012) developed efficient nonparametric predictors for homogeneous pooled data and demonstrated that the optimal rates of convergence can be achieved. The method was shown to have the same convergence rate as in the case of no pooling when the level of pooling is moderate and a different convergence rate from that of an optimal estimator by no more than a logarithmic factor in the setting of "overpooling." This approach improves on the random pooling nonparametric predictor, enables more accurate identification of vulnerable categories of people, and can lead to subsequent studies that can assist individuals who are particularly vulnerable to infection. The authors illustrated the practical performance of the method via simulated examples and an application to the National Health and Nutrition Examination Survey (NHANES) study, a large health and nutrition survey collected in the United States.

23. In order to correct measurement error in epidemiologic studies with information from external calibration samples to provide valid adjusted inferences, Guo et al. (2012) described using summary statistics from an external calibration sample to correct for covariate measurement error. Consider the problem of estimating the regression of an outcome Y on covariates X and Z, where Y and Z are observed, X is unobserved, but a variable W that measures X with error is observed. The authors developed a method that uses summary statistics from the calibration sample to create multiple imputations of the missing values of X in the regression sample, so that the regression coefficients of Y on X and Z and associated standard errors can be estimated using simple multiple imputation combining rules. The authors presented valid statistical inferences under the assumption of a multivariate normal distribution. Simulation studies demonstrated that the method provides better inferences than existing methods, that is, the naive method, classical calibration, and regression calibration, particularly for correction for bias and achieving nominal confidence levels. The method was illustrated with an example using linear regression to examine the relation between serum reproductive hormone concentrations and bone mineral density loss in midlife women in the Michigan Bone Health and Metabolism Study.

24. Consider the case where laboratory assays are combined in order to determine the presence or absence of a poolwise exposure, in lieu of assessing the actual binary exposure status for each member of the pool. Lyles et al. (2012) proposed employing a primary logistic regression model for an observed binary outcome combined with a secondary regression model for exposure using the maximum likelihood method. The authors discussed the applicability of the approach under both cross-sectional and case-control sampling. For longitudinal or repeated measures studies where the binary outcome and exposure are assessed on multiple occasions and within-subject pooling is conducted for exposure assessment, a maximum likelihood approach was developed. The performance of the approaches, along with their computational feasibility, was confirmed by simulation studies, as well as a study of gene–disease association in a population-based case-control study of colorectal cancer (Poynter et al. 2005).

25. Motivated by a nested case-control study of miscarriage and inflammatory factors with highly skewed distributions, Whitcomb et al. (2012) developed a more flexible model than the logistic model for analysis of pooled data in a hybrid design setting for assessment of risk related to biomarkers of exposure when

the association depends on the exposure level. A modified logistic regression was proposed to accommodate nonlinearity because of unequal shape parameters in gamma distributed exposure in case-control studies. Simulation studies were conducted to compare the modified logistic regression approach with existing methods for logistic regression for pooled data considering (a) constant and dose-dependent effects, (b) gamma and lognormal distributed exposure, (c) effect size, and (d) the proportions of biospecimens pooled. It was demonstrated that the modified logistic regression approach allows estimation of odds ratios that vary with exposure level and has minimal loss of efficiency compared with existing approaches when exposure effects are dose invariant. It was shown that the modified model performs similarly to a maximum likelihood estimation approach in terms of bias and efficiency, and provides an easily implemented approach for estimation with pooled biomarker data when effects may not be constant across exposure. The method was illustrated with a study of the role of chemokine levels as indicators of miscarriage.

26. In order to estimate individual-specific probabilities of pooled data in a regression context, McMahan et al. (2013) derived pool-specific misclassification probabilities (sensitivity and specificity) and generalized the regression approach by including individual covariate information. This method extends the hierarchical modeling framework, which relates the continuous response of an assay test to the (latent) antibody concentration in the pool, to include individual covariate information in a regression setting. This approach exploits the information available from underlying continuous biomarker distributions and provides reliable inference in settings where pooling would be most beneficial, and does so even for larger pool sizes. This model formulation is general and can be applied with any test where a continuous biomarker can be measured, with or without error, on individual or pooled specimens. The method was illustrated with hepatitis B data from a study involving Irish prisoners.

27. Perkins et al. (2013) developed asymptotically consistent, efficient estimators for the mean vector and covariance matrix of multivariate normally distributed biomarkers affected by LOD. An approximation for the Fisher information and covariance matrix was developed for the maximum likelihood estimations (MLEs). The method was applied to a receiver operating characteristic curve (see Chapter 8 for details) setting, generating an MLE for the area under the curve for the best linear combination of multiple biomarkers and accompanying confidence interval. Simulation studies were conducted to confirm the good performance of point and confidence interval estimates with bias and root mean squared error and coverage probability presented. The MLEs were shown to be consistent. It was demonstrated that properly addressing LODs can lead to optimal biomarker combinations with increased discriminatory ability. The method was applied to experimental animal, primate, and human studies of association between dioxin and PCBs and endometriosis (Louis et al. 2005) to illustrate how the underlying distribution of multiple biomarkers with LOD can be assessed and display increased discriminatory ability over naïve methods.

16

Calculating Critical Values and p-Values for Exact Tests

16.1 Introduction

Exact tests are well known to be efficient and reliable statistical tools in a variety of applications. The statistical literature has extensively addressed many parametric, semiparametric, and nonparametric exact tests that control Type I error rates given finite sample sizes. In certain scenarios, exact tests control the Type I error rate much less than the desired error rate due to the fact that exact tests have a finite number of error rates given a fixed sample size. There are various examples of exact tests, such as tests for quantiles (Serfling 2009), Fisher's exact test, the exact F-test, the Shapiro–Wilk test of normality, the Wilcoxon signed-rank and rank-sum tests, data-driven rank techniques, several empirical likelihood (EL)–based methods (e.g., Einmahl and McKeague 2003), the density-based EL ratio tests, and t-test-type tests, to name just a few. Many of these tests are readily available using standard statistical software packages, for example, R, SAS, and SPSS. Exact tests are not only useful in the small sample size settings, but are also invaluable in the case of rare events in the large sample setting; for example, see Mudholkar and Hutson (1997) for the case of contingency tables and the inaccuracy of asymptotic methods when there is a large number of zero count cells.

A key and very desirable property of exact tests is that under the null hypothesis, distributions of test statistics for exact tests are independent of the underlying data distributions (Vexler et al. 2014b). For some sets of exact tests called permutation tests, e.g., the Wilcoxon signed-rank test, an additional assumption of exchangeability is required (see Chapter 17). For example, we considered the two-sample t-test with equal variances introduced in Chapter 5. It is well known that when the assumptions of normality regarding the data distribution and homogeneity of variances of observations are satisfied corresponding to the null hypothesis, the test is exact, i.e., the sampling distribution of $t = \left(\bar{X}_1 - \bar{X}_2 \right) \Big/ \left(s_p \sqrt{n_1^{-1} + n_2^{-1}} \right)$ under the true null hypothesis can be given exactly by the t-distribution with degrees of freedom $n_1 + n_2 - 2$ (we refer the reader to Chapter 5 for the notations). However, this same test statistic, t, can be used by simply permuting all of the observations under the null hypothesis to form an exact test, which is as efficient as the normal-based test and only relies on an exchangeability assumption under the null hypothesis; that is, it is in essence distribution-free. In order to present a nonparametric example of exact tests, we assume that it is required to test the distribution function F_Z for symmetry around zero using independent and identically distributed (i.i.d.) data points

$Z_1, ..., Z_n$. In this case, an appropriate test statistic can consist of $\sum_{i=1}^{n}\sum_{j=1}^{n} I\left(Z_i < -Z_j\right)$. Noticing the fact that

$$I(Z_i < -Z_j) = I\left(F_Z\left(Z_i\right) < F_Z(-Z_j)\right) = I(F_Z(Z_i) < 1 - F_Z(Z_j)),$$

where the random variables $F_Z\left(Z_i\right)$, $i = 1, ..., n$, have uniform [0,1] distribution and under H_0: $F_z(x) = 1 - F_Z(-x)$ for all x, the H_0-distribution of the test statistic is independent of the distributions of observations.

Due to the independence of the null distribution of test statistics on the underlying data distributions, the critical values (CVs) of exact tests can be computed exactly, without the need for using asymptotic approximations.

16.2 Methods of Calculating Critical Values of Exact Tests

In this section, we introduce methods that can be used to calculate the critical values of exact tests, including the following three optional procedures: (1) a traditional technique based on Monte Carlo (MC) evaluations, (2) an interpolation method based on a regression technique that uses tabulated critical values of the test statistic, and (3) a Bayesian-type method that uses tabulated critical values of the test as prior information and MC-simulated test statistic values as data. Approach 3 is a hybrid of the MC and the interpolation methods (Vexler et al. 2014b).

16.2.1 Monte Carlo–Based Method

The classical MC strategy is a well-known approach for obtaining accurate approximations for the critical values of exact tests (see, e.g., Metropolis and Ulam [1949] and Rubinstein and Kroese [2011] for details).

The critical values can be calculated by employing data generated from MC simulations, e.g., from a standard normal distribution for the one-sample tests, and from a uniform [0,1] distribution for the two-sample and three-sample tests. For example, the generated values of the test statistic T of an exact test of interest can be used to determine the critical value C_α at the desired significance level α, e.g., $\alpha = 0.05$. Assume that the decision rule is to reject H_0 for large values of the test statistic, T. Then, we can evaluate the required critical value C_α via calculating the $1 - \alpha$ MC quantile of the null distribution of T, that is, applying the notation $\Pr_{H_0}\{T > C_\alpha\} = \alpha$.

Let us consider the specific case of a general one-sample testing problem, that is, testing based on a sample of i.i.d. observations $X_1, ..., X_n$. The critical values can be calculated according to a Monte Carlo form of the equation $\Pr_{H_0}\{T > C_\alpha\} = \Pr_{X_1, ..., X_n \sim norm(0,1)}\{T > C_\alpha|H_0\}$ at the desired significance level α. In the case of the two-sample problem, that is, testing based on data consisting of two samples of i.i.d. observations, say $X_1, ..., X_n$ and $Y_1, ..., Y_m$, the critical value C_α can be estimated as a MC root of the equation $\Pr_{H_0}\{T > C_\alpha\} = \Pr_{X_1, ..., X_n, Y_1, ..., Y_m \sim norm(0,1)}\{T > C_\alpha|H_0\}$. Similarly, the Type I error rate of a K-sample test can be monitored by using the probability statement $\Pr_{H_0}\{T > C_\alpha\} = \Pr_{X_{11},...X_{1n_1},...,X_{k1},...,X_{kn_k} \sim unif(0,1)}\{T > C_\alpha|H_0\}$.

As a more specific example, consider the problem of testing the symmetry of a distribution function about zero based on a sample of i.i.d. observations $X_1, ..., X_n$. The hypothesis of interest in this setting is $H_0: F_X(u) = 1 - F_X(-u)$ for all $-\infty \le u \le \infty$ versus $H_1: F_X(u) \ne 1 - F_X(-u)$

for some $-\infty \leq u \leq \infty$, where the distribution F_X of the observations is unknown. Consider the Wilcoxon signed-rank test for this problem and denote the corresponding test statistic as T. The Wilcoxon signed-rank test for symmetry around zero is to reject the null hypothesis if and only if $T > C_\alpha$, where C_α is the test threshold at the specified significance level α. In order to obtain the critical values, we generate data from a standard normal distribution for a relatively large number of MC repetitions defined as M, for example, $M = 10{,}000$. For the ith ($i = 1, ..., M$) replication of a given MC simulation, we first generate a random sample of size n from a standard normal distribution and calculate the test statistic, say T_i, based on the generated data. Therefore, we can obtain a set of test statistic values $T_1, T_2, ..., T_M$. Let $T_{(1)} < T_{(2)} < ... < T_{(M)}$ denote the corresponding ordered test statistics, that is, a finite set based on the test statistic values $T_1, T_2, ..., T_M$ indexed $1, ..., M$ from lowest to highest. Then for the critical value, the $(1 - \alpha)$th quantile of the simulated values of the test statistic can be obtained as $T_{(\lceil M(1-\alpha) \rceil)}$, where $\lceil x \rceil$ denotes the ceiling function that returns the next integer greater than or equal to x. In other words, at the α level of significance, the critical values can be found as the $(1 - \alpha)$th sample quantile of the test statistic values $T_1, T_2, ..., T_M$ based on MC-simulated data of the sample size n.

In summary, the MC method is very accurate, but the use of the MC technique can be computationally intensive in some testing situations. For example, a relatively large number of MC repetitions, which we define as M, are commonly needed to evaluate critical values that correspond to the 1% significance level, since in this case the 95% confidence interval of such evaluation can be approximated by $\left[0.01 \pm 1.96\sqrt{0.01(1-0.01)/M} \right]$.

16.2.2 Interpolation Method

Another standard method used to obtain the critical values (CVs) or p-value for exact tests is the interpolation technique of relevant critical points based on tabulated values. The interpolation method differs from the MC method in that tables of critical values are calculated beforehand for an exact test of interest for various sample sizes and significance levels, and then the critical value is obtained by interpolation or extrapolation based on tabulated critical values.

In order to conduct the interpolation procedure, the tabulated table of CVs of the test of interest is generated through an MC procedure in the manner described in Section 16.2.1 for the different sample sizes at the different significance levels based on a relatively large number of MC replicate samples of the test statistic. Then we store the tabulated table of CVs generated via the MC procedure, for example, in an Excel table. To be specific, we consider the Wilcoxon signed-rank test for symmetry of one-sample distribution about zero mentioned in Section 16.2.1. Following the MC method, for a sample size n at the α level of significance, the critical values, redefined as $C_{n\alpha}$, can be found as the $100(1 - \alpha)\%$ sample quantile of the test statistic values generated through MC simulations. Then for different sample sizes and different significance levels, the tabulated critical values can be obtained based on the MC method and should be stored for future use.

If the sample size or the significance level of interest does not exist in the tabulated CV table saved beforehand, an appropriate subset of the table data can be selected. Pearson and Hartley (1966) demonstrated the method of interpolation for calculating values within tables. For instance, given a sample of i.i.d. observations $X_1, ..., X_n$, say, the sample size $n = 37$, we consider the Wilcoxon signed-rank test for symmetry of one-sample distribution about zero at the significance level of α. In this case, where a table of critical values is calculated beforehand for $n = 35, 40$ at the 0.05 significance level and the significance level of interest $\alpha = 0.05$, the critical value can be interpolated based on tabulated critical values of $n = 35, 40$ at the 0.05 significance level. If the significance level of interest $\alpha \neq 0.05$, for example, $\alpha = 0.025$, which is not available in the table stored beforehand, then we can obtain the critical value by extrapolating with respect to the significance levels.

In the cases of sample sizes that are not tabulated within fixed tables, an appropriate subset of the table data is selected. Based on extensive MC experiments, Vexler et al. (2014b, 2014c) suggested selecting the data related to sample sizes in the tabulated CV table within a radius of two values around the values of the sample sizes that are needed. For example, if we are interested in the one-sample test based on a sample with size $n = 78$, we can use critical values related to $n = 50, 60, 80$, and 100 to estimate the required critical value.

To outline this method in detail for the case of one sample, we define $C_{n\alpha}$ to be the critical value corresponding to the simple size n and the significance level α. Using the selected table data, we can fit $C_{n\alpha}$ via the regression approximation

$$C_{n\alpha} \cong \beta_0 + \beta_1 n + \beta_2/n + \beta_3 n^2 + \beta_4 \alpha + \beta_5 \alpha^{1/2}$$

or

$$C_{n\alpha} \cong \beta_0 + \beta_1 n + \beta_2/n + \beta_3 n^2 + \beta_4 \alpha + \beta_5 \log (\alpha/(1-\alpha)),$$

using the local maximum likelihood methodology (Fan et al. 1998). In this manner, the coefficients β are estimated yielding estimated values of $C_{n\alpha}$ as a function of n and α.

Similarly for the two- and three-sample tests, we define $C_{nm\alpha}$ and $C_{nmk\alpha}$ to be the critical values corresponding to the sample sizes n, m, k and the significance level α, respectively. Using the selected table data, we fit $C_{nm\alpha}$ and $C_{nmk\alpha}$ via the regression models

$$C_{nm\alpha} \cong \beta_0 + \beta_1 n + \beta_2 m + \beta_3/n + \beta_4/m + \beta_5 n^2 + \beta_6 m^2 + \beta_7 \alpha + \beta_8 \log(\alpha/(1-\alpha)),$$

and

$$C_{nmk\alpha} \cong \beta_0 + \beta_1 n + \beta_2 m + \beta_3 k + \beta_4/n + \beta_5/m + \beta_6/k + \beta_7 n^2 + \beta_8 m^2 + \beta_9 k^2 + \beta_{10} \alpha + \beta_{11} \log (\alpha/(1-\alpha)).$$

In this manner, the coefficients β are estimated yielding estimated values of $C_{nm\alpha}$ and $C_{nmk\alpha}$ as a function of n, m, k, and α. Note that here it is assumed that $C_{n\alpha} = G_1 (n, \alpha)$, $C_{nm\alpha} = G_2 (n, m, \alpha)$, and $C_{nmk\alpha} = G_3(n, m, k, \alpha)$, where the functions G_1, G_2, and G_3 are unknown, but approximated via the equations shown above.

The regression equation with the parameter estimates can be solved backwards for an estimate of the Type I error rate, α, using standard numerical software for solving equations. This is accomplished by plugging the value of the test statistic T based on the observed data for the critical value and the sample sizes of the observed data into the regression equation and solving for α; that is,

$$T = \hat{\beta}_0 + \hat{\beta}_1 n + \hat{\beta}_2 / n + \hat{\beta}_3 n^2 + \hat{\beta}_4 \alpha + \hat{\beta}_5 \log (\alpha / (1-\alpha))$$

should be solved with respect to the significance level α for the one-sample test, for example. Thus, the value obtained for α is an estimate of the p-value for the test. For more details, we refer the reader to Vexler et al. (2014b, 2014c).

As another application of employing the interpolation method to obtain the critical values, we introduce an extension of the method described above proposed by Zhao et al. (2015). This interpolation method proceeds as follows: In order to evaluate critical values of a test for a comparison between two sample distributions, assuming that we have samples with sizes n and m, we define the extensive sample sizes n' and m' such that $n' + m' = n + m$ and the table with CVs has results related to n' and m'. The idea is that it is natural to suppose under the hypothesis that the two samples are from one distribution function that the critical values related to n and m are very close to those obtained using samples with sizes n' and m'. So the data to be selected have been defined as related to the original sample sizes and the extensive sample sizes in the tabulated CV table within a radius of two values around the values of the original sample sizes and the extensive sample sizes that are needed. For example, suppose we have data consisting of two samples with sizes $n = 46$ and $m = 38$ to be tested if both samples are from the same distribution. The original sample sizes are 46 and 38. The extensive sample sizes are n' and m', which $n' + m' = 46 + 38$. So, n' and m' can be the set of numbers $(n', m') = ((30,54), (40,44), (44,40), (30,54), ...)$ that exists in the tabulated CV table. Define $C_{nm\alpha}$ as the critical value corresponding to the sample size n, m and the significant level α. Motivated by the fact that the value of the significance level α, as a probability, should fall within 0 and 1, we consider the logit function of the significance level. Using the selected table data, we fit $C_{nm\alpha}$ on the corresponding sample size n, m and a logit function of the significance level α in the following regression-type model:

$$C_{nm\alpha} \cong \beta_0 + \beta_1(n^{-0.5} + m^{-0.5}) + \beta_2(n^{0.5} + m^{0.5}) + \beta_3\log[\alpha/(1-\alpha)].$$

To obtain an estimate of the p-value, we plugged the value of the test statistic of interest, say T, which is based on the data for the critical value, sample size n, k, into the regression equation and solved for α; that is,

$$T = \hat{\beta}_0 + \hat{\beta}_1(n^{-0.5} + m^{-0.5}) + \hat{\beta}_2(n^{0.5} + m^{0.5}) + \hat{\beta}_3\log[\alpha/(1-\alpha)]$$

should be solved with respect to α for the test of interest. Thus, the value obtained for α is an estimate for the p-value for the test. For more details, we refer the reader to Zhao et al. (2015).

Note that the saved tables have critical values tabulated for a range of sample sizes and significance levels, but are not completed for any set of sample sizes. The applications of the interpolation and extrapolation procedures decrease the accuracy of the estimates of the critical values when actual samples have sample sizes that differ significantly from those used to tabulate the tables. Providing the tables for use by the test increases the speed to execute the test compared with the MC method, but the interpolation method becomes less reliable.

16.2.3 Hybrid Method

16.2.3.1 Introduction of the Method

The MC approach is simple and accurate, but oftentimes computationally intensive. On the other hand, the interpolation method of obtaining relevant critical values (percentiles) based on tabulated values within the testing algorithm is quick and efficient; however, it becomes much less reliable when real data characteristics (e.g., sample sizes) differ from those used to tabulate the critical values.

In this section, we introduce the Bayesian hybrid methods proposed by Vexler et al. (2014b, 2014d). As described in Chapter 6, one may apply empirical likelihood functions to replace parametric likelihood functions in known and well-developed procedures, for example, constructing nonparametric Bayesian inference methods (Vexler et al. 2014d). We refer the reader to Chapter 6 as well as Chapter 7 for more details regarding empirical likelihood and the Bayesian inference, respectively. Lazar (2003), as well as Vexler et al. (2014d), showed that the empirical likelihoods can be used in Bayesian statistical inferences instead of the corresponding parametric likelihoods. This provides nonparametric Bayes procedures. Based on the nonparametric Bayes concept, Vexler et al. (2014b) proposed the Bayesian hybrid method to obtain CVs or p-values of exact tests, considering the incorporation of information from MC simulations and tabulated critical values (Vexler et al. 2014a).

The Bayesian hybrid method considers the tables of tabulated critical values to represent prior information, whereas the likelihood part of the analysis is based on the output of the relevant MC simulations. The key feature of the hybrid method is that if actual data characteristics (e.g., sample sizes) are close to those used in the table of critical values, then relatively few MC simulations are needed to improve the accuracy of p-value calculations. When this is not the case, more MC simulations are necessary.

Consider the following simple illustration. Table 16.1 represents a part of "percentiles of the χ^2-distribution" (Kutner et al. 2005) at 29, 30, 40, and 50 degrees of freedom. Suppose that we are interested in the percentiles of the χ^2-distribution with 35 degrees of freedom and level of significance 0.05. Table 16.1 does not provide an exact percentile in this case. Interpolation between the 30 and 40 degrees of freedom entries or an MC procedure based on randomly generated χ^2 values can accurately approximate the exact (missing and unknown) percentile. In another scenario, suppose we are interested in the case with degrees of freedom 31 and level of significance 0.05. In this case, we could conduct an MC study with fewer replications than required in the previous case (degrees of freedom 35) since the desired percentile is nearer to the tabulated value at degrees of freedom 30. The Bayesian hybrid method calculates the percentile of interest by incorporating the information from Table 16.1 as a prior distribution to improve the accuracy and reduce the computational cost of the simulations.

The two key aspects that need to be addressed for the hybrid method are (1) constructing the functional forms of the prior distribution based on tabulated critical values and (2) developing nonparametric likelihood-type functions from information extracted from MC simulations.

To deal with the first issue, that is, construction of the functional forms of the prior distribution based on tabulated critical values, Vexler et al. (2014b) proposed applying the local maximum likelihood (LML) technique (Fan et al. 1998) to obtain functional forms of

TABLE 16.1

Percentiles of the χ^2-Distribution
(Kutner et al. 2005)

d.f.	Level of Significance		
	0.025	0.050	0.100
29	14.26	16.05	17.71
30	14.95	16.79	18.49
40	22.16	24.43	26.51
50	37.48	40.48	43.19

Note: d.f., degrees of freedom.

prior distributions from tables of critical values. The LML methodology is usually applied to construct functional forms of dependency between variables. For example, in regression, the aim of the LML approach is to explore the association between dependent and independent variables when the regression functions are data driven instead of being limited to a certain presumed form (Fan and Gijbels 1995). The flexibility and relative simplicity of the LML methodology provides a practical solution to the functional forms of the prior distribution based on tabulated critical values.

As for the second problem, that is, construction of likelihood to summarize the data based on MC generations of exact test statistic values, the nonparametric technique of empirical likelihood is used. It is well known that EL is a powerful nonparametric technique of statistical inference (see Chapter 6 for more details) and the EL functions can be used to construct distribution-free Bayesian posterior probabilities (e.g., Lazar 2003).

16.2.3.2 Method

We first formally state the problem related to the development of procedures of computing critical values of exact tests. Let q denote the critical value in general, and it depends on the sample size and the significance level. For instance, suppose for simplicity that we have a two-sample exact test with critical values $q_{n,m}^{1-\alpha}$, where n, m are the respective sample sizes and α is the level of significance. Let the values of $q_{n,m}^{1-\alpha}$ be tabulated for $n \in N$, $m \in M$, and $\alpha \in A$, that is, $q_{n,m}^{1-\alpha} = C_{nm\alpha}$ described in Section 16.2.2, where N and M are sets of integer numbers and A is a set of real numbers from 0 to 1. That is, we have the table defined as $\left\{ q_{n,m}^{1-\alpha} ; n \in N, m \in M, \alpha \in A \right\}$. We are interested in obtaining the critical value $q_{n_0,m_0}^{1-\alpha_0} \notin \left\{ q_{n,m}^{1-\alpha} ; n \in N, m \in M, \alpha \in A \right\}$. Section 16.2.1 introduced the approach based on an MC study for generating values of the test statistic, and Section 16.2.2 described the technique based on interpolation or extrapolation using the table values $\left\{ q_{n,m}^{1-\alpha} ; n \in N, m \in M, \alpha \in A \right\}$. In this section, we introduce the Bayesian hybrid method. The Bayesian hybrid method uses the tables of critical values $\left\{ q_{n,m}^{1-\alpha} ; n \in N, m \in M, \alpha \in A \right\}$ to construct a *prior* distribution for $q_{n_0,m_0}^{1-\alpha_0}$ that will be combined through Bayes's rule with a nonparametric likelihood function based on MC-generated values of the test statistic. Since distributions of test statistic values are unknown, the likelihoods are presented in the EL form. The value of $q_{n_0,m_0}^{1-\alpha_0}$, the $(1-\alpha_0) \times 100\%$ quantile, is then estimated using the posterior expectation of quantiles based on the smoothed EL method.

The algorithm for the Bayesian hybrid method proceeds as follows:

Step 1: Obtain function forms for a prior information based on the tabulated critical values. In order to implement the Bayesian hybrid method to obtain a critical value, we begin by fitting the prior information with a functional form. The tabulated values are assumed to provide prior information regarding the target critical values q. We obtain the prior distribution function $\pi(q)$, with the parameters (μ_0, σ_0), using the local maximum likelihood method (Fan et al. 1998) based on tabulated critical values. Since quantile estimators are commonly, normally distributed when sample sizes are relatively large, the normal function form of $\pi(q)$ can be used, where

$$\pi(q) = \frac{1}{\sqrt{2\pi}\sigma_0} \exp\left\{ -\frac{(q-\mu_0)^2}{2\sigma_0^2} \right\}.$$

To be more specific, we exemplify the details based on a two-sample test. The critical values of the two-sample test have been tabulated. Let α be the level of significance (commonly $\alpha = 0.05$). Suppose that the observed data consists of two samples of sizes $n_0 = 60$ and $m_0 = 47$. We define $q_{nm\alpha}$ to be the critical value corresponding to the sample sizes n_0, m_0 and the significance level α. The data to be selected has been defined to be corresponding sample sizes available in the tables within the radius of two values around the values of the sample sizes that are needed. The selected table data provide critical values around n_0 and m_0 in the form of $q_{nm\alpha}$, where $n = \{40,50,70,90\}$ and $m = \{35,40,50,60\}$. Using the selected table data, we fit $q_{nm\alpha}$ via the regression models, for example, based on the one model we introduced in Section 16.2.2,

$$q_{nm\alpha} = \beta_0 n + \beta_1 m + \beta_2/n + \beta_3/m + \beta_4 n^2 + \beta_5 m^2 + \beta_6 \log\left(\alpha/(1-\alpha)\right) + \varepsilon_{n,m,\alpha}, \varepsilon \sim N\left(0, \sigma_0^2\right).$$

For details about the computation of the table of tabulated values, we refer the reader to Section 16.2.2. Then the estimated regression equation is used to set up μ_0 as

$$\mu_0 = \hat{\beta}_0 n_0 + \hat{\beta}_1 m_0 + \hat{\beta}_2/n_0 + \hat{\beta}_3/m_0 + \hat{\beta}_4 n_0^2 + \hat{\beta}_5 m_0^2 + \hat{\beta}_6 \log\left(\alpha/(1-\alpha)\right),$$

where $\hat{\beta}$ defines the estimator of β. And σ_0 is estimated using the standard regression analysis.

Step 2: Depict the likelihood function based on MC generations of test statistic values and obtain the posterior distribution. The MC generations of test statistic values as data are used to depict the likelihood function. Since distributions of test statistic values are unknown, the likelihoods are presented in the EL form.

We then illustrate the Bayesian approach based on the empirical likelihood. Suppose we have a sample $X_1, X_2, ..., X_t$ of t Monte Carlo realizations of the test statistic values. That is, we survey independent identically distributed observations $X_1, X_2, ..., X_t$. To analyze the test's critical value q_0, we propose a distribution-free Bayesian inference based on empirical likelihood. The classic Bayesian technique provides the posterior probability of q_0: $\Pr\{X_1 \geq q_0\} = \alpha_0$ in the form

$$P(q_0) = \frac{\prod_{i=1}^{t} f\left(X_i|q_0\right) \exp\left(-\left(q_0 - \mu_0\right)^2/(2\sigma_0^2)\right)}{\int_{-\infty}^{\infty} \prod_{i=1}^{t} f\left(X_i|q\right) \exp\left(-\left(q - \mu_0\right)^2/(2\sigma_0^2)\right)dq}, \tag{16.1}$$

where $f(u|q_0)$ is a density function of X_1. The empirical likelihood approach gives the non-parametric form of (16.1) as

$$\hat{P}(q_0) = \frac{\prod_{i=1}^{t} p_i\left(q_0\right) \exp\left(-\left(q_0 - \mu_0\right)^2/(2\sigma_0^2)\right)}{\int_{X_{(1)}}^{X_{(t)}} \prod_{i=1}^{t} p_i\left(q\right) \exp\left(-\left(q - \mu_0\right)^2/(2\sigma_0^2)\right)dq}, \tag{16.2}$$

where $X_{(1)} \leq X_{(2)} \leq \dots \leq X_{(t)}$ are order statistics based on $X_1, \dots, X_t$, and values of $p_i(q)$ should be found to maximize the empirical likelihood $EL(q) = \prod_{i=1}^{t} p_i(q)$ subject to the constraints $\sum_{i=1}^{t} p_i(q) = 1$, $\sum_{i=1}^{t} p_i(q) I(X_i \geq q) = \alpha_0$ (here $I(\cdot)$ is the indicator function). It follows that the point estimator of q_0 can be computed as the posterior mean

$$\hat{q}_0 = \int_{X_{(1)}}^{X_{(t)}} q \hat{P}(q)\, dq = \frac{\int_{X_{(1)}}^{X_{(t)}} q EL(q)\, \pi(q)\, dq}{\int_{X_{(1)}}^{X_{(t)}} EL(q)\, \pi(q)\, dq}$$

$$= \frac{\sum_{j=1}^{t-1} \int_{X_{(j)}}^{X_{(j+1)}} q\, e^{\left[\left(\log(1-\alpha_0)-\log\left(1-\frac{\tau_t(q)}{t}\right)\right)\left(1-\frac{\tau_t(q)}{t}\right)+\left(\log(\alpha_0)-\log\left(\frac{\tau_t(q)}{t}\right)\right)\left(\frac{\tau_t(q)}{t}\right)\right]t-\frac{1}{2\sigma_0^2}(q-\mu_0)^2}\, dq}{\sum_{j=1}^{t-1} e^{\left[\left(\log(1-\alpha_0)-\log\left(\frac{j}{t}\right)\right)\left(\frac{j}{t}\right)+\left(\log(\alpha_0)-\log\left(1-\frac{j}{t}\right)\right)\left(1-\frac{j}{t}\right)\right]t} \int_{X_{(j)}}^{X_{(j+1)}} e^{-\frac{1}{2\sigma_0^2}(q-\mu_0)^2}\, dq} \qquad (16.3)$$

$$= \frac{\sum_{j=1}^{t-1} e^{\left[\left(\log(1-\alpha_0)-\log\left(\frac{j}{t}\right)\right)\left(\frac{j}{t}\right)+\left(\log(\alpha_0)-\log\left(1-\frac{j}{t}\right)\right)\left(1-\frac{j}{t}\right)\right]t} \int_{X_{(j)}}^{X_{(j+1)}} q\, e^{-\frac{1}{2\sigma_0^2}(q-\mu_0)^2}\, dq}{\sum_{j=1}^{t-1} e^{\left[\left(\log(1-\alpha_0)-\log\left(\frac{j}{t}\right)\right)\left(\frac{j}{t}\right)+\left(\log(\alpha_0)-\log\left(1-\frac{j}{t}\right)\right)\left(1-\frac{j}{t}\right)\right]t} \int_{X_{(j)}}^{X_{(j+1)}} e^{-\frac{1}{2\sigma_0^2}(q-\mu_0)^2}\, dq},$$

where $\tau_t(q) = \sum_{i=1}^{t} I\{X_i \geq q\}$.

The following proposition illustrates that the asymptotic result has a remainder term of order $o(t^{-1})$.

Proposition 16.1

Suppose that F, the distribution function of X_1, is twice differentiable at q_0, with $F'(q_0) = f(q_0) > 0$. Then with probability 1,

$$\hat{q}_0 = q_0 + \frac{(1-\alpha_0)-(1-\tau_t(q_0)/t)}{f(q_0)}$$

$$-\left(t\frac{f(q_0)^2 \sigma_0^2}{\alpha_0(1-\alpha_0)} + 1\right)^{-1}\left(q_0 - \mu_0 + \frac{(1-\alpha_0)-(1-\tau_t(q_0)/t)}{f(q_0)}\right) + o(t^{-1}), \quad t \to \infty.$$

For an outline of the proof of Proposition 16.1, we refer the reader to the appendix.

The algorithm to obtain the posterior distribution of the critical value based on MC simulations can be conducted in two stages and repeated until a stopping condition is met.

First, we define the following notations, which are used in the description of the procedures:

- t_k: The number of MC simulations related to stage $k = 1, 2$
- $T_{(1)}^k < T_{(2)}^k < \cdots < T_{(t_k)}^k$: The order statistics based on the test statistic values $T_1^k, T_2^k, \ldots, T_{t_k}^k$, generated on stage k
- The likelihood function on stage k:

$$L_k(q) = \exp\left[t_k F_{k,t_k}(q)\left\{\log(1-\alpha) - \log(F_{k,t_k}(q))\right\} + t_k\left\{1 - F_{k,t_k}(q)\right\}\left\{\log\alpha - \log(1 - F_{k,t_k}(q))\right\}\right]$$

- The EL function on stage k (which has the role of the likelihood function $L_k(q)$): $\max\left\{\prod_{i=1}^{t_k} p_i : \sum_{i=1}^{t_k} p_i = 1, \sum_{i=1}^{t_k} p_i I(T_i < q) = \alpha\right\}$,   where $F_{k,t_k}(q) = \sum_{i=1}^{t_k} I(T_{(i)}^k < q)/t_k$;

- The intervals on stage k:

$$J_k = \left[\max\left\{1, (1-\alpha)t_k - t_k^{1/2}\log(t_k)\right\}, \min\left\{(1-\alpha)t_k + t_k^{1/2}\log(t_k), t_k\right\}\right].$$

Step 2.1: Stage 1 of the MC simulation step ($k = 1$). In the first MC simulation step, t_1 generations (e.g., $t_1 = 200$) of test statistic values are to be conducted as a first stage, and then test statistics $T^1 = (T_1^1, \ldots, T_{t_1}^1)$ based on the generated data are calculated. Next, the posterior expectation of quantiles $\hat{q}_{1,\alpha}$ is calculated. The posterior expectation is given by $E(q \mid y) = \int qL(q \mid y)dq$, where q is the unknown parameter of interest and $L(q \mid y)$ is the likelihood of q given the data. We compute the posterior expectation of quantiles as follows:

$$\hat{q}_{1,\alpha} = \frac{\int_{T_{(1)}^1}^{T_{(t_1)}^1} qL_1(q)\pi(q)dq}{\int_{T_{(1)}^1}^{T_{(t_1)}^1} L_1(q)\pi(q)dq},$$

and then one can show that

$$\hat{q}_{1,\alpha} = \frac{\sum_{j \in J_1} \exp\left\{-\dfrac{t_1}{2\alpha(1-\alpha)}\left(1 - \alpha - \dfrac{j}{t_1}\right)^2\right\}\int_{T_{(j-1)}^1}^{T_{(j)}^1} q\pi(q)dq}{\sum_{j \in J_1} \exp\left\{-\dfrac{t_1}{2\alpha(1-\alpha)}\left(1 - \alpha - \dfrac{j}{t_1}\right)^2\right\}\int_{T_{(j-1)}^1}^{T_{(j)}^1} \pi(q)dq},$$

where

$$\int_{T_{(j-1)}^1}^{T_{(j)}^1} q\pi(q)dq = \sqrt{\frac{\sigma_0^2}{2\pi}}\left[\exp\left\{-\frac{(T_{(j-1)}^1 - \mu_0)^2}{2\sigma_0^2}\right\} - \exp\left\{-\frac{(T_{(j)}^1 - \mu_0)^2}{2\sigma_0^2}\right\}\right] + \mu_0\int_{T_{(j-1)}^1}^{T_{(j)}^1} \pi(q)dq,$$

when the corresponding EL has the role of the likelihood function $L(q)$.

Step 2.2: Stage 2 of the MC simulation step ($k = 2$). During the second stage, t_2 additional generations, say $t_2 = 200$, of the test statistic values are conducted and then test statistics $T^2 = (T_1^2, \ldots, T_{t_2}^2)$ based on simulated data are calculated. We then estimate $f_{2,t_2}(\hat{q}_{1,\alpha})$, an estimate of density function of the test statistic, using the following kernel estimator (see, e.g., Gibbons and Chakraborti [2005] for details):

$$f_{2,t_2}(\hat{q}_{1,\alpha}) = \frac{1}{t_2} \sum_{j=1}^{t_2} \sqrt{\frac{1}{2\pi h^2}} \exp\left\{ -\frac{1}{2h^2}\left(\hat{q}_{1,\alpha} - T_j^2\right)^2 \right\},$$

where $h = 1.06\hat{\sigma}_{t_2} t^{-1/5}$, and $\hat{\sigma}_{t_2}$ is the standard deviation of the test statistics T_j^2. Then, we calculate the estimated variance of $\hat{q}$ as

$$V_1 \equiv \frac{F_{2,t_2}(\hat{q}_{1,\alpha})\left\{1 - F_{2,t_2}(\hat{q}_{1,\alpha})\right\}}{f_{2,t_2}(\hat{q}_{1,\alpha})^2 t_2}.$$

For details of this approximation of the variance, see Serfling (1980).

Step 2.3: Stopping rule of the procedure. To define the stopping rule of the procedure, one can use Proposition 16.1, controlling, for example, the estimated precision $|\hat{q}_0 - q_0|$ based on values of the test statistic obtained in the previous steps of the procedure in the manner mentioned above. Alternatively, we consider the following simple scheme: if $V_1 \leq \sigma_0^2$, then we stop the procedure and calculate, based on the combined values of the test statistics $T_c = (T_1^1, \ldots, T_{t_1}^1, T_1^2, \ldots, T_{t_2}^2)$ and $t_c = t_1 + t_2$, the posterior expectation of the quantiles, $\hat{q}_{c,\alpha}$,

$$\hat{q}_{c,\alpha} = \frac{\int_{T_{(1)}^c}^{T_{(t_c)}^c} q L_c(q)\pi(q)\,dq}{\int_{T_{(1)}^c}^{T_{(t_c)}^c} L_c(q)\pi(q)\,dq} \cong \frac{\sum_{j \in J_c} \exp\left\{ -\frac{t_c}{2\alpha(1-\alpha)}\left(1 - \alpha - \frac{j}{t_c}\right)^2 \right\} \int_{T_{(j-1)}^c}^{T_{(j)}^c} q\pi(q)\,dq}{\sum_{j \in J_c} \exp\left\{ -\frac{t_c}{2\alpha(1-\alpha)}\left(1 - \alpha - \frac{j}{t_c}\right)^2 \right\} \int_{T_{(j-1)}^c}^{T_{(j)}^c} \pi(q)\,dq},$$

where

$$\int_{T_{(j-1)}^c}^{T_{(j)}^c} q\pi(q)\,dq = \sqrt{\frac{\sigma_0^2}{2\pi}}\left[\exp\left\{ -\frac{(T_{(j-1)}^c - \mu_0)^2}{2\sigma_0^2} \right\} - \exp\left\{ -\frac{(T_{(j)}^c - \mu_0)^2}{2\sigma_0^2} \right\} \right].$$

In this case, we reach an estimated value of the variance of the critical values that is comparable with the variance of the critical values found in the table. If the value of the test statistic based on the data, T_0, is greater than $\hat{q}_{c,\alpha}$ then we reject the null.

If $V_1 > \sigma_0^2$, combine T^1 and T^2 into a new T^1, so that the new t_1 is equal to $t_1 + t_2$. Repeat steps 2.2 and 2.3 of the procedure until the stop condition $V_1 \leq \sigma_0^2$ is reached or the number of the new combined values of test statistics, T_1, is greater than 35,000. For more details, we refer the reader to the supplement (Section 16.4) and Vexler et al. (2014b).

Step 3: Decision rule. Reject the null hypothesis if the value of the test statistic based on data, say T_0, is $T_0 > \hat{q}_{c,\alpha}$.

Remark 16.1

If we solve

$$T_0 \cong \frac{\sum_{j \in Jc} \exp\left\{-\dfrac{t_c}{2\alpha(1-\alpha)}\left(1-\alpha-\dfrac{j}{t_c}\right)^2\right\} \int_{T^c_{(j-1)}}^{T^c_{(j)}} q\pi(q)dq}{\sum_{j \in Jc} \exp\left\{-\dfrac{t_c}{2\alpha(1-\alpha)}\left(1-\alpha-\dfrac{j}{t_c}\right)^2\right\} \int_{T^c_{(j-1)}}^{T^c_{(j)}} \pi(q)dq},$$

with respect to α, the solution, $1 - \hat{\alpha}$, gives the estimated p-value.

The hybrid method is to be performed iteratively, and the decision to define sample sizes of Monte Carlo simulations needed to evaluate critical values or p-values depends on the expected quality of the Type I error control.

In summary, the hybrid method combines both interpolation and MC by employing tables as prior and MC as data in a nonparametric Bayesian manner to obtain the posterior expectations of the CVs. In this case, we incorporate the efficiency of the interpolation method and the accuracy of the MC method. The hybrid method can be applied in a broad setting, and is shown to be very efficient in the context of computations of exact tests' critical values and powers (Vexler et al. 2012b, 2014c).

16.3 Available Software Packages

Implementations of methods of calculating critical values of exact tests described in Section 16.2 are easily carried out via the recently developed STATA and R statistical packages.

Vexler et al. (2014c) presented a STATA implementation of the density-based empirical likelihood procedures for testing symmetry of data distributions and *k*-sample comparisons, which are freely available for download at the following link: https://sphhp.buffalo.edu/biostatistics/research-and-facilities/software/stata.html.

Three STATA tables are provided with the command. For the *MC* method, the critical values are obtained by Monte Carlo simulations for each test conducted as described in Section 16.2.1. For the *interpolation* method, the provided tables of critical values are used to obtain the p-value as described in Section 16.2.2. For the *hybrid* method, which is based on the Bayesian approach, the provided tables of critical values are used to obtain initial parameter estimates (μ_0, σ_0) as described in Section 16.2.3. Further, assume the method option is set to interpolation or hybrid. It is noted that the provided tables of critical values are complete for sample sizes of 30 or less, but are incomplete for sample sizes greater than 30. If all the sample sizes are less than 30, then the critical values are directly available in the tables. In this case, the critical values are directly obtained from the appropriate table. If all sample sizes are not less than 30, then the critical values are not directly available in the tables. In this case, the hybrid and interpolation methods are used for obtaining the desired critical values.

Zhao et al. (2015) developed exact parametric and nonparametric likelihood ratio tests for two-sample comparisons in the R statistical software (R Development Core Team 2014).

The developed R package can provide the users outputs of the exact and powerful decision-making mechanisms described above. All test statistics to test for two-sample comparisons are exact, and their null distributions do not depend on the data distributions. In this setting, they provide accurate (not asymptotic) Type I error rates for the density-based EL ratio test, including the traditional MC method, the interpolation method, and the hybrid method. The novel R package is located at the following link: http://cran.r-project.org/web/packages/tsc/index.html.

16.4 Supplement

The issue of numerical methods for calculating critical values and powers of statistical tests is well addressed in the literature. In this section, we outline a methodology by Vexler et al. (2014c) in which the theoretical aspects of the Bayesian hybrid method to compute critical values of exact tests were introduced and examined.

Evaluation of the exact p-value in our context requires statistical inference for quantiles. The inference can be made using the EL technique based on kernel densities. As shown by Chen and Hall (1993), the use of kernel densities to smooth EL significantly improves the performance of the EL ratio tests for quantiles, in terms of relative accuracy. In order to use the data from Monte Carlo generations and tabulated critical values jointly, kernel density estimation within Bayesian-type procedures can be employed. The p-values are linked to the posterior means of quantiles. In this framework, Vexler et al. (2014c) presented relevant information from the Monte Carlo experiments via likelihood-type functions, whereas tabulated critical values are used to reflect prior distributions. The local maximum likelihood technique was used to compute functional forms of prior distributions from statistical tables. Empirical likelihood functions were to replace parametric likelihood functions within the structure of the posterior mean calculations to provide a Bayesian-type procedure with a distribution-free set of assumptions. The authors investigated the asymptotic properties of the nonparametric posterior expectation of quantiles and provided a method to control the accuracy of the p-value evaluations. Based on the theoretical propositions, the minimum number of needed Monte Carlo resamples for the desired level of accuracy based on distances between actual data characteristics (e.g., sample sizes) and characteristics of data used to present corresponding critical values in a table can be obtained.

We focus on the evaluation of the $(1 - \alpha) \times 100\%$ quantile, $\Pr\left(X < q_0^{1-\alpha}\right) = 1 - \alpha$, $\alpha \in (0, 1)$. The algorithm for executing the hybrid procedure is based on the following steps:

1. Obtain the prior distribution with the parameters, for example, the mean and variance parameters (μ_0, σ_0^2), using the local maximum likelihood (LML) method based on tabulated critical values. For the exact form of the prior, we refer the reader to Section 2.2 of the paper of Vexler et al. (2014a).

2. Generate a learning sample (e.g., defining $t = 200$) of the test statistic values under the corresponding null hypothesis using MC simulations.

3. Let X_j ($j = 1, \ldots, t$) denote a realization of the test statistic value at the jth MC iteration when the MC simulations provide in total t generated values of the test

statistic with an unknown density function f. Using the learning sample, estimate $f\left(q_0^{1-\alpha}\right)$, $f'\left(q_0^{1-\alpha}\right)$, $f''\left(q_0^{1-\alpha}\right)$ and $f^{(3)}\left(q_0^{1-\alpha}\right)$ to present $E\tilde{\Delta}(t)$ as a function of t, where

$$
E\tilde{\Delta}(t) = -\frac{f\left(q_0^{1-\alpha}\right)}{\left(1+\dfrac{\alpha(1-\alpha)}{\sigma_0^2 f^2\left(q_0^{1-\alpha}\right)t}\right)}\left\{-\frac{d_2 f'\left(q_0^{1-\alpha}\right)h^2}{2f\left(q_0^{1-\alpha}\right)} - \frac{d_4 f^{(3)}\left(q_0^{1-\alpha}\right)h^4}{24f\left(q_0^{1-\alpha}\right)}\right.
$$

$$
\left. +\frac{\left(d_2\right)^2 f'\left(q_0^{1-\alpha}\right)f''\left(q_0^{1-\alpha}\right)h^4}{4f^2\left(q_0^{1-\alpha}\right)} + \frac{(-1+2\alpha)f\left(q_0^{1-\alpha}\right)}{t}\right\}
$$

$$
-\frac{f\left(q_0^{1-\alpha}\right)}{\left(1+\dfrac{\alpha(1-\alpha)}{\sigma_0^2 f^2\left(q_0^{1-\alpha}\right)t}\right)}\left\{-\frac{\alpha(1-\alpha)f'\left(q_0^{1-\alpha}\right)}{2f^3\left(q_0^{1-\alpha}\right)t} + \frac{\alpha(1-\alpha)\left(\mu_0-q_0^{1-\alpha}\right)}{\sigma_0^2 f^2\left(q_0^{1-\alpha}\right)t}\right\}
$$

$$
-\frac{f'\left(q_0^{1-\alpha}\right)}{2\left(1+\dfrac{\alpha(1-\alpha)}{\sigma_0^2 f^2\left(q_0^{1-\alpha}\right)t}\right)^2}\left\{\frac{\alpha(1-\alpha)}{f^2\left(q_0^{1-\alpha}\right)t}\right\},
$$

$d_v = \int u^v k(u)du$, $v = 2, 4$, and $k(\cdot)$ is a kernel density function. For more details regarding $E\tilde{\Delta}(t)$, we refer the reader to Vexler et al. (2014b).

4. Compare $\left|E\tilde{\Delta}(t)\right|$ with a presumed threshold (e.g., $\upsilon = 0.001$) to compute an appropriate value of t_0 when $\left|E\tilde{\Delta}(t_0)\right| < \upsilon$.

5. Run the MC simulations to obtain t_0 values of the exact test statistic.

6. Use the nonparametric posterior expectation of the $(1 - \alpha)$th quantile or its asymptotic form to obtain the estimator of the quantile of interest, evaluating the critical values.

Proposition 16.2 provides the method from which we can measure the accuracy of the given estimation procedure.

Proposition 16.2

The asymptotic representation of the expectation of the estimated probability at

$$
1 - F\left(\hat{q}_{NP}^{1-\alpha}\right) = \alpha - \left(\hat{q}_{NP}^{1-\alpha} - q_0^{1-\alpha}\right)f\left(q_0^{1-\alpha}\right) - \frac{1}{2}\left(\hat{q}_{NP}^{1-\alpha} - q_0^{1-\alpha}\right)^2 f'\left(q_0^{1-\alpha}\right) - \frac{1}{6}\left(\hat{q}_{NP}^{1-\alpha} - q_0^{1-\alpha}\right)^3 f''\left(q_0^{1-\alpha}\right) + \ldots \text{ is}
$$

$$
E\left\{1 - F\left(\hat{q}_{NP}^{1-\alpha}\right)\right\} = \alpha - E\tilde{\Delta}(t) + o\left(t^{-1}\right),
$$

where $d_v = \int u^v k(u)du$, $v = 2, 4$ and $E\tilde{\Delta}(t)$ is defined below.

In general, the Bayesian hybrid method makes practical applications of exact tests simple and rapid.

16.5 Appendix

Proof of Proposition 16.1

It is clear that by virtue of the definitions (16.2) and (16.3), one can write

$$\hat{q}_0 = \int_{X_{(1)}}^{X_{(t)}} q\hat{P}(q)dp$$

$$= \frac{\sum_{j=1}^{t-1} \exp\left(\left[\left(\log(1-\alpha_0)-\log\left(\frac{j}{t}\right)\right)\left(\frac{j}{t}\right)+\left(\log(\alpha_0)-\log\left(1-\frac{j}{t}\right)\right)\left(1-\frac{j}{t}\right)\right]t\right)\int_{X_{(j)}}^{X_{(j+1)}} qe^{-\frac{1}{2\sigma_0^2}(q-\mu_0)^2} dq}{\sum_{j=1}^{t-1} \exp\left(\left[\left(\log(1-\alpha_0)-\log\left(\frac{j}{t}\right)\right)\left(\frac{j}{t}\right)+\left(\log(\alpha_0)-\log\left(1-\frac{j}{t}\right)\right)\left(1-\frac{j}{t}\right)\right]t\right)\int_{X_{(j)}}^{X_{(j+1)}} e^{-\frac{1}{2\sigma_0^2}(q-\mu_0)^2} dq}$$

(16.4)

Consider the part sum

$$\sum_{1\le j\le(1-\alpha_0)t-t^{1/2}(\log(t))^{1/2}\gamma} \exp\left(\left[\left(\log(1-\alpha_0)-\log\left(\frac{j}{t}\right)\right)\left(\frac{j}{t}\right)+\left(\log(\alpha_0)-\log\left(1-\frac{j}{t}\right)\right)\left(1-\frac{j}{t}\right)\right]t\right)$$

$$\int_{X_{(j)}}^{X_{(j+1)}} q^s \exp\left(-\frac{1}{2\sigma_0^2}(q-\mu_0)^2\right)dq, \quad s=0,1,$$

for $\gamma = \sqrt{2\alpha_0(1-\alpha_0)\upsilon}$ with $\upsilon > 1$. It is clear that the function $(\log(1 - \alpha_0) - \log(u))(u) + (\log(\alpha_0) - \log(1 - u))(1 - u) \le 0$ increases when $u < (1 - \alpha_0)$ and then decreases when $u > (1 - \alpha_0)$, having the maximum value 0 at $u = (1 - \alpha_0)$. That is, we have

$$\sum_{1\le j\le(1-\alpha_0)t-t^{1/2}(\log(t))^{1/2}\gamma} \exp\left(\left[\left(\log(1-\alpha_0)-\log\left(\frac{j}{t}\right)\right)\left(\frac{j}{t}\right)+\left(\log(\alpha_0)-\log\left(1-\frac{j}{t}\right)\right)\left(1-\frac{j}{t}\right)\right]t\right)$$

$$\int_{X_{(j)}}^{X_{(j+1)}} q^s \exp\left(-\frac{1}{2\sigma_0^2}(q-\mu_0)^2\right)dq$$

$$\le \exp\left(\left[\left(\log(1-\alpha_0)-\log\left((1-\alpha_0)-\frac{\gamma(\log(t))^{1/2}}{t^{1/2}}\right)\right)\left((1-\alpha_0)-\frac{\gamma(\log(t))^{1/2}}{t^{1/2}}\right)\right.\right.$$

$$\left.\left.+\left(\log(\alpha_0)-\log\left(\alpha_0+\frac{\gamma(\log(t))^{1/2}}{t^{1/2}}\right)\right)\left(\alpha_0+\frac{\gamma(\log(t))^{1/2}}{t^{1/2}}\right)\right]t\right)$$

$$\sum_{1\le j\le(1-\alpha_0)t-t^{1/2}(\log(t))^{1/2}\gamma} \int_{X_{(j)}}^{X_{(j+1)}} q^s \exp\left(-\frac{1}{2\sigma_0^2}(q-\mu_0)^2\right)dq$$

Using the Taylor expansion of the function

$$
\left(\log(1-\alpha_0) - \log\left((1-\alpha_0) - \frac{\gamma(\log(t))^{1/2}}{t^{1/2}} \right) \right)\left((1-\alpha_0) - \frac{\gamma(\log(t))^{1/2}}{t^{1/2}} \right)
$$

$$
+ \left(\log(\alpha_0) - \log\left(\alpha_0 + \frac{\gamma(\log(t))^{1/2}}{t^{1/2}} \right) \right)\left(\alpha_0 + \frac{\gamma(\log(t))^{1/2}}{t^{1/2}} \right)
$$

with $t^{-1/2}\gamma(\log(t))^{1/2}$ around 0, we have

$$
\left(\log(1-\alpha_0) - \log\left((1-\alpha_0) - \frac{\gamma(\log(t))^{1/2}}{t^{1/2}} \right) \right)\left((1-\alpha_0) - \frac{\gamma(\log(t))^{1/2}}{t^{1/2}} \right)
$$

$$
+ \left(\log(\alpha_0) - \log\left(\alpha_0 + \frac{\gamma(\log(t))^{1/2}}{t^{1/2}} \right) \right)\left(\alpha_0 + \frac{\gamma(\log(t))^{1/2}}{t^{1/2}} \right)
$$

$$
= \frac{-1/2}{\alpha_0(1-\alpha_0)}\left(\frac{\gamma(\log(t))^{1/2}}{t^{1/2}} \right)^2 + o\left(\frac{1}{t^{3/2-\varepsilon}} \right) = -\log(t)\upsilon + o\left(\frac{1}{t^{3/2-\varepsilon}} \right), \quad \varepsilon > 0, t \to \infty.
$$

This implies

$$
\sum_{1 \le j \le (1-\alpha_0)t - t^{1/2}\gamma(\log(t))^{1/2}} \exp\left(\left[\left(\log(1-\alpha_0) - \log\left(\frac{j}{t} \right) \right)\left(\frac{j}{t} \right) + \left(\log(\alpha_0) - \log\left(1 - \frac{j}{t} \right) \right)\left(1 - \frac{j}{t} \right) \right] t \right)
$$

$$
\times \int_{X_{(j)}}^{X_{(j+1)}} q^s \exp\left(-\frac{1}{2\sigma_0^2}(q-\mu_0)^2 \right) dq \tag{16.5}
$$

$$
\le \frac{1}{t^\upsilon} \exp\left(o\left(\frac{1}{t^{1/2-\varepsilon}} \right) \right) \sum_{1 \le j \le (1-\alpha_0)t - t^{1/2}\gamma(\log(t))^{1/2}} \int_{X_{(j)}}^{X_{(j+1)}} q^s \exp\left(-\frac{1}{2\sigma_0^2}(q-\mu_0)^2 \right) dq \to 0, t \to \infty.
$$

In a similar manner to the asymptotic result above, one can show that

$$
\sum_{t-1 \ge (1-\alpha_0)t + t^{1/2}\gamma(\log(t))^{1/2}} \exp\left(\left[\left(\log(1-\alpha_0) - \log\left(\frac{j}{t} \right) \right)\left(\frac{j}{t} \right) + \left(\log(\alpha_0) - \log\left(1 - \frac{j}{t} \right) \right)\left(1 - \frac{j}{t} \right) \right] t \right)
$$

$$
\times \int_{X_{(j)}}^{X_{(j+1)}} q^s \exp\left(-\frac{1}{2\sigma_0^2}(q-\mu_0)^2 \right) dq \tag{16.6}
$$

$$
\le \frac{1}{t^\upsilon} \exp\left(o\left(\frac{1}{t^{1/2-\varepsilon}} \right) \right) \sum_{t-1 \ge (1-\alpha_0)t + t^{1/2}\gamma(\log(t))^{1/2}} \int_{X_{(j)}}^{X_{(j+1)}} q^s \exp\left(-\frac{1}{2\sigma_0^2}(q-\mu_0)^2 \right) dq \to 0, t \to \infty,
$$

$s = 0,1, \ t \to \infty.$

The results (16.5) and (16.6) applied to (16.4) imply

$$
\hat{q}_0 = \int_{X_{(1)}}^{X_{(t)}} q\hat{P}(q)\, dq
$$

$$= \frac{\sum_{j\in J}\exp\left(\left[\left(\log(1-\alpha_0)-\log\left(\frac{j}{t}\right)\right)\left(\frac{j}{t}\right)+\left(\log(\alpha_0)-\log\left(1-\frac{j}{t}\right)\right)\left(1-\frac{j}{t}\right)\right]t\right)\int_{X_{(j)}}^{X_{(j+1)}} q\ e^{-\frac{1}{2\sigma_0^2}(q-\mu_0)^2}\,dq}{\sum_{j\in J}\exp\left(\left[\left(\log(1-\alpha_0)-\log\left(\frac{j}{t}\right)\right)\left(\frac{j}{t}\right)+\left(\log(\alpha_0)-\log\left(1-\frac{j}{t}\right)\right)\left(1-\frac{j}{t}\right)\right]t\right)\int_{X_{(j)}}^{X_{(j+1)}} e^{-\frac{1}{2\sigma_0^2}(q-\mu_0)^2}\,dq}$$

$$+o(t^{-1}),\quad J=\left[(1-\alpha_0)t-t^{1/2}\gamma(\log(t))^{1/2},(1-\alpha_0)t+t^{1/2}\gamma(\log(t))^{1/2}\right].$$

Using again the Taylor expansion of the function $(\log(1-\alpha_0)-\log(u))(u)+(\log(\alpha_0)-\log(1-u))$ $(1-u)$ with u around $1-\alpha_0$ $\left(\text{here } u\in\left[(1-\alpha_0)-t^{-1/2}\gamma(\log(t))^{1/2},(1-\alpha_0)+t^{-1/2}\gamma(\log(t))^{1/2}\right]\right)$, we have

$$\hat{q}_0=\frac{\sum_{j\in J}\exp\left(\frac{-t/2}{\alpha_0(1-\alpha_0)}\left(1-\alpha_0-\frac{j}{t}\right)^2\right)\int_{X_{(j)}}^{X_{(j+1)}} q\ e^{\frac{-1}{2\sigma_0^2}(q-\mu_0)^2}\,dq}{\sum_{j\in J}\exp\left(\frac{-t/2}{\alpha_0(1-\alpha_0)}\left(1-\alpha_0-\frac{j}{t}\right)^2\right)\int_{X_{(j)}}^{X_{(j+1)}} e^{\frac{-1}{2\sigma_0^2}(q-\mu_0)^2}\,dq}+o(t^{-1}),\tag{16.7}$$

$$J=\left[(1-\alpha_0)t-t^{1/2}\gamma(\log(t))^{1/2},(1-\alpha_0)t+t^{1/2}\gamma(\log(t))^{1/2}\right].$$

Consider the integrals $\int_{X_{(j)}}^{X_{(j+1)}} q^s\exp\left(-\frac{1}{2\sigma_0^2}(q-\mu_0)^2\right)dq, s=0,1.$ By virtue of the mean value theorem, we can write

$$\int_{X_{(j)}}^{X_{(j+1)}} q^s\exp\left(-\frac{1}{2\sigma_0^2}(q-\mu_0)^2\right)dq=\left(X_{(j+1)}-X_{(j)}\right)\left(X_{(j)}\right)^s e^{-\frac{1}{2\sigma_0^2}(X_{(j)}-\mu_0)^2}$$

$$+\frac{1}{2}\left(X_{(j+1)}-X_{(j)}\right)^2\left(s-\sigma_0^{-2}(q_\theta)^s(q_\theta-\mu_0)\right)e^{-\frac{1}{2\sigma_0^2}(q_\theta-\mu_0)^2},$$

$$q_\theta=X_{(j+1)}-\theta\left(X_{(j+1)}-X_{(j)}\right),\theta\in(0,1)$$

This equation applied to (16.7) implies

$$\hat{q}_0=\frac{\sum_{j\in J}\exp\left(\frac{-t/2}{\alpha_0(1-\alpha_0)}\left(1-\alpha_0-\frac{j}{t}\right)^2\right)\left(X_{(j+1)}-X_{(j)}\right)X_{(j)}\ e^{-\frac{1}{2\sigma_0^2}(X_{(j)}-\mu_0)^2}}{\sum_{j\in J}\exp\left(\frac{-t/2}{\alpha_0(1-\alpha_0)}\left(1-\alpha_0-\frac{j}{t}\right)^2\right)\left(X_{(j+1)}-X_{(j)}\right)\ e^{-\frac{1}{2\sigma_0^2}(X_{(j)}-\mu_0)^2}}$$

$$+\frac{\sum_{j\in J}\exp\left(\frac{-t/2}{\alpha_0(1-\alpha_0)}\left(1-\alpha_0-\frac{j}{t}\right)^2\right)\frac{1}{2}\left(X_{(j+1)}-X_{(j)}\right)^2\left(1-\sigma_0^{-2}q_\theta(q_\theta-\mu_0)\right)\ e^{-\frac{1}{2\sigma_0^2}(q_\theta-\mu_0)^2}}{\sum_{j\in J}\exp\left(\frac{-t/2}{\alpha_0(1-\alpha_0)}\left(1-\alpha_0-\frac{j}{t}\right)^2\right)\frac{1}{2\sigma_0^2}\left(X_{(j+1)}-X_{(j)}\right)^2(\mu_0-q_\omega)\ e^{-\frac{1}{2\sigma_0^2}(q_\omega-\mu_0)^2}}+o\left(t^{-1}\right),\tag{16.8}$$

$$\omega\in(0,1)$$

To evaluate (16.8), we use the following results:

1. Under the conditions of Proposition 16.1, we have

$$X_{(k)} = q_0 + \frac{k/t - (1 - \tau_t(q_0)/t)}{f(q_0)} + R_{k,t}, \quad R_{k,t} = O\left(t^{-3/4}\left(\log(t)\right)^{(\Delta+1)/2}\right), \quad \Delta > 1/2,$$

$$\tau_t(q) = \sum_{i=1}^{t} I\{X_i \ge q\}, \ k \in J = \left[(1-\alpha_0)t - t^{1/2}\gamma(\log(t))^{1/2}, (1-\alpha_0)t + t^{1/2}\gamma(\log(t))^{1/2}\right]$$

(16.9)

(the Bahadur theorem; see, e.g., Serfling [1980, p. 93]).

2. A Pyke approach (Pyke 1965) expresses the spacings $(X_{(j+1)} - X_{(j)})$, $j \in J$, in the forms of

$$\left(X_{(j+1)} - X_{(j)}\right) = F^{-1}(U_{(j+1)}) - F^{-1}(U_{(j)}) = (U_{(j+1)} - U_{(j)})/f(a_j),$$

where F^{-1} is the inverse function of the distribution F, $U_{(j)}$'s are uniform [0,1] order statistics, a_j lies between $U_{(j+1)}$ and $U_{(j)}$, and the mean value theorem was applied. In this case, we have properties of the spacing $(U_{(j+1)} - U_{(j)})$ presented in Pyke (1965), for example,

$$E(U_{(j+1)} - U_{(j)}) = (n+1)^{-1}, E(U_{(j+1)} - U_{(j)})^2 = 2(n+1)^{-1}(n+2)^{-1},$$

$$\mathrm{cov}\left((U_{(j+1)} - U_{(j)})(U_{(k+1)} - U_{(k)})\right) = -(n+1)^{-2}(n+2)^{-1}, j \ne k,$$

as well as probabilistic properties of $U_{(j+1)}$ presented in David and Nagaraja (2003).

3. The function $u^p \exp(-u^2/a)$ with an integer parameter p and a positive constant a has finite maximum and minimum values at $u = \pm\sqrt{pa/2}$.

By virtue of these results, one can show that

$$\hat{q}_0 = \frac{\sum_{j \in J} \exp\left(\frac{-t/2}{\alpha_0(1-\alpha_0)}\left(1-\alpha_0 - \frac{j}{t}\right)^2\right)(X_{(j+1)} - X_{(j)})\left(q_0 + \frac{j/t - (1-\tau_t(q_0)/t)}{f(q_0)}\right)e^{\frac{-1}{2\sigma_0^2}\left(q_0 + \frac{j/t - (1-\tau_t(q_0)/t)}{f(q_0)} - \mu_0\right)^2}}{\sum_{j \in J} \exp\left(\frac{-t/2}{\alpha_0(1-\alpha_0)}\left(1-\alpha_0 - \frac{j}{t}\right)^2\right)(X_{(j+1)} - X_{(j)}) \, e^{\frac{-1}{2\sigma_0^2}\left(q_0 + \frac{j/t - (1-\tau_t(q_0)/t)}{f(q_0)} - \mu_0\right)^2}}$$

$$+ O\left(t^{-3/4}\left(\log(t)\right)^{(\Delta+1)/2}\right)$$

(16.10)

$$\times \frac{\sum_{j \in J} \exp\left(\frac{-t/2}{\alpha_0(1-\alpha_0)}\left(1-\alpha_0 - \frac{j}{t}\right)^2\right)(X_{(j+1)} - X_{(j)})e^{\frac{-1}{2\sigma_0^2}\left(q_0 + \frac{j/t - (1-\tau_t(q_0)/t)}{f(q_0)} - \mu_0\right)^2}}{\sum_{j \in J} \exp\left(\frac{-t/2}{\alpha_0(1-\alpha_0)}\left(1-\alpha_0 - \frac{j}{t}\right)^2\right)(X_{(j+1)} - X_{(j)}) \, e^{\frac{-1}{2\sigma_0^2}\left(q_0 + \frac{j/t - (1-\tau_t(q_0)/t)}{f(q_0)} - \mu_0\right)^2}}$$

$$+ o(t^{-1}).$$

One can easily show

$$\sum_{j \in J} \exp\left(\frac{-t/2}{\alpha_0(1-\alpha_0)}\left(1-\alpha_0-\frac{j}{t}\right)^2\right) = t\sum_{j \in J} \exp\left(\frac{-t/2}{\alpha_0(1-\alpha_0)}\left(1-\alpha_0-\frac{j}{t}\right)^2\right)\left(\frac{j+1}{t}-\frac{j}{t}\right)$$

$$= O\left(t\int_{-\infty}^{\infty} \exp\left(\frac{-t/2}{\alpha_0(1-\alpha_0)}(1-\alpha_0-u)^2\right)du\right) = O\left(t^{1/2}\right), \quad t \to \infty.$$

Now apply (16.8), (16.10) and (16.9) to (16.7) to obtain

$$\hat{q}_0 = \frac{\displaystyle\sum_{j \in J} e^{\frac{-t/2}{\alpha_0(1-\alpha_0)}\left(1-\alpha_0-\frac{j}{t}\right)^2}\left(q_0+\frac{j/t-(1-\tau_t(q_0)/t)}{f(q_0)}\right)e^{\frac{-1}{2\sigma_0^2}\left(q_0+\frac{j/t-(1-\tau_t(q_0)/t)}{f(q_0)}-\mu_0\right)^2}}{\displaystyle\sum_{j \in J} e^{\frac{-t/2}{\alpha_0(1-\alpha_0)}\left(1-\alpha_0-\frac{j}{t}\right)^2} e^{\frac{-1}{2\sigma_0^2}\left(q_0+\frac{j/t-(1-\tau_t(q_0)/t)}{f(q_0)}-\mu_0\right)^2}} + o(t^{-1})$$

$$= q_0 + \frac{(\tau_t(q_0)/t-1)}{f(q_0)} + \frac{\displaystyle\sum_{j \in J} e^{\frac{-t/2}{\alpha_0(1-\alpha_0)}\left(1-\alpha_0-\frac{j}{t}\right)^2}\frac{j}{f(q_0)t}e^{\frac{-1}{2\sigma_0^2}\left(q_0+\frac{j/t-(1-\tau_t(q_0)/t)}{f(q_0)}-\mu_0\right)^2}}{\displaystyle\sum_{j \in J} e^{\frac{-t/2}{\alpha_0(1-\alpha_0)}\left(1-\alpha_0-\frac{j}{t}\right)^2}e^{\frac{-1}{2\sigma_0^2}\left(q_0+\frac{j/t-(1-\tau_t(q_0)/t)}{f(q_0)}-\mu_0\right)^2}} + o(t^{-1}),$$

$$J = \left[(1-\alpha_0)t-t^{1/2}\gamma(\log(t))^{1/2}, (1-\alpha_0)t+t^{1/2}\gamma(\log(t))^{1/2}\right].$$

Thus, we can conclude that

$$\hat{q}_0 = q_0 + \frac{(\tau_t(q_0)/t-1)}{f(q_0)} + \frac{\displaystyle\sum_{j=-\infty}^{\infty} e^{\frac{-t/2}{\alpha_0(1-\alpha_0)}\left(1-\alpha_0-\frac{j}{t}\right)^2}\frac{j}{f(q_0)t}e^{\frac{-1}{2\sigma_0^2}\left(q_0+\frac{j/t-(1-\tau_t(q_0)/t)}{f(q_0)}-\mu_0\right)^2}}{\displaystyle\sum_{j=-\infty}^{\infty} e^{\frac{-t/2}{\alpha_0(1-\alpha_0)}\left(1-\alpha_0-\frac{j}{t}\right)^2}e^{\frac{-1}{2\sigma_0^2}\left(q_0+\frac{j/t-(1-\tau_t(q_0)/t)}{f(q_0)}-\mu_0\right)^2}} + o(t^{-1})$$

$$= q_0 + \frac{(\tau_t(q_0)/t-1)}{f(q_0)} + \frac{\dfrac{1}{f(q_0)}\displaystyle\sum_{j=-\infty}^{\infty}\int_{j/t}^{(j+1)/t} e^{\frac{-t/2}{\alpha_0(1-\alpha_0)}(1-\alpha_0-u)^2+\frac{-1}{2\sigma_0^2}\left(q_0+\frac{u-(1-\tau_t(q_0)/t)}{f(q_0)}-\mu_0\right)^2}u\,du}{\displaystyle\sum_{j=-\infty}^{\infty}\int_{j/t}^{(j+1)/t} e^{\frac{-t/2}{\alpha_0(1-\alpha_0)}(1-\alpha_0-u)^2+\frac{-1}{2\sigma_0^2}\left(q_0+\frac{u-(1-\tau_t(q_0)/t)}{f(q_0)}-\mu_0\right)^2}du} + o(t^{-1})$$

$$= q_0 + \frac{(\tau_t(q_0)/t-1)}{f(q_0)} + \frac{\dfrac{1}{f(q_0)}\displaystyle\int_{-\infty}^{\infty} e^{\frac{-t/2}{\alpha_0(1-\alpha_0)}(1-\alpha_0-u)^2+\frac{-1}{2\sigma_0^2}\left(q_0+\frac{u-(1-\tau_t(q_0)/t)}{f(q_0)}-\mu_0\right)^2}u\,du}{\displaystyle\int_{-\infty}^{\infty} e^{\frac{-t/2}{\alpha_0(1-\alpha_0)}(1-\alpha_0-u)^2+\frac{-1}{2\sigma_0^2}\left(q_0+\frac{u-(1-\tau_t(q_0)/t)}{f(q_0)}-\mu_0\right)^2}du} + o(t^{-1})$$

$$= q_0 + \frac{(\tau_t(q_0)/t - 1) + (1 - \alpha_0)}{f(q_0)} + \frac{\dfrac{1}{f(q_0)} \displaystyle\int_{-\infty}^{\infty} e^{\frac{-t/2}{\alpha_0(1-\alpha_0)}z^2 + \frac{-1}{2\sigma_0^2}\left(q_0 - \mu_0 + \frac{(1-\alpha_0)-(1-\tau_t(q_0)/t)}{f(q_0)} + \frac{z}{f(q_0)}\right)^2} z\,dz}{\displaystyle\int_{-\infty}^{\infty} e^{\frac{-t/2}{\alpha_0(1-\alpha_0)}z^2 + \frac{-1}{2\sigma_0^2}\left(q_0 - \mu_0 + \frac{(1-\alpha_0)-(1-\tau_t(q_0)/t)}{f(q_0)} + \frac{z}{f(q_0)}\right)^2} dz} + o\!\left(t^{-1}\right).$$

It is clear that row operations to transform the integrals

$$\int_{-\infty}^{\infty} e^{\frac{-t/2}{\alpha_0(1-\alpha_0)}z^2 + \frac{-1}{2\sigma_0^2}\left(q_0 - \mu_0 + \frac{(1-\alpha_0)-(1-\tau_t(q_0)/t)}{f(q_0)} + \frac{z}{f(q_0)}\right)^2} z\,dz \text{ and } \int_{-\infty}^{\infty} e^{\frac{-t/2}{\alpha_0(1-\alpha_0)}z^2 + \frac{-1}{2\sigma_0^2}\left(q_0 - \mu_0 + \frac{(1-\alpha_0)-(1-\tau_t(q_0)/t)}{f(q_0)} + \frac{z}{f(q_0)}\right)^2} dz$$

to the forms of $\int_{-\infty}^{\infty} e^{au - u^2}\,du = \sqrt{\pi} e^{a^2/4}$ and $\int_{-\infty}^{\infty} u e^{au - u^2}\,du = 0.5 a \sqrt{\pi} e^{a^2/4}$ (here a is a constant) complete the proof of Proposition 16.1 (see for details Vexler et al. 2014b).

17

Bootstrap and Permutation Methods

The impact of the bootstrap has transcended both theory and applications. The bootstrap has shown us how to use the power of the computer and iterated calculations to go where theoretical calculations cannot, which introduces a different way of thinking about all of statistics.

G. Casella (2003)

17.1 Introduction

Bootstrap methods and other computationally intensive methods of statistical estimation and inference have a long history dating back to the permutation test introduced in the 1930s by R. A. Fisher. Ever since that time, there has been work toward developing efficient and practical nonparametric models that do not rely on the classical normal-based model assumptions. In the 1940s, Quenouille introduced the method of deleting "one observation at a time" for bias estimation. This method was further developed by Tukey in the 1950s for standard error estimation and coined by him as the jackknife method. This early work was followed by many variants up to the 1970s. The jackknife method was then extended to what is now referred to as the bootstrap method. Even though there were predecessors toward the development of the bootstrap method (e.g., see Hartigan 1969, 1971, 1975), it is generally agreed upon by statisticians that Efron's (1979) paper, in which the term *bootstrap* was coined, in conjunction with the development of high-speed computers, was a cornerstone event toward popularizing this particular methodology. Following Efron's paper, there was an explosion of research on the topic of bootstrap methods. At one time, nonparametric bootstrapping was thought to be a statistical method that would solve almost all problems in an efficient, easy-to-use nonparametric manner. So why do we not have a PROC BOOTSTRAP in SAS, and why are bootstrap methods not used more widely? One answer lies in the fact that there is not a general approach to bootstrapping along the lines of fitting a generalized linear model with normal error terms. Oftentimes, the bootstrap approach to solving a problem requires writing new pieces of sometimes difficult SAS code that only pertains to a specific problem. Another reason for the bootstrap method's failure to take off as a general approach is that it sometimes does not work well in certain situations, and that the method for correcting these deficient procedures is oftentimes difficult or tedious.

In the spirit of Young (1994), who advocates that at its roots the bootstrap method has the attributes of "simplicity" and "general applicability," we aim to provide a nontechnical overview of the utility of the bootstrap methodology and, where applicable, illustrate its use via already built-in SAS PROCs. Since there oftentimes will not be a unique way to carry out the bootstrap procedure in SAS, we attempt to provide different examples of SAS code that contrast simplicity and computational efficiency. It is expected that the reader is familiar with basic statistical models found in most introductory textbooks, for example, regression and analysis of variance. We also explore the power of the bootstrap method for analysts using more complicated models, such as those found in repeated measures or cluster analyses. For a majority of the examples, the reader is expected to understand the basic commands of the DATA step, such as do-loops and the OUTPUT statement, and be familiar with the various statistical PROCs that he or she might use generally given parametric assumptions. Some knowledge of the basic SAS macro language will also be helpful. It is our goal that most of the code provided in this book can be easily modified to handle a variety of problems found in practice.

Our focus is on problems where the simple bootstrap methods are known to work well. However, for important common everyday problems, such as calculating a confidence interval for the correlation coefficient, we provide code that is necessary in small samples in order to obtain more accurate inference. Throughout this book, we contrast the bootstrap results with the standard statistical methodology in order to illustrate the utility of the nonparametric bootstrap approach. Even though the bootstrap method is primarily considered a nonparametric method, it can be used in conjunction with parametric models as well. We also touch on how to utilize the parametric bootstrap method. Common everyday examples where the bootstrap method works well include inference about regression parameters given nonnormal error distributions, calculating standard errors for statistics such as the sample median, and even testing assumptions about normality. More complicated problems where the bootstrap method is a reasonable approach are situations such as repeated measures analyses, where one wishes to treat the correlation structure as a nuisance parameter, as opposed to assuming something unreasonable, or the case where there are unequal numbers of repeated measurements per subject.

There are many well-known "applied" books on bootstrapping. such as Efron and Tibshirani (1993) and Davison and Hinkley (1997), as well as theoretical books such as Shao and Tu (1995). However, these books are not very helpful toward practitioners who wish to code various bootstrapping methods using SAS. The overall goal of this book is to provide the frustrated SAS user a guide toward carrying out bootstrapping methods in SAS in a relatively painless manner, while sketching out the theoretical justifications for the various methods.

The most common use of the bootstrap method is to approximate the sampling distribution of a *statistic*, such as the mean, median, regression slope, or correlation coefficient. Once the sampling distribution has been approximated via the bootstrap method, estimation and inference involving the given statistic follow in a straightforward manner. Note, however, that the bootstrap does not provide exact answers. It provides approximate variance estimates and approximate coverage probabilities for confidence intervals. As with most statistical methods, these approximations improve for increasing sample sizes. The estimated probability distribution of a given statistic based on the bootstrap method is obtained by conditioning on the observed data set and replacing the population distribution function with its estimate in some statistical function, such as the expected value. The method may be carried out using either a parametric or nonparametric estimate of the distribution function. For example, the parametric bootstrap distribution of the sample mean $\bar{x}$ under normality assumptions is given simply by $\hat{F}(x) = \Phi\left(\sqrt{n}(x-\bar{x})/s\right)$, where Φ denotes the probit function, n is the sample size, and $\bar{x}$ and s are the sample mean and sample standard deviation, respectively. The 95% parametric bootstrap confidence interval is given simply by the 2.5th and 97.5th percentiles of $\hat{F}(x)$, or simply $\bar{x} + s \times 1.96/\sqrt{n}$.

This should look familiar to anybody who has opened an introductory statistics book as the approximate normal theory confidence interval for the sample mean.

Oftentimes, the calculations are not so straightforward or we wish to apply the bootstrap method in a nonparametric fashion; that is, we don't wish to constrain ourselves to a parameteric functional form such as the normal distribution when specifying the distribution function $F(x)$. In the majority of cases, we need to approximate the bootstrap method through the generation of *bootstrap replications* of the statistic of interest. Using a resampling procedure, we are able to approximate bootstrap estimates for quantities such as standard errors, p-values, and confidence intervals for a complicated statistic without relying on traditional approximations based on asymptotic normality. The primary focus of this book is on nonparametric bootstrap methods based on resampling techniques programmed using SAS. The general approach applies to both multivariate and univariate data.

As a simple example of the nonparametric bootstrap method, say we have the following: Suppose a researcher wishes to estimate 100% times the coefficient of variation, denoted as $V = 100\% \times \sigma/u$ for the following data set: $x = \{0.25, 0.40, 0.46, 0.27, 2.51, 1.29, 4.11, 6.11, 0.46, 1.37\}$. A moment estimator of V is 100% times the sample standard deviation divided by the sample mean, or $\hat{V} = 100\% \times s / \bar{x}$. For this example, we obtain from PROC UNIVARIATE $\hat{V} = 100\% \times s / \bar{x} = 100 \times 1.98/1.72 = 114.6$. Suppose this same researcher also wants to either calculate the 95% confidence interval for the population coefficient of variation, V, or estimate the standard deviation of the sample coefficient of variation, $\hat{V}$, given the sample data. Even if one assumes an underlying parametric model, such as the gamma distribution, the solution to this task is not trivial. Oftentimes, the only approach is given by an asymptotic approximation, which is often only accurate for very large samples. What we hope to illustrate is that the bootstrap approach provides a simple and theoretically sound solution to this type of problem, as well as many other problems that rely on normality assumptions, asymptotic approximations, or the case where no reasonable solution is built into the software.

To start, let us define some basic statistical quantities that are the basis for nonparametric bootstrapping in univariate sampling. Let $X_1, X_2, \ldots, X_n$ represent an independent and identically distributed (i.i.d.) sample from a continuous population with population distribution function denoted as $F(x)$, that is, notationally $F(x) = \Pr(X < x)$, the area to the left of x under the probability density curve. The basic idea behind the nonparametric bootstrap in the single-sample setting is to use the empirical distribution function defined as $F_n = \sum_{i=1}^{n} I\{x_i \le x\}/n$, in place of $F(x)$ in the calculation of interest, conditional on the data being held "fixed," where I denotes an indicator function that takes the value 1 if $x_i \le x$ and is 0 otherwise. In other words, conditional on the observed data, the empirical probability of observing $X_1 = x_1$ is $1/n$, where X_i denotes the ith random variable and x_i denotes the ith observed data value. For our example data set given in the previous paragraph, $x_1 = 0.25$, $x_2 = 0.40, \ldots, x_{10} = 1.37$, such that $F_n(0.40) = 0.30$; that is, three observations fall below or are equal to 0.40. In contrast, the parametric bootstrap would use a parametric form of F with the parameter estimates in place of the "true" parameter values, for example, assuming normality $\hat{F}(0.4) = \Phi((0.4 - \bar{x})/s) = \Phi((0.4 - 1.72)/1.98) = 0.25$. We touch on the parametric bootstrap elsewhere in the book.

The primary assumption of the bootstrap method is that a statistic $T(F_n(x))$, such as the sample mean, should approximate a population quantity $T(F(x))$ reasonably well in the univariate setting, as well as in the multivariate setting. Theoretically, one may show that the absolute difference between $F_n(x)$ and $F(x)$ grows small as the sample size, n, grows large.

This result is more formally known as the Glivenko–Cantelli theorem and is a principal reason why the bootstrap technique is theoretically sound for most situations found in practice. Note, however, that the convergence of $F_n(x)$ to $F(x)$ does not always imply the convergence of $T(F_n(x))$ to $T(F(x))$, or that the distributional properties of $T(F_n(x))$ are easily estimated using bootstrap methods. Hence, there are instances of bootstrap failure; however, many of these failures are mathematical constructs that one would not encounter in practice; for example, see Shao and Tu (1995) for technical examples. Therefore, in the words of Efron, we can "plug in" $F_n(x)$ for $F(x)$ in some population quantity in order to obtain its estimate.

As an example, suppose that we wish to obtain the bootstrap estimate for the population mean of X, represented as the integral $E(X) = \int x f(x)\,dx = \int x\,dF(x)$, where $F(x)$ is the probability density function. We can show after a simple change of variable that by substituting $F_n(x)$ for $F(x)$ in the integral, we obtain $\int x\,dF_n(x) = \bar{x}$; that is, the bootstrap estimate of the population mean of X turns out to be exactly equal to the sample average. In other words, we calculated the bootstrap estimate of the expected value of X directly. Now what about for more complicated problems, such as the one described above for the coefficient of variation $V = 100\% \times \sigma/u$? How might one calculate the variance of the estimate $\hat{V}$? Using the direct approach of substituting $F_n(x)$ in place of $F(x)$ in some mathematical integral is a difficult, if not mathematically impossible, approach to solving this problem. It turns out, however, that if we sample the data with replacement from $F_n(x)$, an approximate bootstrap solution is relatively straightforward and does not require any knowledge of calculus. This is what most practitioners refer to as the bootstrap method. From this point forward, unless otherwise specified, we will use the term *bootstrapping* to mean the method of resampling from the data (or technically from $F_n(x)$) in order to approximate the distribution of a given statistic. This allows the researcher to solve a variety of complicated problems with statistical accuracy without having to rely on such things as normality assumptions or having to specify complicated variance–covariance structures such as those found in mixed models. The approaches used for single-sample univariate models generally extend to more complicated multivariate models.

Typically data sampled from the original data **x** with replacement are denoted as **x*** in the bootstrap literature; that is, we randomly pick one value of **x**, record it, and replace it, repeating the procedure n times. For example, again denote our sample data set as **x** = {0.25, 0.40, 0.46, 0.27, 2.51, 1.29, 4.11, 6.11, 0.46, 1.37}. If we sample with replacement from **x**, we might obtain a given bootstrap resample of **x*** = {0.25, 0.40, 0.46, 0.27, 2.51, 1.29, 4.11, 6.11, 0.46, 1.37}. Recalculating the coefficient of variation for one bootstrap *replication* based on **x***, we get $\hat{V}^* = 124.9$, different from the observed $\hat{V} = 114.6$. What happens if we repeat this procedure, say, 10,000 times? A histogram of the 10,000 $\hat{V}^*$'s is given in Figure 17.1, followed by summary statistics given by PROC UNIVARIATE in Figure 17.2. The histogram represents an empirical bootstrap estimate of the probability distribution of the statistic $\hat{V}$ based on bootstrap resampling and conditional on the observed data. We see that the estimated distribution of $\hat{V}$ is fairly symmetric, with only a slight skewness to the right. Having obtained an estimate of the distribution, we can then calculate estimates of the variance simply by applying the usual variance formula

$$\frac{1}{B-1}\sum_{i=1}^{B}\left(\hat{V}^* - \sum_{i=1}^{B}\hat{V}^*/B\right)^2,$$
(17.1)

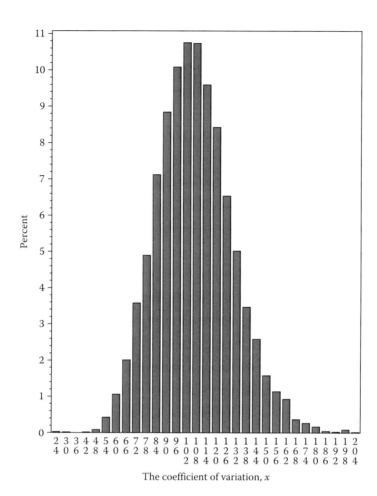

FIGURE 17.1
Bootstrap histogram based on 10,000 replications.

to the resampled values, where B represents the number of bootstrap replications or resamples. For our example $B = 10{,}000$, and from PROC UNIVARIATE in Figure 17.2, the variance estimate is 514.6. What we have just done is to estimate the variance of $\hat{V}$ simply and accurately by applying a computer resampling algorithm using SAS. What we really have done is estimate the value of a complicated mathematical integral via resampling. Note that in addition, we can see from the output information regarding the sample percentiles of the statistic; for example, the estimated 5th and 95th percentiles for V based on $\hat{V}$ are 71.6 and 146.3, respectively. Both the percentile and variance estimates illustrate the high degree of variability of the coefficient of variation for this small sample, and hence the importance of examining these quantities, in addition to relying on the simple point estimate of $\hat{V} = 114.6$ for the purpose of summarizing the data.

The ease of calculation of various sample quantities for a given statistic is the reason why the bootstrap method was so popular when Efron (1979) first developed it. The thinking was that it would change how we carry out statistical inference. As it turns out, things do not always work so well in the bootstrap world, and therefore caution must be used for particular situations. We can extend simple resampling techniques using more sophisticated

The SAS system

The UNIVARIATE procedure
Variable: cv (the coefficient of variation, x)

Moments			
N	10,000	Sum weights	10,000
Mean	106.753833	Sum observations	1067538.33
Std deviation	22.6854201	Variance	514.628287
Skewness	0.35782945	Kurtosis	0.32225676
Uncorrected SS	119109576	Corrected SS	5145768.24
Coeff variation	21.2502161	Std error mean	0.2268542

Basic statistical measures			
Location		Variability	
Mean	106.7538	Std deviation	22.68542
Median	105.5262	Variance	514.62829
Mode	112.5185	Range	181.14325
		Interquartile range	29.95010

Quantiles (Definition 5)	
Quantile	Estimate
100% Max	203.3561
99%	165.0255
95%	146.2990
90%	136.0900
75% Q3	121.0203
50% Median	105.5262
25% Q1	91.0702
10%	78.5930
5%	71.5716
1%	60.0374
0% Min	22.2129

FIGURE 17.2
Summary statistics obtained from bootstrap replications.

bootstrap methods toward creating more accurate confidence intervals and carrying out more exact hypothesis tests in a nonparametric fashion; that is, we will rely on the properties of the empirical distribution function $F_n(x)$ in order to theoretically justify the results, and use the power of SAS to carry out the calculations. The overall difficulty will be to identify the situations where more complicated bootstrap procedures should be used.

The general steps for obtaining basic sample bootstrap quantities are as follows:

1. Determine what you would like to estimate in some unknown continuous population using the appropriate statistic; that is, we wish to estimate the population characteristic θ with the statistic $T(x)$.

2. Generate a *bootstrap sample* of size n from the empirical distribution function $F_n(x)$.

   a. Specifically, draw a sample of size n *with replacement* from the data $x_1, x_2, ..., x_n$.

   b. This provides a single-bootstrap sample $x_1^*, x_2^*, ..., x_n^*$.

3. Calculate a *bootstrap replication* of the statistic of interest $T(x)$, denoted $T(x)^*$, based on the bootstrap sample given by step 2; that is, recalculate $T(x)$ using the resampled x_i^*'s.

4. Repeat steps 2 and 3 B times such that there are now B replications of the $T(x)^*$'s, denoted $T(x)_1^*, T(x)_2^*, ..., T(x)_B^*$. Note that $B \neq n$.

5. The bootstrap mean of the $T(x)^*$'s is given by

$$T(x)^* = \frac{1}{B} \sum_{i=1}^{B} T(x)_i^*$$

6. The variance of $T(x)$ is then given by

$$\frac{1}{B-1} \sum_{i=1}^{B} (T(x)_i^* - T(x)^*)^2$$

For more complicated bootstrap procedures, it will be necessary to carry out double bootstrap resampling plans. The process will follow similarly. Inferential quantities such as confidence intervals for θ and hypothesis testing based on the resampling method described above can be carried out in a variety of ways. These will be discussed in detail in Section 17.3.

17.2 Resampling Data with Replacement in SAS

The majority of nonparametric bootstrap procedures discussed from this point forward rely on the ability to sample from the data with replacement. In this section, we discuss the pieces of code needed to carry out the simple bootstrap in the univariate setting. When we get to more complicated repeated measures and cluster-related data sets elsewhere in the book, we use the code provided below as a jumping-off point. The basic idea is that once you understand the syntax provided in this section, you should be able to easily modify it for most bootstrap-related problems that would be encountered in practice.

It turns out that resampling from the data with replacement can be accomplished relatively easily through the generation of a vector or set of multinomial random variables. The algorithms outlined below are the "front end" for most of bootstrap procedures we intend to discuss. The key to programming the nonparametric bootstrap procedure is to consider carefully how data are managed internally within SAS. The point of the procedures outlined below is to avoid having to create a multitude of arrays or specialized macros, and to try to maximize efficiency, thus making it easier for the novice to carry out the bootstrap procedures. In other instances, we are able to take advantage of PROC SURVEYSELECT, which is an already built-in procedure that allows us to resample the data with replacement. Note, however, for certain problems, one may not be able to avoid using macros or arrays. We deal with a few specialized cases elsewhere in the book.

Let us start with an example data set $x = \{0.5, 0.4, 0.6, 0.2\}$ of size $n = 4$. If we sample from this data set once with replacement, we might obtain a bootstrap replication denoted $x^* = \{0.5, 0.4, 0.6, 0.2\}$. Note that this is equivalent to keeping track of the set of multinomial counts $c = \{2,1,0,1\}$ corresponding to the original data set x as listed and outputting each observation x_i the corresponding c_i number of times, where x_i denotes the ith observation and c_i denotes the corresponding count, for example, $x_2 = 0.4$ and $c_2 = 1$. In other words, sampling with replacement is *exactly* equivalent to generating a set of random multinomial counts with marginal probabilities $1/n$ and outputting the data value for the corresponding number of times. One way to do this in SAS easily and efficiently is to generate random binomial variables conditioned on the margins as described in Davis (1993) and given by the following formula:

$$C_i \sim B\left(n - \sum_{j=0}^{i-1} C_j, \frac{1}{n-i+1}\right) \tag{17.2}$$

for $i = 1, \ldots, n - 1$, where $C_0 = p_0 = 0$ and $C_n = n - \sum_{j=0}^{n-1} C_j$, where $B(n,p)$ denotes a standard binomial distribution. Random binomial variables may be generated using the RANBIN function in SAS. Even though this formula may look intimidating at first glance, it is relatively straightforward to program. Again, note that we are sticking with the convention that a capital C represents a random quantity and a lowercase c represents an observed value. Therefore, in bootstrap parlance, the data x is considered fixed or observed for a given bootstrap resampling procedure, and the multinomial counts C vary randomly every bootstrap replication. The theoretical properties of bootstrap estimators can be examined fairly straightforwardly within this framework by noting that the multinomial counts C are independent of the data X. For our simple example of $n = 4$ observations, we would have for a single-bootstrap resample the following:

1. C_1 is a random binomial variable $B(4,1/4)$.
2. C_2 is a random binomial variable $B(4 - C_1, 1/3)$.
3. C_3 is a random binomial variable $B(4 - C_1 - C_2, 1/2)$.
4. $C_4 = 4 - C_1 - C_2 - C_3$.

We would then want to output the value x_i, C_i number of times for one bootstrap resample. Note that if $n - \sum_{j=0}^{i-1} C_i < 0$, then stop; all subsequent C_i's should be set to 0. The algorithm is easily accomplished in SAS a multiple number of times in a variety of ways. For the first example, let us focus on the most straightforward approach. Let us generate counts for $x = \{0.5, 0.4, 0.6, 0.2\}$, $B = 3$ bootstrap replications without doing anything fancy. We need to generate random binomial variables using the function RANBIN(seed, n, p), where n and p are the parameters of the binomial distribution. The seed dictates the random number stream, and a 0 produces a different random number stream each successive run of the program. Note that there are practical reasons for choosing a non-zero seed, such as the need to recreate a given analysis. In this case, one may choose a positive integer such as 123,453. Seeds less than 0 may also be employed. We refer the reader to see the SAS technical documents for further details.

In order to understand the basic resampling code written below, one must be familiar with the SORT command, in conjunction with the FIRST and LAST commands. In addition, knowledge of the RETAIN command is needed. The function RANBIN is used to generate random binomial variables.

```
data original;
n=4;            /*set the sample size*/
input x_i @@;
do b=1 to 3; /*output the data B times*/
  output;
end;
cards;
0.5 0.4 0.6 0.2
;
proc sort;by b;
```

This first piece of code in `data original` just outputs the same data set three times in a row. We then need to sort the values by b. Now all we do in the next set of code is carry out the generation of multinomial random variables sequentially via a marginal random binomial number generator.

```
data resample;
set original;by b;
retain sumc i; /*need to add the previous
         count to the total */
if first.b then do;
  sumc=0;
  i=1;    /*set counters*/
end;
p=1/(n-i+1); /*p is the probability of a "success"*/

if ^last.b then do;
if n>sumc then c_i=ranbin(0,n-sumc,p); /*generate the binomial variate*/
  else c_i=0;
  sumc=sumc+c_i;
end;
i=i+1;
if last.b then c_i=n-sumc;

proc print;
var b c_i x_i;
```

The statement `else c_i=0` is just a shortcut needed for the cases where we hit the limit of the constraint that $n - \sum_{j=0}^{i-1} C_j$ must be positive. All the other statements are needed for counting purposes and updating the marginal binomial probabilities.

Basically, what we have done is keep track of $n - \sum_{j=0}^{i-1} C_j$ and $\dfrac{1}{n-i+1}$ for $B = 1$, and then we repeated the resampling scheme for $B = 2$ and $B = 3$. The output for a given run is below.

OBS	B	C_I	X_I
1	1	3	0.5
2	1	0	0.4
3	1	0	0.6
4	1	1	0.2
5	2	2	0.5
6	2	0	0.4
7	2	0	0.6
8	2	2	0.2
9	3	1	0.5
10	3	0	0.4
11	3	0	0.6
12	3	3	0.2

What the above program does is basically the nuts and bolts of most univariate boot-strapping procedures. It is easily modified for the multivariate procedures. Note that if there are missing values, they should be eliminated within the first data step.

As an example, consider how the program would work for a simple statistic such as the sample mean $\bar{X} = \sum_{i=1}^{n} X_i/n$. A bootstrap replication of the mean would simply be $\bar{x}^* = \sum_{i=1}^{n} C_i x_i/n$ or, for our example, $\bar{x}_1^* = (3 \times 0.5 + 1 \times 0.2)/4 = 0.426$, or for those who prefer matrix notation, $\bar{x}^* = \mathbf{xc}'/n$. To carry out this process in SAS, simply add the code to the end of the above program:

```
proc means;by b;
var x_i;
weight c_i;
output out=bootstat mean=xbarstar;
```

For the sample mean, we can take advantage of the WEIGHT statement built into PROC MEANS. Since the sample size of $n = 4$ is small, we would basically only need to increase the value of B up to, say, $B = 100$ in this example in order to get a very accurate approximation of the distribution of the sample mean for this data set. Guidelines for the number of resamples will be discussed later. Through the use of the WEIGHT statement, PROC MEANS is "automatically" calculating $\bar{x}^* = \sum_{i=1}^{n} C_i x_i/n$ for each value of B via the BY statement. In a variety of problems, from regression to generalized linear models, we utilize the fact that the WEIGHT utility is built into a number of SAS procedures. From a statistical theory stand-point, in the case of the sample mean, one can easily prove that if $E(\bar{X}) = \mu$, then $E(\bar{X}^*) = \mu$ as well. Note that $E(\bar{X}^*) = E\left(\sum_{i=1}^{n} C_i X_i/n \right) = \sum_{i=1}^{n} E(C_i)E(X_i)/n = \mu$, given $E(C_i) = 1$; that is, remarkably, all bootstrap resampled estimates of the mean are unbiased estimates of μ.

Note that the number of bootstrap replications is typically recommended to be $B = 1000$ or higher for moderately sized data sets (e.g., see Booth and Sarkar, 1998). However, if you can feasibly carry out a higher number of replications, the precision of the boot-strap procedure can only increase; that is, from a theoretical statistical point of view, you can never take too many bootstrap replications. From a practical point of view, you may stretch the memory capacity and speed of your given computer. In general, one should shoot for $B = 1000$. If a value for $B \gg 1000$. can be practically used, then by all means use it. Obviously, the memory requirements for the above algorithm can expand rapidly for moderately sized data sets and values of B around 1000. The above program will run very rapidly; however, it is a "space hog" with respect to disk space.

In some instances, we can keep the code even more simple by replacing the data step resample in the previous approach with PROC SURVEYSELECT, as seen in the following example:

```
proc surveyselect data=original
  method=urs sampsize=4 out=resample;
  by b;

proc print noobs;
var b numberhits x_i;

data restar;set resample;
do ii=1 to numberhits;
  output;
end;
```

The R code is as follows:

```
> resamples <- lapply(1:3, function(i)
+       sample(data, replace = T))
> b1<-c(4, mean(resamples[[1]]), sd(resamples[[1]]), min(resamples[[1]]),
  max(resamples[[1]]))
> names(b1)<-c("N","Mean","Std Dev", "Minimum", "Maximum")
> b2<-c(4,mean(resamples[[2]]),sd(resamples[[2]]),min(resamples[[2]]),max
  (resamples[[2]]))
> names(b2)<-c("N","Mean","Std Dev", "Minimum", "Maximum")
> b3<-c(4,mean(resamples[[3]]),sd(resamples[[3]]),min(resamples[[3]]),max
  (resamples[[1]]))
> names(b3)<-c("N","Mean","Std Dev", "Minimum", "Maximum")
```

method=urs implies unrestricted random sampling with replacement and needs to be specified. Also, note that sampsize=4 corresponds to the sample size of $n = 4$ for this example and needs to be modified manually for different sized data sets. Finally, the output from PROC SURVEYSELECT for this example will look as follows:

b	Number Hits	x_i
1	2	0.5
1	2	0.4
2	1	0.4
2	1	0.6
2	2	0.2
3	1	0.5
3	1	0.4
3	2	0.2

Therefore, there is an additional need to output each observation in the data set resample numberhits times in data set restar. The data from restar are what would then be used in order to calculate the resampled statistic of interest. This approach is slightly more inefficient than the straight generation of conditional multinomial counts, but may be somewhat more straightforward for the novice user. The multinomial approach is what would be recommended if we were carrying out the bootstrap method within PROC IML.

As an alternative to outputting the data set *B* number of times in the input data set, we can use SAS macros, which will carry out the same task as before, albeit somewhat slower. Note, however, that macros tend to be more efficient in terms of space requirements. You do not need to be an expert in macro programming to modify your own programs. The same basic macro language concepts are used throughout the book without too much modification. We refer the reader to see SAS's *Guide to Macro Processing* for further details (SAS Institute 2015). From our point of view, a macro processor basically simplifies repetitive data entry and data manipulation tasks. The macro facility makes it possible to define complex input and output "subroutines." However, with respect to bootstrapping, we need to know only a few basic concepts:

1. All macros have a user-defined macro name, a beginning, and an end.
2. Variables can be passed to macros upon the macro being called.
3. It is possible to repeat a data step over and over again via looping within a macro.
4. Macro variables can be passed to data steps and certain PROCs.

The key macro statements that we use in the bootstrapping program below and throughout the book consist of the following:

1. `%macro multiwt(brep)`: The beginning of the macro is defined by the `%macro` statement. We have chosen to name the macro `multiwt` and pass it the variable named `brep`, which represents the number of bootstrap replications that we have chosen. For this example, the number of bootstrap replications $B = 3$.
2. `%do bsim=1 %to &brep`: The beginning of the macro do-loop; given by the `%do` command. The macro variable `&brep` is given at the macro call. The variable `bsim` is the looping index variable.
3. `b=&bsim`: The macro variable `&bsim` is passed to the data step in order to indicate the current bootstrap resample. An ampersand indicates to the compiler that `bsim` is a macro variable.
4. `%end`: The `%end` closes the macro do-loop.
5. `%mend`: The `%mend` command signifies the end of the macro `multiwt`.
6. `%multiwt(3)`: The command `%multiwt(3)` is the macro call that passes the value of 3 to the macro variable `brep`.

Based on these definitions, we developed a macro version of the bootstrap program contained earlier in this section. In addition, we automatically determine the value for the sample size *n* in this program via the NOBS command. The macro variable `brep` is used to represent the number of bootstrap replications *B*. All that has basically changed compared to the previous code is that we are generating the c's one macro iteration at a time. Later on, we illustrate what additional calculations will be carried out within the macro `multiwt` and what calculations will be carried out outside the scope of the macro.

```
data original;
input x_i @@;
cards;
```

```
0.5 0.4 0.6 0.2
;

data sampsize;
 set original nobs=nobs; /*automatically obtain the sample size*/
 n=nobs;

%macro multiwt(brep);
%do bsim=1 %to &brep;

data resample;
set sampsize;
retain sumc i; /*need to add the previous
                count to the total */
b=&bsim;
if _n_=1 then do;
   sumc=0;
   i=1;
end;
p=1/(n-i+1); /*p is the probability of a "success"*/

if _n_<n then do;
if n>sumc then c_i=ranbin(0,n-sumc,p); /*generate the binomial variate*/
 else c_i=0;
 sumc=sumc+c_i;
end;
i=i+1;
if _n_=n then c_i=n-sumc;

proc append data=resample out=total;

%end;
%mend;
%multiwt(3);

proc print data=total;
var b c_i x_i;
```

The same program may be rewritten using PROC SURVEYSELECT. Note that we had to create a variable called `dummy` in order to automatically input the sample size into PROC SURVEYSELECT. We also no longer have the ability to weight observations. As noted earlier, this may be slightly more inefficient than the previous set of code.

```
data original;
input x_i @@;
dummy=1; /*need a dummy variable for surveyselect*/
cards;
0.5 0.4 0.6 0.2
;

data sampsize;
 set original nobs=nobs;
 _nsize_=nobs; /*control variable for surveyselect*/
 if _n_=1 then output;

%macro multiwt(brep);
```

```
%do bsim=1 %to &brep;

proc surveyselect data=original noprint
 method=urs sampsize=sampsize out=resample;
 strata dummy;

data restar;set resample;
b=&bsim;
do ii=1 to numberhits;
 output;
end;

proc append data=restar out=total;

%end;
%mend;
%multiwt(3);

proc print;
var b x_i;
```

Oftentimes, for simple univariate samples, it is much more efficient in terms of storage issues to use PROC IML in order to carry out the bootstrap resampling methodology. From the *SAS/IML User's Guide*, we have the following description: "SAS/IML software gives you access to a powerful and flexible programming language (Interactive Matrix Language) in a dynamic, interactive environment." (SAS Institute 2015, p. 3). With respect to bootstrap methods, PROC IML is very useful through the efficient use of its array structure. We can use IML in conjunction with other PROCs, macros, or as a stand-alone programming language. Carrying out the multiwt macro from above in a similar fashion using PROC IML consists of the following code:

```
data original;
input x_i @@;
cards;
0.5 0.4 0.6 0.2
;

proc iml;
 use original;
 read all into data;

 /*Create a n by 1 vector of data original
called data*/

 n=nrow(data); /*Calculate the sample size*/
 bootdata=1:n; /*Array to hold one bootstrap resample*/

brep=3;        /*Set the number of bootstrap resamples*/
 do i=1 to brep;
  do j=1 to n;
   index=int(ranuni(0)*n)+1;
   bootdata[j]=data[index];
  end;
  print i bootdata;
 end;

quit;
```

```
/*********Listing File*********/
I BOOTDATA
1 0.5     0.4     0.5     0.5
I BOOTDATA
2 0.4     0.5     0.4     0.5
I BOOTDATA
3 0.6     0.5     0.4     0.2
```

The USE and READ statements simply retrieve SAS data sets and import them into PROC IML. Alternatively, data may be entered directly in PROC IML with a statement such as

```
data={0.5, 0.4, 0.6, 0.2};
```

There are infinitely many possibilities with respect to utilizing this basic IML code. We may want to carry out some calculations within IML or outside IML. We modify the code below for specific cases throughout the book. The main concept is the generation of a random indexing function labeled `index` in the IML code. Basically, we are generating a random integer from 1 to n. This allows us to easily resample from the data `original` using a simple array structure. We see the results for three successive bootstrap resamples with $x_1^* = \{0.5, 0.4, 0.5, 0.5\}$, $x_2^* = \{0.4, 0.5, 0.5, 0.5\}$, and $x_3^* = \{0.6, 0.5, 0.4, 0.2\}$. The only real disadvantage of utilizing PROC IML is that it requires an additional SAS programming skill set.

In later sections, we highlight modifications to the above code for repeated measure designs, clustered data, and even simple two-group comparisons. The appendix includes the program jackboot.sas written by the SAS Institute. We utilize it for more complicated procedures discussed elsewhere in the book.

17.3 Theoretical Quantities of Interest

In this section, we provide a sketch of the common quantities of interest in statistical estimation and outline the corresponding bootstrap statistical theory needed in order to carry out the estimation procedures. These include things such as bias and variance estimation, confidence interval calculations, and the calculation of other inferential quantities, such as bootstrap p-values. For a detailed treatment of bootstrap theory, the reader is referred to Shao and Tu (1995). Again, the ultimate focus is on how to carry out the various bootstrap methods using SAS. As stated earlier, the primary assumption of the bootstrap method is that the function of the empirical distribution, $T(F_n(x))$, should approximate well the same function evaluated using the true distribution, namely, $T(F(x))$; for example, the sample mean is generally the optimal estimator for the expected value or population mean. In order for the more straightforward bootstrap methods to work, the distribution of the statistic $T(F_n(x))$ should be "well behaved" in the univariate as well as in the multivariate setting. There are more specific assumptions to be made with respect to certain statistics that may not have the desired distributional properties. The diagnostics and possible corrective actions for ill-posed problems or ill-behaving statistics are outlined below.

What oftentimes gets lost within the implementation of many bootstrapping procedures, due to the empirical and computational aspects of the method, is the focus of the problem, that is, what is the population quantity that we are estimating? Let us start by reviewing the general notation. Let $T(F(X)) = \theta$ represent the population quantity or parameter that we are interested in, where T is a function, F represents the population cumulative distribution function described earlier, and X denotes a continuous random variable. For example, $T(F(X))$ could represent a population mean, standard deviation, or regression coefficient, or any other population parameter of interest. The basic bootstrap utilizes $T(F_n(x))$ to estimate $T(F(X))$ by plugging in F_n for F. In addition, things such as moment estimators of $E(T(F(x))^k | F(X))$ can be estimated similarly using $E(T(F_n(x))^k | F_n(X))$. Ultimately, the most sophisticated bootstrap methods will not be able to overcome the cases where $T(F_n(x))$ is a poor estimator of $T(F(X))$, for example, estimating inferential quantities involving extreme values. Therefore, careful consideration of the choice of estimator is needed before proceeding with bootstrap methodologies.

There are many instances in which there are a variety of statistics to choose from for estimating the same population quantity. Two important criteria for selecting a statistic are the bias and variance of that statistic. Depending on the problem at hand, other important criteria may include things such as robustness to outliers. A criterion that combines bias and variance quantities into one measure is the mean squared error (MSE). The MSE is defined below. A statistic is defined to be biased if

$$E[T(F_n(X)) | F(X)] = T(F(X)) + b \tag{17.3}$$

that is, the expected value of the statistic $T(F_n(x))$ conditional on the distribution of X has bias given by the value of b. In the ideal situation in which $b = 0$, the statistic is said to be *unbiased*. For example, let $T(F_n(x)) = \bar{x}$ be the sample mean from a continuous population; then $E(T(F_n(X)) | F(X)) = E(X)$ and $b = 0$. This illustrates that $\bar{x}$ is an unbiased estimator of the population mean $E(X)$. If b is known, then it is desirable to define a new statistic $T(F_n(X)) - b$ in order to eliminate the bias. A well-known example of a biased correct statistic is that of the maximum likelihood estimator for the variance σ^2 given a normal population. The maximum likelihood estimator of the variance, $\hat{\sigma}^2 = \sum_{i=1}^{n} (x_i - \bar{x})^2 / n$ has expectation $E[\hat{\sigma}^2 | F(X)] = \sigma^2 - \sigma^2/n$, where $b = -\sigma^2/n$. As it turns out, we do not need to know the bias b in this case in order to make a correction. By applying a simple adjustment, the well-known bias-corrected version $\hat{\sigma}^2 = \sum_{i=1}^{n} (x_i - \bar{x})^2 / (n-1)$ has an expectation of σ^2 with $b = 0$. A bias correction that adds or subtracts a constant amount from a statistic has no impact in terms of increasing or decreasing the variance of the statistic. This is not exactly the case in our normal variance example where we applied a multiplier of $n/(n-1)$ to correct the bias. This multiplicative correction has the impact of inflating the variance of the estimator.

For a large majority of situations, the bias b takes the form $b = c_1/n + c_2/n^2 + ...$, a decreasing function of the sample size n; that is, the bias goes to zero as the sample size n goes to infinity. Since, however, in the real world we sometimes have to deal with small samples, the bias is oftentimes nonnegligible. In these instances, if c_1/n is easily calculated, we might consider an estimator of the form $T(F_n(X)) - c_1/n$, which would have what is termed a first-order bias correction; that is, the bias is of order n^{-2} as opposed to n^{-1} and goes to zero faster as the sample size n goes to infinity. In this case, the estimator $T(F_n(X)) - c_1/n$ is still biased, but will be an improvement over the original estimator $T(F_n(X))$. Other times, c_1/n might be estimable such that a less biased estimator may take the form $T(F_n(X) | F(X)) - \hat{c}_1/n$, where $\hat{c}_1$ is estimated from the data. This first-order estimable type of bias correction is what we can typically handle via bootstrapping. It is important to note that in the bias estimation procedure, the first-order bias term will be minimized by estimating and then subtracting $\hat{c}_1/n$. It will not be eliminated. Since the expectation of the arithmetic average is $E(\bar{x}\,|\,F(X)) = E(X)$, clearly it is an unbiased estimator of the population mean no matter what the true underlying continuous distribution is. What if we were interested in estimating the population median $T(F(X)) = F^{-1}(1/2)$ and again we chose $T(F_n(X)) = \bar{x}$ as the statistic. Under the assumption that the distribution of X is symmetrical and given certain moment conditions, $E[T(F(X))|F(X)] = F^{-1}(1/2)$; that is, $\bar{x}$ is an unbiased estimator of the population median (as well as the mean) in this case. However, if the true distribution of X were asymmetrical or skewed, then in general, $E[T(F(X))|F(X)] = F^{-1}(1/2) + b$; that is, $\bar{x}$ would be a biased estimator of the population median. In this example, it is somewhat clear that you would not want to use $\bar{x}$ to estimate the sample median for all situations. However, you may want to use it in certain instances, say, for example, under the strong assumption that the population has a normal distribution. Bootstrap methods will not overcome the shortcomings of a poor choice of estimator by the analyst. Employing the sample mean to estimate the population median given asymmetry is a poor strategy in terms of bias properties.

In general, the exact form for the value of b cannot be calculated unless we assume something about the distribution of the random variable X. Otherwise, we tend to rely on large sample approximations to approximate the bias. Therefore, if nothing is known a priori about the distribution of X, then a better estimate of the median is possibly $T(F_n(X)) = F_n^{-1}(1/2)$. Note, however, that even the statistic $T(F_n(X)) = F_n^{-1}(1/2)$ is a biased estimator of $T(F(X)) = F^{-1}(1/2)$ given an asymmetrical population. The bias, however, would be much less than that of the sample mean for highly skewed distributions. Now there is a new dilemma. There are other accepted statistics for estimating the median besides $T(F_n(X)) = F_n^{-1}(1/2)$. Many of the simple versions may be calculated in PROC UNIVARIATE by varying the PCTLDEF command. Other versions can be easily programmed in SAS. All have varying degrees of bias in terms of estimating the median. Some are biased even if the population is symmetric, for example, using a single order statistic to estimate the median given an even sample size. Typical estimators of the median include a single order statistic, the average of a small set of interior order statistics, all the way up to kernel estimators, which consist of taking a weighted average of the set of order statistics (e.g., see Sheather and Marron, 1990). If there are so many methods for estimating the median, how does one choose the optimal estimator? Typically, this is done through the examination of the MSE. The MSE is defined as

$$MSE = E\{[T(F_n(X)) - \theta^2\,|\,F(X)\} = \mathrm{var}[T(F_n(X))|F(X)] + b^2, \tag{17.4}$$

and is a joint measure of the variance of the statistic plus its bias squared. If competing statistics are unbiased, then comparing the MSEs reduces to comparing the variance of each estimator and choosing the one with the smaller variance. Even when the quantities b, $\mathrm{var}[T(F_n(X))]$ and the MSE cannot be calculated, they might possibly be estimated via bootstrapping. Note, however, that caution must be taken when considering the corresponding estimators. Only estimators with bias of the form described (a series proportional to terms of order $1/n$) above can be adequately corrected via bootstrap methods. Ultimately, the analyst needs to have at least some basic knowledge of the theoretical properties of the statistic $T(F_n(X))$ before proceeding with any statistical methodology, including bootstrapping; that is, no statistical model can be applied appropriately without certain assumptions being met (approximately).

17.3.1 Bias Estimation

If the bias of a statistic takes the general form $b = c_1/n + c_2/n^2 + \ldots$ described above, then we may estimate a first-order bias correction via bootstrapping. In general, we cannot eliminate bias via bootstrapping, but only reduce it. In order to do this, however, we require some knowledge about the statistic in terms of what it is supposed to be estimating. Hence, some careful thought is needed before utilizing this methodology. An example of a statistic that would be biased in such a way would be the simple estimate of the median given an asymmetrical distribution; that is, average the middle ordered observations if n is even or take the middle ordered observation if n is odd. The median is easily calculated via PROC UNIVARIATE using the default definition. A bootstrap estimator of the bias is then given by replacing $F(X)$ with $F_n(X)$ in Equation 17.3. It takes the form

$$\hat{b} = E[T^*(F_n(X)) \mid F_n(X)] - T(F_n(X)). \tag{17.5}$$

A bootstrap bias-corrected version of the statistic is then given by

$$T(F_n(X)) - \hat{b} = 2T(F_n(X)) - E[T^*(F_n(X)) \mid F_n(X)].$$

Note that this correction does not eliminate the first-order bias term c_1/n. It only reduces the bias by a fractional amount since typically the estimate $\hat{b}$ is itself biased. The bias of the bias reduced estimator $T(F_n(X)) - \hat{b}$ can again be estimated via a second round of bootstrapping, and so on for as many iterations as desired. For each successive round of bootstrap bias reduction, the variance of the new estimator will in general increase; that is, for most statistics, there is in general a bias–variance trade-off that can be quantified through the estimation of the MSE. Because of this property, typically only first-order bias estimation is carried forth via bootstrapping. This property will be discussed below in the variance estimation subsection. The bootstrap estimate of the expectation $E[T(F_n(X)) \mid F_n(X)]$ can be carried out easily via resampling and is given by

$$\bar{T}^*(F_n(X)) = \sum_{i=1}^{B} T_i^*(F_n(X))/B \tag{17.6}$$

where $T_i^*(F_n(X))$ is the statistic recalculated for the ith bootstrap resample and B denotes the number of bootstrap resamples.

As an example, suppose we wish to estimate the median platelet count from $n = 20$ neonates in the intensive care unit, estimate the bias of the sample median, and then calculate a bias-corrected estimate of the median. We will use the simple straightforward resampling program found in Section 17.2 to carry out the bias estimation procedure. What we do within the body of the program is resample from the data set $B = 5000$ times and then calculate the median for each of the 5000 resamples. Note that simple bootstrap estimation of the bias requires a great deal of resamples, especially for nonsmooth statistics such as the median. If possible, we recommend somewhere around $B = 3000$ to $B = 5000$ resamples. More efficient routines exist for a subset of statistics and are given by first averaging the multinomial weights (e.g., see Efron, 1990). This approach, however, does not work well for statistics such as the median that consists of a class of statistics called L-estimators, that is, statistics that are linear combinations of order statistics. Basically, the more efficient routine can be matched by increasing the number of bootstrap replications to $B = 5000$ or $B = 10,000$. The platelet data are read in the DATA step named counts.

```
data counts;
label pl_ct='platelet count';
input pl_ct @@;
cards;
230 222 179 191 103 293 316 520 143 226
225 255 169 204  99 107 280 226 143 259
;

proc univariate noprint data=counts;
var pl_ct;
output out=med median=median;

/***********Begin Standard Resampling Algorithm**********/
data resample;
set counts nobs=nobs;
n=nobs;
do b=1 to 5000; /*output the data B times*/
output;
end;

proc sort;by b;

data boot;
set resample;by b;
retain sumc i; /*need to add the previous
         count to the total */
if first.b then do;
   sumc=0;
   i=1;
end;
p=1/(n-i+1); /*p is the probability of a "success"*/

if ^last.b then do;
if n>sumc then c_i=ranbin(0,n-sumc,p); /*generate the binomial variate*/
 else c_i=0;
 sumc=sumc+c_i;
end;
i=i+1;
if last.b then c_i=n-sumc;

data outboot;
set boot;
if c_i>0 then do;
do i=1 to c_i;
 output;
end;
end;

/*************End Standard Resampling Algorithm************/
```

```
proc univariate noprint;by b;
var pl_ct;
output out=bootmed median=median;
proc means data=bootmed;
var median;
output out=remed mean=bootmed;

data bias;merge med remed;
label
  bc_med='Bias Corrected Median'
  median='Sample Median'
  bootmed='Estimated Expected Value'
  bias='Estimated Bias';
bias=bootmed-median;
bc_med=median-bias;

proc print label noobs;
var median bootmed bias bc_med;
```

Sample Median	Estimated Expected Value	Estimated Bias	Bias Corrected Median
223.5	215.220	-8.2796	231.780

The corresponding R code is as follows:

```
> data<-c(230, 222, 179, 191, 103, 293, 316, 520, 143, 226,
+        225, 255, 169, 204,  99, 107, 280, 226, 143, 259)
> med<-median(data)
> resamples <- lapply(1:5000, function(i)
+       sample(data, replace = T))
> median<-lapply(1:5000, function(i)
+       median(resamples[[i]]))
> vector<-c()
> for (i in 1:5000){
+       vector<-c(vector,median[[i]])
+       i<-i+1
+ }
> output<-c(5000,mean(vector),sd(vector),min(vector),max(vector))
> names(output)<-c("N","Mean","Std Dev", "Minimum", "Maximum")
> output1<-c(med,mean(vector),mean(vector)-med, med-(mean(vector)-med))
> names(output1)<-c('Sample Median','Estimated Expected Value','Estimated
  Bias','Bias Corrected Median')
```

We then estimate the median using PROC UNIVARIATE to be 223.5 from the original data set. This was followed by our core resampling algorithm where we averaged the $B = 5000$ median replications or $T_i^*(F_n(X))$'s output from data step outboot in order to estimate the expected value given by (17.3). The value we obtained for the estimate of the bootstrap expectation was 215.22, which in turn gives us an estimate of the bias of $\hat{b} = -8.28$. Therefore, the bootstrap bias-corrected median turns out to be $223.5 - (-8.28) = 231.78$ or, equivalently, $2 \times 223.50 - 215.22 = 231.78$. These calculations were carried out in the DATA step bias. Note that even though the estimate of 231.78 is less biased than the original estimate of 223.50, it is likely to be more variable. The trade-offs between the two competing estimators can be examined via the MSE. This first requires an estimate of the variance of each estimator (the original and bias-corrected version). If one wishes, we can even correct the bias of the bias-corrected median estimator via another round of double bootstrapping. This will be illustrated in conjunction with the variance estimation example given in the next section.

17.3.2 Variance Estimation, MSE Estimation, and the Double Bootstrap

Variance and MSE estimation for a given statistic are relatively straightforward. It is, however, more complicated to estimate the variance of the bias-corrected statistic $2T(F_n(X)) - E[T^*(F_n(X)) | F_n(X)] = 2T(F_n(X)) - \bar{T}^*(F_n(X))$. This requires a second round of bootstrapping referred to as the double bootstrap in the literature. As you will see, the double bootstrap is a computationally intensive routine when using the most straightforward SAS programming methods. For the simple case, that is, the bootstrap variance estimate of $\text{var}[T^*(F_n(X)) | F_n(X)]$, simply apply the formula

$$\frac{1}{B-1} \sum_{i=1}^{B} [T_i^*(F_n(X)) - \bar{T}^*(F_n(X))]^2,$$

where $\bar{T}^*(F_n(X))$ is given by Equation 17.6 and B again represents the number of bootstrap replications. As described above, the bootstrap estimate of the MSE is simply the bootstrap estimate of the variance plus the bias estimate squared. From our previous example for the median platelet counts we obtained

```
                Analysis Variable : median the median, pl_ct
N          Mean              Std Dev            Minimum            Maximum
-----------------------------------------------------------------------------
5000       215.2204000       18.0331351         125.0000000        280.0000000
-----------------------------------------------------------------------------
```

This gives the bootstrap estimate of the variance for the median to be approximately $\text{var}[T^*(F_n(X)) | F_n(X)] = 18.03^2 = 325.08$ and the MSE estimate to be approximately $325.08 + 8.28^2 = 393.64$. Note that if we reran the program with a random seed, the variance estimates would vary less than 1%. If one wants even more precision in the estimate, then more resamples are needed, that is, increase B.

In order to estimate the variance of the bias-corrected estimate $2T(F_n(X)) - \bar{T}^*(F_n(X))$, we need to implement a second round of bootstrapping. This is easily done using a macro after some modification of the original resampling program. Note, however, that this program is computationally intensive and may run for many hours, depending on the system and the sample size n. We show that by utilizing some preliminary statistical scratch work, we can cut the macro time in half. A more efficient version of this program for our example is given using PROC IML, which ultimately ran in real time for about half an hour on our SUN Ultra 10. This is compared to the original macro, which took many hours. It is important to note that if an explicit equation for the variance of $T(F_n(X))$ exists, for example, the sample mean, we can in general avoid the double-bootstrap routine. This is illustrated with specific procedures elsewhere in the book.

Double bootstrapping is a slight modification of the standard bootstrap described in Section 17.2. It is basically a bootstrap within a bootstrap and consists of an inner and an outer bootstrap "layer." The outer bootstrap is the standard bootstrap resample. The inner bootstrap is a resample of the first set of resampled observations. The algorithm consists of the following steps:

1. As stated earlier, determine what you would like to estimate in some unknown continuous population using the appropriate statistic; that is, we wish to estimate the population characteristic θ with the statistic $T(x)$.

2. Generate a *bootstrap sample* of size n from the empirical distribution function $F_n(x)$.

   a. Specifically, draw a sample of size n *with replacement* from the data $x_1, x_2, ..., x_n$.

   b. This provides a single-bootstrap sample $x_1^*, x_2^*, ..., x_n^*$.

   c. Calculate a *bootstrap replication* of the statistic of interest $T(x)$, denoted $T(x)^*$, by recalculating $T(x)$ using the resampled x_i^*'s.

      i. Now for the inner bootstrap, draw a sample of size n *with replacement* from the outer bootstrap data $x_1^*, x_2^*, ..., x_n^*$.

      ii. This provides a single-bootstrap inner sample $x_1^{**}, x_2^{**}, ..., x_n^{**}$.

      iii. Calculate the bootstrap resample statistic of interest from the inner bootstrap sample and denote it $T(x)^{**}$.

      iv. repeat steps i and ii B_2 times.

3. Repeat step 2 B_1 times such that there are now B_1 replications of the $T(x)^*$'s, denoted $T(x)_1^*, T(x)_2^*, ... T(x)_B^*$, and $B_1 \times B_2$ double-bootstrapped $T(x)^{**}$'s, denoted by the double subscript $T(x)_{ij}^{**}$, where $i = 1, 2, ..., B_1$ and $j = 1, 2, ..., B_2$.

4. The bootstrap mean of the $T(x)^*$'s is given as before by

$$\overline{T}(x)^* = \frac{1}{B_1} \sum_{i=1}^{B} T(x)_i^*$$

5. The variance of $T(x)$ is then given by

$$\frac{1}{B_1 - 1} \sum_{i=1}^{B_1} (T(x)_i^* - \overline{T}(x)^*)^2$$

6. The bootstrap mean of the $T(x)^{**}$'s is given by

$$\overline{T}(x)^{**} = \frac{1}{B_1 B_2} \sum_{i=1}^{B_1} \sum_{j=1}^{B_2} T(x)_{ij}^{**}$$

7. The variance estimate is then given by

$$\frac{1}{B_1 B_2 - 1} \sum_{i=1}^{B_1} \sum_{j=1}^{B_2} (T(x)_{ij}^{**} - \overline{T}(x)^{**})^2$$

Now with respect to estimating the variance of the bias-corrected bootstrap estimator $T(F_n(X)) - \hat{b}$, it is important to note that within the bootstrap estimation procedure,

$$\text{var}[T(F_n(X)) - \hat{b} \mid F_n(X)] = \text{var}[2T(F_n(X)) - T^*(F_n^*(X)) \mid F_n(X)]$$

is estimated by plugging in $F_n^*(X)$ for $F_n(X)$ in the above equation such that the variance of $T(F_n(X)) - \hat{b}$ is given by

$$\text{var}[T^*(F_n^*(X)) \mid F_n^*(X)],$$

conditional on the x's. This is true because with respect to the original statistic, $T(F_n(X))$ is a constant within the inner layer of bootstrapping conditional on $F_n^*(X)$. This simplifies the calculations somewhat.

For our example, we will now estimate the statistic of interest, and its bias-corrected version, along with the corresponding standard deviations, and MSEs of each estimator. The most straightforward approach is to reuse the macro presented earlier, by basically cutting and pasting it so that we repeat it within a double do-loop. This is the most computationally intensive approach for carrying out the double bootstrap in SAS; however, it is also the most straightforward. Therefore, if you do not mind letting your program run overnight or in the background, this approach is fine. If time or CPU costs are critical, this approach should be avoided if double bootstrapping is needed. Within the double-bootstrap example we also utilize a few additional SAS commands and PROCs:

1. Within the `options` command, utilize the `nonotes` and `nosource` commands. This is one way to suppress a large log file during successive macro loops. The log file would grow for thousands of pages if kept unchecked.
2. We utilize PROC APPEND to stack the output data set. Every time, through the macro loop, we can add an element to a given data set via PROC APPEND.
3. PROC DATASETS is useful for deleting data sets from the current loop. This saves some space during the execution of the program.

Note that within the execution of the current program, I decided to "fix" the random number seeds to b1+100 and b2+100. This simply guarantees that the results are consistent over time. This is important if the results need to be reconstructed for some future purpose; for example, the Food and Drug Administration (FDA) might wish to examine the program results.

Even though the macro programs that follow pertaining to our example may look terribly daunting, they basically consist of the following skeleton. There is an outer loop and an inner loop indexed by the macro variables `bsim1` and `bsim2`. This is given by the sketch below, followed by the first version of the program:

```
data counts; /*READ IN DATA*/
data sampsize; /*DETERMINE SAMPLE SIZE*/

%macro multiwt(brep1,brep2); /*OUTER LOOP*/
%do bsim1=1 %to &brep1; /*outer bootstrap layer*/
  data resample; /*RESAMPLE BREP1 NUMBER OF TIMES*/
```

```
     proc univariate /*CALCULATE THE MEDIAN FROM BREP1
                      NUMBER OF RESAMPLES*/
     proc append data=med1 out=first; /*APPEND THE RESULT*/

     %do bsim2=1 %to &brep2; /*INNER LOOP*/

     data resample2; /*RESAMPLE FROM THE RESAMPLE BREP2 NUMBER OF TIMES*/
     proc univariate noprint data=double; /*CALCULATE THE RESAMPLE
       MEDIAN*/
     proc append data=med2 out=second; /*APPEND THE RESULT*/
 %end;
%end;

%mend; /*MACRO END*/
%multiwt(5000,100);

proc means data=first; /*RESULTS OF INNER AND OUTER LOOP*/
proc means data=second;
```

Now what follows is the full program with the basic resampling program based on multinomial weights inserted.

```
data counts;
label pl_ct='platelet count';
input pl_ct @@;
cards;
230 222 179 191 103 293 316 520 143 226
225 255 169 204  99 107 280 226 143 259
;

data sampsize;
 set counts nobs=nobs;
 n=nobs;

%macro multiwt(brep1,brep2);
%do bsim1=1 %to &brep1; /*outer bootstrap layer*/

/***********Begin Standard Resampling Algorithm**********/

data resample;
set sampsize;
retain sumc i; /*need to add the previous
                count to the total */

b1=&bsim1;
if _n_=1 then do;
 sumc=0;
 i=1;
end;
p=1/(n-i+1); /*p is the probability of a "success"*/

if _n_<n then do;
if n>sumc then c_i=ranbin(b1+100,n-sumc,p); /*generate the binomial
  variate*/
 else c_i=0;
 sumc=sumc+c_i;
```

```
end;
i=i+1;
if _n_=n then c_i=n-sumc;


data main;set resample;
if c_i>0 then do;
do i=1 to c_i;
 output;
 end;
end;


proc univariate noprint data=main;
var pl_ct;
output out=med1 median=median;


proc append data=med1 out=first;


%do bsim2=1 %to &brep2; /*inner bootstrap layer*/
/**********Begin Standard Inner Resampling Algorithm**********/


data resample2;
set main;
retain sumc2 i2; /*need to add the previous
                   count to the total */

b2=&bsim2;
if _n_=1 then do;
  sumc2=0;
  i2=1;
end;
p2=1/(n-i2+1); /*p is the probability of a "success"*/


if _n_<n then do;
 if n>sumc2 then
  c2_i=ranbin(b2+100,n-sumc2,p2); /*generate the binomial variate*/
 else c2_i=0;
 sumc2=sumc2+c2_i;
end;
i2=i2+1;
if _n_=n then c2_i=n-sumc2;


data double;set resample2;
if c2_i>0 then do;
do i=1 to c2_i;
 output;
 end;
end;
proc univariate noprint data=double;
var pl_ct;
output out=med2 median=median;
```

```
proc append data=med2 out=second;
%end;
%end;
/***********End Double Bootstrap Resampling Algorithm***********/

%mend;
%multiwt(5000,100);

proc means data=first;
var median;

proc means data=second;
var median;
```

The MEANS Procedure
Analysis Variable : median the median, pl_ct

N	Mean	Std Dev	Minimum	Maximum
5000	217.2425000	18.3955055	138.0000000	293.0000000

The MEANS Procedure
Analysis Variable : median the median, pl_ct

N	Mean	Std Dev	Minimum	Maximum
500000	213.9920790	26.2817476	99.0000000	520.0000000

Recall that the sample median for our example was $T(F_n) = 223.5$. The corresponding expectation and variance estimates from this run of the program are $E[T^*(F_n(X))|F_n(X)] = 217.2$ and $var[T^*(F_n(X))|F_n(X)] = 338.4$, slightly different from the previous run of the program given earlier where $E[T^*(F_n(X))|F_n(X)] = 215.2$ and $var[T^*(F_n(X))|F_n(X)] = 393.6$. If we ran the program $B = 10,000$ times, the discrepancy between runs would be less. The size of B then becomes a decision for the analyst with respect to efficiency and computational accuracy versus computational speed versus the application (exploratory or confirmatory). The bias-corrected estimate of the median based on this run is $2T(F_n) - E[T^*(F_n(X))|F_n(X)] = 2 \times 223.5 - 217.2 = 229.8$, with variance given by the inner bootstrap layer of $var[T^{**}(F_n(X))|F_n^*(X)] = 26.28^2 = 690.6$ The bias of the more complicated bias-corrected median $2T(F_n) - E[T^*(F_n(X))|F_n(X)]$ turns out to be calculated as $E[T^{**}(F_n(X))|F_n^*(X)] - 2E[T^*(F_n(X))|F_n(X)] + T(F_n) = 213.99 - 2 \times 217.24 + 223.5 = 3.0$. So as we expect, the bias of the new estimator is much less than the original median, 3.0 versus 6.3, respectively. However, the variance is close to twice as large. The MSE given by Equation 17.4 for the median $T(F_n)$ is then given by $338.4 + 6.3^2 = 378.1$ versus the MSE of $2T(F_n) - E[T^*(F_n(X))|F_n(X)]$, which is equal to $690.6 + 3.0^2 = 699.6$. If MSE is the overall criterion for the choice of estimator, then clearly the straight sample mean is the appropriate choice. If bias reduction is more important, the bootstrap bias-corrected version of the median may be more appropriate. Ultimately, it depends on the specific problem under consideration.

As noted before, the basic double-bootstrap program can run for hours for a small sample size. A slightly more efficient program with respect to storage is given below.

The modifications consist of doing some preliminary calculations. For each of the sets of inner subsamples we do not store every single $T^{**}(F_n(X))$; instead, we calculate the sum and sums of squares $T^{**}(F_n(X))$ after the completion of each of the outer loops indexed by bsim1 in the sample program. Notationally, these sums would correspond to $\sum_{i=1}^{B_2} T(x)_{ij}^{**}$ and $\sum_{i=1}^{B_2} (T(x)_{ij}^{**})^2$, respectively. In the sample program, these quantities are given by the variables median and median _ sq and are appended at the end of each run through the B_1 outer loop. This allows us to store far fewer elements over the run of the program, and hence cuts the run time in half. After the completion of the macro, we then can calculate the overall estimated mean and variance of $T^{**}(F_n(X))$ through some standard algebraic formulas given in the program by

```
exp_median2=s2/(&brep1*&brep2);
var2=(s2_sq-(&brep1*&brep2)*exp_median2**2)/(&brep1*&brep2-1);,
```

where s2 and s2 _ sq correspond to adding $\sum_{i=1}^{B_2} T(x)_{ij}^{**}$ and $\sum_{i=1}^{B_2} (T(x)_{ij}^{**})^2$ over the entirety of the B_1 runs. The point of this example carries throughout bootstrapping. A little up-front hard work in terms of programming can lead to substantial gains in computational efficiency. These programs can be used over and over again with a variety of different statistics. Note, however, that in practical terms, the most efficient way to double-bootstrap in SAS is via PROC IML.

```
data counts;
label pl_ct='platelet count';
input pl_ct @@;
cards;
230 222 179 191 103 293 316 520 143 226
225 255 169 204  99 107 280 226 143 259
;

data sampsize;
 set counts nobs=nobs;
 n=nobs;

%macro multiwt(brep1,brep2);
%do bsim1=1 %to &brep1; /*outer bootstrap layer*/

/**********Begin Standard Outer Resampling Algorithm**********/

data resample;
set sampsize;
retain sumc i; /*need to add the previous
        count to the total */
b1=&bsim1;
if _n_=1 then do;
 sumc=0;
 i=1;
end;
p=1/(n-i+1); /*p is the probability of a "success"*/
```

```
if _n_<n then do;
 if n>sumc then c_i=ranbin(b1+100,n-sumc,p); /*generate the binomial
 variate*/
 else c_i=0;
 sumc=sumc+c_i;
end;
i=i+1;
if _n_=n then c_i=n-sumc;

data main;set resample;
if c_i >0 then do;
do i=1 to c_i;
 output;
 end;
end;

proc univariate noprint data=main;
var pl_ct;
output out=med1 median=median;

%do bsim2=1 %to &brep2; /*inner bootstrap layer*/

/***********Begin Standard Inner Resampling Algorithm**********/

data resample2;
set main;
retain sumc2 i2; /*need to add the previous
                    count to the total */
b2=&bsim2;
if _n_=1 then do;
 sumc2=0;
 i2=1;
end;
p2=1/(n-i2+1); /*p is the probability of a "success"*/

if _n_<n then do;
 if n>sumc2 then
   c2_i=ranbin(b2+100,n-sumc2,p2); /*generate the binomial variate*/
 else c2_i=0;
 sumc2=sumc2+c2_i;
end;
i2=i2+1;
if _n_=n then c2_i=n-sumc2;

data double;set resample2;
if c2_i>0 then do;
do i=1 to c2_i;
 output;
 end;
end;

proc univariate noprint data=double;
var pl_ct;
output out=med2 median=median;
```

```
data square;set med2;
median_sq=median**2; /*Get sums and sums of squares
                        from the inner bootstrap*/

proc append data=square out=second;
%end;

proc means data=second noprint;
var median median_sq;
output out=inn sum=median2 median2_sq;

proc datasets;
delete second;

data all;merge inn med1;

proc append data=all out=reduce;
%end;

/*********End Double Resampling Standard Resampling Algorithm*********/

proc means data=reduce;
var median;

proc means data=reduce noprint;
var median2 median2_sq;
output out=final2 sum=s2 s2_sq;

data dvar;set final2; /*Calculate inner bootstrap mean and variance*/
exp_median2=s2/(&brep1*&brep2);
var2=(s2_sq-(&brep1*&brep2)*exp_median2**2)/(&brep1*&brep2-1);
std2=sqrt(var2);

proc print;
var exp_median2 var2 std2;

%mend;
%multiwt(5000,100);
```

What follows is a third more efficient iteration of the double-bootstrap resampling program now rewritten using PROC IML. What we basically did was translate the first example program into PROC IML code. The reader is referred to the SAS/IML manual for details. The data are read in exactly as before and stored in a vector called data within PROC IML. The resampled values from the inner and outer loops are stored in the vectors bootdata1 and bootdata2. The key is the resampling algorithm. It consists of first generating a random uniform number via the built-in RANUNI function and applying the function int(ranuni(0)*n)+1. This function generates a random integer from 1 to n, and facilitates sampling with replacement from the data. The rank command is specific with respect to calculating the median. The commands

```
 e_med1=sum(boot1)/brep1;
 e_med2=sum(boot2)/(brep1*brep2);
```

```
var1=(boot1`*boot1-brep1*e_med1**2)/(brep1-1);
var2=(boot2`*boot2-brep1*brep2*e_med2**2)/(brep1*brep2-1);
```

correspond to the mean and variance calculations for $T^{**}(F_n(X))$ and $T^{*}(F_n(X))$, respectively, described in items 4–7 in the bootstrap algorithm overview above.

```
data counts;
label pl_ct='platelet count';
input pl_ct @@;
cards;
230 222 179 191 103 293 316 520 143 226
225 255 169 204  99 107 280 226 143 259
;

proc iml;
 use counts;
 read all into data;

/*Create a n by 1 vector of data counts
called data*/

n=nrow(data); /*Calculate the sample size*/
bootdata1=(1:n)`; /*Initialize array for holding
                  one bootstrap resample*/
bootdata2=(1:n)`; /*Initialize array for holding
                  one bootstrap resample for inner loop*/

brep1=5000; /*Set the number of bootstrap resamples*/
brep2=100; /*Set the number of bootstrap resamples*/

boot1=(1:brep1)`;
boot2=(1:brep1*brep2)`;

in2=0;
do i1=1 to brep1;
 do j1=1 to n;
  index=int(ranuni(0)*n)+1;
  bootdata1[j1]=data[index];
 end;
 rankd1=rank(bootdata1);

 med1=0;
 if n/2=int(n/2) then do; /*Median for even n*/
  do k1=1 to n;
   if rankd1[k1]=n/2 | rankd1[k1]=n/2+1 then med1=med1+bootdata1[k1]/2;
  end;
 end;
 else do;     /*Median for odd n*/
  do k1=1 to n;
   if rankd1[k1]=(n+1)/2 then med1=bootdata1[k1];
  end;
 end;

 do i2=1 to brep2;
  in2=in2+1;
```

```
  do j2=1 to n;
   index=int(ranuni(0)*n)+1;
   bootdata2[j2]=bootdata1[index];
   end;
  rankd2=rank(bootdata2);

 med2=0;
 if n/2=int(n/2) then do; /*Median for even n*/
  do k2=1 to n;
   if rankd2[k2]=n/2 | rankd2[k2]=n/2+1 then med2=med2+bootdata2[k2]/2;
  end;
 end;
 else do;      /*Median for odd n*/
    do k2=1 to n;
      if rankd2[k2]=(n+1)/2 then med2=bootdata2[k2];
    end;
 end;

 boot2[in2]=med2;

 end;
 boot1[i1]=med1;
end;

e_med1=sum(boot1)/brep1;
 e_med2=sum(boot2)/(brep1*brep2);

 var1=(boot1`*boot1-brep1*e_med1**2)/(brep1-1);
 std1=sqrt(var1);

 var2=(boot2`*boot2-brep1*brep2*e_med2**2)/(brep1*brep2-1);
 std2=sqrt(var2);

print e_med1 var1 std1 e_med2 var2 std2;

quit;
```

E_MED1	VAR1	STD1	E_MED2	VAR2	STD2
214.8392	333.12047	18.251588	212.90634	759.23504	27.55422

We see that from this run of the IML version of the program that we obtain the estimates $E[T^*(F_n(X))|F_n(X)] = 214.8$ and $\text{var}[T^*(F_n(X))|F_n(X)] = 333.1$. The other quantities may be calculated similar to before.

If the double bootstrap becomes too computationally intensive, other strategies exist, such as jackknifing (delete one observation at a time) the variance of the inner loop as opposed to resampling.

17.4 Bootstrap Confidence Intervals

Confidence interval estimation is in general the most widely used application of the bootstrap method. Multiple approaches will be discussed in this section. We will start with the straightforward percentile method and work our way through more complicated methods such as the bias-corrected methods. For moderate to large samples, all of the methods provide accurate coverage with the relatively same results. However, for small samples of $n < 50$, careful consideration of the methodology is warranted. For samples of size $n < 10$, most nonparametric bootstrap intervals either are unstable or have poor coverage properties. The choice of method becomes one of simplicity versus accuracy of the interval. Our general recommendation would be to use the bootstrap percentile-t method. Within this section, we will deal with the simple single-sample cases. Note, however, that the approach for the single-sample case in general carries over to more complicated data structures. Specific examples, such as the correlation coefficient, will be tackled in their own dedicated section.

17.4.1 Percentile Method

The percentile method is very straightforward and consists of simply using the basic bootstrap resampling algorithm from Section 17.2 and sorting the B resampled values of the statistic of interest, the $T^*(F_n(X))$'s, and then obtaining the lower $\alpha/2$th percentile and the upper $1 - \alpha/2$th percentile from the bootstrap distribution; for example, a 95% bootstrap percentile interval would simply consist of obtaining the 2.5th and 97.5th percentile values of the statistic after B resamples. The simplicity of this method gives it its great popularity. Theoretically, one may show that as the sample size goes to infinity, the coverage probability of the percentile interval converges to $1 - \alpha$. The rate of this convergence is, however, slower than some of the more complicated methods discussed below. Therefore, even though this approach has the correct large sample properties, it may produce intervals with severe undercoverage in the small finite sample setting (e.g., see Polansky, 2000). In other words, the confidence intervals will be narrower than expected when the sample size is small ($n < 50$).

More formally, denote the ordered resampled statistics from B bootstrap resamples as $T^*_{(1)}(F_n(X)) \leq T^*_{(2)} (F_n(X)) \leq \dots T^*_{(B)} (F_n(X))$. Then the $(1 - \alpha) \times 100\%$ approximate two-sided confidence interval is defined as the interval

$$(T^*_{(l)}(F_n(X)), T^*_{(u)} (F_n(X))) \tag{17.7}$$

where the indices corresponding to the lower and upper bounds are given by $l = \lfloor B\alpha/2 \rfloor$ and $u = \lfloor B(1 - \alpha/2) \rfloor$, and $\lfloor \cdot \rfloor$ denotes the floor function. The floor function may be calculated via the INT function in SAS. We can also make use of the already built-in functionality of PROC UNIVARIATE with respect to the calculation of percentile intervals. Note that one-sided intervals are calculated similarly simply by letting $l = \lfloor B\alpha \rfloor$ for a one-sided lower bound or by letting $u = \lfloor B(1 - \alpha) \rfloor$ for a one-sided upper bound.

The theoretical quantities that we are approximating via resampling are percentiles of the statistic given by an expectation–minimization expression

$$\inf_{\theta \in R} E\left\{ |T(F_n(X)) - \theta| + (2\alpha - 1)(T(F_n(X)) - \theta) | F_n \right\}, \tag{17.8}$$

where inf denotes the infimum (minimum). The complicated expression at (17.8) is a more formal way of defining a percentile for a given statistic in terms of its expectation. Obviously, for most practical situations, direct calculation of (17.8) is infeasible, or possibly even unnecessary given the accuracy of the resampling approach under certain conditions.

However, for certain statistics such as the sample median equation, (17.8) can be implemented via PROC NLP. Some specific examples follow later in the text.

Let us illustrate the bootstrap percentile confidence interval method using CD4 counts obtained from newborns infected with HIV. Suppose that we are interested in calculating the 95% confidence interval for the CD4 count data using a less standard measure, but more robust measure of location, say the α-trimmed mean statistic. The trimmed mean statistic is defined so as to "slice off" α percent of the extreme observations from both tails of the empirical distribution. For symmetric distributions, this statistic has the same expectation as does the sample mean. For asymmetric distributions, the trimmed mean will be less influenced by observations in the tail; that is, in general its expectation will be to the right or left of that of the sample mean in a direction opposite that of the tail. The median is a specific case of the trimmed mean as $\alpha \to 1/2$ in a limit. One may calculate the trimmed mean within SAS's PROC UNIVARIATE using the TRIMMED command along with its approximate 95% confidence interval under the assumption that the data are sampled from a symmetric population. The actual trimmed mean statistic is given as

$$T(F_n(X)) = \bar{x}_\alpha = \frac{1}{n-2k} \sum_{i=k+1}^{n-k} x_{(i)}, \tag{17.9}$$

where $x_{(i)}$ denotes the ith ordered observation, α denotes the trimming proportion, and $k = \lfloor n\alpha \rfloor$. The function $\lfloor \cdot \rfloor$ again denotes the floor function. Suppose we specify for our example the trimming proportion of $\alpha = 0.5$. It implies that $k = \lfloor 44.05 \rfloor = 2$ observations are trimmed from each tail. Given that this trimming strategy seems very straightforward, we need to step back and ask, "What is the population parameter that we are estimating?" It is very important to have an understanding of what you are estimating prior to carrying out any bootstrap estimation procedure. The α-trimmed mean statistic is an estimator of the population trimmed mean

$$E_\alpha(X) = \frac{1}{1-2\alpha} \int_{F^{-1}(\alpha)}^{F^{-1}(1-\alpha)} x \, dF,$$

that is, the population parameter in this instance is $E_\alpha(X)$, not the expected value of X, $E(X)$. For the specific case where the distribution is symmetric about the mean, $E_\alpha(X) = E(X)$. This is not the case for asymmetric distributions. Therefore, in this case our goal is to obtain a 95% confidence interval for $E_\alpha(X)$.

Within the program corresponding to our example, the CD4 count data from $n = 44$ subjects are read into data step `original`. The histogram of the original data set is given by Figure 17.3. Therefore, the assumption of symmetry appears to be violated with respect to the calculation of a confidence interval for $E_\alpha(X)$ using the built-in SAS routine. As an alternative to what is provided in PROC UNIVARIATE, we can calculate the bootstrap percentile confidence interval nonparametrically and compare the results. Note that the "guts" of the sample program is the same as what we have been utilizing throughout for simple bootstrapping. Within the simple bootstrap algorithm, we can calculate the trimmed mean in PROC UNIVARIATE using the `trimmed` command and output the value via SAS's Output Delivery System (ODS) to the data set `tr`; that is, there is no real additional programming to be done other than to use the already built-in calculations within PROC UNIVARIATE. The lower and upper bootstrap percentiles are then calculated and output via a separate run of PROC UNIVARIATE using the command `pctlpts=2.5 97.5 pctlpre=p`.

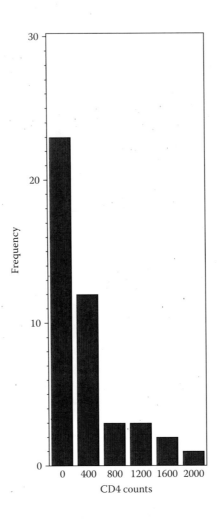

FIGURE 17.3
Histogram of CD4 counts.

For our example data set, the trimmed mean and its standard deviation (of the trimmed mean) turned out to be $\bar{x}_{.05} = 304.9 \pm 76.8$ compared to the sample mean $\bar{x} = 377.7 \pm 74.3$. The difference between the two statistics again illustrates the asymmetry in the data and reinforces the fact that the built-in confidence interval procedure should probably be avoided. For this example, the 95% semiparametric confidence interval for the trimmed mean, as calculated in PROC UNIVARIATE under an asymmetry assumption, turned out to be (149.3, 460.6). For $B = 1000$ resamples, the indices for the percentile interval are $l = \lfloor 10,000 \times 0.025 \rfloor = 250$ and $u = \lfloor 10,000 \times 0.975 \rfloor = 9750$. Therefore, the 95% bootstrap interval would be the 250th and 9750th ordered resampled values or, namely, $(T^*_{(250)}(F_n(X)), T^*_{(9750)}(F_n(X)))$. After $B = 10,000$ resamples, the 95% bootstrap percentile interval was calculated as (181.8, 466.0). The histogram of all $B = 10,000$ resampled $T^*_{(i)}(F_n(X))$'s are given by Figure 17.4. As you can see, there is a large difference with respect to the lower bound, indicating that the built-in interval calculated in PROC UNIVARIATE may not be appropriate for this data set given its asymmetry, and that possibly some transformation to symmetry is first necessary prior to its implementation. Also note that the percentile

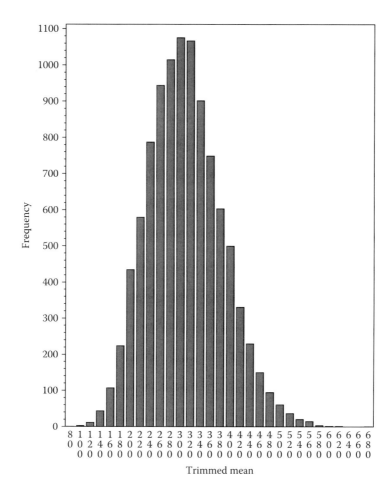

FIGURE 17.4

Bootstrap percentile histogram based on 10,000 replications.

interval is not constrained to be symmetric about the statistic $\bar{x}_{0.05} = 304.9$, thus making it much more flexible with respect to underlying assumptions. Given the moderately large sample size of $n = 44$ and the smoothness of the trimmed mean statistic, as illustrated in the histogram of the replications in Figure 17.4, we should feel fairly confident about the coverage accuracy of the bootstrap percentile confidence for this example. We will compare this interval with other more complicated bootstrap methods given later on. At the minimum, the percentile method is useful for examining the assumptions of parametric or semiparametric methods in terms of their validity. As noted earlier, in general the bootstrap-t method is what we would recommend. It is described in the next section.

```
data original;
label x_i='CD4 counts';
input x_i @@;
cards;
1397 471 64 1571 663 1128 719 407
480 1147 362 2022 10 175 494 31
202 751 30 27 118 8 181 1432 31 18
```

```
105 23 8 70 12 504 252 0 100 4
545 226 390 230 28 5 0 176
;

proc univariate trimmed=.05;
var x_i;
ods listing select trimmedmeans;

/***********Begin Standard Resampling Algorithm**********/

data sampsize;
 set original nobs=nobs;
 n=nobs;
do b=1 to 10000; /*output the data B times*/
 output;
end;

proc sort data=sampsize;by b;

data resample;
set sampsize;by b;
retain sumc i; /*need to add the previous
                count to the total */
if first.b then do;
   sumc=0;
   i=1;
end;
p=1/(n-i+1); /*p is the probability of a "success"*/

if ^last.b then do;
 if n>sumc then c_i=ranbin(0,n-sumc,p); /*generate the binomial variate*/
 else c_i=0;
 sumc=sumc+c_i;
end;
i=i+1;
if last.b then c_i=n-sumc;

data main;set resample;
if c_i >0 then do;
do i=1 to c_i;
 output;
 end;
end;

/*************End Standard Resampling Algorithm****************/

/***********Calculate 10000 Trimmed Means**********/
proc univariate trimmed=.05;by b;
var x_i;
ods listing close;
ods output trimmedmeans=tr;

/***********Calculate Percentile Interval**********/
proc univariate data=tr noprint;
var mean;
output out=quantile pctlpts=2.5 97.5 pctlpre=p;
```

```
/***********Print Results***********/

proc print data=quantile;

title '95% Bootstrap Percentile Confidence Interval';
```

The R code is as follows:

```
> data<-c(1397, 471, 64, 1571, 663, 1128, 719, 407,
+         480, 1147, 362, 2022, 10, 175, 494, 31,
+         202, 751, 30, 27, 118, 8, 181, 1432, 31, 18,
+         105, 23, 8, 70, 12, 504, 252, 0, 100, 4,
+         545, 226, 390, 230, 28, 5, 0, 176)
> data_sort<-sort(data)
> resamples <- lapply(1:1000, function(i)
+       sample(data, replace = T))
> each_mean<-lapply(1:1000, function(i)
+       mean(resamples[[i]]))
> vector<-c()
> for (i in 1:1000){
+       vector<-c(vector,each_mean[[i]])
+       i<-i+1
+ }
> quantile(vector,c(0.025,0.975))
      2.5%   97.5%
243.0193 530.7216
```

17.4.2 Bootstrap-*t* Method

Theoretically, the bootstrap-*t* method is only slightly more complicated than the percentile method. In terms of maintaining the same computational simplicity as that of the percentile interval, a readily available estimator of the standard deviation of the statistic $T^*(F_n(X))$ following each bootstrap replication is required. For example, if we were calculating an interval based on the sample mean, the estimate of the standard deviation of $T^*(F_n(X)) = \bar{x}^*$ would simply be $s^*/\sqrt{n}$, where s^* is the sample standard deviation of the resampled x^* 's. It turns out that there are quite a few statistics already built into SAS that have the property of a readily available standard deviation estimate, which in turn makes the bootstrap-*t* method straightforward in a variety of settings. Specific examples such as regression coefficients will be examined in further detail in later sections. If the standard deviation is not easily calculated, we need to utilize the more computationally intensive double-bootstrap procedure described earlier in Section 17.3.2.

The advantage of the bootstrap-*t* method over the percentile method is that it can be shown theoretically to have more accurate coverage properties in the small to moderate sample setting; that is, this approximate interval converges to the appropriate coverage levels at a faster rate than the percentile interval. A disadvantage of the bootstrap-*t* method is that it sometimes becomes unstable if the sample size is too small, for example, $n < 10$. In these situations, some type of smoothing is needed. The primary assumption with respect to utilizing the bootstrap-*t* method is that the statistic $T(F_n(X))$ should be independent of its variance estimator (at least approximately). Given that the large majority of statistics in use in practice can be shown to be asymptotically normally distributed, this assumption generally holds in practice. For statistics such as the sample proportion, we immediately know that direct use of the bootstrap-*t* approach is not appropriate. In these instances, more statistic-specific methods are needed; for example, a variance-stabilizing transformation might be utilized. The variance-stabilized bootstrap-t method is described later in this section.

The general idea behind the bootstrap-t approach is that we estimate the percentiles of sampling distribution of the standardized statistic

$$t = \frac{T(F_n(X)) - E[T(F_n(X)) \mid F_n]}{\sqrt{\text{var}[T(F_n(X)) \mid F_n]}}$$

using the corresponding bootstrap estimator

$$t^* = \frac{T^*(F_n(X)) - T(F_n(X))}{\sqrt{\text{var}[T^*(F_n(X)) \mid F_n^*]}} \tag{17.10}$$

For example, for the case of the mean, we get the familiar $t = \sqrt{n}(\bar{x} - u)/s$ estimated by $t^* = \sqrt{n}(\bar{x}^* - \bar{x})/s^*$. The bootstrap-$t$ method is an improvement over the percentile method in the sense that the approximated sampling distribution of $T(F_n(X))$ is centered and scaled more precisely.

For a given resample, denote the bias-corrected rescaled version of the statistic $T^*(F_n(X))$ as

$$S^*(F_n(X), F_n^*(X)) = T(F_n(X)) - \frac{\sqrt{\text{var}[T(F_n(X)) \mid F_n]}}{\sqrt{\text{var}[T^*(F_n(X)) \mid F_n^*]}} [T^*(F_n(X)) - T(F_n(X))] \tag{17.11}$$

Even though this expression is ugly looking, for specific cases it simplifies quite nicely. For the sample mean example with $T(F_n(X)) = \bar{x}$, we get

$$S^*(F_n(X), F_n^*(X)) = \bar{x} - \frac{s}{s^*}(\bar{x}^* - \bar{x}),$$

where the $\sqrt{n}$ factors cancel out with respect to the standard deviation estimators. Note that it can be easily shown for the case $T(F_n(X)) = \bar{x}$ that $E(S^*(F_n(X), F_n^*(X))) = E(X)$; that is, for this specific case, $E(S^*(F_n(X), F_n^*(X)))$ is an unbiased estimator of the population mean. Calculation of confidence intervals is similar to what was done in the bootstrap percentile interval calculation. Let the B ordered $S^*(F_n(X), F_n^*(X))$'s be denoted as $S_{(1)}^*(\cdot) \le S_{(2)}^*(\cdot) \le ... \le S_{(B)}^*(\cdot)$. The bootstrap-$t$ interval is then given by

$$(S_{(l)}^*(F_n(X), F_n^*(X)), S_{(u)}^*(F_n(X), F_n^*(X))) \tag{17.12}$$

where again the indices corresponding to the lower and upper bounds are given by $l = \lfloor B\alpha/2 \rfloor$ and $u = \lfloor B(1 - \alpha/2) \rfloor$, and $\lfloor \cdot \rfloor$ denotes the floor function. As always, the larger the value for B, the less the Monte Carlo error will be introduced into the estimation procedure. A diagnostic plot of the $T(F_n^*(X))$ versus the $\sqrt{\text{var}[T^*(F_n(X)) \mid F_n^*]}$ is useful for assessing the assumption that these two quantities are approximately independent.

If a readily available estimate for the bootstrap variance quantity $\text{var}[T^*(F_n(X)) \mid F_n^*]$ is available, there is only one additional step to carry out in SAS compared to the simple percentile interval. We need to merge the values of $T(F_n(X))$ and $\sqrt{\text{var}[T(F_n(X)) \mid F]}$ based on the statistics of interest to each successive bootstrap iteration and then calculate $S^*(F_n(X), F_n^*(X))$.

A quick-and-dirty strategy for merging the variables in SAS is to create a dummy variable used solely for the purpose of linking quantities such as $T(F_n(X))$ and the $T^*(F_n(X))$'s.

Example 17.1: Bootstrap-*t* Interval for the Trimmed Mean

Let us revisit our example from the percentile interval section involving the trimmed mean $\bar{x}_\alpha$. As you recall, we were interested in measures of location for CD4 count data. Previously, we calculated 95% bootstrap confidence intervals for $E_{0.05}(X)$ and $E_{0.25}(X)$ based on the trimmed means $T(F_n(X)) - \bar{x}_{0.05}$ and $T(F_n(X)) - \bar{x}_{0.25}$, respectively. In order to recalculate these intervals for the same data set using the bootstrap-*t* method, compared to the percentile interval approach, we need some additional programming steps. These are given in the example SAS program below.

The first step in modifying the existing programs is to create a dummy variable used to merge bootstrap quantities labeled `dummy`. For this example, `dummy=1` for every data and resample value. To calculate the trimmed mean and its standard deviation, we utilize the ODS with the command `ods output trimmedmeans=trbase` in conjunction with PROC UNIVARIATE. This allowed us to output the trimmed mean and standard deviation to the data set `trbase` within our sample program. It is important to note that the standard deviation estimate is labeled as the standard error in SAS; that is, what is calculated is the standard error estimate for X and the standard deviation for the statistic $\bar{X}_\alpha$.

After outputting the trimmed mean and its standard deviation from PROC UNIVARIATE, we reassigned them new variable names within the data set `rename`. This was necessary so that values were not overwritten when merged with the bootstrap resampled trimmed means and standard deviations of the same name. As with the original trimmed mean calculation, the bootstrap resampled statistics were also calculated using PROC UNIVARIATE and output using ODS to data set `combine`. In addition, within data set `combine` we calculated the $S^*(F_n(X), F_n^*(X))$'s defined at (17.11), needed in order to calculate the interval. The bootstrap-*t* interval based on the ordered $S^*(F_n(X), F_n^*(X))$'s was then processed via PROC UNIVARIATE. We also recalculated the percentile interval within this program for comparison. The intervals were distinguished by the percentile prefixes `pp` and `pt`, for the percentile and bootstrap-*t* methods, respectively.

The sampling distribution for $S^*(F_n(X), F_n^*(X))$ is given in Figure 17.5. Compared to the sampling distribution for $T(F_n(X))$ given in Figure 17.4, we see that the sampling distribution for $S^*(F_n(X), F_n^*(X))$ is slightly more skewed and has a bigger spread. This is to be expected since percentile-based sampling distributions are notorious for not being properly scaled. The diagnostic plot of $T(F_n^*(X))$ versus the $\sqrt{\mathrm{var}[T^*(F_n(X))|F_n^*]}$ given in Figure 17.6 indicates that the trimean statistic and its standard deviation estimator are approximately independent. Care must be taken when interpreting these plots in the sense that for a given realization of the data, dependence may be simply due to a spurious result in conjunction with the discreteness of the bootstrap procedure. In most cases, some careful thought about the statistical theory underlying the test statistic is in order. If you truly have a reason to believe that the independence assumption is not met, one may resort to variance-stabilizing techniques. The will be illustrated later in this section. The apparent clustering within the diagnostic plot is due to the discrete nature of the bootstrap procedure; that is, there is a finite sample of possible values after resampling.

For our example run, $B = 10,000$ resamples were used. The 95% interval turned out to be (179.9, 471.1) compared to the previous run given in the earlier section of (181.8, 466.0). This gives you an idea of how much the intervals might change from successive runs, even with $B = 10,000$ resamples. The bootstrap-*t* 95% confidence interval turned out to

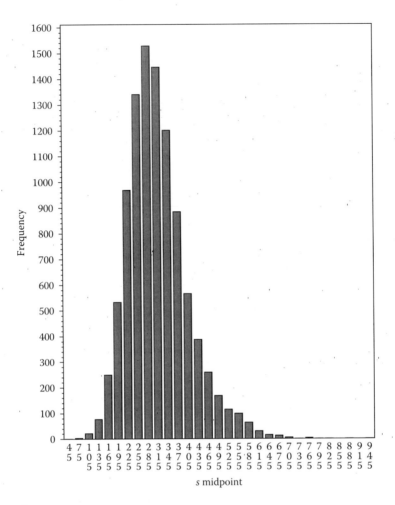

FIGURE 17.5
Bootstrap-*t* histogram based on 10,000 replications, $\alpha = 0.05$.

be $(S^*_{(250)}(\cdot), S^*_{(9750)}(\cdot)) = (170.5, 537.1)$. Recall also that the semiparametric interval built into SAS, calculated under the assumption of symmetry, yielded the interval of (149.3, 460.6). Given the apparent skewness in our example CD4 count data set, the bootstrap-*t* interval may be shown to be theoretically preferable to the semiparametric interval calculated by SAS in this instance. We will discuss its comparison to the percentile interval within the context of the variance-stabilized method in the next section. The bootstrap-*t* interval for this example is reflective of the skewness of the original data set and is wider than the percentile method since it was scaled more appropriately. Also, notice how the bootstrap-*t* interval is shifted slightly to the right compared to the semiparametric interval, again due to the asymmetry of the original data set.

Note that the symmetry assumption may be relaxed somewhat if the trimming proportion is increased. Let us examine the effect of the choice of trimming proportion as well; for example, say we wished to use a more robust measure of location. We can rerun the example with a trimming proportion of $\alpha = 0.25$, compared to $\alpha = 0.05$ above; that is, in this case we will eliminate 25% of the extreme observations from either tail of the distribution prior to estimating the mean. For our CD4 count data, $\bar{x}_{0.25} = 210.1 \pm 61.5$

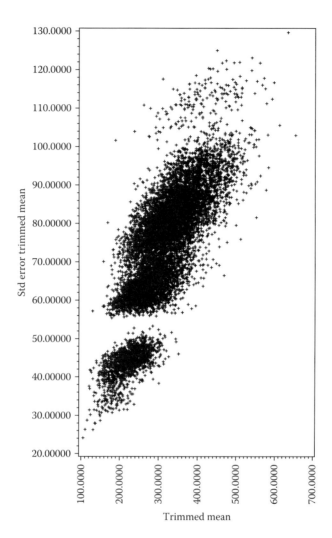

FIGURE 17.6
Diagnostic plot for bootstrap-t, $\alpha = 0.05$.

compared to $\bar{x}_{0.05} = 304.9 \pm 76.8$, and $\bar{x} = 377.7 \pm 74.3$. The confidence intervals in turn for $\bar{x}_{0.25}$ were (108.0, 351.1), (99.3, 397.2), and (82.3, 338.0) for the percentile, bootstrap-t, and semiparametric methods, respectively. The intervals are not too dissimilar. In general, the more trimming that takes place, the more we can relax the assumption of an underlying symmetrical distribution. The histogram of the resampled $\bar{x}^*_{0.25}$'s is given in Figure 17.7, and is slightly more symmetric than that of the current run of the $\bar{x}^*_{0.05}$'s given in Figure 17.5. The diagnostic plot given by Figure 17.8 again illustrates the approximate independence between the bootstrap mean and variance resample estimators, where again the clusters are due to the discreteness of the bootstrap distribution. The independence assumption will be revisited in Section 17.4.3.

```
data original;
label x_i='CD4 counts';
input x_i @@;
  dummy=1; /*define a dummy variable to merge on*/
```

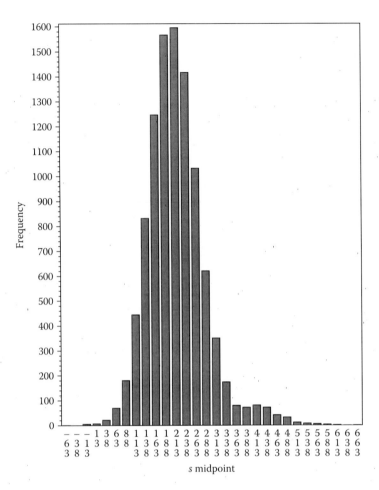

FIGURE 17.7
Bootstrap-*t* histogram based on 10,000 replications, $\alpha = 0.25$.

```
cards;
1397 471 64 1571 663 1128 719 407
480 1147 362 2022 10 175 494 31
202 751 30 27 118 8 181 1432 31 18
105 23 8 70 12 504 252 0 100 4
545 226 390 230 28 5 0 176
;


proc univariate trimmed=.05;by dummy;
var x_i;
ods listing select trimmedmeans;
ods output trimmedmeans=trbase; /*output trimmed mean and standard
deviation*/


data rename;set trbase; /*re-label the variables*/
keep dummy tbase stdbase;
tbase=mean;
stdbase=stdmean;
```

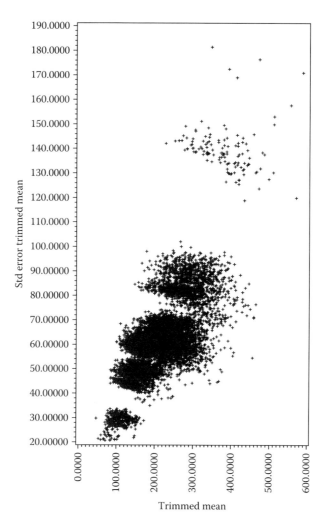

FIGURE 17.8
Diagnostic plot for bootstrap-*t*, α = 0.25.

```
/**********Begin Standard Resampling Algorithm**********/

data sampsize;
 set original nobs=nobs;
 n=nobs;
do b=1 to 10000; /*output the data B times*/
 output;
end;

proc sort data=sampsize;by b;

data resample;
set sampsize;by b;
retain sumc i; /*need to add the previous
                count to the total */
if first.b then do;
  sumc=0;
  i=1;
end;
```

```
p=1/(n-i+1); /*p is the probability of a "success"*/

if ^last.b then do;
  if n>sumc then c_i=ranbin(0,n-sumc,p); /*generate the binomial variate*/
  else c_i=0;
  sumc=sumc+c_i;
end;
i=i+1;
if last.b then c_i=n-sumc;

data main;set resample;
if c_i >0 then do;
do i=1 to c_i;
  output;
end;
end;

/*************End Standard Resampling Algorithm*************/
proc univariate trimmed=.05;by dummy b;
var x_i;
ods output trimmedmeans=tr;

data combine;merge tr rename;by dummy;
s=tbase-stdbase*(mean-tbase)/stdmean;

proc gplot data=combine;
plot stdmean*mean;

proc gchart;
vbar s;

proc univariate data=combine noprint;
var mean s;
output out=quantile pctlpts=2.5 97.5 pctlpre=pp pt;

proc print data= quantile;
title '95% Bootstrap Percentile and t Confidence Intervals';
```

17.4.3 Variance-Stabilized Bootstrap-*t* Method

Within the example diagnostic plots generated from the bootstrap-*t* example, and given by Figures 17.6 and 17.8, it could be argued that there is some evidence of dependence between $T^*(F_n(X))$ and $\sqrt{\mathrm{var}[T(F_n(X))|F_n]}$. In practical terms, there is no formal test of dependence between $T^*(F_n(X))$ and $\sqrt{\mathrm{var}[T(F_n(X))|F_n]}$ given the complicated structure of the resampling approach. A computationally intensive bootstrap procedure could be used on a case-by-case basis. However, in most instances, a bootstrap test for independence would be infeasible. In other instances, the functional relationship between $T^*(F_n(X))$ and $\sqrt{\mathrm{var}[T(F_n(X))|F_n]}$ may be known exactly, for example, the sample proportion and its standard deviation. A dependent structure between $T^*(F_n(X))$ and $\sqrt{\mathrm{var}[T(F_n(X))|F_n]}$ would in general indicate that the bootstrap-*t* method would perform poorly in terms of coverage probabilities compared to more complicated approaches.

If the functional form between $T^*(F_n(X))$ and $\sqrt{\mathrm{var}[T(F_n(X))|F_n]}$ is known, we can simply calculate confidence intervals using the bootstrap-*t* method on the variance-stabilized scale, and then back-transform the interval; for example, if we were interested in calculating a confidence interval for the geometric mean, we would first calculate a confidence interval based on the sample mean of the log-transformed data values using the bootstrap-t method and then back-transform the confidence interval by simply exponentiating the lower and upper bounds of the interval.

If graphical evidence of dependence does exist between $T^*(F_n(X))$ and $\sqrt{\text{var}[T(F_n(X))|F_n]}$, and the functional form of the dependence is unknown, but may be approximated well, we may wish to utilize the variance-stabilized bootstrap-t for confidence interval calculation. The key to this approach is to define a function g that approximately captures the dependence relationship between the pairs $T^*(F_n(X))$ and $\sqrt{\text{var}[T(F_n(X))|F_n]}$; that is, we are interested in the functional relationship of the form $\sqrt{\text{var}[T(F_n(X))|F_n]} \approx g[T^*(F_n(X))]$. In order for the variance stabilization method to have any utility, the function g should be nonlinear, and in general will depend on the problem at hand. The choice of g may be as simple or as complex as the analyst deems necessary. It is important to note that just like any other statistical approach based on data transformations, different choices of g will lead to different bootstrap solutions. Hence, care must be taken when interpreting the results based on the final selection of g.

The steps that need to be followed in order to carry out the variance-stabilized bootstrap-t routine are as follows:

1. Define a function g of the form $\sqrt{\text{var}[T(F_n(X))|F_n]} = g[T^*(F_n(X))]$, which best approximates the relationship between the first B resampled pairs of $T^*(F_n(X))$'s and $\sqrt{\text{var}[T(F_n(X))|F_n]}$'s. The functional form for g could be as simple as $g(x) = \beta_0 + \beta_1 x$ or as complex as needed, for example, a higher-order polynomial relationship.

2. Estimate the parameters used to define g using the appropriate estimation method. If we chose $g(x) = \beta_0 + \beta_1 x + \beta_2 x^2$ to be a quadratic function, we could simply estimate β_0, β_1, and β_2 through a least-squares regression of $\sqrt{\text{var}[T(F_n(X))|F_n]}$ on $T^*(F_n(X))$. Denote the estimated function as $\hat{g}$. Note that the choice of estimation method may ultimately impact the overall results.

3. The function $\hat{h}(y) = \int^y 1/\hat{g}(x)dx$ (the approximation of $h(y) = \int^y 1/g(x)dx$ needs to be calculated directly or through a numerical integration technique; for example, if we chose the functional $\hat{g}(x) = \hat{\beta}_0 + \hat{\beta}_1 x$, then $\hat{h}(y) = \log(\hat{\beta}_0 + \hat{\beta}_1 y)/\hat{\beta}_1$. Note that the variables x and y used in this illustration are simply dummy variables used to define the functions. Also note that the integration constant can be ignored.

4. Now generate an additional B pairs of $T^*(F_n(X))$'s. through the use of the standard resampling algorithm.

5. Apply the function $\hat{h}$ to the $T^*(F_n(X))$'s; that is, calculate the B values of the function $\hat{h}[S^*(F_n(X))]$.

6. Next let

$$S^*(F_n(X), F_n^*) = \hat{h}(T) - \frac{\hat{g}(T^*)}{\sqrt{\text{var}[T^*(F_n(X))|F_n^*]}}\left[\hat{h}(T^*) - \hat{h}(T)\right], \tag{17.13}$$

where $T = T(F_n(X))$ and $T^* = T^*(F_n(X))$. This is a slight modification of what was presented in Equation 17.13 due to the variance stabilization; that is, $\sqrt{\text{var}[\hat{h}(T)]}$ is considered to be approximately constant.

7. Calculate the bootstrap-t $(1-\alpha) \times 100\%$ confidence interval based on the B ordered $\hat{h}[S^*(F_n(X))]'s$, $\hat{h}[S^*(F_n(X))]_{(1)}, \hat{h}[S^*(F_n(X))]_{(2)}, \ldots, \hat{h}[S^*(F_n(X))]_{(B)}$, and given by

$$\left(\hat{h}[S^*(F_n(X))]_{(l)}, \hat{h}[S^*(F_n(X))]_{(u)}\right) \qquad (17.14)$$

where the lower and upper bounds are given by $l = \lfloor B\alpha/2 \rfloor$ and $u = \lfloor B(1-\alpha/2) \rfloor$, and $\lfloor \cdot \rfloor$ denotes the floor function.

8. Now back-transform the interval by applying the inverse function, $\hat{h}^{-1}(y)$, to the lower and upper bounds, namely, $\hat{h}[S^*(F_n(X))]_{(l)}$ and $\hat{h}[S^*(F_n(X))]_{(u)}$, in order to obtain the variance-stabilized confidence interval for $E[T^*(F_n(X))$.

It is important to note that if the function $1/g(x)$ is not easily integrated, the majority of the steps listed above need to be calculated numerically, and thus implementation in SAS or any other software package becomes labor-intensive. If you wish to carry out the more complicated numerical methods, PROC IML would typically need to be employed. Hence, like most statistical problems, one needs to balance the need to carry out a specific technique versus the practicality of the problem at hand; for example, maybe a simple percentile interval would suffice if the sample size is moderately large.

Example 17.2: Variance Stabilized Bootstrap-t Interval for the Trimmed Mean

In order to illustrate and contrast this technique to the previous methods, we again revisited our CD4 count example for the 5% trimmed mean, $\bar{x}_{0.05}$, where the goal was to generate a 95% confidence interval for $E(\bar{x}_{0.05})$. An examination of Figure 17.6 does not offer immediate clues regarding a complex functional form of g. It would, however, appear that we might be able to assume without too much of a stretch that a simple correlational structure between $T'(F_n(X))$'s and $\sqrt{\text{var}[T(F_n(X))|F_n]}$'s may be approximately correct. Hence, a linear function of the form $g(x) = \beta_0 + \beta_1 x$ should work reasonably well. As described in the steps above, the approximate variance-stabilizing transformation would then be $h(\bar{x}^*_{0.05}) = \log(\hat{\beta}_0 + \hat{\beta}_1 \bar{x}^*_{0.05})/\hat{\beta}_1$, where $\hat{\beta}_0$ and $\hat{\beta}_1$ will be estimated by regressing the first B resampled standard deviations of the trimmed mean on the $\bar{x}^*$'s. Again, in general, a closed-form solution for this method may not be available. In these instances, the programming becomes complicated and problem specific.

The SAS program below follows the outline described above for carrying out the variance-stabilized bootstrap-t method. The one little trick that was used was to define twice B equal to the variable `brep` within the very first data step `original`. Within this program, the variable `brep` was set to 10,000 replications, meaning that the first 5000 resampled trimmed means and their standard deviation estimates will be used to obtain the estimates $\hat{\beta}_0$ and $\hat{\beta}_1$ for the function $\hat{g}$, while the second 5000 resampled trimmed means will be used to calculate the variance-stabilized bootstrap-t interval. Note also that the variable `brep` is also used as a dummy variable upon which to merge various data elements.

Once 10,000 pairs of the $T'(F_n(X))$'s and $\sqrt{\text{var}[T(F_n(X))|F_n]}$'s are generated, we need to split them into two data sets. This is done within the program at the data steps named `split1` and `split2`. The values in the data set `split1` are then used to obtain the estimates $\hat{\beta}_0$ and $\hat{\beta}_1$ via PROC REG and output to the data set `tranparm`. The estimates in data set `tranparm` are then merged with the second 5000 resampled pairs given in data set `split2` to form data step `transform`, where the function $S^*(F_n(X), F_n^*(X))$ at (17.13) is calculated and given the variable name `sstar`. The 5000 $S^*(F_n(X), F_n^*(X))$'s are then fed into PROC UNIVARIATE, from which we obtain the 2.5th and 97.5th percentiles' corresponding to $S^*(F_n(X))_{(l)}$ and $S^*(F_n(X))_{(u)}$ to form a 95% confidence interval on the transformed scale. Finally, the values are output into data set `quantile` and set into data step `backtrans`, where the function h^{-1} is applied. The results of the interval calculations are output printed at the end of the program via PROC PRINT.

For our example, we obtained the 95% variance-stabilized bootstrap-t interval for the 5% trimmed mean as (183.0, 525.7), compared to the bootstrap-t interval of (170.5, 537.1) and the percentile interval of (179.9, 471.1). Under the assumption that we chose the appropriate functional form for g, the interval (183.0, 525.7) is the most appropriate. If g is *incorrectly specified*, then the intervals based on the variance stabilization procedure may be *biased*.

```
data original;
label x_i='CD4 counts';
input x_i @@;
  brep=10000; /*define a dummy variable to merge on
         and set the number of bootstrap
         replications*/
cards;
1397 471 64 1571 663 1128 719 407
480 1147 362 2022 10 175 494 31
202 751 30 27 118 8 181 1432 31 18
105 23 8 70 12 504 252 0 100 4
545 226 390 230 28 5 0 176
;
proc univariate trimmed=.05;by brep;
var x_i;
ods listing select trimmedmeans;
ods output trimmedmeans=trbase;

data rename;set trbase;
keep brep tbase;
tbase=mean;

data sampsize;
 set original nobs=nobs;
 n=nobs;
do b=1 to brep; /*output the data B times*/
 output;
end;

proc sort data=sampsize;by b;

data resample;
set sampsize;by b;
retain sumc i; /*need to add the previous
                count to the total */
if first.b then do;
sumc=0;
i=1;
end;
p=1/(n-i+1); /*p is the probability of a "success"*/

if ^last.b then do;
```

```
if n>sumc then c_i=ranbin(0,n-sumc,p); /*generate the binomial
variate*/
else c_i=0;
sumc=sumc+c_i;
end;
i=i+1;
if last.b then c_i=n-sumc;

data main;set resample;
if c_i >0 then do;
do i=1 to c_i;
  output;
end;
end;
/***********End Standard Resample Algorithm***********/


proc univariate trimmed=.05;by brep b;
var x_i;
ods output trimmedmeans=tr;
ods listing close;

data combine;merge tr rename;by brep;


/***************Split Sample***************/

data split1;set combine;
bmean=mean;
if b<=brep/2 then output;


/***********Split 2 contains second B resamples***********/
data split2;set combine;

mean_star=mean;
std_star=stdmean;
if b>brep/2 then output;


/**Estimate a Simple Variance Stabilizing
Transformation*************/

proc reg data=split1 outest=tranparm;by brep;
model stdmean=bmean;

/*****Calculate S* ****************************/
data transform;merge split2 tranparm;by brep;

newmean=log(intercept+bmean*mean_star)/bmean;
neworig=log(intercept+bmean*tbase)/bmean;
newstd=std_star/sqrt((intercept+bmean*mean_star)**2);
s_star= neworig-(newmean-neworig)/newstd;

proc univariate data=transform noprint;
var s_star;
output out=quantile pctlpts=2.5 97.5 pctlpre=new;


/********Back Transform the Intervals********/
data backtrans;merge quantile tranparm;
lower=(exp(bmean*new2_5)-intercept)/bmean;
```

```
upper=(exp(bmean*new97_5)-intercept)/bmean;

proc print data=backtrans;
title '95% Bootstrap Percentile Confidence Interval';
var lower upper;
ods printer ps file='var_stab_ci.ps';
```

17.4.4 Bootstrap-*t* Method via Double Bootstrapping

If an estimator of the variance of the statistic of interest, $T(F_n(X))$, is not readily available, then we will need to utilize the double-bootstrap methodology described in Section 17.4.2 in order to carry out the bootstrap-*t* method. The basic idea is to implement the double bootstrap to obtain a measure of scale not only for the original statistic, $T(F_n(X))$, but also for the resampled statistics, $T^*(F_n(X))$. The double-bootstrap method is in general computationally intensive. For most cases, we recommend the use of PROC IML. The guts of the PROC IML routine used in this section are provided in Section 17.3.2.

Let us continue with our example involving CD4 counts. Suppose that instead of using the trimmed mean statistic defined in (17.9) to estimate a measure of location, we instead wish to utilize Tukey's trimean defined as

$$T(F_n(X)) = \hat{Q}(1/4)/4 + \hat{Q}(1/2)/2 + \hat{Q}(3/4)/4, \tag{17.15}$$

where $\hat{Q}(\cdot)$ denotes the sample quantile function (inverse of the distribution function). We see from (17.15) that Tukey's trimean is a robust measure of location consisting of a weighted average of the upper and lower quartiles, and the median. Unfortunately, there is no readily available estimator of the variance of Tukey's trimean already built into SAS or easily programmed, except under certain parametric assumptions. Therefore, if we wish to use this alternate well-known statistic as a basis of our bootstrap-*t* interval, we need to carry out a much more computationally intensive double-bootstrap routine. The most efficient way of doing this is through the use of PROC IML. If you are uncomfortable using PROC IML, we have provided a less efficient and more time-consuming SAS macro-based program in the appendix. The program in the appendix essentially does the same thing as the IML program presented in this section. Note, however, that depending on the specific operating system, the macro-based program may run many hours, compared to many minutes for the IML-based program.

As in the earlier examples involving the trimmed mean, we need to calculate the following quantities: $T(F_n(X))$, $T^*(F_n(X))$, $\sqrt{\text{var}[T(F_n(X))\,|\,F_n]}$, and $\sqrt{\text{var}[T^*(F_n(X))\,|\,F_n^*]}$. However, unlike the last example, we need to calculate these quantities, with the exception of $T(F_n(X))$, via the double-bootstrap resampling algorithm.

The actual syntax of the IML program provided in this section is only a slight modification (specific to this example) of what was described earlier in Section 17.2. The first part of the program simply reads in the data and feeds them into PROC IML. Then within PROC IML, we first need to program the calculation for Tukey's trimean. This involves utilizing the sample quantile function defined for this example as $\hat{Q}(u) = X_{(\lfloor nu \rfloor + 1)}$, where $X_{(i)}$ denotes the *i*th-order statistic. In order to calculate the quantile function, we need to sort or rank the actual data values. That is done through the utilization of the `sort`, `int`, and `rank` functions within PROC IML. Prior to the outer bootstrap loop indexed by `brep1`, we calculate Tukey's trimean and assign it the name `tukey`. Within the outer bootstrap loop, we calculate $T'(F_n(X))$ and $\sqrt{\text{var}[T(F_n(X))|F_n]}$ given by the variables `tukey1` and `std1`, respectively. Recall that the resampling mechanism is carried out through the generation of random uniform variates, which are then truncated. Within our program, we utilize the statement `index=int(ranuni(0)*n)+1`. The function assigned to `index` generates random integers from 1 to n. If for some regulatory purpose the rerun of this program needs to be reproducible, we need to work out a strategy with respect to choice of seeds.

In the inner bootstrap loop indexed by `brep2`, we calculated $T'(F_n(X))$ and $\sqrt{\text{var}[T^*(F_n(X))|F_n^*]}$ given by the variables `tukey2` and `std2`, respectively. The calculation of $T^*(F_n(X))$ is necessary for the calculation of $\sqrt{\text{var}[T^*(F_n(X))|F_n^*]}$. Once we exit the inner bootstrap loop, we are essentially back to what is done in the more simple bootstrap procedures; that is, the added layer of complexity entails the inner loop. We then calculate t^* described in (17.10). It saves a few programming steps to first obtain the standardized portion of t^* upon exiting the inner loop, which in this program is given as `zboot[i1]=(tukey1-tukey)/std2`, and then store the values in the array labeled `zboot`. Then s^* defined in (17.11) is given by `sstar=tukey+std1*zboot` and sorted. As described in the earlier part of the section, the 95% bootstrap confidence interval is found by sorting `sstar`, calculated in this program as `sstar=tukey+std1*zboot`, and finding the lower 2.5th and upper 97.5th quantiles given by the variables called `lower` and `upper`.

Recall that for our CD4 count data, $\bar{x}_{0.25} = 210.1 \pm 61.5$ compared to $\bar{x}_{0.05} = 304.9 + 76.8$, and $\bar{x} = 377.7 \pm 74.3$. The bootstrap-t 95% confidence intervals in turn for $\bar{x}_{0.05}$ and $\bar{x}_{0.25}$ were (170.5, 537.1) and (99.3, 397.2), respectively. For our double-bootstrap routine, we used $B_1 = 5000$ outer resample loops and $B_2 = 100$ inner resample loops. One run of the program utilizing Tukey's trimean (TRI) produced an estimate of $TRI = 223.5 \pm 68.3$ with a corresponding 95% bootstrap-t confidence interval of (98.9, 352.3). A post hoc examination of the various estimators indicates that Tukey's trimean was more efficient than both $\bar{x}_{0.05}$ and $\bar{x}_{0.25}$, thus producing a narrower confidence interval. Not surprisingly, since both TRI and $\bar{x}_{0.25}$ primarily utilize the inner 50% of the data, they produced similar results. As it pertains to this example, it is important to understand that if the assumption of symmetry is violated, then the underlying population parameter of interest varies for each statistic utilized in our examples; that is, the confidence intervals need to be interpreted differently across each statistic since they correspond to different population parameters. One alternative in terms of comparing the intervals across statistics would be to first choose a symmetrizing transformation and then calculate the intervals.

```
data original;
label x_i='CD4 counts';
input x_i @@;
cards;
1397 471 64 1571 663 1128 719 407
480 1147 362 2022 10 175 494 31
202 751 30 27 118 8 181 1432 31 18 command
105 23 8 70 12 504 252 0 100 4
545 226 390 230 28 5 0 176
;
```

```
proc iml;
 use original;
 read all into data;

 /*Create a n by 1 vector of data counts called data*/
 n=nrow(data); /*Calculate the sample size*/

 sort=data;
 sort[rank(data),]=data;
 data=sort;

tukey=data[int(n/4)+1]/4+data[int(n/2)+1]/2+data[int(3*n/4)+1]/4;
print tukey; /*Calculate Tukey's Trimean*/

 bootdata1=(1:n)`; /*Initialize array for holding
                      one bootstrap resample*/
 bootdata2=(1:n)`; /*Initialize array for holding
                      one bootstrap resample for inner loop*/

 brep1=5000; /*Set the number of bootstrap resamples*/
 brep2=100; /*Set the number of bootstrap resamples*/

boot1=(1:brep1)`;
boot2=(1:brep2)`;
zboot=(1:brep1)`;
tboot=(1:brep1)`;

in2=0;
do i1=1 to brep1;
 do j1=1 to n;
  index=int(ranuni(0)*n)+1;
  bootdata1[j1]=data[index];
 end;
sort1=bootdata1;
sort1[rank(bootdata1),]=bootdata1;
bootdata1=sort1;
tukey1=bootdata1[int(n/4)+1]/4+bootdata1[int(n/2)+1]/2
  +bootdata1[int(3*n/4)+1]/4;

/*Calculate Tukey's Trimean called tukey1 from outer loop*/

do i2=1 to brep2;
 do j2=1 to n;
  index=int(ranuni(0)*n)+1;
  bootdata2[j2]=bootdata1[index];
 end;
  sort2=bootdata2;
  sort2[rank(bootdata2),]=bootdata2;
  bootdata2=sort2;
  tukey2=bootdata2[int(n/4)+1]/4+bootdata2[int(n/2)+1]/2
      +bootdata2[int(3*n/4)+1]/4;
```

```
/*Calculate Tukey's Trimean called tukey2 from inner loop*/

 boot2[i2]=tukey2;

 end;

/*******************Exit inner bootstrap loop*******************/
 e_tukey2=sum(boot2)/(brep2);
 var2=(boot2`*boot2-brep2*e_tukey2**2)/(brep2-1);
 std2=sqrt(var2);
/*Estimate mean and variance of tukey2*/
 boot1[i1]=tukey1;
 zboot[i1]=(tukey1-tukey)/std2;
/*Calculate standard bootstrap ``z-score''*/
end;

/*******************Exit outer bootstrap loop*******************/
 e_tukey1=sum(boot1)/brep1;
 var1=(boot1`*boot1-brep1*e_tukey1**2)/(brep1-1);
 std1=sqrt(var1);
/*Estimate mean and variance of tukey1*/
sstar=tukey+std1*zboot;

/*Calculate sstar*/
print e_tukey1 var1 std1 e_tukey2 var2 std2;

 sortp=sstar;
 sortp[rank(sstar),]=sstar;
 sstar=sortp;

alpha=.05;

lower=sstar[int(brep1*alpha/2)+1];
upper=sstar[int(brep1*(1-alpha/2))+1];

print lower upper;
quit;
```

17.4.5 Bias-Corrected Method

The bias-corrected (BC) method corrects for the bias of coverage when the distribution of the statistic is not nearly symmetric.

In the percentile method, the $(1 - \alpha) \times 100\%$ approximate two-sided confidence interval is defined as

$$\left(T^*_{(l)}(F_n(X)), T^*_{(u)}(F_n(X)) \right),$$ (17.16)

where the lower and upper bounds are given by $l = \lfloor B\alpha/2 \rfloor$ and $u = \lfloor B(1-\alpha/2) \rfloor$. In the bias-corrected method, the same equation will be used, the only difference being that the lower and upper bounds of the confidence interval are adjusted by $\hat{z}_0$, the bias correction, as follows:

$$l = \lfloor B\Phi(2\hat{z}_0 + z_{\alpha/2}) \rfloor$$

$$u = \lfloor B\Phi(2\hat{z}_0 + z_{1-\alpha/2}) \rfloor \qquad (17.17)$$

where

$$\hat{z}_0 = \Phi^{-1}\{\Pr[T^*_{(i)}(F_n(X)) < \hat{T}(F_n(X))]\}, i = 1, 2, ..., B$$

$$z_{\alpha/2} = \Phi^{-1}(\alpha/2), z_{1-\alpha/2} = \Phi^{-1}(1 - \alpha/2) \qquad (17.18)$$

Here, Φ can be any cumulative distribution function (CDF) and Φ^{-1} is the inverse function of the CDF. Usually, a CDF from the standard normal distribution is used.

To obtain the confidence interval, let $g(\cdot)$ be a function that is monotonically increasing. Let

$$\phi = g(T(F_n(X))), \qquad (17.19)$$

$$U = g(\hat{T}^*(F_n(X))). \qquad (17.20)$$

If there exists a $g(\cdot)$ such that the following equation holds,

$$U \sim N(\phi - \hat{z}_0\sigma(\phi), \sigma^2(\phi)), \qquad (17.21)$$

we obtain the confidence limit for ϕ:

$$\hat{\phi}_\alpha = u + \hat{z}_0\sigma(u) + z_\alpha\sigma(u), \qquad (17.22)$$

where z_α is the αth quantile of the standard normal distribution.

In addition, the CDF can be calculated from the following equation:

$$\hat{G}(T^*_\alpha(F_n(X))) = \Pr^*\left(U^* < \hat{\phi}_\alpha\right)$$

$$= \Phi\left(\frac{\hat{\phi}_\alpha - u}{\sigma(u)} + \hat{z}_0\right) \qquad (17.23)$$

$$= \Phi\left(2\hat{z}_0 + z_\alpha\right)$$

The steps to calculate the bias-corrected confidence interval are summarized below:

1. Perform *B bootstrap replications.* Sort them into order:

$$T^*_{(1)}(F_n(X)), T^*_{(2)}(F_n(X)), ..., T^*_{(B)}(F_n(X))$$

2. Find the statistic $\hat{T}(F_n(X))$ from the original data.

3. Calculate $\hat{z}_0 = \Phi^{-1}(p/B)$, where $p = \sum_{i=1}^{B} I(T^*_{(i)}(F_n(X)) \leq \hat{T}(F_n(X)))$ and I is the indicator function (note in the SAS code below that $\hat{z}_0$ is denoted as b).

4. Calculate $l = \lfloor B\Phi(2\hat{z}_0 + z_{\alpha/2}) \rfloor$, $u = \lfloor B\Phi(2\hat{z}_0 + z_{1-\alpha/2}) \rfloor$.

5. Find $T^*_{(l)}(F_n(X))$ and $T^*_{(u)}(F_n(X))$. The bias-corrected confidence interval is then $\left(T^*_{(l)}(F_n(X)), T^*_{(u)}(F_n(X)) \right)$.

The example below is to calculate the 95% confidence interval for Tukey's trimean:

```
**************************************************;
******Bias Corrected Percentile Method******;
**************************************************;

* Read in the same data file as used for variance estimation on Page 54;
* The program below estimates the trimean and its confidence interval;

data counts;
label pl_ct='platelet count';
input pl_ct @@;
cards;
1397 471 64 1571 663 1128 719 407
480 1147 362 2022 10 175 494 31
202 751 30 27 118 8 181 1432 31 18
105 23 8 70 12 504 252 0 100 4
545 226 390 230 28 5 0 176
;

proc iml;
use counts;
read all into data;

*reset print;

n=nrow(data);
brep=5000; * Number of Bootstrap replications;

total=n*brep;
bootdata=j(total,3, 0);

* Create bootstrap replications;
do i=1 to total;
  index=int(ranuni(0)*n)+1;
  bootdata[i,1]=data[index];
  bootdata[i,2]=int(((i-1)/n)+1; * This is the number of
replications;
end;

call sortndx(ndx, bootdata, {2, 1});
        * Sort data by replication number and values;
  bootdata=bootdata[ndx,];

do i=1 to total;
```

```
   bootdata[i,3]=mod(i,n) + (mod(i,n)=0)*n;
        * This is the order of each replicated data;
end;

* Find trimmed mean;

subset=bootdata[loc(bootdata[,3]=int(n/4)+1|bootdata[,3]=int(n/2)+1
        |bootdata[,3]=int(3*n/4)+1),1];
matrix1=I(brep);
matrix2={0.25 0.5 0.25};
matrix3=matrix1 @ matrix2;
tukey = matrix3 * subset;

call sort(tukey, {1});
tukey=tukey;

* Find trimmed mean for the original data;
call sortndx(ndx, data, {1});
data=data[ndx,];
trimmean=1/4 * data[int(n/4)+1,1] + 1/2 * data[int(n/2)+1, 1]
        + 1/4 * data[int(n*3/4) +1,1];

*Calculate b;
subset = tukey[loc(tukey[,1] <= trimmean),];
p=nrow(subset)/brep;
b=quantile('NORMAL', p); * b=z_0;

* Calculate confidence interval;
alpha=0.05;
z_alpha_2 = quantile('NORMAL', alpha/2);
Q_l=int(brep*probnorm(2*b + z_alpha_2));
Q_u=int(brep*probnorm(2*b - z_alpha_2));

if Q_l=0 then Lower=0;
 else Lower=tukey[Q_l];
Upper=tukey[Q_u];

CI=trimmean||p||b||Lower||Upper;
colname={'trimmean' 'P' 'b' 'lower' 'upper'};
print CI[colname=colname];

quit;
```

Based on 5000 replications, the estimated confidence interval is

Trimean	P	b	Lower	Upper
223.5	0.4388	−0.154012	112.25	386.75

If the statistic $T(F_n(X))$ cannot be estimated directly, a double-bootstrap strategy may be needed.

The macro version of the SAS program is

```
data original;
label x_i='CD4 counts';
```

```
input x_i @@;
dummy=1; /*define a dummy variable to merge on*/
cards;
1397 471 64 1571 663 1128 719 407
480 1147 362 2022 10 175 494 31
202 751 30 27 118 8 181 1432 31 18
105 23 8 70 12 504 252 0 100 4
545 226 390 230 28 5 0 176
;

ods listing close;

proc univariate trimmed=.05;by dummy;
var x_i;
ods listing select trimmedmeans;
ods output trimmedmeans=trbase;

data rename;set trbase;
keep dummy tbase ;
tbase=mean;

ods printer ps file='trim_BC.ps';

data sampsize;
set original nobs=nobs;
n=nobs;
do b=1 to 10000; /*output the data B times*/
output;
end;

proc sort data=sampsize;by b;

data resample;
set sampsize;by b;
retain sumc i; /*need to add the previous
        count to the total */
if first.b then do;
  sumc=0;
  i=1;
end;
p=1/(n-i+1); /*p is the probability of a "success"*/

if ^last.b then do;
if n>sumc then c_i=ranbin(0,n-sumc,p); /*generate the binomial variate*/
else c_i=0;
sumc=sumc+c_i;
end;
i=i+1;
if last.b then c_i=n-sumc;

data main;set resample;
if c_i >0 then do;
do i=1 to c_i;
output;
end;
end;
```

```
proc univariate trimmed=.05;by dummy b;
var x_i;
ods output trimmedmeans=tr;

data combine;merge tr rename;by dummy;
ind=0;
if mean<tbase then ind=1;

proc means mean noprint;
var ind;
output out=bias mean=phat;

%macro bc;

data percents;set bias;
alpha=0.05;
z0=probit(phat);
lower=100*probnorm(2*z0+probit(alpha/2));
upper=100*probnorm(2*z0+probit(1-alpha/2)); /*need percentiles*/
call symput('lll',lower);
call symput('uuu',upper);

proc univariate noprint pctldef=4 data=combine;
var mean;
output out=quantile pctlpts= &lll &uuu pctlpre=p;

%mend;
%bc;
proc print;
ods listing;
```

The 95% confidence interval is (179.92, 471.49).

17.4.6 Bias-Corrected and Accelerated Method

Compare to the percentile method, the bias-corrected method shows substantial improvement of the coverage by correcting for the lack of symmetry of the distribution of the statistic. However, it does not consider the situation where the shape of the distribution may change with $T(F_n(X))$. The bias-corrected and accelerated (BCa) method is a strategy to further correct the variation of shape.

Similar to the bias-corrected method, in the bias-corrected and accelerated method, we need to recalculate the lower and upper bounds of the confidence interval such that

$$l = B\Phi\left(\hat{z}_0 + \frac{\hat{z}_0 + z_{\alpha/2}}{1 - \hat{a}(\hat{z}_0 + z_{\alpha/2})}\right)$$

$$u = B\Phi\left(\hat{z}_0 + \frac{\hat{z}_0 + z_{1-\alpha/2}}{1 - \hat{a}(\hat{z}_0 + z_{1-\alpha/2})}\right) \tag{17.24}$$

In these forms, $\hat{z}_0$ is still called the bias correction as defined previously. $\hat{a}$ is called acceleration, which is associated with the shape of the distribution of the statistic. One of the ways to calculate the acceleration is via the *jackknife* method:

$$\hat{a} = \frac{\sum_{i=1}^{B}\left(\hat{T}^{(\cdot)}(F_n(X)) - \hat{T}^{(i)}(F_n(X))\right)^3}{6\left\{\sum_{i=1}^{B}\left(\hat{T}^{(\cdot)}(F_n(X)) - \hat{T}^{(i)}(F_n(X))\right)^2\right\}^{3/2}} \tag{17.25}$$

where $\hat{T}^{(i)}(F_n(X))$, $i = 1, 2, ..., B$, are estimates of $T(F_n(X))$ when $T_i^*(F_n(X))$ is omitted, and $\hat{T}^{(\cdot)}(F_n(X))$ is the average of $\hat{T}^{(i)}(F_n(X))$. More complicated methods can be used to calculate the acceleration (see Efron and Tibshirani, 1993).

To obtain the confidence interval, we again need to find a monotonically increasing function $g(\cdot)$ such that

$$U \sim N\left(\phi - \hat{z}_0(1 + \hat{a}\phi), (1 + \hat{a}\phi)^2\right) \tag{17.26}$$

The confidence limit can then be calculated as

$$\hat{\phi}_a = u + \sigma(u)\frac{\hat{z}_0 + z_\alpha}{1 - \hat{a}(\hat{z}_0 + z_\alpha)}$$

where z_α is the αth quantile of the standard normal distribution.

The calculation of CDF is then

$$\hat{G}\left(T_\alpha^*(F_n(X))\right) = \Pr^*(U^* < \hat{\phi}_\alpha)$$

$$= \Phi\left(\frac{\hat{\phi}_\alpha - u}{\sigma(u)} + \hat{z}_0\right) \tag{17.27}$$

$$= \Phi\left(\hat{z}_0 + \frac{\hat{z}_0 + z_\alpha}{1 - \hat{a}(\hat{z}_0 + z_\alpha)}\right)$$

The steps to calculate the BCa confidence interval are

1. Eliminate one of the observations of the data, and then calculate the statistic of interest $\hat{T}^{(i)}(F_n(X))$, $i = 1, 2, ..., B$.
2. Calculate $\hat{a}$ using the equation above.
3. Perform *B bootstrap replications*. Sort them into order:

$$T_{(1)}^*(F_n(X)), T_{(2)}^*(F_n(X)), ..., T_{(B)}^*(F_n(X))$$

4. Find the statistic $\hat{T}(F_n(X))$ from the original data.

5. Calculate $\hat{z}_0 = \Phi^{-1}(p/B)$, where $p = \sum_{i=1}^{B} I(T_{(i)}^*(F_n(X))) \leq \hat{T}(F_n(X))$ and I is the indicator function (note in the SAS code below that $\hat{z}_0$ is denoted as b).

6. Calculate l, u using the equations above.

7. Find $T_{(l)}^*(F_n(X))$ and $T_{(u)}^*(F_n(X))$. The bias-corrected and accelerated confidence interval is then $(T_{(l)}^*(F_n(X)), T_{(u)}^*(F_n(X)))$.

The steps to calculate the BCa confidence interval are the same as those to calculate the BC confidence interval; the only difference exists in the use of acceleration $\hat{a}$.

```
***************************************************;
*******Bias Corrected and Accelerated Method*******;
***************************************************;
* Read in the same data file as used for variance estimation on Page 54;
* The program below estimates the trimean and its confidence interval;

data counts;
label pl_ct='platelet count';
input pl_ct @@;
cards;
1397 471 64 1571 663 1128 719 407
480 1147 362 2022 10 175 494 31
202 751 30 27 118 8 181 1432 31 18
105 23 8 70 12 504 252 0 100 4
545 226 390 230 28 5 0 176
;

proc iml;
use counts;
read all into data;

*reset print;

n=nrow(data);
brep=500; * Number of Bootstrap replications;

total=n*brep;
bootdata=j(total,3, 0);

* Create bootstrap replications;
do i=1 to total;
 index=int(ranuni(0)*n)+1;
 bootdata[i,1]=data[index];
 bootdata[i,2]=int((i-1)/n)+1; * This is the number of replications;
end;

call sortndx(ndx, bootdata, {2, 1});
       * Sort data by replication number and values;
bootdata=bootdata[ndx,];

do i=1 to total;
 bootdata[i,3]=mod(i,n) + (mod(i,n)=0)*n;
```

```
        * This is the order of each replicated data;
end;

* Calculate a;
call sort(data, {1});
col=(1:n)`;
data_perm=data||col;

do i=1 to n;
 permut=data_perm[loc(data_perm[,2] ^= i),];
  col2=(1:n-1)`;
 permut=permut||col2;
 trim_perm=1/4 * permut[int((n-1)/4)+1,1] + 1/2 *
   permut[int((n-1)/2)+1, 1]
       + 1/4 * permut[int((n-1)*3/4) +1,1];
 perm_a=perm_a//trim_perm;
end;
print perm_a;

a_vector=perm_a||col||col||col;
a_vector[,4] = a_vector[+,1]/n;
a_vector[,2] = (a_vector[,1] - a_vector[,4])##3;
a_vector[,3] = (a_vector[,1] - a_vector[,4])##2;
a=a_vector[+,2] /6/a_vector[+,3]##1.5; *a;

* Find trimmed mean;
subset=bootdata[loc(bootdata[,3]=int(n/4)+1|bootdata[,3]=int(n/2)+1
       |bootdata[,3]=int(3*n/4)+1),1];
matrix1=I(brep);
matrix2={0.25 0.5 0.25};
matrix3=matrix1 @ matrix2;
tukey = matrix3 * subset;

call sort(tukey, {1});
tukey=tukey;

* Find trimmed mean for the original data;
call sortndx(ndx, data, {1});
data=data[ndx,];
trimmean=1/4 * data[int(n/4)+1,1] + 1/2 * data[int(n/2)+1, 1]
       + 1/4 * data[int(n*3/4) +1,1];

*Calculate b;
subset = tukey[loc(tukey[,1] <= trimmean),];
p=nrow(subset)/brep;
b=fuzz(quantile('NORMAL', p)); * b=z_0;

* Calculate confidence interval;
alpha=0.05;
z_alpha_2=quantile('NORMAL', alpha/2);
Q_l=int(brep *probnorm(b + (z_alpha_2 + b)/(1 - a * (z_alpha_2 + b))));
Q_u=int(brep*probnorm(b + (- z_alpha_2 + b)/(1 - a * (- z_alpha_2
   + b))));
```

```
if Q_l=0 then Lower=0;
 else Lower=tukey[Q_l];
Upper=tukey[Q_u];

CI=trimmean||p||a||b||Lower||Upper;
colname={'trimmean' 'P' 'a' 'b' 'lower' 'upper'};
print CI[colname=colname];
quit;
```

Based on 5000 replications, the estimated confidence interval is

Trimean	P	a	b	Lower	Upper
223.5	0.4348	−0.011665	−0.164167	116	376.25

The BCa method produces a narrower confidence interval than the BC method. A macro version of the SAS program is

```
data original;
 label x_i='platelet count';
 input x_i@@;
 dummy=1;
 cards;
1397 471 64 1571 663 1128 719 407
480 1147 362 2022 10 175 494 31
202 751 30 27 118 8 181 1432 31 18
105 23 8 70 12 504 252 0 100 4
545 226 390 230 28 5 0 176
;

* The trimmed mean of the original data;
proc univariate data=original trimmed=.05;by dummy;
var x_i;
ods listing select trimmedmeans;
ods output trimmedmeans=trbase;
quit;

data rename;set trbase;
keep dummy tbase ;
tbase=mean;

ods printer ps file='trim_BC.ps';

data sampsize;
set original nobs=nobs;
n=nobs;
do b=1 to 10000; /*output the data B times*/
output;
end;

proc sort data=sampsize;by b;

*Bootstrap sampling;
data resample;
set sampsize;by b;
```

```
retain sumc i; /*need to add the previous
        count to the total */
if first.b then do;
sumc=0;
i=1;
end;
p=1/(n-i+1); /*p is the probability of a "success"*/

if ^last.b then do;
if n>sumc then c_i=ranbin(0,n-sumc,p); /*generate the binomial variate*/
else c_i=0;
sumc=sumc+c_i;
end;
i=i+1;
if last.b then c_i=n-sumc;

data main;set resample;
if c_i >0 then do;
do i=1 to c_i;
output;
end;
end;
run;

* The estimated trimmed mean of the Bootstrap samples;
proc univariate data=main trimmed=.05;by dummy b;
var x_i;
ods output trimmedmeans=tr;
run;

data combine;merge tr rename;by dummy;
ind=0;
if mean<tbase then ind=1;
run;

* Calculating z0, the bias;
proc means data=combine mean noprint;
var ind;
output out=bias mean=phat;
run;

* Calculating a, the acceleration;
data temp;
set original;
id=_n_;
run;

%macro jackknife();
%do i=1 %to 44;
dm "log;clear;output;clear";
proc univariate data=temp trimmed=.05;by dummy;
var x_i;
```

```
where id ne &i;
ods output trimmedmeans=jack;
run;

proc append data=jack out=jackknife;
run;
%end;
%mend;
%jackknife;

proc means data=jackknife noprint;
var mean;
by dummy;
output out=summary mean=mean_trimean;
run;

data jk;
merge jackknife summary;
by dummy;
num=( mean_trimean - mean )**3;
den=( mean_trimean - mean )**2;
keep mean mean_trimean num den;
run;

proc means data=jk;
var num den;
output out=summary sum=sum_num sum_den;
run;

data bias;
merge bias summary;
ahat=sum_num/6/sum_den**1.5;
run;

%macro bc;

data percents;set bias;
alpha=0.05;
z0=probit(phat);
lower=100*probnorm(z0 + (z0 + probit(alpha/2))
 /(1 - ahat*(z0 +probit(alpha/2) )));
upper=100*probnorm(z0 + (z0 + probit(1-alpha/2))
 /(1 - ahat*(z0 +probit(1-alpha/2) )));
/*need percentiles*/
call symput('lll',lower);
call symput('uuu',upper);

proc univariate noprint pctldef=4 data=combine;
var mean;
output out=quantile pctlpts= &lll &uuu pctlpre=p;
run;
%mend;
%bc;

proc print;
```

```
run;
ods listing;
```

The 95% confidence interval is (186.09, 482.38).
The R code is as follows:

```
> data<-c(1397, 471, 64, 1571, 663, 1128, 719, 407,
+         480, 1147, 362, 2022, 10, 175, 494, 31,
+         202, 751, 30, 27, 118, 8, 181, 1432, 31, 18,
+         105, 23, 8, 70, 12, 504, 252, 0, 100, 4,
+         545, 226, 390, 230, 28, 5, 0, 176)
> library(boot)
> my.mean = function(x, indices) {
+    return( mean( x[indices] ) )
+ }
> time.boot = boot(data, my.mean, 5000)
> boot.ci(time.boot,type="bca")
BOOTSTRAP CONFIDENCE INTERVAL CALCULATIONS
Based on 5000 bootstrap replicates

CALL :
boot.ci(boot.out = time.boot, type = "bca")

Intervals :
Level         BCa
95%      (253.1, 550.7 )
Calculations and Intervals on Original Scale
```

17.4.7 Calibration of the Intervals

The confidence intervals obtained from the approaches in the previous section may have undesired coverage probabilities that are caused by the random errors in the sampling–resampling algorithm, the skewed distribution of the data, and so on. To address this issue, calibration of the intervals can be performed by adjusting the nominal significance level α using double-bootstrap methods.

The confidence interval based on the percentile method is again given as an example to describe the bootstrap calibration method. As denoted before, the $(1-\alpha)\times 100\%$ confidence interval using the percentile method is

$$\left(T^*_{(l)}(F_n(X)), T^*_{(u)}(F_n(X))\right),\tag{17.28}$$

where the lower and upper bounds are given by $l=\lfloor B\alpha/2\rfloor$ and $u=\lfloor B(1-\alpha/2)\rfloor$.

In the bootstrap calibration method, α is replaced with $\hat{q}(\alpha)$ such that the estimated coverage probability is close to α, where $\hat{q}(\alpha)$ is the adjusted significance level. Steps for the bootstrap calibration method for the confidence interval obtained from the percentile method are

1. Generate a *bootstrap sample* of size n from the empirical distribution function $F_n(x)$.
   a. Specifically, draw a sample of size n *with replacement* from the data $x_1, ..., x_n$.
   b. This provides a single-bootstrap sample $x^*_1, ..., x^*_n$.

   c. Calculate a *bootstrap replication* of the statistic of interest $T(x)$, denoted $T(x)^*$, by recalculating $T(x)$ using the resampled x_i's.

      i. Now for the inner bootstrap, draw a sample of size n *with replacement* from the outer bootstrap data $x_1^*, ..., x_n^*$.

      ii. This provides a single-bootstrap inner sample $x_1^{**}, ..., x_n^{**}$.

      iii. Calculate the bootstrap resample statistic of interest from the inner bootstrap sample and denote it $T(x)^{**}$.

      iv. Repeat steps i and ii B_2 times.

2. Repeat step 1 B_1 times such that there are now B_1 replications of the $T(x)^*$'s, denoted $T(x)_1^*, ..., T(x)_{B_1}^*$, and $B_1 \times B_2$ double-bootstrapped $T(x)^{**}$'s, denoted by the double subscript $T(x)_{ij}^{**}$, where $i = 1, ..., B_1$ and $j = 1, ..., B_2$.

3. Sort $T(x)_1^*, ..., T(x)_{B_1}^*$ into order $T_{(1)}(x)^*, ..., T_{(B_1)}(x)^*$.

4. Calculate the confidence interval using the percentile method. In this step, only the B_1 replications of the $T(x)^*$'s will be used:

   a. Define the significance level α.

   b. Calculate $l = \lfloor B\alpha/2 \rfloor$ and $u = \lfloor B(1 - \alpha/2) \rfloor$.

   c. Obtain the $(1 - \alpha) \times 100\%$ confidence interval: $(T_{(l)}(x)^*, T_{(u)}(x)^*)$.

5. Calculate the estimated coverage of the confidence interval obtained in the above step:

$$p = \sum_{i=1}^{B_1} \sum_{j=1}^{B_2} I\left(T(x)_{ij}^{**} \in \left(T_{(l)}(x)^*, T_{(u)}(x)^*\right)\right) \Big/ (B_1 B_2) \tag{17.29}$$

6. If p is not close to $1 - \alpha$, adjust the significance level α by $\hat{q}(\alpha)$ and repeat steps 4 and 5 until the calculated coverage probability is close to $1 - \alpha$.

The example below is to calculate the 95% confidence interval for Tukey's trimean based on the percentile method, and then calibrate it using the double-bootstrap method.

```
data counts;
label pl_ct='platelet count';
input pl_ct @@;
cards;
1397 471 64 1571 663 1128 719 407
480 1147 362 2022 10 175 494 31
202 751 30 27 118 8 181 1432 31 18
105 23 8 70 12 504 252 0 100 4
545 226 390 230 28 5 0 176
;

proc iml;
 use counts;
 read all into data;
 *reset print;

 /*Create an n by 1 vector of data counts
 called data*/

 n=nrow(data); /*Calculate the sample size*/
```

```
* Find trimmed mean for the original data;
call sortndx(ndx, data, {1});
ndx=data[ndx,];
trimmean=1/4 * ndx[int(n/4)+1,1] + 1/2 * ndx[int(n/2)+1, 1] + 1/4 *
    ndx[int(n*3/4) +1,1];

bootdata1=j(n,1,0); /*Initialize array for holding
        one bootstrap resample*/
bootdata2=j(n,1,0); /*Initialize array for holding
        one bootstrap resample for inner loop*/

brep1=5000; /*Set the number of bootstrap resamples*/
brep2=50; /*Set the number of bootstrap resamples*/

boot1=j(brep1, 1, 0);
boot2=j(brep1*brep2, 1, 0);

in2=0;
do i1=1 to brep1;
 do j1=1 to n;
  index=int(ranuni(0)*n)+1;
  bootdata1[j1]=data[index];
end;

 call sort(bootdata1, {1}); *sort data;
 bootdata1=bootdata1;

 *Trimmed mean at each out loop;
 trimmean_out=1/4 * bootdata1[int(n/4)+1,1] + 1/2 * bootdata1[int(n/2)+1,1]
      + 1/4 * bootdata1[int(n*3/4) +1,1];

 *Trimmed mean at each inner loop;
 do i2=1 to brep2;
 in2=in2+1;
  do j2=1 to n;
    index=int(ranuni(0)*n)+1;
    bootdata2[j2]=bootdata1[index];
    end;

  call sort(bootdata2, {1});

  trimmean_in=1/4 * bootdata2[int(n/4)+1,1] + 1/2*
bootdata2[int(n/2)+1,1]
    + 1/4 * bootdata2[int(n*3/4) +1,1];

  boot2[in2]=trimmean_in;

  end;
  boot1[i1]=trimmean_out;
 end;

 *print boot1 boot2;

 call sort(boot1, {1});

 * Adjust the significance level, and calculate the confidence interval;
 alpha=0.05;
 do until (abs(coverage-0.95)<0.01);
 z_alpha_2 = quantile('NORMAL', alpha/2);
 Q_l=int(brep1*probnorm(z_alpha_2));
 Q_u=int(brep1*probnorm(-z_alpha_2));
```

```
   if Q_l=0 then Lower=0;
   else Lower=boot1[Q_l];
   Upper=boot1[Q_u];

   CI = lower@j(brep1*brep2, 1, 1) ||upper@j(brep1*brep2, 1, 1)
        ||boot2|| j(brep1*brep2, 1, 1);
   CI [,4] =( CI[,1] <= CI[,3] & CI[,3]<= CI[,2]);
   coverage=CI[+, 4] / brep2/brep1;
   alpha=alpha+ sign(coverage - 0.95)*0.0001;
   final = trimmean||alpha||lower||upper||coverage;
end;
   print final [colname={"trimmean" "alpha" "lower" "upper" "coverage"}];
   quit;
```

Based on $B_1 = 5000$, $B_2 = 50$, the estimated confidence interval is (98.25, 511.75).

Trimean	α	Lower	Upper	Coverage
223.5	0.0091	98.25	511.75	0.940928

17.5 Simple Two-Group Comparisons

A staple of introductory statistical textbooks is the two-sample t-test and the corresponding confidence interval for the difference between two means. The usual assumptions involve sampling from two continuous normal populations. In addition to the normality assumption, we generally assume a common variance between the two groups such that the t-test has the exact level α. In the case of unequal variances and normally distributed data, the t-test based on modifying the degrees of freedom or some other variant is only an approximate test. What if we are interested in comparing group means when we know in advance that the populations are nonnormal and the variances are not equal between the groups? For that matter, the two groups may not even have the same underlying distribution. The bootstrap methodology allows one approach toward solving this problem and extends easily to other quantities of interest, such as comparing two medians.

It is interesting to note that simple two-group comparisons of other population quantities, such as the median or geometric mean, are not included in introductory statistical textbooks. The reasoning for this is simple: the statistical theory for developing these tests is usually complex and generally relies on large sample approximations that may be highly inaccurate in small to even somewhat large sample sizes. The same bootstrap approach toward comparing two-group means holds for two-group comparison of medians, geometric means, variances, proportions, and so forth. This same idea will hold for more complex situations, such as comparing two correlation coefficients.

In this section, we focus on illustrating simple two-group comparisons via the percentile method and the bootstrap-t method for calculating confidence intervals. We also show how to invert these intervals into statistical tests such that an approximate p-value may be calculated. The more complex bootstrap methods are illustrated within the context of some regression examples in the next section.

17.5.1 Summary Statistics

The bread-and-butter procedure for descriptive statistics in SAS is PROC UNIVARIATE. This procedure calculates several of the commonly used univariate sample statistics. The idea illustrates how to utilize PROC UNIVARIATE for two-group bootstrap comparisons in a straightforward manner in conjunction with PROC SURVEYSELECT. Note that our approach for these two-group examples in this section is not necessarily the most efficient. It should, however, be one of the more straightforward approaches in terms of minimizing the number of programming statements. Generally, the most efficient way to carry out these problems is via PROC IML. We illustrate the use of PROC IML for use in bootstrapping with respect to the more complex regression setting.

The key to this relatively straightforward two-group bootstrapping process based on the percentile method is the ability to resample from each group with replacement. This can be done via PROC SURVEYSELECT in conjunction with a BY statement. The resampled values are then sent to PROC UNIVARIATE and the statistic of interest is calculated, again by group, as directed through the BY statement. The values of the statistic are output and the differences are calculated and sorted. The confidence interval is then calculated based on the ordered resampled values as described in Section 17.4, again utilizing PROC UNIVARIATE. The bootstrap-t approach is slightly more complicated and requires a double-looping structure through the data. For the percentile approach, we utilize the simple base SAS commands and then redo the example using the SAS macro language. The bootstrap-t approach is then be illustrated using the SAS macro language with inner and outer macro do-loops.

Our first example deals with comparing two groups in terms of week 13 pABG levels in women randomized to receive 400 or 800 mg of folate supplementation. Note that there are only 12 subjects per treatment arm. We used a small sample size in order to illustrate this example more easily. As was described earlier, large sample sizes provide more accurate bootstrap approximations. The first version of this example illustrates a straightforward approach toward comparing the means and medians between the two treatment groups via a 95% confidence interval for the difference in means or medians, respectively. We then illustrate how to modify the program to get an approximate bootstrap p-value for the two-sided test for comparing the equality of both the means and medians for the two groups. Even though we are comparing means and medians for this example, we could just as easily compare trimmed means or some other statistic that is already built into PROC UNIVARIATE.

For this example, our population quantities of interest are a function of the difference between measures of central tendency. If we use the notation of Section 17.3 and denote the 400 mg group as 0 and the 800 mg group as 1, the population quantity of interest for the difference of means is given by $E[T(F(X_1)) - T(F(X_0))]$, or simply $u_1 - u_0$, while the population quantity of interest for the difference of medians is given by $E[T(F(X_1)) - T(F(X_0))]$, or simply $F_1^{-1}(1/2) - F_0^{-1}(1/2)$, where $F(\cdot)$ denotes the cumulative distribution function. The estimators of the population quantities are then simply given by plugging in the empirical distribution function $F_n(\cdot)$ for the population quantity $F(\cdot)$ to arrive at the difference between sample means or sample medians, respectively.

For the example code given below, we read the data using data step `original` and also set the number of bootstrap resamples to $B = 1000$ within the same data step. This approach is somewhat inefficient in the sense that 1000 replicates of the original data set are created. This approach to programming becomes infeasible for much larger data sets. For larger data sets, the macro approach given next would be one alternative.

The next step is to sample with replacement using PROC SURVEYSELECT in conjunction with the STRATA command. The STRATA command indicates to PROC SURVEYSELECT to sample with replacement within each bootstrap replication b and treatment arm `group`. For each observation, PROC SURVEYSELECT generates the variable `numberofhits`, which indicates the number of times that the observation was resampled within a given bootstrap replication. We now need to create the bootstrap resamples using the variable `numberofhits`. Note that the command `sampsize` needs to be set equal to the sample size per group. If there is an unequal number of subjects per group, more programming is needed in terms of utilizing two runs of PROC SURVEYSELECT per group. This is illustrated in an example later in the section.

To do this, we output the individual observations from PROC SURVEY SELECT `numberofhits` times via the data step `restar` to form each bootstrap resample, where `numberofhits` is a SAS label given to a variable created within PROC SURVEY SELECT indicating the number of times a given SAS observation should be resampled per bootstrap replication. This is followed simply by calculating the bootstrap resampled means and medians via PROC UNIVARIATE. These values are output to data set `difference`, where the bootstrap resampled difference of the group means or medians is calculated. The final step is to simply calculate the bootstrap 95% confidence intervals by obtaining the lower 2.5th percentile and upper 97.5th percentile of the $B = 1000$ differences. This is accomplished using PROC UNIVARIATE in conjunction with the PCTLDEF command.

For this example, the 95% confidence for the mean difference was (0.77, 3.93). This is compared to the classical 95% confidence interval for mean differences calculated within PROC TTEST and based on strict assumptions, which turned out to be (0.54, 4.16). The 95% confidence for the median differences was (0.33, 3.78). This example illustrates how for certain underlying assumptions, mean and median differences may have similar properties.

This example is easily modified in terms of comparing other summary statistics that are built into PROC UNIVARIATE, such as trimmed or Winsorized means. All that needs to be modified are the choice of statistics output via the PROC UNIVARIATE `output` statement.

```
proc format;
value gform 0='400mg'
      1='800mg';

data original;
input group pabg13 @@;
do b=1 to 1000; /*Set the number of boostrap resamples*/
output;
end;
format group gform.;
cards;
0 3.9 0 7.4 0 6.8 0 6.2 0 8.2 0 4.8
0 9.9 0 6.0 0 5.0 0 4.0 0 4.0 0 7.0
1 7.5 1 6.8 1 11.6 1 8.5 1 9.5 1 5.0
1 7.0 1 8.5 1 14.0 1 8.0 1 7.0 1 8.0
;

proc sort;by b;

proc surveyselect data=original
method=urs sampsize=12 out=resample noprint;
```

```
strata b group; /*sample with replacement
        within bootstrap resample and
        treatment group*/

data restar;set resample;
keep b group pabg13;
do ii=1 to numberhits;
output; /*Output the resampled observation*/
end; /*numberofhits times*/

proc univariate noprint;by b group;
var pabg13;
output out=tstar mean=mean median=median; /*calculate the
        resampled statistic
        per treatment group*/

data difference;set tstar;by b group;
keep diff_mean diff_median;
diff_mean=mean-lag(mean);
diff_median=median-lag(median); /*calculate the mean and median*/
if last.b then output;      /*differences between groups*/

proc univariate;
var diff_mean diff_median;
output out=quantile pctlpts=2.5 97.5 pctlpre=mean median;

proc print; /*print the 95% percentile confidence intervals
        for the mean and median*/
```

17.5.2 Bootstrap p-Values

In order to calculate the approximate bootstrap-based p-values for the two-sided tests for comparing means, $H_0: u_1 = u_0$, and comparing medians, $H_0 : F_1^{-1}(1/2) = F_0^{-1}(1/2)$, we need to obtain an empirical approximation to the null distribution for each test statistic based on the differences via bootstrapping.

Once this distribution is estimated, the next step is to count how many extreme resampled values there were compared to the observed mean or median differences, assuming the null hypothesis is true. This will require a slight modification of the program used to calculate the percentile confidence intervals. In terms of the theoretical notation, we need to center the bootstrap resampled statistics around the average value to get the B values given by $C^* = [T_1^*(F_n(X)) - T_0^*(F_n(X))] - [\bar{T}_1^*(F_n(X)) - \bar{T}_0^*(F_n(X))]$. We then count the number of C^*'s that are more extreme than the original observed test statistic, $T(F_n(X))$. In this example, $T(F_n(X))$ is differences between either means or medians between the two groups. We also need to assume that the null distribution is somewhat symmetrical about the average bootstrap value $\bar{T}_1^*(F_n(X)) - \bar{T}_0^*(F_n(X))$ for our test to approximately hold. In terms of SAS programming, this requires a few additional merging operations compared to the confidence interval approach and becomes a little more tedious with respect to the direct programming approach. Those more advanced in macro language programming skills may take advantage of the SYMPUT and SYMGET functions in terms of streamlining the programming statements. Note that exact p-values for these two tests can also be calculated via permutation testing, as described in Section 17.8.

The first feature of this program is the creation of a variable `dummy` within data step `original`. This variable will be used for some simple merging operations. As with the confidence interval approach, we utilize PROC UNIVARIATE to first calculate the resampled statistics per group. The differences between the means and medians are again calculated within the data step `difference`.

What is slightly changed from the confidence interval program is that we now need to obtain the averages of the bootstrap difference of the resampled values, $\bar{T}_1^*(F_n(X)) - \bar{T}_0^*(F_n(X))$; that is, there will be $B = 1000$ differences that need to be averaged. We can use PROC UNIVARIATE to do this as well, and then merge the average values with every one of the original resampled values, $T_1^*(F_n(X)) - T_0^*(F_n(X))$. This is carried forth within the data step `count` using `dummy` as the merge variable. Within the same merge, we also include the observed mean and median differences $\bar{T}_1(F_n(X)) - \bar{T}_0(F_n(X))$. Ultimately, we need to create a variable that is centered around the observed test statistic (difference of the means or medians). This creates the null distribution. Note that even though this seems complicated and tedious, the same program can then be reused over and over again for similar types of problems.

In our SAS program below, the centered bootstrap value C^* for the means is given by `diff_mean_star-mean_star` and for the medians is given by `diff_median_star-median_star`. The final step for a two-sided test is to determine how extreme the observed statistic $T_1(F_n(X)) - T_0(F_n(X))$ is compared to the empirical null distribution of the C^*'s. This is done by calculating the proportion of times by which the absolute values of the centered resampled values $\left| \bar{T}_1^*(F_n(X)) - \bar{T}_0^*(F_n(X)) \right|$ are larger than the absolute values of the observed statistic $|T_1(F_n(X)) - T_0(F_n(X))|$ and creating an indicator variable. This is done within data step `count` using the indicator variables `indmean` and `indmedian` for each test, respectively. The absolute value function in the corresponding if–then statement facilitates the two-sided comparison within one if–then statement; that is, we reduce the counting of the extreme observations in both tails to using one if–then statement, as opposed to an if–then statement for each of the left and the right tail of the null distribution.

The final p-values are calculated in PROC MEANS and are based on averaging the indicator variable `indmean` or `indmedian` coded within the data step `count`. For our example we obtain $p = 0.013$ for the standard t-test, $p = 0.004$ for the bootstrap test for means, and $p = 0.039$ for the bootstrap test for medians. These results are consistent with the results of our bootstrap percentile confidence intervals, where the 95% mean and median confidence intervals did not contain 0.

```
proc format;
value gform 0='400mg'
        1='800mg';

data original;
input group pabg13 @@;
dummy=1; /*use dummy to merge various data elements*/
format group gform.;
cards;
0 3.9 0 7.4 0 6.8 0 6.2 0 8.2 0 4.8
0 9.9 0 6.0 0 5.0 0 4.0 0 4.0 0 7.0
1 7.5 1 6.8 1 11.6 1 8.5 1 9.5 1 5.0
1 7.0 1 8.5 1 14.0 1 8.0 1 7.0 1 8.0
;

proc univariate noprint;by dummy group;
var pabg13;
```

```
output out=t mean=mean median=median; /*calculate the statistic
per treatment group*/

data difft;set t;by dummy group;
keep dummy diff_mean diff_median;
diff_mean=mean-lag(mean);
diff_median=median-lag(median); /*calculate the mean and median*/
if last.dummy then output;      /*differences between groups*/

data original2;set original;
do b=1 to 1000; /*Set the number of boostrap resamples*/
output;
end;

proc sort;by dummy b;

proc surveyselect data=original2
method=urs sampsize=12 out=resample noprint;
strata b group;      /*sample with replacement
        within bootstrap resample and
        treatment group*/

data restar;set resample;
keep dummy b group pabg13;
do ii=1 to numberhits;
output;         /*Output the resampled observation*/
end;            /*numberofhits times*/

proc univariate noprint;by dummy b group;
var pabg13;
output out=tstar mean=mean median=median; /*calculate the
        resampled statistic
        per treatment group*/

data difference;set tstar;by dummy b group;
keep dummy diff_mean_star diff_median_star;
diff_mean_star=mean-lag(mean);
diff_median_star=median-lag(median); /*calculate the mean and median*/
if last.b then output;      /*differences between groups*/

proc univariate noprint;by dummy;
var diff_mean_star diff_median_star;
output out=average mean=mean_star median_star; /*calculate the
        average of the
        bootstrap resamples*/

data count; merge difference average difft;by dummy;
    /*count the number of extreme*/
indmean=0;                  /* bootstrap resamples*/
cstar_mean=diff_mean_star-mean_star;
if abs(cstar_mean)>abs(diff_mean) then indmean=1;

indmedian=0;
cstar_median=diff_median_star-median_star;
if abs(cstar_median)>abs(diff_median) then indmedian=1;

proc means;
title 'approximate bootstrap p-values';
var indmean indmedian;
```

The R code is as follows:

```
> data<-c( 3.9, 7.4, 6.8, 6.2, 8.2, 4.8,
+           9.9, 6.0, 5.0, 4.0, 4.0, 7.0,
+           7.5, 6.8, 11.6, 8.5, 9.5, 5.0,
+           7.0, 8.5, 14.0, 8.0, 7.0, 8.0)
> group1<-c(mean(data[1:12]),median(data[1:12]))
> group2<-c(mean(data[13:24]),median(data[13:24]))
> diff<-abs(group1-group2)
>
> resamples1 <- lapply(1:1000, function(i)
+     sample(data[1:12], replace = T))
> resamples2 <- lapply(1:1000, function(i)
+     sample(data[13:24], replace = T))
> resm1<-lapply(1:1000, function(i)
+     c(mean(resamples1[[i]]),median(resamples1[[i]])))
> resm2<-lapply(1:1000, function(i)
+     c(mean(resamples2[[i]]),median(resamples2[[i]])))
>
> diff2<- lapply(1:1000, function(i)
+     abs(resm1[[i]]-resm2[[i]])
+ )
> average_v<-average_v1<-c()
> for (i in 1:1000){
+     average_v<-c(average_v,diff2[[i]][1])
+     i<-i+1
+ }
> for (i in 1:1000){
+     average_v1<-c(average_v1,diff2[[i]][2])
+     i<-i+1
+ }
> avg_mean<-mean(average_v)
> avg_median<-mean(average_v1)
> cstar_mean<-cstar_median<-c()
> for (i in 1:1000){
+     cstar_mean<-c(cstar_mean,(diff2[[i]][1]-avg_mean))
+     i<-i+1
+ }
> for (i in 1:1000){
+     cstar_median<-c(cstar_median,(diff2[[i]][2]-avg_median))
+     i<-i+1
+ }
> p<-sum(1*(abs(cstar_mean)>diff[1]))/1000
> p1<-sum(1*(abs(cstar_median)>diff[2]))/1000
```

17.5.3 Using the SAS Macro Language for Calculating Percentile Intervals

The next stage in our formulation is to rework our program for calculating the percentile intervals using the SAS macro language. This will give a jumping-off point for calculating the more precise bootstrap-*t* intervals and provides a slightly different programming perspective. You may want to refer to Section 17.3 for a more detailed description of the SAS macro code needed for bootstrapping.

As we mention throughout this text, one simple tip when utilizing the SAS macro language with respect to bootstrapping is to incorporate the nonotes option within the options statement. This can be implemented once you are sure that the program is running properly given only a small number of *B* bootstrap resamples. The only other major modification is that we now utilize a single macro do-loop in conjunction with PROC APPEND, as opposed to outputting data set original, b number of times, as in the previous section.

The beginning of the macro is given by the command %macro diffboot, where we chose the name diffboot. We did not choose to pass any parameters when we called diffboot within this example. The more experienced programmers may wish to do so within more elaborate programs. The macro command %do b=1 %to 1000 indicates that we will resample 1000 times. The loop is closed by the command %end. The macro version of the two-group comparison of the means and medians uses much less memory, but may run slower. We suggest that you may need to code in this manner if the input data set is large, where outputting a large data set *B* number of times would be clearly infeasible. The end of the macro is given by the command %mend. The macro is called by the command %diffboot and can be run multiple times with multiple calls if so desired. After each pass through the macro, the mean and median resampled differences are concatenated to the data set alldiffs via PROC APPEND. The 95% intervals are then calculated as before using PROC UNIVARIATE in conjunction with the PCTLDEFS command.

For this example, the 95% confidence for the mean difference was (0.72917, 4.02917), compared to our first run of the earlier version of the program, which was (0.67083, 4.01667). The 95% confidence for the median difference was (0.225, 3.85), compared to our first run of (0.3, 4). This illustrates that even if the value of *B* is as high as 1000 resamples, there is some element of imprecision. To obtain a higher degree of precision, simply increase the number of resamples to some feasible number based on your specific operating system and time constraints.

```
proc format;
value gform 0='400mg'
        1='800mg';

data original;
input group pabg13 @@;
format group gform.;
cards;
0 3.9 0 7.4 0 6.8 0 6.2 0 8.2 0 4.8
0 9.9 0 6.0 0 5.0 0 4.0 0 4.0 0 7.0
1 7.5 1 6.8 1 11.6 1 8.5 1 9.5 1 5.0
1 7.0 1 8.5 1 14.0 1 8.0 1 7.0 1 8.0
;

%macro diffboot;
%do b=1 %to 1000; /*choose the number of resamples*/

proc surveyselect data=original
method=urs sampsize=12 out=resample noprint;
strata group; /*sample with replacement
                within bootstrap resample and
                treatment group*/
```

```
data restar;set resample;
keep group pabg13;
do ii=1 to numberhits;
output; /*Output the resampled observation*/
end; /*numberofhits times*/

proc univariate noprint;by group;
var pabg13;
output out=tstar mean=mean median=median; /*calculate the
                                             resampled statistic
                                             per treatment group*/

data difference;set tstar;by group;
keep diff_mean diff_median;
diff_mean=mean-lag(mean);
diff_median=median-lag(median); /*calculate the mean and median*/
if _n_=2 then output;      /*differences between groups*/

proc append data=difference out=alldiffs;

%end;
%mend;
%diffboot;

proc univariate data=alldiffs;
var diff_mean diff_median;
output out=quantile pctlpts=2.5 97.5 pctlpre=mean median;

proc print; /*print the 95% percentile confidence intervals
             for the mean and median*/
```

17.5.4 Using the SAS Macro Language for Calculating Bootstrap-*t* Intervals

Even though the bootstrap-*t* interval is relatively straightforward to understand conceptionally, it is somewhat difficult to program using the SAS macro language in conjunction with standard SAS code. More advanced programmers with experience in macro language coding may be able to utilize the SYMPUT and SYMGET functions in order to streamline the program. As you recall from Section 17.3, the bootstrap-*t* method for confidence interval generation generally requires the double bootstrap, described in detail in Section 17.3.2. In order to rework our example for calculating the 95% confidence intervals for the mean and median differences, we need to calculate the version of the statistic $S^*(F_n(X), F_n^*(X))$ described in Equation 17.11 as

$$S^*(F_n(X), F_n^*(X)) = T(F_n(X)) - \frac{\sqrt{\text{var}[T(F_n(X)) \,|\, F_n]}}{\sqrt{\text{var}[T^*(F_n(X)) \,|\, F_n^*]}} [T^*(F_n(X)) - T(F_n(X))], \quad (17.30)$$

where now the quantities of interest specific to our example are based on mean or median differences between the two groups and have the form $T_1(F_n(X)) - T_0(F_n(X))$ for the observed statistic or $T_1^*(F_n(X)) - T_0^*(F_n(X))$ for the resampled version of the statistic. Even though this quantity looks daunting mathematically, it is basically a scaled and bias-corrected version of the original resample statistic $T_1^*(F_n(X))$. Recall that the quantities that make up S^* come from both an inner and an outer bootstrap loop, as well as the original value of the test statistic. Therefore, we need to merge a variety of quantities together from various stages of the program. This becomes a little tricky the first time programming this type of problem. Note, however, the same base code can be utilized over and over again for a variety of problems.

Therefore, within our program we have to calculate and keep track of four key quantities, which then have to be merged together in a specific fashion. The skeleton of our program given below consists of an inner and an outer bootstrap loop within the macro labeled diffboot. There are $B_1 = 1000$ outer resamples and $B_2 = 100$ inner resamples. The skeleton is as follows:

1. `%macro diffboot(outer,inner);`.
2. Calculate $T_1(F_n(X)) - T_0(F_n(X))$ for the mean and median difference.
3. `%do b1=1 %to &outer;`.
4. Calculate $T_1^*(F_n(X)) - T_0^*(F_n(X))$.
5. `%do b2=1 %to &inner;`.
6. Calculate $T_1^{**}(F_n(X)) - T_0^{**}(F_n(X))$.
7. `%end;`.
8. Calculate the standard deviation of $T_1^*(F_n(X)) - T_0^*(F_n(X))$ using the inner resamples $T_1^{**}(F_n(X)) - T_0^{**}(F_n(X))$.
9. Merge quantities from the inner loop.
10. `%end;`.
11. `%mend;`.
12. Calculate the standard deviation of $T_1(F_n(X)) - T_0(F_n(X))$.
13. Merge quantities via the variable dummy.

More complex macros are possible, which would eliminate some of the merge steps. In these instances, we suggest utilizing the SYMPUT and SYMGET functions.

Our full-blown program given below follows the conventions laid out in Section 17.3. Basically, we are reusing the percentile program twice. The same code from the simpler percentile program is used in an inner and an outer loop. As before, PROC SURVEYSELECT is used for the resampling for both the inner and outer bootstrap loops. The values of $T_1(F_n(X)) - T_0(F_n(X))$ for the observed mean and median differences are given by the variables diff _ mean and diff _ median, respectively. The values of the resampled statistics $T_1^*(F_n(X)) - T_0^*(F_n(X))$ for the mean and median differences are given by the variables diff _ mean1 and diff _ median1, respectively. Similarly, the values of the standard deviation of $T_1(F_n(X)) - T_0(F_n(X))$ for the observed mean and median differences are given by the variables sdiff _ mean1 and sdiff _ median1, respectively, while the values of the resampled statistic standard deviation $T_1^*(F_n(X)) - T_0^*(F_n(X))$ for the mean and median differences based on $T_1^{**}(F_n(X)) - T_0^{**}(F_n(X))$ are given by the variables sdiff _ mean2 and sdiff _ median2, respectively.

All these quantities are eventually merged into the data step labeled standardize following an intermediate merge at data step in _ out, where the inner- and outer-loop quantities are first merged. Within the data step standardize the values of $S^*(F_n(X), F_n^*(X))$ corresponding to the bias-corrected and standardized mean difference resampled values and the bias-corrected and standardized median difference resampled values are finally calculated. The final step for calculating the 95% bootstrap-t intervals is to pass the values of the respective $S^*(F_n(X), F_n^*(X))$'s to PROC UNIVARIATE and then simply calculate the upper and lower 2.5th percentiles via the PCTLDEF command.

```
proc format;
value gform 0='400mg'
1='800mg';

data original;
input group pabg13 @@;
format group gform.;
cards;
0 3.9 0 7.4 0 6.8 0 6.2 0 8.2 0 4.8
0 9.9 0 6.0 0 5.0 0 4.0 0 4.0 0 7.0
1 7.5 1 6.8 1 11.6 1 8.5 1 9.5 1 5.0
1 7.0 1 8.5 1 14.0 1 8.0 1 7.0 1 8.0
;

proc univariate noprint data=original;by group;
var pabg13;
output out=tstar mean=mean median=median; /*calculate the
                                            original statistic
                                            per treatment group*/
data difference;set tstar;by group;
keep diff_mean diff_median;
diff_mean=mean-lag(mean);
diff_median=median-lag(median); /*calculate the mean and median*/
if _n_=2 then output;       /*differences between groups*/

%macro diffboot(outer,inner); /*macro for double bootstrap
                                resampling*/
%do b1=1 %to &outer;

proc surveyselect data=original
method=urs sampsize=12 out=resample1 noprint;
strata group;         /*generate bootstrap resample*/

data restar1;set resample1;
keep group pabg13;
do ii=1 to numberhits;
output;        /*Output the resampled observation*/
end;          /*numberofhits times*/

proc univariate noprint data=restar1;by group;
var pabg13;
output out=tstar1 mean=mean median=median; /*calculate the
                                             resampled statistic
                                             per treatment group*/

data difference1;set tstar1;by group;
keep diff_mean1 diff_median1;
diff_mean1=mean-lag(mean);
diff_median1=median-lag(median); /*calculate the mean and median*/
if _n_=2 then output;       /*differences between groups*/

%do b2=1 %to &inner;
```

```
proc surveyselect data=restar1
method=urs sampsize=6 out=resample2 noprint;
strata group;            /*sample with replacement
                           within bootstrap resample and
                           treatment group*/

data restar2;set resample2;
keep group pabg13;
do ii=1 to numberhits;
output;        /*Output the resampled observation*/
end;         /*numberofhits times*/
proc univariate noprint data=restar2;by group;
var pabg13;
output out=tstar2 mean=mean median=median; /*calculate the
                                            resampled statistic
                                            per treatment group*/

data difference2;set tstar2;by group;
keep diff_mean2 diff_median2;
diff_mean2=mean-lag(mean);
diff_median2=median-lag(median); /*calculate the mean and median*/
if _n_=2 then output;      /*differences between groups*/

proc append data=difference2 out=alldiffs2;

%end; /*closer inner do-loop*/

proc means data=alldiffs2 noprint;
var diff_mean2 diff_median2;
output out=innstats std=sdiff_mean2 sdiff_median2;

data in_out;merge difference difference1 innstats;
drop _type_ _freq_;
dummy=1;

proc append data=in_out out=alldiffs1;
%end; /*close outer do-loop*/
%mend;
%diffboot(1000,100); /*pass the values for b1 and b2*/

proc means data=alldiffs1 noprint;by dummy;
var diff_mean1 diff_median1;
output out=outstats std=sdiff_mean1 sdiff_median1;

data standardize;merge alldiffs1 outstats;by dummy;
tstar_mean=diff_mean-sdiff_mean1*(diff_mean1-diff_mean)/sdiff_mean2;
tstar_median=diff_median-
sdiff_median1*(diff_median1-diff_median)/sdiff_median2;

proc univariate data=standardize;
var tstar_mean tstar_median;
output out=quantile pctlpts=2.5 97.5 pctlpre=mean median;

proc print; /*print the 95% bootstrap-t confidence intervals
             for the mean and median*/
```

For our example, the 95% bootstrap-*t* confidence intervals for the mean and median differences turned out to be (1.30722, 3.30574) and (0.70395, 2.80934), respectively. This is compared to our first run of the straight percentile interval approach, which gave 95% confidence intervals for the mean and median differences of (0.72917, 4.02917) and (0.225, 3.85), respectively.

17.5.5 Repeated Measures and Clustered Data

When dealing with repeated measures or clustered data, there is only a subtle difference in terms of SAS programming as it pertains to calculating percentile confidence intervals or bootstrap-*t* confidence intervals. The only functional change is that we now resample vectors or clusters of observations, as opposed to individual observations. The key assumption for our next example is that the vectors of observations are independent and the observations within clusters come from some common underlying distribution, for example, a standard random effects model assumption. Say, for example, we had three repeated measures per subject and were interested in comparing the difference in mean response between two treatment groups across all measures. We would now simply resample the vector of three observations for a given subject within a treatment group, as opposed to the individual observations. The data vectors are independent between subjects, even though the individual observations are correlated within subject. The same theoretical argument holds as before; only now we are plugging in the multivariate version of the empirical distribution function, $F_n(\cdot)$, for its population counterpart, $F_n(\cdot)$, in some population quantity. The same idea for repeated measures data holds for clustered data as well when the clustering units are considered independent from one another.

The approach is pretty straightforward in terms of programming percentile-based intervals in SAS in conjunction with PROC SURVEYSELECT. There are some subtle programming steps that are needed to extend our bootstrap-*t* program from the previous section in terms of linking the number of resamples to the original data set and the subsampled data set within the inner bootstrap loop.

We illustrate both approaches using the data set contained in the appendix. The data have three columns. The first column corresponds to the subject sample, the second column is the G-CSF treatment type, and the last column is the outcome, villous area. Note that this data set is somewhat small in terms of the number of subject samples for these methods to be highly accurate. This example will illustrate the bootstrap method for clustered data in the sense that there are multiple and unequal numbers of observations per subject sample, and the fact that there is no temporal relationship. For illustration purposes, we wish to calculate 95% confidence intervals for both the mean and median differences between groups using all the observations. For this example, the sampling units are labeled x1='Sample Name'. There are $n_1 = 5$ observations for the untreated group and $n_2 = 8$ observations for the treated group labeled as x2='G-CSF Type'. In the program given below, we need to do a few key things different from the univariate case:

1. Create an index variable for each cluster of observations for use in PROC SURVEYSELECT.

2. Use PROC SURVEYSELECT separately for each treatment group. This is due to the fact that there are an unequal number of subjects per treatment group.

3. Merge the index variables back to the original data set and then output the data `numberhits` times.

In our program below, the data are read in using data set a. The data are then sorted by treatment group variable x2 and then subject sample x1. From there, we create two "indexing" data sets, a1 and a2, for use in separate runs of PROC SURVEYSELECT. The output from each run of PROC SURVEYSELECT produces the data sets resamp1 and resamp2, which contain the key variable numberhits described in detail in previous examples. The data sets resamp1 and resamp2 are stacked and then merged back to the original data set a. At this stage, we are at the same point as our earlier programming involving univariate data.

We simply output each cluster of observations numberhits times, noting that we need to account for the times when numberhits is missing (set to ·) with a simple if–then statement. This is done in data step restar. From this point forward, we calculate the mean and median differences from the resampled clusters of observations within the data step difference. Those values are stored through each successive bootstrap resample carried out within the macro labeled diffboot with $B = 1000$. The data are stored in data step alldefs via PROC APPEND through each loop of the macro. Then as before, we simply obtain the lower 2.5th and upper 97.5th percentiles for the variables diff _ mean and diff _ median to obtain our 95% confidence interval.

For this example, we end up with a 95% confidence for the mean difference between group 2 and group 1 of (−3650.31, 1141.81) and a median difference between group 2 and group 1 of (−4178.59, 1627.49), respectively, indicating no significant differences between the two groups in terms of either means or medians. Note that even though we did not examine the within-cluster correlation structure, it is accounted for in the confidence interval generation simply by resampling clusters, as opposed to individual observations. Thus, we have illustrated how the bootstrap approach provides a very powerful tool for nonparametrically dealing with correlated data structures in a straightforward and easy-to-use method.

```
proc format;
value gcsf 1='untreated'
      2='heat-treated';

data a;
infile 'area.dat';
label x1='Sample Name'
     x2='G-CSF Type'
     x3='Area (um^2)';
input x1 $ x2 x3;
format x2 gcsf.;

proc sort;by x2 x1;

proc freq;by x2;
tables x1;

data a1 a2;set a;by x2 x1;
keep x1 x2;
if x2=1 and first.x1 then output a1; /*create subject indices*/
if x2=2 and first.x1 then output a2; /*for each treatmentgroup*/
```

```
%macro diffboot;
%do b=1 %to 1000;

proc surveyselect data=a1
method=urs out=resamp1 sampsize=5 noprint; /*resample number */
strata x2 ;            /*for first group*/

proc surveyselect data=a2
method=urs out=resamp2 sampsize=8 noprint; /*resample number */
strata x2;            /*for second group*/

data resample;set resamp1 resamp2; /*set the resample datasets*/

data restar;merge a resample;by x2 x1; /*merge back to original data*/
keep x1 x2 x3;
if numberhits^=. then do;
do ii=1 to numberhits;
 output;        /*Output the resampled observation*/
end;           /*numberofhits times*/
end;

proc univariate noprint;by x2;
var x3;
output out=tstar mean=mean median=median; /*calculate the
                                  resampled statistic
                                  per treatment group*/

data difference;set tstar;by x2;
keep diff_mean diff_median;
diff_mean=mean-lag(mean);
diff_median=median-lag(median); /*calculate the mean and median*/
if _n_=2 then output;       /*differences between groups*/

proc append data=difference out=alldiffs;

%end;
%mend;
%diffboot;

proc univariate data=alldiffs;
var diff_mean diff_median;
output out=quantile pctlpts=2.5 97.5 pctlpre=mean median;

proc print; /*print the 95% percentile confidence intervals
            for the mean and median*/
```

The bootstrap-*t* confidence interval was somewhat complex in terms of SAS programming for the univariate setting. It is made even slightly more complex in repeated measures or clustered data settings. A strong understanding of data merging is necessary in order to carry out the calculations. As was laid out previously, within our program we have to calculate four key quantities, which then have to be merged together in a specific fashion, as in the univariate setting. The skeleton of our program given below consists of an inner and an outer bootstrap loop within the macro labeled `diffboot`.

1. `%macro diffboot(outer,inner);`.
2. Calculate $T_1 (Fn(X)) - T_2 (Fn(X))$ for the mean and median difference.
3. `%do b1=1 %to &outer;`.
4. Calculate $T_1^*(F_n(X)) - T_0^*(F_n(X))$.
5. `%do b2=1 %to &inner;`.
6. Calculate $T_1^{**}(F_n(X)) - T_0^{**}(F_n(X))$.
7. `%end;`.
8. Calculate the standard deviation of $T_1^*(F_n(X)) - T_0^*(F_n(X))$ from the values $T_1^{**}(F_n(X)) - T_0^{**}(F_n(X))$.
9. Merge quantities from the inner loop.
10. `%end;`.
11. `%mend;`.
12. Calculate the standard deviation of $T_1 (F_n(X)) - T_0 (F_n(X))$.
13. Merge quantities via the variable `dummy`.

The additional layer of work for the bootstrap-*t* interval extends the ideas in the previous program for our clustered data percentile confidence interval. Similar to the percentile approach, we need to do a few key things within the outer bootstrap layer different from in the univariate case:

1. Create an index variable for each cluster of observations for use in PROC SURVEYSELECT.
2. Use PROC SURVEYSELECT separately for each treatment group. This is due to the fact that there are an unequal number of subjects per treatment group.
3. Merge the index variables back to the original data set and then output the data `numberhits` times.

In addition, we need to do the exact set of steps given by 1–3 above within the inner bootstrap layer while carefully merging the index variable back to the inner resampled data set.

The example program given below extends our percentile interval program given above to the bootstrap-*t* approach. As before, we read the data into data step a. We then calculate the sample means and median for each treatment group via PROC UNIVARIATE. The differences between the group means and medians are then calculated in the data step `difference`. We will eventually need to merge these values to obtain S^*, ultimately calculated in the data step `standardize`. As you recall, the resampling procedure for the bootstrap-*t* involves an inner and an outer loop. These are contained within the macro `diffboot` and indexed by the macro variables `b1` and `b2`. Within the inner and outer loops, we utilize PROC SURVEYSELECT separately for each treatment group. The indices for the outer loop are contained in data steps `a1` and `a2`, while the indices for the inner loop are contained in data steps `r1` and `r2`, respectively. Within the outer loop, we stack the output from each of the runs of PROC SURVEYSELECT in the data step `resample1`, and within the inner loop, we stack the output from each of the runs of PROC SURVEYSELECT in the data step `resample2`, respectively. Finally, we merge the `resample1` to data step a and `resample2` to data step `restar1`. Recall that data step contains the original data, while data step restar1 contains the resampled data from the outer bootstrap loop. At this point, we can calculate the individual components that make up having the form described earlier and given as

$$S^*(F_n(X), F_n^*(X)) = T(F_n(X)) - \frac{\sqrt{\text{var}[T(F_n(X)) \,|\, F_n]}}{\sqrt{\text{var}[T^*(F_n(X)) \,|\, F_n^*]}} [T^*(F_n(X)) - T(F_n(X))]. \quad (17.31)$$

The final complicated set of merges involve piecing together S^*. This is done with two sets of merges within data step in _ out within the outer loop and finally within data step `standardize` outside the outer loop. The 95% bootstrap-t intervals are then calculated using PROC UNIVARIATE in conjunction with the PCTLDEF command. Note that the bootstrap percentile interval can also be calculated using this bootstrap-t interval program for comparison purposes simply by including the variables *diff_mean*1 and *diff_median*1 in the run of PROC UNIVARIATE at the end of the program.

For this example, we end up with the 95% bootstrap-t intervals of (–3564.63, 431.82) and (–5386.33, –370.29) for the mean and median differences, respectively. This is compared to (–3650.31, 1141.81) and (–4178.59, 1627.49) for the mean and median 95% intervals. It is important to note that both these intervals are likely on the anticonservative side since the total number of subjects is small. This is true even though there is a large number of observations. In practice, one should have at least 20–30 subjects per treatment group for the results to have the approximate confidence level desired.

Is it worth going to the extra trouble of programming the bootstrap-t interval when the percentile approach is much simpler. If the sample size is large ($n > 50$ per group), both methods should give similar results. For smaller sample sizes (20–50 per group), we recommend that the bootstrap-t method be used. Both approaches start to fall apart in terms of maintaining the appropriate confidence level if the sample size is much smaller, but still provide reasonable methods for obtaining descriptive quantities such as standard errors. One may wish to consider the parameteric bootstrap as an alternative.

```
proc format;
value gcsf 1='untreated'
       2='heat-treated';

data a;
infile 'area.dat';
label x1='Sample Name'
      x2='G-CSF Type'
      x3=' Area (um^2)';
input x1 $ x2 x3;
format x2 gcsf.;

proc sort;by x2 x1;

proc univariate noprint data=a;by x2;
var x3;
output out=tstar mean=mean median=median; /*calculate the
                              original statistic
                              per treatment group*/
```

```
data difference;set tstar;by x2;
keep diff_mean diff_median;
diff_mean=mean-lag(mean);
diff_median=median-lag(median); /*calculate the mean and median*/
if _n_=2 then output; /*differences between groups*/

data a1 a2;set a;by x2 x1;
keep x1 x2;
if x2=1 and first.x1 then output a1; /*create subject indices*/
if x2=2 and first.x1 then output a2; /*for each treatmentgroup*/

%macro diffboot(outer,inner); /*macro for double bootstrap
                              resampling*/

%do b1=1 %to &outer;

proc surveyselect data=a1
method=urs out=resamp1 sampsize=5 noprint; /*resample number */
strata x2 ;            /*for first group*/

proc surveyselect data=a2
method=urs out=resamp2 sampsize=8 noprint; /*resample number */
strata x2; /*for second group*/

data resample1;set resamp1 resamp2; /*set the resample datasets*/

data restar1;merge a resample1;by x2 x1; /*merge back to original data*/
keep x1 x2 x3 ii;
if numberhits^=. then do;
do ii=1 to numberhits;
 output;       /*Output the resampled observation*/
end;         /*numberofhits times*/
end;

proc univariate noprint data=restar1;by x2;
var x3;
output out=tstar1 mean=mean median=median; /*calculate the
                                 resampled statistic
                                 per treatment group*/

data difference1;set tstar1;by x2;
keep diff_mean1 diff_median1;
diff_mean1=mean-lag(mean);
diff_median1=median-lag(median); /*calculate the mean and median*/
if _n_=2 then output; /*differences between groups*/

proc sort data=restar1;by x2 x1 ii;

data r1 r2;set restar1;by x2 x1 ii;
keep ii x1 x2;
if x2=1 and first.ii then output r1;
if x2=2 and first.ii then output r2;

%do b2=1 %to &inner;
```

```
proc surveyselect data=r1
method=urs out=resamp1 sampsize=5 noprint;
strata x2 ;

proc surveyselect data=r2
method=urs out=resamp2 sampsize=8 noprint;
strata x2 ;

data resample2;set resamp1 resamp2; /*set the resample datasets*/

data restar2;merge restar1 resample2;by x2 x1 ii; /*merge back to */
keep x1 x2 x3;                     /*resampled data from*/
if numberhits^=. then do;          /*outer loop*/
do ii=1 to numberhits;
 output;               /*Output the resampled observation*/
end;                /*numberofhits times*/
end;

proc univariate noprint data=restar2;by x2;
var x3;
output out=tstar2 mean=mean median=median; /*calculate the
                                     resampled statistic
                                     per treatment group*/

data difference2;set tstar2;by x2;
keep diff_mean2 diff_median2;
diff_mean2=mean-lag(mean);
diff_median2=median-lag(median); /*calculate the mean and median*/
if _n_=2 then output;       /*differences between groups*/

proc append data=difference2 out=alldiffs2;

%end; /*closer inner do-loop*/

proc means data=alldiffs2 noprint;
var diff_mean2 diff_median2;
output out=innstats std=sdiff_mean2 sdiff_median2;

data in_out;merge difference difference1 innstats;
drop _type_ _freq_;
dummy=1;

proc append data=in_out out=alldiffs1;

%end; /*close outer do-loop*/
%mend;
%diffboot(1000,100); /*pass the values for b1 and b2*/

proc means data=alldiffs1 noprint;by dummy;
var diff_mean1 diff_median1;
output out=outstats std=sdiff_mean1 sdiff_median1;

data standardize;merge alldiffs1 outstats;by dummy;
tstar_mean=diff_mean-sdiff_mean1*(diff_mean1-diff_mean)/sdiff_mean2;
tstar_median=diff_median-
sdiff_median1*(diff_median1-diff_median)/sdiff_median2;
```

```
proc univariate data=standardize;
var tstar_mean tstar_median;
output out=quantile pctlpts=2.5 97.5 pctlpre=mean median;

proc print; /*print the 95% bootstrap-t confidence intervals
        for the mean and median*/
```

17.5.6 Censored Data

Bootstrap methodology for censored data, most notably survival data, does not differ too much from the uncensored case under some standard assumptions. In the right-censored data setting, let the observed random variable be denoted as $T_i = \min(X_i, C_i)$, $i = 1, 2, ..., n$, where X_i is the ith survival time and C_i is the ith censoring time. The true failure time X_i is known only if $X_i \leq C_i$. The data of interest for a single group are given by the pair (Y_i, δ_i), where $\delta_i = 1$ if $X_i \leq C_i$ (uncensored) and $\delta_i = 0$ if $X_i > C_i$ (censored). In the case that the C_i's can be considered random variables, standard bootstrap sampling of the pairs (Y_i, D_i) with replacement is applicable for one group or more than one group; that is, the same bootstrap techniques used throughout the text for the uncensored examples apply here. We will not deal with more complicated censoring patterns in this text, which require a more specialized treatment with respect to bootstrap methods.

SAS has several procedures to deal with survival data analysis. The procedure that deals with nonparametric survival methods, PROC LIFETEST, produces estimates of the survival curve via Kaplan–Meier estimates. One may also compare overall survival nonparametrically between two or more groups of survival curves within PROC LIFETEST using either the log-rank, Wilcoxon, or likelihood ratio tests. Sample quartiles are also part of the standard output. What if one was not interested in differences in overall survival between two groups, but was more interested in differences between specific quartiles, such as the median? One approach to examining these differences is via the generation of bootstrap confidence intervals.

Our example will make use of the well-known product–limit estimator introduced by Kaplan and Meier (1958), with the empirical survival function estimator defined as

$$
S_n(t) = \begin{cases} \displaystyle\prod_{T_{(j)} \leq t} \left(\frac{n-j}{n-j+1}\right)^{\delta_{(j)}}, & T < T_{(n)} \\ 0, & t \geq T_{(n)} \end{cases} \tag{17.32}
$$

where $T_{(1)} \leq T_{(2)} \leq \cdots \leq T_{(n)}$ are the order statistics corresponding to the i.i.d. sample of n failure or censoring times $T_1, T_2, ..., T_n$, and $\delta_{(1)}, \delta_{(2)}, ..., \delta_{(n)}$ are censoring indicators corresponding to the ordered T_i's, respectively. A value of $\delta_{(i)} = 1$ indicates that $T_{(i)}$ is uncensored, while a value of $\delta_{(i)} = 0$ indicates that $T_{(i)}$ is censored.

One important thing to note is that by definition, we make $\hat{S}_n(t)$ at (17.32) a proper estimator of the survivor function; that is, the estimated survival function is defined to take on values from 0 to 1 even if the last observation is censored. The version of $\hat{S}_n(t)$ used in PROC LIFETEST is not defined to be a proper survivor function if the last observation is censored. The reason that it is important to utilize the version defined at (17.32) is that even though the specific quartiles may be estimable given some fraction of the data being censored, these same quartiles may not be estimable within a given bootstrap resample. More obvious to note is that if there is a substantial amount of censoring, no bootstrap method will work particularly well for calculating confidence intervals for the upper quartiles. In terms of SAS programming, we simply need to tweak the data if the largest observed time is censored by defining it to be uncensored.

The data for our example program consist of time-to-event data in weeks for two different treatment (pristane vs. phosphate-buffered saline [PBS]) groups in terms of change in disease status. Our interest is to calculate the 95% confidence interval for the median differences. The programming follows the same approach as our other two-group comparison examples given in the beginning of this section. We did utilize the ODS in terms of suppressing the output for each run of the bootstrap macro via the ods listing close command. We also used the ODS output command to output the sample medians from PROC LIFETEST. The censoring variable for our example is given by censor, and the time-to-event variable is labeled as time. The only subtle part to this programming is to define the last observation from each run of PROC LIFETEST to be uncensored. This is done within data steps fixed1 and fixed2 by forcing the variable censor to take the value 1 for the largest value of time for a given resample and making sure that it is larger than the next smallest possibly censored observation. For this, we use a simple ad hoc approach of adding time/100000000 to the largest resampled value. This does not impact the statistical inference at all, but does ensure that the last observation is uncensored if there is a tie to the next-to-last observation that may be uncensored.

For our example, the 95% interval for the median difference between PBS and pristane turned out to be (2, 5) weeks, indicating a significant difference between the groups.

```
proc format;
value gform 0='pristane'
           1='PBS';

data a;
label time='time to death';
input group time censor @@;
format group gform.;
cards;
0 1 1 0 2 1 0 4 1 0 4 1
0 4 1 0 4 1 0 5 1 0 5 1
0 6 1 0 7 1 0 6 0 1 3 1
1 4 1 1 5 1 1 6 1 1 7 1
1 8 1 1 9 1 1 6 0 1 6 0
1 6 0 1 7 0 1 7 0 1 8 0
1 8 0 1 8 0 1 9 0
;

proc lifetest data=a ;
time time*censor(0);       /*Calculate original estimates*/
strata group;

data b0 b1;set a;
if group=0 then output b0;
if group=1 then output b1;
```

```
ods listing close;

%macro diffboot;
%do b=1 %to 1000;

proc surveyselect data=b0
method=urs out=resamp0 sampsize=11 noprint; /*resample number */
strata group;                    /*for first group*/

proc surveyselect data=b1
method=urs out=resamp1 sampsize=16 noprint; /*resample number */
strata group;                    /*for second group*/

data resample0;set resamp0; /*set the resample datasets*/
do ii=1 to numberhits;
 output;      /*Output the resampled observation*/
end;          /*numberofhits times*/

proc sort data=resample0;by group time;

data fixed0;set resample0;by group time;
if last.group and censor=0 then do;
censor=1;
time=time+time/100000000;
end;          /*set the last observation
              as uncensored*/

data resample1;set resamp1; /*set the resample datasets*/
do ii=1 to numberhits;
 output;      /*Output the resampled observation*/
end;          /*numberofhits times*/

proc sort data=resample1;by group time;

data fixed1;set resample1;by group time;
if last.group and censor=0 then do;
censor=1;
time=time+time/100000000;
end;          /*set the last observation
              as uncensored*/

proc lifetest data=fixed0;
time time*censor(0);
ods output quartiles=q0;   /*calculate the resampled quartiles*/

data med0;set q0;
keep median0;
if percent=50 then do;
median0=estimate;   /*output the median value*/
output;
end;

proc lifetest data=fixed1;
time time*censor(0);
```

```
ods output quartiles=q1; /*calculate the resampled quartiles*/

data med1;set q1;
keep median1;
if percent=50 then do;
median1=estimate;   /*output the median value*/
output;
end;

data difference;merge med0 med1;
keep diff_median;
diff_median=median1-median0; /*calculate the median
                             differences between groups*/
proc append data=difference out=alldiffs;

%end;
%mend;
%diffboot;

proc univariate data=alldiffs;
var diff_median;
output out=quantile pctlpts=2.5 97.5 pctlpre=median;

ods listing;

proc print; /*print the 95% percentile confidence intervals
for the median*/
```

17.6 Simple Regression Modeling

Let us start with one of the oldest statistical models, the simple linear regression model, which takes the form

$$Y_i = \beta_0 + \beta_1 x_i + \varepsilon_i$$

where Y_i is the response variable, β_0 is the intercept parameter, β_1 is the slope parameter, and ε_i is taken to be some random error term with mean 0 and variance σ_i^2. Oftentimes one assumes a simpler form with homoscedastic error terms, that is, $\sigma_i^2 = \sigma^2$. In certain instances, x_i may be considered a fixed constant, while in other models, x_i may be considered a random quantity; the latter model is oftentimes referred to as a correlational model. The method of bootstrapping is dictated by whether x_i is considered fixed or random. We focus on what is called the paired bootstrap method as the general procedure to use, whether or not x_i is considered fixed or random. Theoretically, the paired bootstrap can be shown to be a more robust approach to bootstrapping simple regression models. We will outline an alternative method based on bootstrapping residuals at the end of the section.

In the simple regression model described above, there are typically two pieces of analysis that one wishes to carry out:

1. Estimate β_0 and β_1 and calculate their respective standard errors.
2. Make inferences about β_1 via either confidence intervals or hypothesis testing.

No assumptions regarding the error terms ε_i are needed to carry out the descriptive statistical task of estimating β_0 and β_1; that is, we are basically calculating a mean and standard error. The most well-known method of estimation is through the use of least squares, which minimizes the quantity

$$\sum_{i=1}^{n}\left(Y_i - (\beta_0 + \beta_1 x_i)\right)^2$$

with respect to both β_0 and β_1. This is easily carried out within a variety of SAS routines, such as PROC REG, PROC GLM, or PROC MIXED. With respect to inference about β_1, typically it is assumed that the error terms ε_i are i.i.d. normally distributed with mean 0 and variance σ^2. Note, however, that more complex error structures can be accommodated via PROC MIXED under normality assumptions. If the error terms are not normally distributed, a tricky question, especially in small samples, is whether a variety of well-known "artificial" remedies exist, such as transformations and weighted least squares. What the bootstrap procedure allows us to do is obtain valid inferences involving β_1 simply by nonparametrically using the properties of the empirical distribution of the error terms. The primary assumption about the ε_i for the paired bootstrap is that they are i.i.d. and continuous. The "restriction" regarding homoscedasticity of the error terms may be relaxed. It is important to note that if the error terms were truly normally distributed, the results of the bootstrap method in terms of generating inferences would not be very much different than the classical results. The standard error estimates are slightly different for the paired bootstrap compared to the least-squares-based variance estimates.

Possibly even more interesting is to realize that the bootstrap method allows the user to consider inference via other minimization methods, such as minimizing the absolute deviations

$$\sum_{i=1}^{n}\left|Y_i - (\beta_0 + \beta_1 x_i)\right|$$

The minimization can be accomplished easily using PROC NLP. This method is a so-called robust regression and is oftentimes referred to as least-median, median, or least-absolute deviation regression (e.g., see Rousseeuw, 1984). This is basically an extension of estimating the simple sample median conditional on some covariate x_i, similar to least squares being an extension of estimating the simple sample mean given x_i. About the only practical way of carrying out inferential methods for least-median regression is through the use of the bootstrap. In other words, the bootstrap method provides the user the option of using more modern and robust methods of regression in terms of being able to estimate standard errors and carry out inferences.

Let us start exploring these concepts with a simple example. Below is an output listing of data examining the calculated adherence of cromolyn, a certain asthma medication, as a function of a child's age in years. Let us suppose we are interested in regressing adherence (COMP) on age (AGE).

```
                           Subject
            Obs    Drug        Age    Adherence
            1      Cromolyn    4      0.0
            2      Cromolyn    8      32.0
            3      Cromolyn    1      100.0
            4      Cromolyn    2      14.1
            5      Cromolyn    2      83.3
            6      Cromolyn    8      12.6
            7      Cromolyn    10     45.1
            8      Cromolyn    1      65.8
            9      Cromolyn    1      37.3
            10     Cromolyn    7      16.7
```

The code for the simple regression of adherence on age is given simply as follows:

```
proc reg;
model comp=age;
```

We see from a simple scatterplot in Figure 17.9 that a child's adherence rate appears to drop somewhat as a function of age. From PROC REG (see Figure 17.10) we get $\hat{\beta}_0 = 59.3$

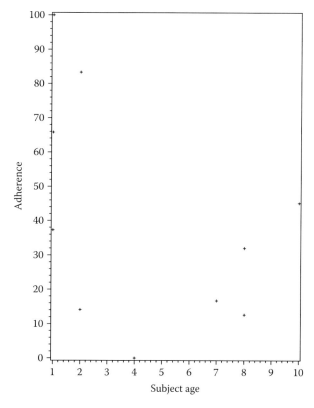

FIGURE 17.9
Scatterplot of adherence by age.

The SAS system

The REG procedure
model: MODEL1
Dependent variable: comp adherence

Analysis of variance					
Source	DF	Sum of squares	Mean square	F value	Pr > F
Model	1	1981.87878	1981.87878	2.03	0.1922
Error	8	7815.65022	976.95628		
Corrected total	9	9797.52900			

Root MSE	31.25630	R^2	0.2023
Dependent mean	40.69000	Adj R^2	0.1026
Coeff var	76.81568		

Parameter estimates						
Variable	Label	DF	Parameter estimate	Standard error	t Value	Pr > |t|
Intercept	Intercept	1	59.33261	16.40174	3.62	0.0068
Age	Subject age	1	−4.23696	2.97477	−1.42	0.1922

FIGURE 17.10
Regression output.

and $\hat{\beta}_1 = -4.2$; that is, compliance drops on average −4.2% for every year the child's age increases within the constraints of this simple linear model. Is age a significant factor? According to the model based on normally distributed homoscedastic error terms, $p = 0.19$, not significant at the traditional $\alpha = 0.05$ level. The corresponding 95% confidence interval for β_1 is given by $\hat{\beta}_1 \pm s.e.(\beta_1)t_{\alpha/2,n-2}$ or (−11.1, 2.6). How valid is this inference? From the histogram of the studentized residuals in Figure 17.11, it is hard to say anything about the normality assumption. A formal test of normality would be somewhat meaningless in terms of power given the small sample size. What alternatives are there when normality assumptions are questionable or quite wrong?

For regression models, the simple percentile method for constructing a confidence interval for β_1 in conjunction with paired bootstrapping tends to work reasonably well. What we need to do is resample the pairs of data (Y_i, x_i) with replacement via a simple modification of the resampling program outlined in Section 17.2. For the first piece of code starting with data original, we manually set $n = 10$, read in the data set, and output it $B = 5000$ times; that is, we resample from the pairs of data (Y_i, x_i) 5000 times in sets of $n = 10$. Next, we generate the multinomial weights via the data set resample.

```
data original;
drop drug;
label comp='Calculated adherence';
```

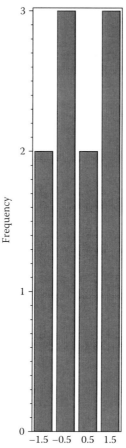

FIGURE 17.11
Residual plot.

```
n=10; /*set the sample size*/
input drug $ age comp;
do b=1 to 5000; /*output the data B times*/
output;
end;
cards;
Cromolyn 4 0.0
Cromolyn 8 32.0
Cromolyn 1 100.0
Cromolyn 2 14.1
Cromolyn 2 83.3
Cromolyn 8 12.6
Cromolyn 10 45.1
Cromolyn 1 65.8
Cromolyn 1 37.3
Cromolyn 7 16.7
;
```

```
proc sort;by b;

data resample;
set original;by b;
retain sumc i; /*need to add the previous
     count to the total */
if first.b then do;
 sumc=0;
 i=1;
end;
p=1/(n-i+1); /*p is the probability of a "success"*/

if ^last.b then do;
if n>sumc then c_i=ranbin(0,n-sumc,p); /*generate the binomial variate*/
else c_i=0;
sumc=sumc+c_i;
end;
i=i+1;
if last.b then c_i=n-sumc;
```

Then we employ PROC REG to rerun the regression 5000 times weighted by the multinomial weights c _ i, and output the bootstrap resample estimate $\hat{\beta}_i^*$ via the outest command. Note that by default, the variable age corresponds to $\hat{\beta}_i^*$ following the PROC REG procedure. Then we simply use PROC MEANS to estimate the standard error of $\hat{\beta}_1$ and PROC UNIVARIATE to obtain the 95% confidence interval. PROC MEANS was used for the summary simply to streamline the output. Note that the command pctldef=4 simply interpolates the percentiles and provides a slight smoothing to the bootstrap procedure. Setting pctlpts=2.5 corresponds to obtaining the 2.5th percentile of the 5000 resampled $\hat{\beta}_i^*$'s.

```
proc reg noprint outest=bests;by b;
model comp=age;
weight c_i;

proc means data=bests;
var age;

proc univariate data=bests pctldef=4;
var age;
output out=ci pctlpts=2.5 97.5 pctlpre=p;
```

From the output we see that the bootstrap estimate of the standard error via paired resampling for $\hat{\beta}_1$ is 3.80, compared to 2.97 for the normal-based model assuming homoscedastic error terms. Note that the term *standard deviation* of the resampled values is the standard error of the estimate. The 95% confidence interval for β_1 is (–11.2, 4.2) compared to the slightly narrower interval (–11.1, 2.6) from the standard normal-based model under more restrictive assumptions. In this case, the overall conclusions do not change much; note, however, that the error estimates are slight larger.

```
proc print;
title '95% Confidence Interval for the Slope';
```

```
      Analysis Variable : AGE

  N       Mean        Std Dev        Minimum       Maximum
--------------------------------------------------------------
5000    -4.5982695    3.7965199     -44.3800000   10.4032258
--------------------------------------------------------------
          95% Confidence Interval for the Slope
          OBS            P2_5        P97_5
           1           -11.2320     4.17287
```

The R code is as follows:

```
> age<-c(4,8,1,2,2,8,10,1,1,7)
> comp<-c(0.0,32.0,100.0,14.1,83.3,12.6,45.1,65.8,37.3,16.7)
> data<-matrix(cbind(age,comp),nrow=10,ncol=2)
> boot.huber <- function(data, indices){
+      data <- data[indices,] # select obs. in bootstrap sample
+      mod <- lm(data[,2] ~ data[,1])
+      coefficients(mod)[2] # return coefficient vector
+}
> duncan.boot <- boot(data, boot.huber, 5000)
> boot.ci(boot.out = duncan.boot)
BOOTSTRAP CONFIDENCE INTERVAL CALCULATIONS
Based on 5000 bootstrap replicates

CALL:
boot.ci(boot.out = duncan.boot)

Intervals:
Level  Normal          Basic
95% (-10.297, 2.641 ) ( -9.202, 2.220 )

Level  Percentile      BCa
95% (-10.694, 0.728 ) (-10.086, 1.176 )
Calculations and Intervals on Original Scale
```

As an alternative, let us redo the analysis using a slightly more complex bootstrap-*t* method with smoothed multinomial counts as described in Section 17.3. Again, the practical reason for smoothing the weights for small sample sizes is to avoid regressions for "extreme" resamples that consist of all of the same pair data; for example, for this data set, a given resample could consist of $(y^*, x^*) = \{(32,8), (32,8), \ldots, (32,8)\}$ which yields a regression model that is not of full rank. The smoothing itself in conjunction with the percentile bootstrap confidence interval should not be used in conjunction with every type of bootstrap method. However, the bootstrap-*t* method in conjunction with smoothing rescales the confidence interval based on the least-squares estimate of the variance, thus providing the appropriately scaled confidence interval. For statistics that are ratios of more basic statistics, such as regression coefficients, smoothing is preferable in order to avoid things such as division by 0. As described earlier, the smoothed counts are given simply as $w_i = c_i - (c_i - 1)/n$. Note that theoretically, one can show that $E(w_i) = E(c_i) = 1$. All we have done to modify the resampling code is to add the line $w\_i = c\_i - (c\_i - 1)/n^{**}2$ in data step `resample`.

```
data resample;
set original;by b;
retain sumc i; /*need to add the previous
                count to the total */
```

```
if first.b then do;
   sumc=0;
   i=1;
end;
p=1/(n-i+1);  /*p is the probability of a "success"*/

if ^last.b then do;
if n>sumc then c_i=ranbin(0,n-sumc,p); /*generate the binomial variate*/
   else c_i=0;
   sumc=sumc+c_i;
end;
i=i+1;
if last.b then c_i=n-sumc;
w_i=c_i-(c_i-1)/n**2;
```

Next, as described in Section 17.3, we need to output not only $\hat{\beta}_1^*$, but also the corresponding estimate of the standard error. This is accomplished via the `outseb` command in conjunction with the `outest` command. We then need the statistic $t^* = \left(\beta_1^* - \hat{\beta}_1\right)/s.e.(\beta_1^*)$, that is, the standardized bootstrap replication. The $B = 5000$ t^*'s basically generate a nonparametric null distribution, as opposed to a table of z or t values commonly found at the end of most introductory statistics books. Note that $\hat{\beta}_1 = -4.236957$ was manually entered into `data standard`. If one wished, he or she could modify the program such that the manual steps could be carried out automatically. The reason for leaving this piece out is for illustration purposes only.

```
proc reg noprint outseb outest=bests;by b;
model comp=age;
weight w_i;

data standard;set bests;by b;
retain betastar;
beta1=-4.236957;
if first.b then betastar=age;
t=(lag(age)-beta1)/age;
if last.b then output;
```

As described earlier, a simple diagnostic tool with respect to the bootstrap-t is to examine the correlation between $\hat{\beta}_1^*$ and $s.e.\left(\hat{\beta}_1^*\right)$. We see from the output that $r = -0.25$; that is, a slight correlation between the estimators indicates that the bootstrap-t procedure should provide somewhat reasonable results. Finally, the bootstrap-t 95% confidence interval is given by $\left(\hat{\beta}_1 - s.e.(\hat{\beta}_1)t_{0.975}^*, \hat{\beta}_1 - s.e.(\hat{\beta}_1)t_{0.025}^*\right)$ or simply $(-10.0, 0.5)$, where $t_{0.975}^* = 1.94$ and $t_{0.025}^* = -1.58$ are given by the PROC UNIVARIATE output below. The bootstrap-t generates a slightly different confidence interval relative to the bootstrap percentile method and, if feasible, should be the preferred method to use compared to the simple percentile method.

```
proc corr;
var age;
with betastar;

proc univariate pctldef=4 plot;
var t;
output out=ci pctlpts=2.5 97.5 pctlpre=p;
```

```
proc print;
title 'Lower and Upper Percentiles Needed for CI';
```

```
 Pearson Correlation Coefficients / Prob > |R| under Ho: Rho=0
 / N = 5000
                              AGE
            BETASTAR     -0.25497
                          0.0001
      Lower and Upper Percentiles Needed for CI
            OBS      P2_5      P97_5
             1    -2.16637    2.90127
```

A bootstrap p-value can be computed within the framework of the program given above. To test H_0: $\beta_1 = b_1$ versus H_1: $\beta_1 \neq b_1$, simply calculate the test statistics $T = (\beta_1 - b_1)/s.e.(\beta_1)$ and compare them to the percentiles of t^* exactly the same way that you would use Student's t-distribution in the traditional sense. For example, to test H_0: $\beta_1 = 0$ versus H_1: $\beta_1 \neq 0$, add the following code:

```
proc sort data=standard;by t;
proc print;
var t;
```

We know from the original PROC REG output that $T = -1.424$. From PROC PRINT, we get a subset of the output from observation 444 to observation 453 (out of all 5000):

```
        444 -1.43261
        445 -1.43216
        446 -1.43054
        447 -1.42732
        448 -1.42459
        449 -1.42362
        450 -1.42232
        451 -1.42218
        452 -1.41945
        453 -1.41837
```

We see that –1.424 falls between the 448th and 449th observation out of $B = 5000$ observations. This implies that the p-value for the two-sided test is simply $P^* = 448 \times 2/5000 = 0.1792$, compared to 0.1922 under normality assumptions. One could interpolate between the 448th and 449th observation for a very slight refinement of the result.

In order to carry out a different method of regression, such as least absolute deviation regression, as described above, we need to use a general-purpose minimization routine. Overall, PROC NLP is a powerful tool that can be used to solve many nonstandard problems. Due to some I/O restrictions on PROC NLP, we need to use the macro `multiwt` to carry out the procedure. As before, we will resample the data $B = 5000$ times with replacement and run PROC NLP via the macro.

```
data original;
drop drug;
label comp='Calculated adherence';
input drug $ age comp;
cards;
Cromolyn 4    0.0
Cromolyn 8   32.0
```

```
Cromolyn 1     100.0
Cromolyn 2      14.1
Cromolyn 2      83.3
Cromolyn 8      12.6
Cromolyn 10     45.1
Cromolyn 1      65.8
Cromolyn 1      37.3
Cromolyn 7      16.7
;

data sampsize;
set original nobs=nobs;
n=nobs;
```

Note that data step `sampsize` is just a quick and dirty example of a way to automatically generate the sample size $n = 10$, as opposed to manually entering the value.

```
%macro multiwt(brep);
%do bsims=1 %to &brep;

data resample;
set sampsize;
retain sumc i; /*need to add the previous
                 count to the total */
if _n_=1 then do;
  sumc=0;
  i=1;
end;
p=1/(n-i+1); /*p is the probability of a "success"*/

if _n_<n then do;
if n>sumc then c_i=ranbin(0,n-sumc,p); /*generate the binomial variate*/
  else c_i=0;
  sumc=sumc+c_i;
end;
i=i+1;
if _n_=n then c_i=n-sumc;
w_i=c_i-(c_i-1)/n;
```

Again, note that we will utilize the smoothed counts $w_i = c_i - (c_i-1)/n$. This means that for a given bootstrap resample, we need to minimize the weighted least absolute deviations given by

$$\sum_{i=1}^{n} w_i |Y_i - (\beta_0 + \beta_1 x_i)|$$

This is easily done via PROC NLP setting `f=w_i*abs(comp-(beta0+beta1*age));`, using the code below. We can then output the parameter estimates using the `outest` command. The purpose of the data step `standard` is to separate out the parameter estimate from additional output created by the `outest` command. Now all that is left to do for this example is to obtain estimates for $\hat{\beta}_0$ and $\hat{\beta}_1$ and their corresponding standard errors. In addition, let us say that we want to calculate the 95% bootstrap confidence interval.

This is easily carried out as before using PROC MEANS and PROC UNIVARIATE. Note that PROC MEANS was used in conjunction with PROC UNIVARIATE simply because of the smaller amount of output. On a technical note, because we are minimizing the absolute deviations, least absolute deviation regression may not produce unique estimates for β_0 and β_1; that is, there is a set of values for β_0 and β_1 that may satisfy the minimization of $\sum_{i=1}^{n} |Y_i - (\beta_0 + \beta_1 x_i)|$, with respect to β_0 and β_1. A more stable estimate would be to use the bootstrap means as the estimates, for example, $\hat{\beta}_1 = \sum_{i=1}^{B} \hat{\beta}_{1i}^* / B$. From the output below, we then have $\hat{\beta}_0 = 2.91$ with corresponding standard error 7.74 and $\hat{\beta}_1 = 2.99$ with corresponding standard error 1.56. The 95% bootstrap confidence interval β_1 is then given by PROC UNIVARIATE as (–0.26, 4.41). As expected in small data sets, the results of this method differ quite a bit from least-squares regression. However, the 95% interval for β_1 still contains a 0, indicating nonsignificance. We will leave it up to the reader to decide which method of regression may be more appropriate.

```
proc nlp data=resample outest=bests noprint;
minimize f;
parms beta0 beta1 ;
f=w_i*abs(comp-(beta0+beta1*age));

data standard;set bests;
if_type_='PARMS' then output;

proc append data=standard out=total;

%end;
%mend;
%multiwt(5000);

proc means data=total;
var beta0 beta1;

proc univariate pctldef=4 noprint data=total;
var beta1;
output out=ci pctlpts=2.5 97.5 pctlpre=p;

proc print;
title '95% Confidence Interval for the Slope';
```

Variable	N	Mean	Std Dev	Minimum
BETA0	5000	2.9075251	7.7424433	-22.7494598
BETA1	5000	2.9875508	1.5587234	-16.6241488

Variable	Maximum
BETA0	133.0690410
BETA1	6.7849456

95% Confidence Interval for the Slope

OBS	P2_5	P97_5
1	-0.25516	4.40828

17.7 Relationship between Empirical Likelihood and Bootstrap Methodologies

For a comprehensive overview of bootstrap methodologies, see the encyclopedia entry "bootstrap methods" (Vexler et al. 2014f). In order to tie EL methods to bootstrap methodology, we first provide some basic background. For this purpose and without loss of generality, we focus on the univariate case. In the univariate nonparametric setting, let $\theta = t(F)$ denote the parameter of interest and denote the corresponding nonparametric estimator as $\hat{\theta} = t(F_n)$, where we define the function $F_n(x) = \sum_{i=1}^{n} I\{x_i \leq x\}/n$. A straightforward example of these types of functionals is the population mean given as $\theta = \int x\,dF$ and the corresponding estimator $\hat{\theta} = \int x\,dF_n = \sum_{i=1}^{n} x_i/n$. The distribution of $\hat{\theta} - \theta$ contains all of the information necessary for assessing the precision of $\hat{\theta}$. In certain rare instances, the distribution of $\hat{\theta} - \theta$ or certain statistical measures of interest, such as the mean of $\hat{\theta}$, can be found directly (e.g., see Ernst and Hutson, 2003). A classic example of direct calculation of the distribution of $\hat{\theta} - \theta$ is the case where $\theta = F^{-1}(u)$ represents the population quantile and $\hat{\theta} = x_{[nu]+1:n}$ is the $([nu] + 1)$ st-order statistic, such that $[\cdot]$ denotes the integer part. In practice, the distribution of $\hat{\theta} - \theta$ is generally approximated via Monte Carlo resampling with replacement from F_n. Since F_n is the nonparametric maximum likelihood estimator of F, we are essentially using a form of the nonparametric maximum likelihood within the bootstrap methodology in order to estimate the statistical functional $\theta = t(F)$. EL methods are generally constructed to focus on hypothesis testing, with confidence interval estimation carried forth through test inversion. Bootstrap methods are generally focused more on confidence interval generation. As described in the "bootstrap methods" entry, several extensions and modifications to bootstrap methods have been developed. Alternative and smoothed versions based on quantile functions are also available in order to develop more accurate coverage of confidence intervals (e.g., see Hutson, 2002). An example of exact bootstrap methods used in clinical practice was based on the method developed by Hutson (2007) for comparing medians between two groups. Wiest et al. (2010) used this exact bootstrap median test to compare changes in S1 neural responses during tactile discrimination learning.

Parametric bootstrap methods follow similarly. Assume the functional of interest is given by $\theta = t(F_\mu)$, where F_μ is a defined parametric form of a data distribution, for example, a normal distribution, and the parameters that define F_μ, given by μ, may be p-dimensional. Then the estimator of interest is given by $\hat{\theta} = t(F_{\hat{\mu}})$, where in the simplest case $\hat{\theta} = \hat{\mu}$ and μ is one-dimensional. If direct calculation is not feasible, then resampling with replacement from $F_{\hat{\mu}}$ is used to generate bootstrap resamples by generating a sample of n random $U(0,1)$ variables $u_1, u_2, ..., u_n$ such that a resampled bootstrap data value is given as $x_i^* = F_{\hat{\mu}}^{-1}(u_i)$, $i = 1, 2, ..., n$.

The direct linkage between EL methods and bootstrap methodologies is through a specific technique developed by Efron (1981), who coined the term *nonparametric tilting*, which now is referred to as *bootstrap tilting*. In fact, one could make the case that bootstrap tilting is essentially one of the forerunners to nonparametric EL methods. As we outline the procedure for bootstrap tilting, we note that this is an approach developed by Efron (1981) for hypothesis testing via bootstrap methodology with an eye toward improved type I error control, compared to more straightforward bootstrap resampling schemes.

The general bootstrap tilting approach as given as follows: Suppose we are interested in testing H_0: $\theta = \theta_0$ or, equivalently, written in terms of the notation of statistical functionals,

$H_0: t(F) = t(F_0)$ versus $H_0: t(F) > t(F_0)$, as opposed to confidence interval generation. The idea behind tilting is to use a nonparametric estimate of F_0 relative to maintaining the Type I error control; that is, minimize statistical functional-based distances such as $\left| P\left(t\left(\hat{F}_0 \right) > t(F_0) \right) - \alpha \right|$ under H_0 for a desired α level such as 0.05. This approach implies using a form of the empirical estimator constrained under H_0 and having the form $F_{0,n}(x) = \sum_{i=1}^{n} w_{0,i} I\{x_i \le x\}$. The $w_{0,i}$'s are chosen to minimize the distance from $w_i = 1/n$, $i = 1, 2, ..., n$, under the null hypothesis constraint $t\left(\hat{F}_0 \right) = \theta_0$ and constraints on the weights of $\sum_{i=1}^{n} w_{0,i} = 1$ given all $w_{0,i} > 0$, $i = 1, 2, ..., n$. One approach for determining the weights is via the Kullback–Leibler distance (e.g., see Efron, 1981). Other distance measures, such as those based on entropy concepts, may also be used. The weights obtained using the Kullback–Leibler distance-based approach are identical to those obtained via the EL method described in this entry. Once the $w_{0,i}$'s are determined, the null distribution can be estimated via Monte Carlo resampling B times from $\hat{F}_0$. In rare cases, the null distribution may be obtained directly, for example, when the parameter of interest is the population quantile given as $\theta = F^{-1}(u)$. The approximate bootstrap p-value estimated via Monte Carlo resampling is given as $\left(\hat{\theta}_0^*\text{'s} > \theta_0 \right)/B$, where $\hat{\theta}_0^*$ denotes the estimator obtained from a bootstrap resample from $\hat{F}_0$. For the specific example, $\theta = t(F) = \int x \, dF$ is the mean and the weights $w_{0,i}$ are chosen to minimize the Kullback–Leibler distance $D(w, w_0) = \sum_{i=1}^{n} w_{0,i} \log(n w_{0,i})$ subject to the constraints $\sum_{i=1}^{n} w_{0,i} x_i = \theta_0$, $\sum_{i=1}^{n} w_{0,i} = 1$, and all $w_{0,i} > 0$, $i = 1, 2, ..., n$. Parametric alternatives follow similarly to those described relative to confidence interval generation given above; that is, resample from $F_{\hat{\mu}_0}$, where $\hat{\mu}_0$ is estimated under H_0. An interesting example of use of the bootstrap tilting approach in clinical trials is illustrated in Chuang and Lai (2000) relative to estimating confidence intervals for trials with group sequential stopping rules where a natural pivot does not exist.

17.8 Permutation Tests

Permutation tests, oftentimes known as exact tests or rerandomization tests, offer a practical alternative to the bootstrap methodology. Whereas bootstrap methods are based on sampling from the data with replacement, permutation methods can loosely be thought of as sampling from the data without replacement and then relabeling the observations. Computationally, bootstrap methods lend themselves more easily to the nonparametric generation of confidence intervals, while permutation tests are generally associated with hypothesis tests and the generation of an exact p-value. Both methods can handle the dual problem (hypothesis tests and confidence intervals); however, in general, bootstrap methods are associated with confidence interval generation. We will only provide a brief introduction to the permutation method. For a more detailed discussion, see Good (1995).

Just as we discussed in Section 17.3, exact bootstrap quantities may be attained with some difficulty. Fortunately, we also illustrated that the Monte Carlo approach to bootstrap methods yields highly accurate approximations when compared to the exact approach. The same idea holds for permutation tests. In a few instances, such as the

Wilcoxon rank-sum test, the exact permutation approach is feasible for small sample sizes. For larger samples, the Monte Carlo approach yields fairly accurate approximations to the exact results. In fact, SAS has many permutation-based methods built in as an option. These include the exact and Monte Carlo permutation methods for many of the statistics utilized in the PROCs FREQ, UNIVARIATE, NPAR1WAY, and LOGISTIC. For other methods, such as a permutation version of the Student's *t*-test, we illustrate how to program the Monte Carlo version in SAS.

17.8.1 Outline of Permutation Theory

The most basic and elegant idea of permutation testing can be traced back to R. A. Fisher in the 1930s. When this method is considered in the context of a randomized experiment, the permutation test generally should be the test of choice. In other contexts, such as epidemiological studies, certain assumptions regarding the underlying stochastic processes need to be made. Classical statistical tests such as Student's two-sample *t*-test rely on strict assumptions; for example, samples are drawn from two independent continuous normally distributed populations, and strictly speaking should be thought of as approximations to a permutation-based *t*-test. The reality in most statistical experiments, such as a clinical trial, is that experimental units are not sampled from some underlying population, but selected and then randomized to an experimental condition. The randomization process ensures that inferences based on population methods are approximately correct. Note, however, that inferences based on permutation methods in the same setting are exact; that is, the Type I error is controlled at level α. Note that due to the discreteness of the permutation test, the exactness of the test depends on the choice of α; that is, the test may be conservative in some settings if we choose the traditional $\alpha = 0.05$. This is because for a given sample size n, the number of exact p-values generated by the permutation method over all realizations of an experiment is finite. Even more importantly, the assumptions regarding permutation-based methods are less restrictive than population-based test statistics. Permutation tests fall into a class of methods termed semiparametric methods.

For example, the permutation version of Student's two-sample *t*-test does *not* rely on the assumption of normality. Yet the interpretation of the classic Student's two-sample *t*-test and the permutation version are similar. Both compare differences between group means using a standardized test statistic. Not only that, but they utilize the exact same test statistic, namely, $t = (\bar{x} - \bar{y})/s_{\text{pooled}}\sqrt{1/n_1 + 1/n_2}$. The key assumption in permutation testing is the notion of exchangeability. In general terms, exchangeability implies that if the null hypothesis is true, for example, no differences in means, then the underlying distributions of the two groups corresponding to random variables X and Y are equivalent. Therefore, it would be valid to carry out a permutation Student's *t*-test on highly skewed data under the assumption that if the group means were the same, each probability distribution would be equivalent versus the alternative that the distribution for one of the groups shifts by some constant amount. If the exchangeability assumption is violated, permutation tests still have good Type I error control. In general, the penalty for gross violations of exchangeability is loss of statistical power. More interesting to note is that permutation tests have similar properties in terms of statistical power even when the parametric test assumptions are met. For example, the powers to detect differences in treatment means under normality are very similar when a permutation test is used versus the classic two-sample *t*-test. The p-values will be almost identical as well. In other words, there is no real penalty for using a permutation-based two-sample *t*-test even when the strict normality assumption is met. The choice of test statistic for use in permutation testing depends on interpretation; that is, are you interested in average differences, median differences, general shift alternatives, and so forth? In fact, the test statistic used in the classical *t*-test takes the form $t = (\bar{x} - \bar{y}) / s_{\text{pooled}} \sqrt{1/n_1 + 1/n_2}$, more based on historical limitations due to the need in earlier years to use standardized tables now found in the back of textbooks. As we illustrate in our examples, the beauty of the permutation test is that it can be based simply on the differences of the means, $s = (\bar{x} - \bar{y})$.

We will sketch out the basic theory using a two-group comparison as an example. Similar arguments hold for multivariate comparisons, one-sample comparisons, and so forth. We will illustrate these methods via example below. Say we are interested in comparing mean values of some active treatment (Y) versus mean values of placebo control (X) using a two-sample *t*-test. Let $X_1, ..., X_m$ and $Y_1, ..., Y_n$ constitute i.i.d. samples from normal distributions. Suppose that the clinical trial consists of $N = m + n$ subjects drawn at random from the population to which the treatment could be applied. The active treatment is given to the first *n* randomly selected subjects, while the placebo control is given to next *m* randomly selected subjects. The effect of the active treatment can be considered the sum of two components, namely, the effect of the *i*th subject and the effect of the *i*th treatment given. Call these effects U_i and V_i, respectively.

Assume that the U_i and V_i are independently distributed. The *V*'s have a normal distribution, either $N(\eta, \sigma^2)$ or $N(\xi, \sigma^2)$, depending on whether the treatment is active or placebo. Also assume that the subject effect, U_i, comes from a random sample from $N(u, \sigma_1^2)$, where

$$E(X) = E(U + V(placebo)) = u + \xi$$

$$E(Y) = E(U + V(active)) = u + \eta$$

$$\text{var}(X) = \text{var}(Y) = \sigma^2 + \sigma_1^2$$

Under these restrictive assumptions, we can test $H_0: \eta = \xi$ using the standard two-sample *t*-test.

What happens under actual experimental conditions? The subjects for a clinical trial are generally not selected randomly from a population. The subjects may come from a certain hospital, they may be volunteers, and so forth. The *U*'s are now unknown fixed constants, say u_i. They are not randomly distributed $N(u, \sigma_1^2)$. Now the joint density of the $m + n$ measurements is

$$\frac{1}{\left(\sqrt{2\pi}\sigma\right)^{m+n}} \exp\left[-\frac{1}{2\sigma^2}\left(\sum_{i=1}^{m}(x_i - u_i - \xi)^2 + \sum_{i=1}^{m}(y_j - u_{m+j} - \eta)^2\right)\right]$$

It is clearly *impossible* to distinguish between $H_0: \eta = \xi$ and the alternative, say $H_1: \eta > \xi$. Data that could serve as a basis for testing whether the treatment has an effect can be obtained through the fundamental device of *randomization* and hence permutation testing (e.g., see Lehmann and Romano 2006).

If the $N = m + n$ treatments are assigned at random, there are $N!$ assignments each with probability $1/N!$ of being chosen. Now the *N* measurements are distributed $N(\xi + u_{j_i}, \sigma^2)$ ($i = 1, ..., m$) or $N(\eta + u_{j_i}, \sigma^2)$ ($i = m + 1, ..., m+n$), depending on whether the assignment was for placebo control or active treatment, respectively. The overall joint density (over all possible randomizations) is now given by

$$\frac{1}{N!} \sum_{j_1,\dots,j_N} \frac{1}{\left(\sqrt{2\pi}\sigma\right)^N} \exp\left[-\frac{1}{2\sigma^2}\left(\sum_{i=1}^{m}(x_i - u_{j_i} - \xi)^2 + \sum_{i=1}^{n}(y_j - u_{j_{m+i}} - \eta)^2 \right) \right],$$

where the outer summation extends over all $N!$ permutations $j_1, \dots, j_N$ of $(1, \dots, N)$. Under the hypothesis $\eta = \xi$ (no treatment effect) $E(\bar{X} - \bar{Y}) = 0$ under H_0.

Without randomization, a set of y's that is large relative to the x's could be explained entirely in terms of the unit effects u_i, for example, confounding effects and selection bias. If the u_i's are assigned to the x's and y's at random, they will be balanced (over all possible randomizations). Therefore, a marked superiority of the treatment under the null hypothesis becomes very unlikely. This permits the construction of an α-level test that $\eta = \xi$, whose power exceeds α against all alternatives $\eta - \xi > 0$. The actual power of such a test will, however, depend not only on the alternative value of $\eta - \xi$, which measures the effect of treatment, but also on the unit effects of u_i. If the intersubject variability is large relative to the treatment variability, there will be little or no power to detect any given alternative $\eta - \xi$. If the intersubject variability is large, the power can be increased via stratification or blocking. Randomization is then applied within the groups.

Therefore, very simply, a permutation test of the two-group comparison consists of the following steps:

1. Define the null hypothesis in terms of some measureable characteristic of interest, for example, the mean, median, or a proportion.
2. Determine the test statistic, which best captures differences between the groups in terms of departures from the null hypothesis.
3. Calculate the value of the test statistic with respect to the original group assignments.
4. Compute the test statistic over all possible relabeling of the groups (or approximate this process via Monte Carlo simulation); that is, relabel an observation in one group as being in the other group. Do this until you have exhausted all possible permutations for the relabeling.
5. Use the distribution of the permuted test statistics to calculate the exact p-value; that is, the exact p-value is simply the number of permuted values of the test statistic that are more extreme than the observed test statistic.

If you can master the examples given in this section, more complicated problems, such as repeated measures or clustered data, follow suit.

17.8.2 Two-Sample Methods

Two-sample comparisons are generally the most widely used permutation methods. They are relatively straightforward to carry out in SAS or may even be built into various procedures such as PROC NPAR1WAY. One popular permutation test that is not built into SAS is the permutation version of Student's t-test. We will carry out an example using SAS macro language to illustrate the Monte Carlo approach to the two-sample permutation t-test and then compare it to the exact Wilcoxon rank-sum test. Following this, we will also illustrate a very efficient method to compare means via PROC IML.

Suppose that we randomly assign treatments to two groups 1 and 2 and that we are interested in testing a simple null hypothesis H_0: $u_1 \neq u_2$ versus a simple two-sided alternative H_1: $u_1 \neq u_2$ about the group means via a permutation test. We also wished that our test mirrored the classic two-sample Student's t-test if the data were truly normally distributed. If the overall sample size was $N = n_1 + n_2$ corresponding to the two groups, then we would choose our test statistics to be $t = (\bar{x}_1 - \bar{x}_2)/s_{\text{pooled}}\sqrt{1/n_1 + 1/n_2}$. We would then need to calculate t over every possible permutation (relabeling) of the two groups and denote those values as the t^*'s. Once that is accomplished, the exact p-value corresponding to the two-sided test is given by the proportion of times that the permuted value $|t^*|$ was larger than the observed value of $|t|$, where $|\cdot|$ denotes the absolute value function. One-sided tests will consist of counting the number of times that t is either less than the t^*'s or greater than the t^*'s, depending on the direction of the alternative hypothesis of interest. In general, directly programming the exact approach for such a problem is rather complex. Fortunately, we can carry out an accurate Monte Carlo approximation to the permutation test rather quickly and easily. Basically, we are rerandomizing the observed data to a new set of treatment assignments in proportion to the original treatment assignment numbers over multiple simulations. This approach easily extends to the regression setting where we simply reorder the rows of the design matrix over all possible permutations.

Our first example comes from a study carried out by Fishbein et al. (2000) examining the pharmacokinetic and pharmacodynamic effects of a nicotine nasal inhaler versus placebo following a single dose. The investigators were interested in comparing several parameters between the nicotine group and the placebo group. One such parameter was the peak percent change in heart rate over the course of time.

The two SAS variables of interest are `maxhr` and `treat`. They are read into `data a`, after which a standard two-sample t-test is carried out via PROC TTEST. We can also utilize PROC TTEST as a component of the Monte Carlo simulation of the permutation version of the t-test. This means that we need to randomly reassign the values of `treat` to the observed values for `maxhr` and calculate the t-test statistic over and over. This is done within the simple macro `permute` 10,000 times.

Basically what is needed is to generate a random uniform number denoted by the SAS variable u in our example program. We then sort the values of the dependent variable `maxhr` by u and relabel the first $n/2$ observations as placebo and the second $n/2$ observations as nicotine. Note that if there were an uneven number of observations between the two groups, a slightly different programming statement would be needed to ensure the proper proportion of relabels that correspond to the original assignment. The permuted treatment values are given by the SAS variable `ptreat` in order to distinguish the permuted tests from the original calculation. We then simply calculate the t-test `mccount` number of times and store the values in the data set `pttests` via PROC APPEND.

We ran this program with 10,000 replications. The variable dummy was created in order to merge the original t-test result with the 10,000 simulated values. The two-sided approximation to the exact permutation-based p-value is given by utilizing the if–then statement `if abs(obs _ tvalue)<abs(tvalue) then ind=1;`. For one-sided tests, we may use `if obs _ tvalue<abs(tvalue then ind=1;` or `if obs _ tvalue>abs(tvalue then ind=1;`, depending on the direction of the alternative hypothesis. Note that for this example we need to assume that the permutation version of the null distribution is symmetrical for a two-sided alternative. This is not the case for less restrictive one-sided alternatives; that is, for a two-sided alternative, we need to assume that the null distributions are symmetrical for both groups.

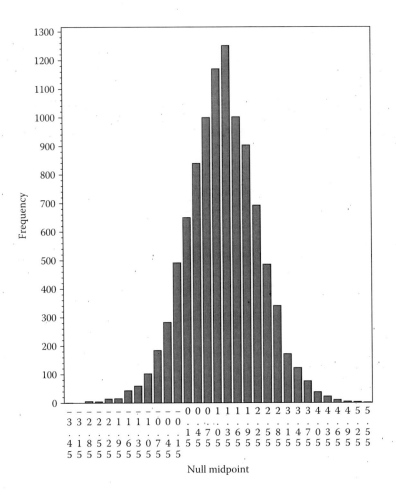

FIGURE 17.12
Permutation distribution under the null hypothesis based on 10,000 Monte Carlo simulations.

For our example, the observed t value was –1.24. We also plotted the null distribution of the permutation t-statistic as seen in Figure 17.12. Upon close inspection, the distribution looks to be somewhat close to the textbook t-distribution one might expect under standard parameteric assumptions. For this example, the permutation p-value is the proportion of observations less than –1.24 in the left tail of the null distributions, in addition to the proportion of observations greater than 1.24 in the right tail of the distribution. As it turns out, the mean of the placebo group was 15.1 and the mean of the nicotine group was 21.5, respectively. The classic two-sample t-test yielded a p-value of 0.23, while the permutation test yielded a similar p-value of 0.23. Note that the interpretations of the two tests are similar with respect to inferences involving mean differences, yet the permutation test is much less restrictive in terms of overall assumptions; that is, the observed data do *not* necessarily need to be normally distributed in order for the permutation t-test to be valid.

```
proc format;
value tform 0='Placebo'
            1='Nicotine';
```

```
data a;
label maxhr='Max percent change'; /* Read in data*/
input treat      maxHR @@;
dummy=1;
format treat tform.;
cards;
0 25.18 0 24.81 0 48.87
0 19.51 0 11.63 0 19.20
0 14.43 0 11.60 0 22.96
0 32.43 1 18.24 1 38.50
1 32.14 1 25.44 1 26.25
1 46.08 1 44.83 1 17.43
1 17.96 1 24.93
;

proc ttest;by dummy; /*Calculate Observed t-value*/
class treat;
var maxhr;
ods output ttests=ttests;

data observe;set ttests; /*Output t-value based
                           on pooled deviations*/
keep dummy obs_tvalue;
obs_tvalue=tvalue;
if method='Pooled' then output;

%macro permute(mccount); /*Monte Carlo Macro*/
                         /*mcount is the number of simulations*/
%do ii=1 %to &mccount;

data permute;set a nobs=nobs;
n=nobs/2;
u=ranuni(0);       /*generate a random uniform to
                     create a sampling with
                     replacement algorithm*/
proc sort data=permute;by u;

data relabel;set permute;by u;
drop n u ;
if _n_<=n then ptreat=0; /*relabel the observations*/
 else ptreat=1;

proc ttest data=relabel;by dummy; /*calculate the t-value*/
class ptreat;                     /*for the relabelled values*/
var maxhr;
ods output ttests=ttests;
ods listing close;

data pobserve;set ttests;
keep dummy tvalue;
if method='Pooled' then output;

proc append data=pobserve out=pttests; /*store the t-values*/
%end;
```

```
%mend;
%permute(10000);            /*set the number of resamples*/

data exactp;merge pttests observe;by dummy;
ind=0;
if abs(obs_tvalue)<abs(tvalue) then ind=1; /*count the fraction*/
null=tvalue-obs_tvalue; /*t-values greater than
                        the observed t-value
                        and examine null distribution*/

proc means n mean;
title 'Monte Carlo Approximation for the';
title ' exact two-sided p-value';
var ind;
```

The R code is as follows:

```
> Placebo=c(25.18, 24.81, 48.87, 19.51, 11.63, 19.20, 14.43, 11.60,
  22.96, 3 2.43)
> Nicotine<-c(18.24,38.50,32.14, 25.44, 26.25, 46.08, 44.83, 17.43,
  17.96, 2 4.93)
> t.test_obs<-t.test(Placebo,Nicotine)$statistic
> resamples_p <- lapply(1:10000, function(i)
+       sample(Placebo, replace = T))
> resamples_n<- lapply(1:10000, function(i)
+       sample(Nicotine, replace = T))
> t_test<-lapply(1:10000, function(i)
+       t.test(resamples_p[[i]],resamples_n[[i]])$statistic)
> vector<-c()
> for (i in 1:10000){
+       vector<-c(vector,abs(t_test[[i]]))
+ }
> sum<-0
> for (i in 1:10000){
+       if (((vector[i]>1.24)||(vector[i]< -1.24))=="TRUE") sum<-sum+1
+       i<-i+1+
+ }
```

The same programming approach above can be used to compare medians, trimmed means, and so forth, via a permutation test. Hence, the reason for illustrating the macro-based version of a permutation test is so the user can modify it for other test statistics of interest, such as comparing medians. As it turns out for the specific case of the two-sample *t*-test, a very straightforward approach is available. We can obtain the exact p-value simply using PROC FREQ with the exact option for the Pearson correlation by noting the one-to-one correspondence between a regression slope p-value and the Pearson correlation p-value; that is, a two-sample *t*-test can be written in the form of a linear model $Y_i = \beta_0 + \beta_1 x_i + \varepsilon_i$ where the x_i are coded as indicator variables consisting of 0's or 1's, depending on the treatment assignment. The ODS output system was used to suppress the table typically generated in PROC FREQ and to direct SAS to output only the exact p-value based on 10,000 Monte Carlo simulations. The key command in PROC FREQ is given by exact pcorr/mc n=10000. The estimated permutation p-value from one run of this program was $p = 0.23$. We will illustrate in later examples that PROC FREQ can be used for general linear regression models as well.

```
proc format;
value tform 0='Placebo'
            1='Nicotine';

data a;
label maxhr='Max percent change'; /* Read in data*/
input treat      maxHR @@;
format treat tform.;
cards;
0 25.18 0 24.81 0 48.87
0 19.51 0 11.63 0 19.20
0 14.43 0 11.60 0 22.96
0 32.43 1 18.24 1 38.50
1 32.14 1 25.44 1 26.25
1 46.08 1 44.83 1 17.43
1 17.96 1 24.93
;

proc means;
class treat; /*calculate summary statistics*/
var maxhr;

proc freq;
tables maxhr*treat/agree;
exact pcorr/mc n=10000; /*suppress table for
                           continuous outcome*/
ods select pearsoncorr pearsoncorrtest
pearsoncorrmc; /*calculate exact p-value for
                  two-sample t-test*/
```

We redid our nicotine example from above using the exact Wilcoxon rank-sum procedure. The example program gives both the exact method and the approximation to the exact method. Both are built-in routines in SAS. For the exact method, simply specify the command `exact wilcoxon;` in PROC NPAR1WAY. For the approximate method, use the command `exact wilcoxon/mc n=10000;`, where mc stands for Monte Carlo and n determines the number of simulations. Note that for moderate to large sample sizes, the purely exact method will not be feasible. Remember that the Wilcoxon rank-sum test is for shift alternatives with the same general assumption that the two groups are exchangeable under the null hypothesis. For our example, the asymptotic, exact, and Monte Carlo approximations to the exact p-value turned out to be 0.22, 0.22, and 0.23, respectively—comparable to our *t*-test results. The choice between the permutation *t*-test and the Wilcoxon rank-sum tests depends on the parameter of interest. Note that it just happened that the p-values coincided so closely for this example between the three methods. In may be that for a given problem, the p-values obtained via each method could vary dramatically. In general, the choice of test statistic should be in line with the parameter of interest, for example, mean, median, or correlation. Knowing the general approach to permutation testing allows the analyst to line up the test to the parameter of interest using a relatively robust semiparametric approach.

```
proc npar1way wilcoxon; /*exact method*/
class treat;
var maxhr;
exact wilcoxon;
```

```
proc npar1way wilcoxon; /*Monte Carlo approximation*/
class treat;
var maxhr;
exact wilcoxon/mc n=10000;
```

As we have seen throughout the book, PROC IML provides a useful and efficient way to carry out computationally intensive statistical methods in SAS. We will rework our current example using PROC IML in conjunction with standard linear model matrix algebra. For the more advanced programmer, PROC IML provides a flexible approach to customized programming SAS.

It is well known that differences between two group means can be estimated within a linear models or regression framework. In this version of our example, our permutation-based test statistics will simply be the difference of the treatment means as estimated by a regression slope from a simple linear model similar to our utilization of PROC FREQ exact Pearson correlation values in the above example. This is done easily by using the indicator variable that denotes our treatment; that is, the SAS variable treat is coded as 0 or 1, corresponding to placebo or treatment, respectively. We can take advantage of the simple regression of maximum percent change in heart rate on treatment to efficiently perform a permutation test for mean differences. The basic notion is that we need to permute the rows of the design matrix in the linear regression setting and then calculate the slope over each permutation of the design matrix. This program is important in the sense that it provides the framework for more involved multiple regression problems and extends beyond standard linear models.

The first step is to get the data into PROC IML and broken into the $n \times 1$ outcome vector Y and the $n \times 2$ design matrix x through some simple manipulations. The intercept and slope are estimated by the classic least-squares method by equation $(x'x)^{-1} x'Y$ and denoted betahat in the program. The slope is the second element of the 2×1 matrix betahat. We then permute the rows of x over mc number of times, calculate $(x'x)^{-1} x'Y$ each time, and denote these values as pbetahat. They key to the program is the code given by

```
do i=1 to n;
 puni[i]=ranuni(0);
  index[i]=i;
end;

sort0=index;
sort0[rank(puni)]=index; /*permute the index 1 to n*/
```

where we shuffle the integers 1 to sample size n using a random uniform number generator. This vector is given by the SAS variable sort0. We then create the permuted design matrix using the sort0 variable using the following code:

```
do i=1 to n;
 px(|i,|)=x(|sort0[i],|); /*permute the rows of the design
matrix*/
 end;
```

The rest is simply counting up the extreme values of the slopes. This program ran very fast compared to the SAS macro-based version of the program and yielded a p-value of 0.23. Note that this test is slightly different than the permutation *t*-test in the sense that we did not standardize the test statistics. We simply needed to calculate the mean difference (slope) over all permutations.

```
data a;
label maxhr='Max percent change'; /* Read in data*/
input treat maxHR @@;
int=1;
cards;
0 25.18 0 24.81 0 48.87
0 19.51 0 11.63 0 19.20
0 14.43 0 11.60 0 22.96
0 32.43 1 18.24 1 38.50
1 32.14 1 25.44 1 26.25
1 46.08 1 44.83 1 17.43
1 17.96 1 24.93
;

proc iml;
use a;
read all into data; /*read DATA A into matrix data*/

n=nrow(data); /*determine total sample size*/
y=data(|,1|); /*create vector of outcomes*/
x=data(|,3|)||data(|,2|); /*create design matrix*/

betahat=inv(x`*x)*x`*y;
betahat1=betahat[2]; /*mean contrast estimate*/

mc=10000; /*set the number of Monte Carlo simulations*/
ct=0;     /*initiate counter for p-value calculation*/
do ii=1 to mc;

 puni=(1:n)`;
 index=(1:n)`; /*intiate vectors used for permutations*/
 do i=1 to n;
   puni[i]=ranuni(0);
   index[i]=i;
 end;

 sort0=index;
 sort0[rank(puni)]=index; /*permute the index 1 to n*/

 px=x;
 do i=1 to n;
   px(|i,|)=x(|sort0[i],|); /*permute the rows of the design
matrix*/
 end;

 pbetahat=inv(px`*px)*px`*y;
 pbetahat1=pbetahat[2]; /*permutation mean contrast estimate*/

 if abs(betahat1)<abs(pbetahat1) then
  ct=ct+1; /*count extreme permutations*/
end;
```

```
pvalue=ct/mc;
print mc betahat1 pvalue; /*output mean difference and exact p-value*/
```

17.8.3 Correlation and Regression

The permutation tests for both the Pearson and Spearman correlation coefficients are readily built into SAS's PROC FREQ. Even though PROC FREQ is traditionally thought of as a categorical data analysis routine, we can utilize it to analyze correlation coefficients even if the assumed underlying distribution is continuous. The reason that PROC FREQ is useful in this context for continuous data is simply that the permutation test itself is basically a discrete test. As was mentioned in the *t*-test example, the only basic issue about using PROC FREQ is the suppression of a possibly large cross-tabulation table. This is easily done by making use of the ODS.

Our example comes from a study by Ignatz et al. (2002) examining various associations in neonates, where for one research question we were simply interested in testing whether the Pearson correlation between x1='Gestational Age' and x2='Platelet Count' is 0 under the null hypothesis versus a two-sided alternative. We first use the standard asymptotic approach that is a component of PROC CORR, followed by the exact permutation approach built into PROC FREQ. For this example, we need to utilize the Monte Carlo approximation because of the computational infeasibility of carrying out the exact test directly. Note the ODS command line of ods select pearsoncorr pearsoncorrtest pearsoncorrmc; controls the output from PROC FREQ. The approximate asymptotic p-value was 0.98 and was basically equivalent to two decimal points to the exact p-value of 0.98.

```
data a;
label
x1='Gestational Age'
x2='Platelet Count';
input x1 x2 @@;
cards;
41   192  27   162  26   310
40   258  40   224  28   172
30   213  33   173  33   271
28   345  25   210  28   274
40   168  39   208  27   345
31   162  27   263  25   191
25   205  31   378  39   369
30   186  31   158  35   278
40   235  39   202  35   353
28   335  35   301  27   215
29   170  25   209  31   276
32   184  28   159  31   189
31   258  31   200  27   351
27   422  27   182  25   161
;

proc corr data=a pearson;
var x1;
with x2;

proc freq;
tables x1*x2/agree;
```

```
exact pcorr/mc n=10000; /*suppress table for
                        continuous outcome*/
ods select pearsoncorr pearsoncorrtest
pearsoncorrmc;
```

For standard least-squares linear regression models, we can take advantage of the same built-in routine in PROC FREQ that we used for the Pearson correlation coefficient for inferences regarding the regression coefficient. Denote the traditional linear model as $Y_i = \beta_0 + \beta_1 x_{1i} + \beta_2 x_{2i} + \cdots + \beta_p x_{pi} + \varepsilon_i$. If one wished to calculate the exact p-value for testing whether a regression slope in a simple linear regression model was 0 in a one-sided or two-sided test, we could utilize PROC FREQ, as well as calculate the permutation-based p-value and attach it to the regression estimate obtained from PROC REG. This is due to the one-to-one correspondence between tests for regression slopes from simple linear regression and tests for the Pearson correlation coefficient. For more complex regression models, there are two approaches that we will illustrate for a permutation-based approach.

Our next example comes from a large study by Bailey et al. (2002) examining homocysteine levels as a function of various factors such as vitamin B12 levels. We will skip the programming steps. Our goal is to illustrate the permutation approach for the regression of homocysteine levels on B12 levels. Our SAS variables are labeled as `thcy` and `b12` for homocysteine and B12 levels, respectively. Our data were read into the data set labeled read. We first carried out our simple regression using PROC REG of the form $Y_i = \beta_1 + \beta_0 x_{1i} + \varepsilon_i$, where again the outcome variable Y corresponds to `thcy` and the regressor x corresponds to `b12`. Our results came out to be $\hat{\beta}_0 = 7.65$ and $\hat{\beta} = -.002$, respectively. The normal-based test of H_0: $\beta_1 = 0$, two-sided, gave a p-value of 0.0017. In order to get the permutation-based p-value, we again can simply utilize PROC FREQ with the code `exact pcorr` and suppress the PROC FREQ table. This is again due to the one-to-one relationship between tests for correlation coefficients and regression slopes in least-squares regression. We used 10,000 Monte Carlo simulations and obtained the approximate permutation p-value of 0.0023—very similar to the standard analysis. If one wanted to test a more general hypothesis of the form H_0: $\beta_1 = b_1$, then simply convert the problem to that of a correlation coefficient simply by standardizing the Y and x values by the mean and standard deviation and reformulating the null hypothesis about the standardized values.

```
proc reg data=read;
model thcy=b12;

proc freq data=read;
tables thcy*b12 /agree;
exact pcorr/mc n=10000; /*suppress table for
                        continuous outcome*/
ods select pearsoncorr pearsoncorrtest
pearsoncorrmc;
```

Our next set of examples deal with a more general approach to permutation testing for regression models via either a SAS macro or PROC IML. Even though we stick with a simple linear regression model in order to illustrate the concept, the SAS approach given below extends to a variety of generalized linear models. Hence, if you can follow this approach, the results can be extended to other models, such as a Poisson regression model and nonlinear regression models. The basic concept is that the outcome variable Y for a variety of models can be written as a function of covariates or regressors taking the form

$g(Y) = x'\beta$, where the function $g(\cdot)$ is applied to each element of the vector Y, x denotes the $p + 1 \times n$ design matrix, and β denotes the $p + 1 \times 1$ vector of regression parameters. For a simple linear regression of the form $Y_i = \beta_0 + \beta_1 x_{1i}\, \varepsilon_i$, we have the design matrix taking the form

$$x' = \begin{pmatrix} 1 & x_{11} \\ 1 & x_{12} \\ \cdot & \cdot \\ \cdot & \cdot \\ \cdot & \cdot \\ 1 & x_{1n} \end{pmatrix}.$$

Additional regressors or covariates simply mean that we need to add extra columns to the design matrix. In the simple linear regression case, the function $g(\cdot)$ is the identity function $g(t) = t$. The programming goal of the more general approach consists of permuting the rows of x' and then estimating the regression coefficients over all permutations. The same approach holds for various methods such as nonlinear regression. The test of the form H_0: $\beta_1 = 0$ then requires that we only examine how extreme the original estimate $\hat\beta_1$ is with respect to the permutation-based estimates of β_1. Our first example revisits the data set used in Section 17.5, where we wish to regress calculated drug adherence on the age of the subject.

As before, we read the original data into the data set a. Our aim is to regress x1='Calculated adherence' on x2='Age'. In this case, permutation of the design matrix simply means that we have to permute the variable x2 and merge it back to the x1 stored in data set a in the original order. The rows of the design matrix are permuted with the macro permute in the data step labeled permute2 in conjunction with PROC SORT. This is done simply by sorting the values of x2 based on the random uniform number u. This process is finalized in the data step labeled newp, where we merge the permuted values of x2 with the original values of x1. We then regress the original values of x1 on the permuted values of x2 mccount number of times within the macro labeled permute. The final step is to merge the original regression estimate output into data set hold and rename the data set observe with the 10,000 permuted values of the slope estimates contained in perms. As with previous examples, we created the variable dummy simply for merging purposes. The final step is to count how many values from the permutation regressions are more extreme than the observed slope estimate in order to estimate the permutation p-value. This is done in the data step labeled exactp. Our results show that $\hat\beta_0 = 59.23$ and $\hat\beta_1 = -4.24$. The standard linear model's p-value for the test H_0: $\beta_1 = 0$ was 0.19. The approximate permutation p-value turned out to be $p = 0.20$. If we wished to work with some other nonlinear model, the same approach would hold with routines such as PROC NLIN, PROC NLMIXED, and PROC NLP. Simply permute the rows of the design matrix, redo the regression, and output the regression slopes as seen below. The PROC IML version of this program is provided in the appendix.

```
data a;
drop drug;
label x1='Calculated adherence'
      x2='Age';
```

```
input drug $ x2 x1;
dummy=1;
cards;
Cromolyn 4      0.0
Cromolyn 8     32.0
Cromolyn 1    100.0
Cromolyn 2     14.1
Cromolyn 2     83.3
Cromolyn 8     12.6
Cromolyn 10    45.1
Cromolyn 1     65.8
Cromolyn 1     37.3
Cromolyn 7     16.7
;


proc reg data=a outest=hold;by dummy;
model x1=x2;

data observe;
set hold;
keep dummy beta1;
beta1=x2;

data permute1;set a;
drop x2;
%macro permute(mccount); /*Monte Carlo Macro*/
                      /*mcount is the number of simulations*/
%do ii=1 %to &mccount;

data permute2;set a;
drop x1;
u=ranuni(0);


proc sort;by u;

data newp;
merge permute1 permute2;

proc reg noprint outest=parms;by dummy;
model x1=x2;

proc append data=parms out=perms;

%end;
%mend;
%permute(10000);    /*set the number of resamples*/

data exactp;merge perms observe;by dummy;
ind=0;
if abs(beta1)<abs(x2) then ind=1;      /*count the fraction*/
                               /*slopes greater than
                               the observed slope*/
```

```
proc means n mean;
title 'Monte Carlo Approximation for the';
title 'exact two-sided p-value';
var ind;
```

17.9 Supplement

1. Feuerverger et al. (1999) provide a nice overview and show the second-order relative accuracy, on bounded sets, of the Studentized bootstrap, exponentially tilted bootstrap, and nonparametric likelihood tilted bootstrap, for means and smooth functions of means.

2. Carpenter (1999) explores the theoretical and practical implications of using bootstrap test inversion to construct confidence intervals. In the presence of nuisance parameters, they show that the coverage error of such intervals is $O(n^{-1/2})$, which may be reduced to $O(n^{-1})$ if a Studentized statistic is used.

3. Polansky (2000) presents techniques for stabilizing bootstrap-t intervals for small samples. His methods are motivated theoretically and investigated through simulations.

4. Hall and Wilson (1991) provide and overview two guidelines for nonparametric bootstrap hypothesis testing. The first recommends that resampling be done in a way that reflects the null hypothesis, even when the true hypothesis is distant from the null. The second guideline argues that bootstrap hypothesis tests should employ methods that are already recognized as having good features in the closely related problem of confidence interval construction. Violation of the first guideline can seriously reduce the power of a test. Sometimes this reduction is spectacular, since it is most serious when the null hypothesis is grossly in error. The second guideline is of some importance when the conclusion of a test is equivocal. It has no direct bearing on power, but improves the level accuracy of a test.

5. Krishnamoorthy et al. (2007) propose parametric boostrap testing of the equality of several normal means when the variances are unknown and arbitrary. Even though several tests are available in the literature, none of them perform well in terms of Type I error probability under various sample size and parameter combinations. The parametric boostrap approach is compared with three existing location-scale invariant tests: the Welch test, the James test, and the generalized F (GF) test.

6. Lin et al. (2015) explore the accuracy of the chi-square tests through an extensive simulation study and then propose their bootstrap versions that appear to work better than the asymptotic chi-square tests. The bootstrap tests are useful even for small-cell frequencies, as they maintain the nominal level quite accurately.

7. Djogbenou et al. (2015) consider bootstrap inference in a factor-augmented regression context where the errors could potentially be serially correlated. This makes the bootstrap applicable to forecasting contexts where the forecast horizon is greater than 1. They propose and justify two residual-based approaches, a block

wild bootstrap and a dependent wild bootstrap. Their simulations document improvement in coverage rates of confidence intervals for the coefficients when using block wild bootstrap or dependent wild bootstrap relative to both asymptotic theory and the wild bootstrap when serial correlation is present in the regression errors.

8. Kleiner et al. (2014) introduce the "bag of little bootstraps" (BLB) for massively big data sets, which is a new procedure that incorporates features of both the bootstrap and subsampling to yield a robust, computationally efficient means of assessing the quality of estimators. The BLB is well suited to modern parallel and distributed computing architectures and furthermore retains the generic applicability and statistical efficiency of the bootstrap. They demonstrate the BLB's favorable statistical performance via a theoretical analysis elucidating the procedure's properties, as well as a simulation study comparing the BLB with the bootstrap, the m out of n bootstrap, and subsampling. In addition, they present results from a large-scale distributed implementation of the BLB demonstrating its computational superiority on massive data, a method for adaptively selecting the BLB's tuning parameters, an empirical study applying the BLB to several real data sets, and an extension of the BLB to time series data.

9. Cheng et al. (2013) provide a theoretical justification of using the cluster bootstrap for the inferences of the generalized estimating equations (GEEs) for clustered or longitudinal data. Under the general exchangeable bootstrap weights, we show that the cluster bootstrap yields a consistent approximation of the distribution of the regression estimate and a consistent approximation of the confidence sets. They also show that a computationally more efficient one-step version of the cluster bootstrap provides asymptotically equivalent inference.

17.10 Appendix: Bootstrap-*t* Example Macro

```
options nonotes nosource;

data original;
label x_i='CD4 counts';
input x_i @@;
cards;
1397 471 64 1571 663 1128 719 407
480 1147 362 2022 10 175 494 31
202 751 30 27 118 8 181 1432 31 18
105 23 8 70 12 504 252 0 100 4
545 226 390 230 28 5 0 176
;

proc univariate noprint;
var x_i;
output out=stat median=median q1=q1 q3=q3;

data tukey;set stat;
trimean=q1/4+median/2+q3/4;
```

```
proc print;
title "Tukey's Trimean";
var trimean;

data sampsize;
 set original nobs=nobs;
 n=nobs;

%macro multiwt(brep1,brep2);

%do bsim1=1 %to &brep1; /*outer bootstrap layer*/

/**********Begin Standard Outer Resampling Algorithm**********/

data resample;
set sampsize;
retain sumc i; /*need to add the previous
                count to the total */
b1=&bsim1;
if _n_=1 then do;
 sumc=0;
 i=1;
end;
p=1/(n-i+1); /*p is the probability of a "success"*/

if _n_<n then do;
 if n>sumc then c_i=ranbin(b1+100,n-sumc,p); /*generate the binomial
 variate*/
   else c_i=0;
   sumc=sumc+c_i;
end;
i=i+1;
if _n_=n then c_i=n-sumc;

data main;set resample;
if c_i >0 then do;
do i=1 to c_i;
 output;
end;
end;

proc univariate noprint data=main;
var x_i;
output out=tri1_a median=median q1=q1 q3=q3;

data tri1;set tri1_a;
drop q1 median q3;
trimean=q1/4+median/2+q3/4;

%do bsim2=1 %to &brep2; /*inner bootstrap layer*/

/**********Begin Standard Inner Resampling Algorithm**********/
```

```
data resample2;
set main;
retain sumc2 i2; /*need to add the previous
                  count to the total */
b2=&bsim2;
if _n_=1 then do;
 sumc2=0;
 i2=1;
end;
p2=1/(n-i2+1); /*p is the probability of a "success"*/

if _n_<n then do;
 if n>sumc2 then
 c2_i=ranbin(b2+100,n-sumc2,p2); /*generate the binomial
variate*/
   else c2_i=0;
   sumc2=sumc2+c2_i;
end;
i2=i2+1;
if _n_=n then c2_i=n-sumc2;

data double;set resample2;
if c2_i>0 then do;
do i=1 to c2_i;
 output;
end;
end;

proc univariate noprint data=double;
var x_i;
output out=tri2_a median=median q1=q1 q3=q3;

data tri2;set tri2_a;
drop median q1 q3;
trimean=q1/4+median/2+q3/4;

data square;set tri2;
trimean_sq=trimean**2; /*Get sums and sums of squares
                        from the inner bootstrap*/

proc append data=square out=second;

%end;

proc means data=second noprint;
var trimean trimean_sq;
output out=inn sum=trimean2 trimean2_sq;

proc datasets;
 delete second;

data all;merge inn tri1;

proc append data=all out=reduce;

%end;
```

```
/********End Double Resampling Standard Resampling Algorithm*******/

/*******************Calculate t-star*******************/

data summary;set reduce;
dummy=1;
trimean2=trimean2/&brep2;
var2=(trimean2_sq-&brep2*trimean2**2)/(&brep2-1);
std2=sqrt(var2);

proc means data=summary noprint;by dummy;
var trimean;
output out=std std=std1;

proc print;
title 'Variance of Trimean';
var std1;

data tstar;merge summary std;by dummy;
sstar=trimean-std1*(trimean2-trimean)/std1;

%mend;
%multiwt(5000,100);

/*****************Calculate Bootstrap=t Interval*****************/

proc univariate data=tstar noprint;
var trimean sstar;
output out=quantile pctlpts=2.5 97.5 pctlpre=p t;

/***********************Print Results***********************/

proc print data=quantile;
title '95% Bootstrap Percentile and t Confidence Intervals';
```

References

Airola, A., Pahikkala, T., Waegeman, W., De Baets, B., and Salakoski, T. (2011). An Experimental Comparison of Cross-Validation Techniques for Estimating the Area under the ROC Curve. *Computational Statistics and Data Analysis* 55(4): 1828–1844.

Aitchison, J., Hebbema, J. D. F., and Kay, J. W. (1977). A Critical Comparison of Two Methods of Statistical Discriminant Analysis. *Applied Statistics* 26: 15–25.

Aitkin, M. (1991). Posterior Bayes Factors. *Journal of the Royal Statistical Society: Series B (Methodological)* 53(1): 111–142.

Akritas, M. G., and Van Keilegom, I. (2001). Ancova Methods for Heteroscedastic Nonparametric Regression Models. *Journal of the American Statistical Association* 96(453): 220–232.

Albers, W., Boon, P. C., and Kallenberg, W. (1997). The Asymptotic Behavior of Tests for Normal Means Based on a Variance Pre-Test. *Journal of Statistical Planning and Inference* 88(1): 47–57.

Albers, W., Boon, P. C., and Kallenberg, W. C. (2000). Size and Power of Pretest Procedures. *Annals of Statistics* 28(1): 195–214.

Albert, P. S., Harel, O., Perkins, N., and Browne, R. (2010). Use of Multiple Assays Subject to Detection Limits with Regression Modeling in Assessing the Relationship between Exposure and Outcome. *Epidemiology (Cambridge, Mass.)* 21(Suppl. 4): S35–S43.

Alfredas, R., and Charles, S. (2004). Holder Norm Test Statistics for Epidemic Change. *Journal of Statistical Planning and Inference* 126(2): 495–520.

Aly, E.-E. A. A., and Bouzar, N. (1992). On Maximum Likelihood Ratio Tests for the Change-Point Problem. Technical Report 7. Department of Mathematical Science Center, University of Alberta.

Andersen, E. B. (1970). Asymptotic Properties of Conditional Maximum-Likelihood Estimators. *Journal of the Royal Statistical Society: Series B (Methodological)* 32(2): 283–301.

Anderson, T. W., and Darling, D. A. (1952). Asymptotic Theory of Certain Goodness of Fit Criteria Based on Stochastic Processes. *Annals of Mathematical Statistics* 23(2): 193–212.

Anderson, T. W., and Darling, D. A. (1954). A Test of Goodness of Fit. *Journal of the American Statistical Association* 49(268): 765–769.

Andrews, D. W., Lee, I., and Ploberger, W. (1996). Optimal Changepoint Tests for Normal Linear Regression. *Journal of Econometrics* 70(1): 9–38.

Anscombe, F. J. (1973). Graphs in Statistical Analysis. *American Statistician* 27(1): 17–21.

Arizono, I., and Ohta, H. (1989). A Test for Normality Based on Kullback-Leibler Information. *American Statistician* 43(1): 20–22.

Armitage, P. (1975). *Sequential Medical Trials*. John Wiley & Sons, New York.

Armitage, P. (1981). Importance of Prognostic Factors in the Analysis of Data from Clinical Trials. *Controlled Clinical Trials* 1(4): 347–353.

Armitage, P. (1991). Interim Analysis in Clinical Trials. *Statistics in Medicine* 10(6): 925–937.

Armitage, P., McPherson, C., and Rowe, B. (1969). Repeated Significance Tests on Accumulating Data. *Journal of the Royal Statistical Society: Series A (General)* 132(2): 235–244.

Armstrong, D. (1994). *Free Radicals in Diagnostic Medicine: A Systems Approach to Laboratory Technology, Clinical Correlations, and Antioxidant Therapy*. Springer Science & Business Media, New York.

Aroian, L. A. (1968). Sequential Analysis, Direct Method. *Technometrics* 10(1): 125–132.

Aroian, L. A., and Robison, D. (1969). Direct Methods for Exact Truncated Sequential Tests of the Mean of a Normal Distribution. *Technometrics* 11(4): 661–675.

Ashby, D. (2006). Bayesian Statistics in Medicine: A 25 Year Review. *Statistics in Medicine* 25(21): 3589–3631.

Auh, S., and Sampson, A. R. (2006). Isotonic Logistic Discrimination. *Biometrika* 93(4): 961–972.

Austin, P. C., Mamdani, M. M., Juurlink, D. N., and Hux, J. E. (2006). Testing Multiple Statistical Hypotheses Resulted in Spurious Associations: A Study of Astrological Signs and Health. *Journal of Clinical Epidemiology* 59(9): 964–969.

Azzalini, A., and Bowman, A. (1990). A Look at Some Data on the Old Faithful Geyser. *Applied Statistics* 39(3): 357–365.

Azzalini, A., and Dalla Valle, A. (1996). The Multivariate Skew-Normal Distribution. *Biometrika* 83(4): 715–726.

Baggerly, K. A. (1998). Empirical Likelihood as a Goodness-of-Fit Measure. *Biometrika* 85(3): 535–547.

Bai, J., and Perron, P. (2003). Computation and Analysis of Multiple Structural Change Models. *Journal of Applied Econometrics* 18(1): 1–22.

Bailey, L. B., Duhaney, R. L., Maneval, D. R., Kauwell, G. P., Quinlivan, E. P., Davis, S. R., Cuadras, A., Hutson, A. D., and Gregory, J. F. (2002). Vitamin B-12 Status Is Inversely Associated with Plasma Homocysteine in Young Women with C677t and/or A1298c Methylenetetrahydrofolate Reductase Polymorphisms. *Journal of Nutrition* 132(7): 1872–1878.

Bakeman, R. (1997). *Observing Interaction: An Introduction to Sequential Analysis.* Cambridge University Press, New York.

Bakeman, R., and Quera, V. (1995). Log-Linear Approaches to Lag-Sequential Analysis When Consecutive Codes May and Cannot Repeat. *Psychological Bulletin* 118(2): 272–284.

Bakeman, R., and Robinson, B. F. (2013). *Understanding Log-Linear Analysis with ILOG: An Interactive Approach.* Psychology Press, Hillsdale, NJ.

Baker, S. G., Schuit, E., Steyerberg, E. W., Pencina, M. J., Vickers, A., Moons, K. G., Mol, B. W., and Lindeman, K. S. (2014). How to Interpret a Small Increase in AUC with an Additional Risk Prediction Marker: Decision Analysis Comes Through. *Statistics in Medicine* 33(22): 3946–3959.

Bakir, S. T. (2004). A Distribution-Free Shewhart Quality Control Chart Based on Signed-Ranks. *Quality Engineering* 16(4): 613–623.

Balakrishnan, N., Johnson, N. L., and Kotz, S. (1994). *Continuous Univariate Distributions.* Wiley, New York.

Balakrishnan, N., and Lai, C.-D. (2009). *Continuous Bivariate Distributions.* Springer Science & Business Media, New York.

Ball, P. (2011). *Shapes: Nature's Patterns: A Tapestry in Three Parts.* Oxford University Press, New York.

Bamber, D. (1975). The Area above the Ordinal Dominance Graph and the Area below the Receiver Operating Characteristic Graph. *Journal of Mathematical Psychology* 12(4): 387–415.

Bandos, A. I., Rockette, H. E., and Gur, D. (2005). A Permutation Test Sensitive to Differences in Areas for Comparing ROC Curves from a Paired Design. *Statistics in Medicine* 24(18): 2873–2893.

Banerjee, M., and Wellner, J. A. (2001). Likelihood Ratio Tests for Monotone Functions. *Annals of Statistics* 29(6): 1699–1731.

Bantis, L. E., Nakas, C. T., and Reiser, B. (2014). Construction of Confidence Regions in the ROC Space after the Estimation of the Optimal Youden Index-Based Cut-Off Point. *Biometrics* 70(1): 212–223.

Barbieri, M. M., Liseo, B., and Petrella, L. (2000). Miscellanea. Bayes Factors for Fieller's Problem. *Biometrika* 87(3): 717–723.

Bargmann, E., and Ghosh, S. P. (1964). Non-central Statistical Distribution Programs for a Computer Langugage. (IBN Research Report RC-1231).

Barlow, R. E. (1968). Likelihood Ratio Tests for Restricted Families of Probability Distributions. *Annals of Mathematical Statistics* 39(2): 547–560.

Barnard, F. R. (1927). One Picture Is Worth Ten Thousand Words. *Printers' Ink* 114–115.

Barnard, G. A. (1946). Sequential Tests in Industrial Statistics. *Journal of the Royal Statistical Society* 8(Suppl.): 1–26.

Barnett, V. (1975). Probability Plotting Methods and Order Statistics. *Applied Statistics* 24(1): 95–108.

Barry, D., and Hartigan, J. A. (1993). A Bayesian Analysis for Change Point Problems. *Journal of the American Statistical Association* 88(421): 309–319.

Bartholomew, D. (1961). Ordered Tests in the Analysis of Variance. *Biometrika* 48(3/4): 325–332.

Bartky, W. (1943). Multiple Sampling with Constant Probability. *Annals of Mathematical Statistics* 14(4): 363–377.

Barton, D. E., and Mallows, C. L. (1965). Some Aspects of the Random Sequence. *Annals of Mathematical Statistics* 36(1): 236–260.

Basu, A. (1983). Identifiability. *Encyclopedia of Statistical Sciences* 4: 2–6.

Bauer, P., and Kohne, K. (1994). Evaluation of Experiments with Adaptive Interim Analyses. *Biometrics* 50(4): 1029–1041.

Baum, C. W., and Veeravalli, V. V. (1994). A Sequential Procedure for Multihypothesis Testing. *IEEE Transactions on Information Theory* 40(6): 1994–2007.

Baumgartner, W., Weiß, P., and Schindler, H. (1998). A Nonparametric Test for the General Two-Sample Problem. *Biometrics* 54(3): 1129–1135.

Bayes, T. (1763). An Essay toward Solving a Problem in the Doctrine of Chances. *Philosophical Transactions of the Royal Society of London* 53: 376–398.

Beeton, M., Yule, G., and Pearson, K. (1900). Data for the Problem of Evolution in Man. V. On the Correlation between Duration of Life and the Number of Offspring. *Proceedings of the Royal Society of London* 67: 159–179.

Bell, C., and Doksum, K. (1967). Distribution-Free Tests of Independence. *Annals of Mathematical Statistics* 38(2): 429–446.

Bembom, O., and van der Laan, M. J. (2007). Statistical Methods for Analyzing Sequentially Randomized Trials. *Journal of the National Cancer Institute* 99(21): 1577–1582.

Bender, R. (1999). Quantitative Risk Assessment in Epidemiological Studies Investigating Threshold Effects. *Biometrical Journal* 41(3): 305–319.

Benjamini, Y., and Hochberg, Y. (1995). Controlling the False Discovery Rate: A Practical and Powerful Approach to Multiple Testing. *Journal of the Royal Statistical Society: Series B (Methodological)* 57(1): 289–300.

Berger, J. O. (1980). *Statistical Decision Theory: Foundations, Concepts, and Methods.* Springer-Verlag, New York.

Berger, J. O. (1985). *Statistical Decision Theory and Bayesian Analysis.* Springer-Verlag, New York.

Berger, J. O., and Delampady, M. (1987). Testing Precise Hypotheses. *Statistical Science* 2(3): 317–335.

Berger, J. O., and Pericchi, L. R. (1996). The Intrinsic Bayes Factor for Model Selection and Prediction. *Journal of the American Statistical Association* 91(433): 109–122.

Berger, J. O., and Sellke, T. (1987). Testing a Point Null Hypothesis: The Irreconcilability of P Values and Evidence. *Journal of the American Statistical Association* 82(397): 112–122.

Berger, J. O., and Wolpert, R. L. (1988). *The Likelihood Principle.* 2nd ed. Institute of Mathematical Statistics, Hayward, CA.

Berger, J. O., Wolpert, R. L., Bayarri, M., DeGroot, M., Hill, B. M., Lane, D. A., and LeCam, L. (1988). The Likelihood Principle. *Lecture Notes—Monograph Series* 6: iii–199.

Berk, R. H. (1973). Some Asymptotic Aspects of Sequential Analysis. *Annals of Statistics* 1(6): 1126–1138.

Berk, R. H. (1975). Locally Most Powerful Sequential Tests. *Annals of Statistics* 3(2): 373–381.

Bernardo, J. M., and Smith, A. F. M. (1994). *Bayesian Theory.* Wiley, Toronto.

Berwick, M., Begg, C. B., Fine, J. A., Roush, G. C., and Barnhill, R. L. (1996). Screening for Cutaneous Melanoma by Skin Self-Examination. *Journal of the National Cancer Institute* 88(1): 17–23.

Betensky, R. A. (1997). Conditional Power Calculations for Early Acceptance of H0 Embedded in Sequential Tests. *Statistics in Medicine* 16(4): 465–477.

Betensky, R. A. (1998). Multiple Imputation for Early Stopping of a Complex Clinical Trial. *Biometrics* 54(1): 229–242.

Bhat, K., and Rao, K. A. (2007). On Tests for a Normal Mean with Known Coefficient of Variation. *International Statistical Review* 75(2): 170–182.

Bhattacharya, P., Gastwirth, J., and Wright, A. (1982). Two Modified Wilcoxon Tests for Symmetry about an Unknown Location Parameter. *Biometrika* 69(2): 377–382.

Bhattacharyya, G., and Johnson, R. A. (1968). Nonparametric Tests for Shift at an Unknown Time Point. *Annals of Mathematical Statistics* 39(5): 1731–1743.

Bhattacharyya, G., Johnson, R. A., and Neave, H. (1970). Percentage Points of Some Non-Parametric Tests for Independence and Empirical Power Comparisons. *Journal of the American Statistical Association* 65(330): 976–983.

Bhuchongkul, S. (1964). A Class of Nonparametric Tests for Independence in Bivariate Populations. *Annals of Mathematical Statistics* 35(1): 138–149.

Bickel, P., Chibishov, D., and Van Zwet, W. (1981). On the Efficiency of First and Second Order. *International Statistical Review* 49(2): 169–175.

Birnbaum, M. (2012). A Statistical Test of Independence in Choice Data with Small Samples. *Judgment and Decision Making* 7(1): 97–109.

Bland, J. M., and Altman, D. G. (1998). Bayesians and Frequentists. *BMJ* 317: 1151–1160.

Bleistein, N., and Handelsman, R. A. (1975). *Asymptotic Expansions of Integrals*. Courier Corporation, New York.

Blest, D. C. (1999). Choice and Order: An Extension to Kendall's Tau. *Journal of the Royal Statistical Society: Series D (The Statistician)* 48(2): 227–237.

Bloch, D. A., Lai, T. L., and Tubert-Bitter, P. (2001). One-Sided Tests in Clinical Trials with Multiple Endpoints. *Biometrics* 57(4): 1039–1047.

Blum, J. R., Kiefer, J., and Rosenblatt, M. (1961). Distribution Free Tests of Independence Based on the Sample Distribution Function. *Annals of Mathematical Statistics* 36(2): 485–498.

Bock, M., Diaconis, P., Huffer, F., and Perlman, M. (1987). Inequalities for Linear Combinations of Gamma Random Variables. *Canadian Journal of Statistics* 15(4): 387–395.

Bolboaca, S.-D., and Jäntschi, L. (2006). Pearson versus Spearman, Kendall's Tau Correlation Analysis on Structure-Activity Relationships of Biologic Active Compounds. *Leonardo Journal of Sciences* 5(9): 179–200.

Booth, J. G., and Sarkar, S. (1998). Monte Carlo Approximation of Bootstrap Variances. *American Statistician* 52(4): 354–357.

Borovkov, A. A. (1999). Asymptotically Optimal Solutions in the Change-Point Problem. *Theory of Probability and Its Applications* 43(4): 539–561.

Bowman, A., and Foster, P. (1993). Adaptive Smoothing and Density-Based Tests of Multivariate Normality. *Journal of the American Statistical Association* 88(422): 529–537.

Box, G. E. (1976). Science and Statistics. *Journal of the American Statistical Association* 71(356): 791–799.

Box, G. E. (1980). Sampling and Bayes' Inference in Scientific Modelling and Robustness. *Journal of the Royal Statistical Society: Series A (General)* 143(4): 383–430.

Box, G. E., and Cox, D. R. (1964). An Analysis of Transformations. *Journal of the Royal Statistical Society: Series B (Methodological)* 26(2): 211–252.

Box, G. E., Hunter, W. G., and Hunter, J. S. (1978). *Statistics for Experimenters*. John Wiley, New York.

Box, G. E., and Tiao, G. C. (2011). *Bayesian Inference in Statistical Analysis*. John Wiley & Sons, New York.

Bradley, E. L. (1985). Overlapping Coefficient. *Encyclopedia of Statistical Sciences* 6: 546–547.

Branscum, A. J., Johnson, W. O., Hanson, T. E., and Gardner, I. A. (2008). Bayesian Semiparametric ROC Curve Estimation and Disease Diagnosis. *Statistics in Medicine* 27(13): 2474–2496.

Braun, J. V., Braun, R., and Müller, H.-G. (2000). Multiple Changepoint Fitting via Quasilikelihood, with Application to DNA Sequence Segmentation. *Biometrika* 87(2): 301–314.

Bravo, F. (2003). Second-Order Power Comparisons for a Class of Nonparametric Likelihood-Based Tests. *Biometrika* 90(4): 881–890.

Breiman, L. (1968). *Probability*. Addison-Wesley, Reading, MA.

Bretz, F., Hothorn, T., and Westfall, P. (2010). *Multiple Comparisons Using R*. CRC Press, Boca Raton, FL.

Brodsky, E., and Darkhovsky, B. S. (1993). *Nonparametric Methods in Change Point Problems*. Kluwer Academic Publishers: Dordrecht.

Brooks, S. P., and Roberts, G. O. (1998). Assessing Convergence of Markov Chain Monte Carlo Algorithms. *Statistics and Computing* 8(4): 319–335.

Brown, R. L., Durbin, J., and Evans, J. M. (1975). Techniques for Testing the Constancy of Regression Relationships over Time. *Journal of the Royal Statistical Society: Series B (Methodological)* 37(2): 149–192.

Browne, R. H. (2010). The T-Test P Value and Its Relationship to the Effect Size and P (X > Y). *American Statistician* 64(1): 30–33.

Bruce, M. L., Ten Have, T. R., Reynolds III, C. F., Katz, I. I., Schulberg, H. C., Mulsant, B. H., Brown, G. K., McAvay, G. J., Pearson, J. L., and Alexopoulos, G. S. (2004). Reducing Suicidal Ideation and Depressive Symptoms in Depressed Older Primary Care Patients: A Randomized Controlled Trial. *JAMA* 291(9): 1081–1091.

Brumback, L. C., Pepe, M. S., and Alonzo, T. A. (2006). Using the ROC Curve for Gauging Treatment Effect in Clinical Trials. *Statistics in Medicine* 25(4): 575–590.

Buckland, S. T., Anderson, D. R., Burnham, K. P., and Laake, J. L. (2005). Distance Sampling. In *Encyclopedia of Biostatistics*, ed. P. Armitage and T. Colton. Wiley, Chichester, UK.

Burman, C. F., and Sonesson, C. (2006). Are Flexible Designs Sound? *Biometrics* 62(3): 664–669.

Buse, A. (1982). The Likelihood Ratio, Wald, and Lagrange Multiplier Tests: An Expository Note. *American Statistician* 36(3a): 153–157.

Campbell, G. (1994). Advances in Statistical Methodology for the Evaluation of Diagnostic and Laboratory Tests. *Statistics in Medicine* 13(5–7): 499–508.

Canner, P. L. (1975). A Simulation Study of One- and Two-Sample Kolmogorov-Smirnov Statistics with a Particular Weight Function. *Journal of the American Statistical Association* 70(349): 209–211.

Cao, R., and Van Keilegom, I. (2006). Empirical Likelihood Tests for Two-Sample Problems via Nonparametric Density Estimation. *Canadian Journal of Statistics* 34(1): 61–77.

Capon, J. (1961). Asymptotic Efficiency of Certain Locally Most Powerful Rank Tests. *Annals of Mathematical Statistics* 32(1): 88–100.

Carlin, B. P., and Chib, S. (1995). Bayesian Model Choice via Markov Chain Monte Carlo Methods. *Journal of the Royal Statistical Society: Series B (Methodological)* 57(3): 473–484.

Carlin, B. P., and Louis, T. A. (1997). Bayes and Empirical Bayes Methods for Data Analysis. *Statistics and Computing* 7(2): 153–154.

Carlin, B. P., and Louis, T. A. (2011). *Bayesian Methods for Data Analysis*. CRC Press, Boca Raton, FL.

Carlstein, E. (1988). Nonparametric Change-Point Estimation. *Annals of Statistics* 16(1): 188–197.

Carpenter, J. (1999). Test Inversion Bootstrap Confidence Intervals. *Journal of the Royal Statistical Society: Series B (Statistical Methodology)* 61(1): 159–172.

Carpenter, J., and Bithell, J. (2000). Bootstrap Confidence Intervals: When, Which, What? A Practical Guide for Medical Statisticians. *Statistics in Medicine* 19(9): 1141–1164.

Carroll, R. J., Ruppert, D., Stefanski, L. A., and Crainiceanu, C. M. (2012). *Measurement Error in Nonlinear Models: A Modern Perspective*. CRC Press, Boca Raton, FL.

Carroll, R. J., Spiegelman, C. H., Lan, K. G., Bailey, K. T., and Abbott, R. D. (1984). On Errors-in-Variables for Binary Regression Models. *Biometrika* 71(1): 19–25.

Caussinus, H., and Mestre, O. (2004). Detection and Correction of Artificial Shifts in Climate Series. *Journal of the Royal Statistical Society: Series C (Applied Statistics)* 53(3): 405–425.

Chan, K. C. G. (2012). Uniform Improvement of Empirical Likelihood for Missing Response Problem. *Electronic Journal of Statistics* 6: 289–302.

Chan, N. H., Chen, S. X., Peng, L., and Yu, C. L. (2009). Empirical Likelihood Methods Based on Characteristic Functions with Applications to Lévy Processes. *Journal of the American Statistical Association* 104(488): 1621–1630.

Chang, M. N. (1989). Confidence Intervals for a Normal Mean Following a Group Sequential Test. *Biometrics* 45(1): 247–254.

Chapman, D. G. (1958). A Comparative Study of Several One-Sided Goodness-of-Fit Tests. *Annals of Mathematical Statistics* 29(3): 655–674.

Chen, C.-H., Härdle, W. K., and Unwin, A. (2007). *Handbook of Data Visualization*. Springer-Verlag, Berlin.

Chen, C. W., Chan, J. S., Gerlach, R., and Hsieh, W. Y. (2011). A Comparison of Estimators for Regression Models with Change Points. *Statistics and Computing* 21(3): 395–414.

Chen, H., and Chen, J. (2000). Bahadur Representations of the Empirical Likelihood Quantile Processes. *Journal of Nonparametric Statistics* 12(5): 645–660.

Chen, J., Chen, S. Y., and Rao, J. (2003a). Empirical Likelihood Confidence Intervals for the Mean of a Population Containing Many Zero Values. *Canadian Journal of Statistics* 31(1): 53–68.

Chen, J., Conigrave, K. M., Macaskill, P., Whitfield, J. B., and Irwig, L. (2003b). Combining Carbohydrate-Deficient Transferrin and Gamma-Glutamyltransferase to Increase Diagnostic Accuracy for Problem Drinking. *Alcohol and Alcoholism* 38(6): 574–582.

Chen, J., and Gupta, A. K. (2011). *Parametric Statistical Change Point Analysis: With Applications to Genetics, Medicine, and Finance.* Springer, New York.

Chen, L. (1995). Testing the Mean of Skewed Distributions. *Journal of the American Statistical Association* 90(430): 767–772.

Chen, S. X. (1994). Comparing Empirical Likelihood and Bootstrap Hypothesis Tests. *Journal of Multivariate Analysis* 51(2): 277–293.

Chen, S. X. (1996). Empirical Likelihood Confidence Intervals for Nonparametric Density Estimation. *Biometrika* 83(2): 329–341.

Chen, S. X., and Hall, P. (1993). Smoothed Empirical Likelihood Confidence Intervals for Quantiles. *Annals of Statistics* 21(3): 1166–1181.

Chen, X., Vexler, A., and Markatou, M. (2015). Empirical Likelihood Ratio Confidence Interval Estimation of Best Linear Combinations of Biomarkers. *Computational Statistics and Data Analysis* 82: 186–198.

Cheng, G., Yu, Z., and Huang, J. Z. (2013). The Cluster Bootstrap Consistency in Generalized Estimating Equations. *Journal of Multivariate Analysis* 115: 33–47.

Cheng, J., Small, D., Tan, Z., and TenHave, T. R. (2009). Efficient Nonparametric Estimation of Causal Effects in Randomized Trials with Noncompliance. *Biometrika* 96: 19–36.

Chernoff, H., and Zacks, S. (1964). Estimating the Current Mean of a Normal Distribution Which Is Subjected to Changes in Time. *Annals of Mathematical Statistics*: 35(3): 999–1018.

Cheung, Y. K. (2008). Simple Sequential Boundaries for Treatment Selection in Multi-Armed Randomized Clinical Trials with a Control. *Biometrics* 64(3): 940–949.

Choi, S., Hall, W., and Schick, A. (1996). Asymptotically Uniformly Most Powerful Tests in Parametric and Semiparametric Models. *Annals of Statistics* 24(2): 841–861.

Chrzanowski, M. (2014). Weighted Empirical Likelihood Inference for the Area under the ROC Curve. *Journal of Statistical Planning and Inference* 147: 159–172.

Chu, C.-S. J., Hornik, K., and Kaun, C.-M. (1995). Mosum Tests for Parameter Constancy. *Biometrika* 82(3): 603–617.

Chuang, C.-S., and Lai, T. L. (2000). Hybrid Resampling Methods for Confidence Intervals. *Statistica Sinica* 10(1): 1–32.

Claeskens, G., and Hjort, N. L. (2004). Goodness of Fit via Non-Parametric Likelihood Ratios. *Scandinavian Journal of Statistics* 31(4): 487–513.

Claeskens, G., Jing, B. Y., Peng, L., and Zhou, W. (2003). Empirical Likelihood Confidence Regions for Comparison Distributions and ROC Curves. *Canadian Journal of Statistics* 31(2): 173–190.

Clarkson, E., Denny, J., and Shepp, L. (2009). ROC and the Bounds on Tail Probabilities via Theorems of Dubins and F. Riesz. *Annals of Applied Probability: An Official Journal of the Institute of Mathematical Statistics* 19(1): 467.

Clayton, D. (1992). Models for the Analysis of Cohort and Case-Control Studies with Inaccurately Measured Exposures. In *Statistical Models for Longitudinal Studies of Health*, ed. J. H. Dwyer, F. Manning, P. Lippert, and H. Hoffmeister, 301–331. Oxford University Press, Oxford.

Clemens, J., Savarino, S., Abu-Elyazeed, R., Safwat, M., Rao, M., Wierzba, T., Svennerholm, A. M., Holmgren, J., Frenck, R., Park, E., and Naficy, A. (2004). Development of Pathogenicity-Driven Definitions of Outcomes for a Field Trial of a Killed, Oral Vaccine against Enterotoxigenic *Escherichia coli* in Egypt: Application of an Evidence-Based Method. *Journal of Infectious Diseases* 189: 2299–2307.

Cleveland, W. S. (1993). *Visualizing Data.* AT&T Bell Laboratories, Murray Hill, NJ.

Cochran, W. G. (1968). Errors of Measurement in Statistics. *Technometrics* 10(4): 637–666.

Cody, R. (2007). *Learning SAS by Example: A Programmer's Guide.* SAS Institute, Cary, NC.

Cohen, J. (1969). *Statistical Power Analysis for the Behavioral Sciences.* Academic Press, New York.

Coin, D. (2008). A Goodness-of-Fit Test for Normality Based on Polynomial Regression. *Computational Statistics and Data Analysis* 52(4): 2185–2198.

Cole, B. F., Gelber, R. D., and Goldhirsch, A. (1993). Cox Regression Models for Quality Adjusted Survival Analysis. *Statistics in Medicine* 12(10): 975–987.

Committee for Proprietary Medicinal Products (CFPM). (2002). Points to Consider on Multiplicity Issues in Clinical Trials. European Agency for the Evaluation of Medicinal Products (EMEA), London.

Conover, W. (1965). Several K-Sample Kolmogorov-Smirnov Tests. *Annals of Mathematical Statistics* 36(3): 1019–1026.

Cook, N. R., Rosner, B. A., Chen, W., Srinivasan, S. R., and Berenson, G. S. (2004). Using the Area under the Curve to Reduce Measurement Error in Predicting Young Adult Blood Pressure from Childhood Measures. *Statistics in Medicine* 23(22): 3421–3435.

Cook, R. D., and Johnson, M. E. (1981). A Family of Distributions for Modelling Non-Elliptically Symmetric Multivariate Data. *Journal of the Royal Statistical Society: Series B (Methodological)* 43(2): 210–218.

Cook, R. D., and Weisberg, S. (1999). *Applied Regression Including Computing and Graphics.* Wiley, New York.

Cook, T. D. (2002). P-Value Adjustment in Sequential Clinical Trials. *Biometrics* 58(4): 1005–1011.

Cooke, T., and Peake, M. (2002). The Optimal Classification Using a Linear Discriminant for Two Point Classes Having Known Mean and Covariance. *Journal of Multivariate Analysis* 82(2): 379–394.

Copas, J., and Corbett, P. (2002). Overestimation of the Receiver Operating Characteristic Curve for Logistic Regression. *Biometrika* 89(2): 315–331.

Cordy, C. B., and Thomas, D. R. (1997). Deconvolution of a Distribution Function. *Journal of the American Statistical Association* 92(440): 1459–1465.

Cox, C. P., and Roseberry, T. D. (1966). A Note on the Variance of the Distribution of Sample Number in Sequential Probability Ratio Tests. *Technometrics* 8(4): 700–704.

Cox, D., and Hinkley, D. (1974). *Theoretical Statistics.* Chapman-Hall, London.

Cox, D. R., and Snell, E. J. (1981). *Applied Statistics—Principles and Examples.* CRC Press, Boca Raton, FL.

Crawley, M. J. (2012). *The R Book.* John Wiley & Sons, Chichester, UK.

Crupi, V., Chater, N., and Tentori, K. (2012). New Axioms for Probability and Likelihood Ratio Measures. *British Journal for the Philosophy of Science* 64(1): 189–204.

Csörgö, M., and Horváth, L. (1997). *Limit Theorems in Change-Point Analysis.* Wiley, New York.

Csorgo, S. (1986). Testing for Normality in Arbitrary Dimension. *Annals of Statistics* 14(2): 708–723.

Cutler, S., Greenhouse, S., Cornfield, J., and Schneiderman, M. (1966). The Role of Hypothesis Testing in Clinical Trials: Biometrics Seminar. *Journal of Chronic Diseases* 19(8): 857–882.

Czajkowski, M., Gill, R., and Rempala, G. (2008). Model Selection in Logistic Joinpoint Regression with Applications to Analyzing Cohort Mortality Patterns. *Statistics in Medicine* 27(9): 1508–1526.

Daniel, C. (1959). Use of Half-Normal Plots in Interpreting Factorial Two-Level Experiments. *Technometrics* 1(4): 311–341.

Daniels, H. (1945). The Statistical Theory of the Strength of Bundles of Threads. I. *Proceedings of the Royal Society of London A: Mathematical, Physical and Engineering Sciences* 183(995): 405–435

Daniels, H. (1950). Rank Correlation and Population Models. *Journal of the Royal Statistical Society: Series B (Methodological)* 12(2): 171–191.

Daniels, M. J., and Hogan, J. W. (2008). *Missing Data in Longitudinal Studies: Strategies for Bayesian Modeling and Sensitivity Analysis.* CRC Press, Boca Raton, FL.

Darbellay, G., and Vajda, I. (2000). Entropy Expressions for Multivariate Continuous Distributions. *IEEE Transactions on Information Theory* 46(2): 709–712.

Darkhovskh, B. (1976). A Nonparametric Method for the A Posteriori Detection of the "Disorder" Time of a Sequence of Independent Random Variables. *Theory of Probability and Its Applications* 21(1): 178–183.

DasGupta, A. (2008). *Asymptotic Theory of Statistics and Probability.* Springer, New York.

Dass, S. C., and Berger, J. O. (2003). Unified Conditional Frequentist and Bayesian Testing of Composite Hypotheses. *Scandinavian Journal of Statistics* 30(1): 193–210.

David, H. A. (1998). First (?) Occurrence of Common Terms in Probability and Statistics—A Second List, with Corrections. *American Statistician* 52(1): 36–40.

David, H. A., and Nagaraja, H. N. (2003). *Order Statistics*. John Wiley, New York.

David, H. T. (1958). A Three-Sample Kolmogorov-Smirnov Test. *Annals of Mathematical Statistics* 29(3): 842–851.

Davies, O. L. (1954). The Design and Analysis of Industrial Experiments. *Statistics Neerlandica* 9(4): 189–207.

Davies, O. L., and Box, G. E. P. (1956). *The Design and Analysis of Industrial Experiments*. Oliver and Boyd, London.

Davis, C. S. (1993). The Computer Generation of Multinomial Random Variates. *Computational Statistics and Data Analysis* 16(2): 205–217.

Davison, A. (1986). Approximate Predictive Likelihood. *Biometrika* 73(2): 323–332.

Davison, A. C., and Hinkley, D. V. (1997). *Bootstrap Methods and Their Application*. Cambridge University Press, Cambridge.

Dawid, A. P., and Skene, A. M. (1979). Maximum Likelihood Estimation of Observer Error-Rates Using the EM Algorithm. *Applied Statistics* 28(1): 20–28.

De Bruijn, N. G. (1970). *Asymptotic Methods in Analysis*. Dover Publications, Inc. New York.

De Santis, F., and Spezzaferri, F. (1997). Alternative Bayes Factors for Model Selection. *Canadian Journal of Statistics* 25(4): 503–515.

DeGroot, M. H. (2005). *Optimal Statistical Decisions*. John Wiley & Sons, Hoboken, NJ.

Delaigle, A., and Hall, P. (2012). Nonparametric Regression with Homogeneous Group Testing Data. *Annals of Statistics* 40(1): 131–158.

DeLong, E. R., DeLong, D. M., and Clarke-Pearson, D. L. (1988). Comparing the Areas under Two or More Correlated Receiver Operating Characteristic Curves: A Nonparametric Approach. *Biometrics* 44(3): 837–845.

Delwiche, L. D., and Slaughter, S. J. (2012). *The Little SAS Book: A Primer: A Programming Approach*. SAS Institute, Cary, NC.

DeMets, D. L., and Ware, J. H. (1980). Group Sequential Methods for Clinical Trials with a One-Sided Hypothesis. *Biometrika* 67(3): 651–660.

DeMets, D. L., and Ware, J. H. (1982). Asymmetric Group Sequential Boundaries for Monitoring Clinical Trials. *Biometrika* 69(3): 661–663.

Deming, W. E. (1943). *Statistical Adjustment of Data*. Wiley, New York.

Dempster, A. P., and Schatzoff, M. (1965). Expected Significance Level as a Sensitivity Index for Test Statistics. *Journal of the American Statistical Association* 60(310): 420–436.

Desmond, R. A., Weiss, H. L., Arani, R. B., Soong, S.-J., Wood, M. J., Fiddian, P. A., Gnann, J. W., and Whitley, R. J. (2002). Clinical Applications for Change-Point Analysis of Herpes Zoster Pain. *Journal of Pain and Symptom Management* 23(6): 510–516.

Desquilbet, L., and Mariotti, F. (2010). Dose-Response Analyses Using Restricted Cubic Spline Functions in Public Health Research. *Statistics in Medicine* 29(9): 1037–1057.

DiCiccio, T. J., Hall, P., and Romano, J. P. (1989). Comparison of Parametric and Empirical Likelihood Functions. *Biometrika* 76(3): 465–476.

DiCiccio, T. J., Kass, R. E., Raftery, A., and Wasserman, L. (1997). Computing Bayes Factors by Combining Simulation and Asymptotic Approximations. *Journal of the American Statistical Association* 92(439): 903–915.

DiCiccio, T. J., Martin, M. A., and Stern, S. E. (2001). Simple and Accurate One-Sided Inference from Signed Roots of Likelihood Ratios. *Canadian Journal of Statistics* 29(1): 67–76.

Ding, A. A., and Wang, W. (2004). Testing Independence for Bivariate Current Status Data. *Journal of the American Statistical Association* 99(465): 145–155.

Djogbenou, A., Gonçalves, S., and Perron, B. (2015). Bootstrap Inference in Regressions with Estimated Factors and Serial Correlation. *Journal of Time Series Analysis* 36(3): 481–502.

Dmitrienko, A., Chuang-Stein, C., and D'Agostino, R. B. (2007). *Pharmaceutical Statistics Using SAS: A Practical Guide*. SAS Institute, Cary, NC.

Dmitrienko, A., Molenberghs, G., Chuang-Stein, C., and Offen, W. (2005). *Analysis of Clinical Trials Using SAS: A Practical Guide*. SAS Institute, Cary, NC.

Dmitrienko, A., Tamhane, A. C., and Bretz, F. (2010). *Multiple Testing Problems in Pharmaceutical Statistics.* CRC Press, New York.

Dodge, H. F., and Romig, H. (1929). A Method of Sampling Inspection. *Bell System Technical Journal* 8(4): 613–631.

Doksum, K. (1974). Empirical Probability Plots and Statistical Inference for Nonlinear Models in the Two-Sample Case. *Annals of Statistics* 2(2): 267–277.

Doksum, K. A., and Sievers, G. L. (1976). Plotting with Confidence: Graphical Comparisons of Two Populations. *Biometrika* 63(3): 421–434.

Domhof, S., and Langer, F. (2002). *Nonparametric Analysis of Longitudinal Data in Factorial Experiments.* Wiley-Interscience, New York.

Dong, L. B., and Giles, D. E. (2007). An Empirical Likelihood Ratio Test for Normality. *Communications in Statistics—Simulation and Computation* 36(1): 197–215.

Drummond, G. B., and Vowler, S. L. (2011). Show the Data, Don't Conceal Them. *Journal of Physiology* 589(8): 1861–1863.

Dubins, L. E. (1962). On Extreme Points of Convex Sets. *Journal of Mathematical Analysis and Applications* 5(2): 237–244.

Duin, R. P. W. (1976). On the Choice of Smoothing Parameters for Parzen Estimators of Probability Density Functions. *IEEE Transactions on Computers* 25(11): 1175–1179.

Dumbgen, L. (1991). The Asymptotic Behavior of Some Nonparametric Change-Point Estimators. *Annals of Statistics* 19(3): 1471–1495.

Durbin, J., and Stuart, A. (1951). Inversions and Rank Correlation Coefficients. *Journal of the Royal Statistical Society: Series B (Methodological)* 13(2): 303–309.

Dwass, M. (1960). *Some K-Sample Rank-Order Tests.* Stanford University Press, Stanford, CA.

Eales, J. D., and Jennison, C. (1992). An Improved Method for Deriving Optimal One-Sided Group Sequential Tests. *Biometrika* 79(1): 13–24.

Eddy, D. M. (1989). The Confidence Profile Method: A Bayesian Method for Assessing Health Technologies. *Operations Research* 37(2): 210–228.

Edelman, D. (1989). A Candidate for Locally Most Powerful Sequential T Test. *Biometrika* 76(1): 197–201.

Edwards, A. L. (1976). *An Introduction to Linear Regression and Correlation.* W.H. Freeman, San Francisco.

Edwards, L. J., Stewart, P. W., MacDougall, J. E., and Helms, R. W. (2006). A Method for Fitting Regression Splines with Varying Polynomial Order in the Linear Mixed Model. *Statistics in Medicine* 25(3): 513–527.

Efron, B. (1967). The Two Sample Problem with Censored Data. In *Proceedings of the Fifth Berkeley Symposium on Mathematical Statistics and Probability.* Prentice-Hall: Englewood Cliffs, NJ.

Efron, B. (1979). Bootstrap Methods: Another Look at the Jackknife. *Annals of Statistics* 7(1): 1–26.

Efron, B. (1981). Nonparametric Standard Errors and Confidence Intervals. *Canadian Journal of Statistics/La Revue Canadienne de Statistique* 9(2): 139–158.

Efron, B. (1982). *The Jackknife, the Bootstrap and Other Resampling Plans.* Society for Industrial and Applied Mathematics, Philadelphia.

Efron, B. (1983). Estimating the Error Rate of a Prediction Rule: Improvement on Cross-Validation. *Journal of the American Statistical Association* 78(382): 316–331.

Efron, B. (1986a). How Biased Is the Apparent Error Rate of a Prediction Rule? *Journal of the American Statistical Association* 81(394): 461–470.

Efron, B. (1986b). Why Isn't Everyone a Bayesian? *American Statistician* 40(1): 1–5.

Efron, B. (1990). More Efficient Bootstrap Computations. *Journal of the American Statistical Association* 85(409): 79–89.

Efron, B., and Morris, C. (1972). Limiting the Risk of Bayes and Empirical Bayes Estimators. Part II. The Empirical Bayes Case. *Journal of the American Statistical Association* 67(337): 130–139.

Efron, B., and Tibshirani, R. J. (1993). *An Introduction to the Bootstrap.* CRC Press, Boca Raton, FL.

Eilertsen, A., Qvigstad, E., Andersen, T., Sandvik, L., and Sandset, P. (2006). Conventional-Dose Hormone Therapy (Ht) and Tibolone, but Not Low-Dose Ht and Raloxifene, Increase Markers of Activated Coagulation. *Maturitas* 55(3): 278–287.

Einmahl, J. H., and McKeague, I. W. (2003). Empirical Likelihood Based Hypothesis Testing. *Bernoulli* 9(2): 267–290.

Elffers, H. (1980). On Interpreting the Product Moment Correlation Coefficient*. *Statistica Neerlandica* 34(1): 3–11.

Embrechts, P., McNeil, A., and Straumann, D. (2002). Correlation and Dependence in Risk Management: Properties and Pitfalls. In *Risk Management: Value at Risk and Beyond*, ed. M. A. H. Dempster, 176–223. Cambridge University Press, Cambridge.

Emerson, S. C., and Owen, A. B. (2009). Calibration of the Empirical Likelihood Method for a Vector Mean. *Electronic Journal of Statistics* 3: 1161–1192.

Emerson, S. C., Rudser, K. D., and Emerson, S. S. (2011). Exploring the Benefits of Adaptive Sequential Designs in Time-to-Event Endpoint Settings. *Statistics in Medicine* 30(11): 1199–1217.

Emerson, S. S., Kittelson, J. M., and Gillen, D. L. (2005). Bayesian Evaluation of Group Sequential Clinical Trial Designs. *Statistics in Medicine* 26(7): 1431–1449.

Emerson, S. S., Kittelson, J. M., and Gillen, D. L. (2007). Frequentist Evaluation of Group Sequential Clinical Trial Designs. *Statistics in Medicine* 26(28): 5047–5080.

Eng, J. (2005). Receiver Operating Characteristic Analysis: A Primer1. *Academic Radiology* 12(7): 909–916.

Epps, T. W., and Pulley, L. B. (1983). A Test for Normality Based on the Empirical Characteristic Function. *Biometrika* 70(3): 723–726.

Ernst, M. D., and Hutson, A. D. (2003). Utilizing a Quantile Function Approach to Obtain Exact Bootstrap Solutions. *Statistical Science* 18(2): 231–240.

Evans, M., Guttman, I., and Olkin, I. (1992). Numerical Aspects in Estimating the Parameters of a Mixture of Normal Distributions. *Journal of Computational and Graphical Statistics* 1(4): 351–365.

Evans, M., and Swartz, T. (1995). Methods for Approximating Integrals in Statistics with Special Emphasis on Bayesian Integration Problems. *Statistical Science* 10(3): 254–272.

Everitt, B. S., and Palmer, C. (2010). *Encyclopaedic Companion to Medical Statistics*. John Wiley & Sons, Hoboken, NJ.

Fagerland, M. W., and Sandvik, L. (2009a). Performance of Five Two-Sample Location Tests for Skewed Distributions with Unequal Variances. *Contemporary Clinical Trials* 30(5): 490–496.

Fagerland, M. W., and Sandvik, L. (2009b). The Wilcoxon–Mann–Whitney Test under Scrutiny. *Statistics in Medicine* 28(10): 1487–1497.

Fan, J., Farmen, M., and Gijbels, I. (1998). Local Maximum Likelihood Estimation and Inference. *Journal of the Royal Statistical Society: Series B (Statistical Methodology)* 60(3): 591–608.

Fan, J., and Gijbels, I. (1995). Data-Driven Bandwidth Selection in Local Polynomial Fitting: Variable Bandwidth and Spatial Adaptation. *Journal of the Royal Statistical Society: Series B (Methodological)* 57(2): 371–394.

Fan, J., and Jiang, J. (2007). Nonparametric Inference with Generalized Likelihood Ratio Tests. *Test* 16(3): 409–444.

Fan, J., Zhang, C., and Zhang, J. (2001). Generalized Likelihood Ratio Statistics and Wilks Phenomenon. *Annals of Statistics* 29(1): 153–193.

Fan, J. Q. (1991). Asymptotic Normality for Deconvolution Kernel Density Estimators. *Sankhyā* 53(A): 97–110.

Faraggi, D., and Reiser, B. (2002). Estimation of the Area under the ROC Curve. *Statistics in Medicine* 21(20): 3093–3106.

Faraggi, D., Reiser, B., and Schisterman, E. F. (2003). ROC Curve Analysis for Biomarkers Based on Pooled Assessments. *Statistics in Medicine* 22(15): 2515–2527.

Farcomeni, A., and Ventura, L. (2012). An Overview of Robust Methods in Medical Research. *Statistical Methods in Medical Research* 21(2): 111–133.

Fawcett, T. (2006). An Introduction to ROC Analysis. *Pattern Recognition Letters* 27(8): 861–874.

Fears, T. R., Benichou, J., and Gail, M. H. (1996). A Reminder of the Fallibility of the Wald Statistic. *American Statistician* 50(3): 226–227.

Fellingham, S., and Stoker, D. (1964). An Approximation for the Exact Distribution of the Wilcoxon Test for Symmetry. *Journal of the American Statistical Association* 59(307): 899–905.

Feng, P., Zhou, X.-H., Zou, Q.-M., Fan, M.-Y., and Li, X.-S. (2012). Generalized Propensity Score for Estimating the Average Treatment Effect of Multiple Treatments. *Statistics in Medicine* 31(7): 681.

Ferger, D. (1994). On the Power of Nonparametric Changepoint-Tests. *Metrika* 41(1): 277–292.

Feuerverger, A., Robinson, J., and Wong, A. (1999). On the Relative Accuracy of Certain Bootstrap Procedures. *Canadian Journal of Statistics* 27(2): 225–236.

Fieller, E. C., Hartley, H. O., and Pearson, E. S. (1957). Tests for Rank Correlation Coefficients. I. *Biometrika* 44(3/4): 470–481.

Fienberg, S. E. (1979). Graphical Methods in Statistics. *American Statistician* 33(4): 165–178.

Finner, H., and Roters, M. (2001). On the False Discovery Rate and Expected Type I Errors. *Biometrical Journal* 43(8): 985–1005.

Fishbein, L., O'Brien, P., Hutson, A., Theriaque, D., Stacpoole, P., and Flotte, T. (2000). Pharmacokinetics and Pharmacodynamic Effects of Nicotine Nasal Spray Devices on Cardiovascular and Pulmonary Function. *Journal of Investigative Medicine: The Official Publication of the American Federation for Clinical Research* 48(6): 435–440.

Fisher, L. D. (1998). Self-Designing Clinical Trials. *Statistics in Medicine* 17(14): 1551–1562.

Fisher, M., Cheung, K., Howard, G., and Warach, S. (2006). New Pathways for Evaluating Potential Acute Stroke Therapies. *International Journal of Stroke* 1(2): 52–58.

Fisher, N., and Switzer, P. (2001). Graphical Assessment of Dependence: Is a Picture Worth 100 Tests? *American Statistician* 55(3): 233–239.

Fisher, R. A. (1925). *Statistical Methods for Research Workers*. Genesis Publishing, Edinburgh.

Fisher, R. A. (1936a). *Statistical Methods for Research Workers*. Genesis Publishing, Edinburgh.

Fisher, R. A. (1936b). The Use of Multiple Measurements in Taxonomic Problems. *Annals of Eugenics* 7(2): 179–188.

Fisher, R. A., and Yates, F. (1938). *Statistical Tables for Biological, Agricultural and Medical Research*. Oliver and Boyd, London.

Fisher, R. A., and Yates, F. (1949). *Statistical Tables for Biological, Agricultural and Medical Research*. Oliver and Boyd, London.

Food and Drug Administration (FDA). (1988). *Guideline for the Format and Content of the Clinical and Statistical Sections of New Drug Applications*. FDA, U.S. Department of Health and Human Services, Rockville, MD.

Ford, I., Titterington, D., and Wu, C. (1985). Inference and Sequential Design. *Biometrika* 72(3): 545–551.

Fréchet, M. (1951). *Les Espaces Abstrait Et Leur Théorie Considérée Comme Introduction À L'analyse Générale*. Gauthier-Villars, Paris.

Fredricks, G. A., and Nelsen, R. B. (2007). On the Relationship between Spearman's Rho and Kendall's Tau for Pairs of Continuous Random Variables. *Journal of Statistical Planning and Inference* 137(7): 2143–2150.

Freedman, D. (2009). *Statistical Models: Theory and Practice*. Cambridge University Press, Oxford.

Freeman, H. A., Friedman, M., Mosteller, F., and Wallis, W. A. (1948). *Sampling Inspection*. McGraw-Hill, New York.

Freidlin, B., and Korn, E. L. (2002). A Comment on Futility Monitoring. *Controlled Clinical Trials* 23(4): 355–366.

Freiman, J. A., Chalmers, T. C., Smith Jr., H., and Kuebler, R. R. (1978). The Importance of Beta, the Type II Error and Sample Size in the Design and Interpretation of the Randomized Control Trial. Survey of 71 "Negative" Trials. *New England Journal of Medicine* 299(13): 690–694.

Frömke, C., Hothorn, L. A., and Kropf, S. (2008). Nonparametric Relevance-Shifted Multiple Testing Procedures for the Analysis of High-Dimensional Multivariate Data with Small Sample Sizes. *BMC Bioinformatics* 9(1): 54.

Fu, L., and Wang, Y.-G. (2012). Statistical Tools for Analyzing Water Quality Data. *Water Quality Monitoring and Assessment*, ed. K. Voudouris and D. Voutsa, 143–168. Intech, Rijeka, Croatia.

Fuller, W. A. (2009). *Measurement Error Models*. John Wiley & Sons, New York.

Ganocy, S. J. (2003). Estimation Problems from Data with Change Points. PhD thesis, Case Western Reserve University.

Gao, F., Xiong, C., Yan, Y., Yu, K., and Zhang, Z. (2008). Estimating Optimum Linear Combination of Multiple Correlated Diagnostic Tests at a Fixed Specificity with Receiver Operating Characteristic Curves. *Journal of Data Science* 6(1): 105–123.

Gardener, M. (2012). *Beginning R: The Statistical Programming Language*. John Wiley & Sons, Mississauga, ON.

Gavit, P., Baddour, Y., and Tholmer, R. (2009). Use of Change-Point Analysis for Process Monitoring and Control. *BioPharm International* 22(8).

Gelfand, A. E., and Dey, D. K. (1994). Bayesian Model Choice: Asymptotics and Exact Calculations. *Journal of the Royal Statistical Society: Series B (Methodological)* 56(3): 501–514.

Gelman, A., Carlin, J. B., Stern, H. S., Dunson, D. B., Vehtari, A., and Rubin, D. B. (2013). *Bayesian Data Analysis*. 3rd ed. CRC Press, Boca Raton, FL.

Gelman, A., Carlin, J. B., Stern, H. S., and Rubin, D. B. (2003). *Bayesian Data Analysis*. 2nd ed. CRC Press, Boca Raton, FL.

Gelman, A., and Rubin, D. B. (1992a). Inference from Iterative Simulation Using Multiple Sequences. *Statistical Science* 7(4): 457–472.

Gelman, A., and Rubin, D. B. (1992b). A Single Series from the Gibbs Sampler Provides a False Sense of Security. *Bayesian Statistics* 4: 625–631.

Genest, C., and Boies, J.-C. (2003). Detecting Dependence with Kendall Plots. *American Statistician* 57(4): 275–284.

Genest, C., and Nešlehová, J. (2009). Analytical Proofs of Classical Inequalities between Spearman's P and Kendall's T. *Journal of Statistical Planning and Inference* 139(11): 3795–3798.

Genest, C., and Rivest, L.-P. (1993). Statistical Inference Procedures for Bivariate Archimedean Copulas. *Journal of the American Statistical Association* 88(423): 1034–1043.

Genz, A., and Kass, R. E. (1997). Subregion-Adaptive Integration of Functions Having a Dominant Peak. *Journal of Computational and Graphical Statistics* 6(1): 92–111.

Geweke, J. (1989). Bayesian Inference in Econometric Models Using Monte Carlo Integration. *Econometrica: Journal of the Econometric Society* 57(6): 1317–1339.

Ghosh, B. (1969). Moments of the Distribution of Sample Size in a SPRT. *Journal of the American Statistical Association* 64(328): 1560–1575.

Ghosh, M. (1995). Inconsistent Maximum Likelihood Estimators for the Rasch Model. *Statistics and Probability Letters* 23(2): 165–170.

Gibbons, J. D. (1986). P Values. *Encyclopedia of Statistical Sciences* 7: 366–368.

Gibbons, J. D., and Chakraborti, S. (2005). *Nonparametric Statistical Inference*. 4th ed. Marcel Dekker, New York.

Gibbons, J. D., and Chakraborti, S. (2010). *Nonparametric Statistical Inference*. CRC Press, Boca Raton, FL.

Gibbons, J. D., and Pratt, J. W. (1975). P-Values: Interpretation and Methodology. *American Statistician* 29(1): 20–25.

Gill, R. D., Keiding, N., and Andersen, P. K. (1997). *Statistical Models Based on Counting Processes*. Springer, New York.

Gillespie, B. W., Chen, Q., Reichert, H., Franzblau, A., Hedgeman, E., Lepkowski, J., Adriaens, P., Demond, A., Luksemburg, W., and Garabrant, D. H. (2010). Estimating Population Distributions When Some Data Are Below a Limit of Detection by Using a Reverse Kaplan-Meier Estimator. *Epidemiology* 21(4): S64–S70.

Gilovich, T., Vallone, R., and Tversky, A. (1985). The Hot Hand in Basketball: On the Misperception of Random Sequences. *Cognitive Psychology* 17(3): 295–314.

Gnanadesikan, R., and Lee, E. T. (1970). Graphical Techniques for Internal Comparisons amongst Equal Degree of Freedom Groupings in Multiresponse Experiments. *Biometrika* 57(2): 229–237.

Gnedenko, B., and Korolyuk, V. (1951). On the Maximum Discrepancy between Two Empirical Distributions. *Doklady Akademii Nauk SSSR* 80: 525–528.

Godambe, V. P. (1991). *Estimating Functions*. Clarendon Press, Oxford.

Goering, H. K., and Van Soest, P. J. (1970). *Forage Fiber Analyses (Apparatus, Reagents, Procedures, and Some Applications)*. USDA Agriculture Handbook 379. U.S. Government Printing Office, Washington, DC.

Gombay, E. (1994). Testing for Change-Points with Rank and Sign Statistics. *Statistics and Probability Letters* 20(1): 49–55.

Gombay, E. (2001). U-Statistics for Change under Alternatives. *Journal of Multivariate Analysis* 78(1): 139–158.

Gombay, E., and Horvath, L. (1994). An Application of the Maximum Likelihood Test to the Change-Point Problem. *Stochastic Processes and Their Applications* 50(1): 161–171.

Gombay, E., and Horvath, L. (1996). On the Rate of Approximations for Maximum Likelihood Tests in Change-Point Models. *Journal of Multivariate Analysis* 56(1): 120–152.

Gönen, M., Johnson, W. O., Lu, Y., and Westfall, P. H. (2005). The Bayesian Two-Sample T Test. *American Statistician* 59(3): 252–257.

Good, I. (1992). The Bayes/Non-Bayes Compromise: A Brief Review. *Journal of the American Statistical Association* 87(419): 597–606.

Good, P. (1995). *Permutation Tests*. Springer, New York.

Goodman, L. A., and Kruskal, W. H. (1979). *Measures of Association for Cross Classifications*. Springer, New York.

Goodman, S. N. (1999a). Toward Evidence-Based Medical Statistics. 1. The P Value Fallacy. *Annals of Internal Medicine* 130(12): 995–1004.

Goodman, S. N. (1999b). Toward Evidence-Based Medical Statistics. 2. The Bayes Factor. *Annals of Internal Medicine* 130(12): 1005–1013.

Gordon, L., and Pollak, M. (1997). Average Run Length to False Alarm for Surveillance Schemes Designed with Partially Specified Pre-Change Distribution. *Annals of Statistics* 25(3): 1284–1310.

Gordon Lan, K., Simon, R., and Halperin, M. (1982). Stochastically Curtailed Tests in Long-Term Clinical Trials. *Sequential Analysis* 1(3): 207–219.

Gössl, C., and Kuechenhoff, H. (2001). Bayesian Analysis of Logistic Regression with an Unknown Change Point and Covariate Measurement Error. *Statistics in Medicine* 20(20): 3109–3121.

Govindarajulu, Z. (1968). Distribution-Free Confidence Bounds for P (X<Y). *Annals of the Institute of Statistical Mathematics* 20(1): 229–238.

Graubard, B. I., and Korn, E. L. (1987). Choice of Column Scores for Testing Independence in Ordered 2 x K Contingency Tables. *Biometrics* 43(2): 471–476.

Greaney, V., and Kellaghan, T. (1984). *Equality of Opportunity in Irish Schools: A Longitudinal Study of 500 Students*. Educational Company, Dublin.

Green, D. M., and Swets, J. A. (1966). *Signal Detection Theory and Psychophysics*. Wiley, New York.

Green, P. J. (1990). On Use of the EM for Penalized Likelihood Estimation. *Journal of the Royal Statistical Society: Series B (Methodological)* 52(3): 443–452.

Greenland, S. (1993). Methods for Epidemiologic Analyses of Multiple Exposures: A Review and Comparative Study of Maximum-Likelihood, Preliminary-Testing, and Empirical-Bayes Regression. *Statistics in Medicine* 12(8): 717–736.

Gretton, A., Fukumizu, K., Teo, C. H., Song, L., Schölkopf, B., and Smola, A. J. (2008). A Kernel Statistical Test of Independence. *Advances in Neural Information Processing Systems*.

Gretton, A., and Györfi, L. (2010). Consistent Nonparametric Tests of Independence. *Journal of Machine Learning Research* 11: 1391–1423.

Grimmett, G., and Stirzaker, D. (1992). *Probability and Random Processes*. Oxford University Press, Oxford.

Gu, M., Dong, X., Zhang, X., Wang, X., Qi, Y., Yu, J., and Niu, W. (2012). Strong Association between Two Polymorphisms on 15q25.1 and Lung Cancer Risk: A Meta-Analysis. *PLoS One* 7(6): e37970.

Guan, Z. (2004). A Semiparametric Changepoint Model. *Biometrika* 91(4): 849–862.

Guan, Z. (2007). Semiparametric Tests for Change-Points with Epidemic Alternatives. *Journal of Statistical Planning and Inference* 137(6): 1748–1764.

Guan, Z., and Zhao, H. (2005). A Semiparametric Approach for Marker Gene Selection Based on Gene Expression Data. *Bioinformatics* 21(4): 529–536.

Guggenberger, P., and Smith, R. J. (2005). Generalized Empirical Likelihood Estimators and Tests under Partial, Weak, and Strong Identification. *Econometric Theory* 21(04): 667–709.

Guo, Y., and Little, R. J. (2011). Regression Analysis with Covariates That Have Heteroscedastic Measurement Error. *Statistics in Medicine* 30(18): 2278–2294.

Guo, Y., Little, R. J., and McConnell, D. S. (2012). On Using Summary Statistics from an External Calibration Sample to Correct for Covariate Measurement Error. *Epidemiology* 23(1): 165–174.

Gupta, A. (1952). Estimation of the Mean and Standard Deviation of a Normal Population from a Censored Sample. *Biometrika* 39(3/4): 260–273.

Gupta, R. C., Ghitany, M., and Al-Mutairi, D. (2013). Estimation of Reliability from a Bivariate Log-Normal Data. *Journal of Statistical Computation and Simulation* 83(6): 1068–1081.

Gurevich, G. (2006). Nonparametric Amoc Changepoint Tests for Stochastically Ordered Alternatives. *Communications in Statistics—Theory and Methods* 35(5): 887–903.

Gurevich, G. (2007). Retrospective Parametric Tests for Homogeneity of Data. *Communications in Statistics—Theory and Methods* 36(16): 2841–2862.

Gurevich, G., and Vexler, A. (2005). Change Point Problems in the Model of Logistic Regression. *Journal of Statistical Planning and Inference* 131(2): 313–331.

Gurevich, G., and Vexler, A. (2010). Retrospective Change Point Detection: From Parametric to Distribution Free Policies. *Communications in Statistics—Simulation and Computation* 39(5): 899–920.

Gurevich, G., and Vexler, A. (2011). A Two-Sample Empirical Likelihood Ratio Test Based on Samples Entropy. *Statistics and Computing* 21(4): 657–670.

Habbema, J. D. F., Hermans, J., and Broek, K. V. D. (1974). A Step-Wise Discriminant Analysis Program Using Density Estimation. *Compstat* 101–110.

Habibi, R. (2011). Cusum Procedure Using Transformed Observations. *Applied Mathematical Sciences* 5(43): 2177–2185.

Haccou, P., and Meelis, E. (1988). Testing for the Number of Change Points in a Sequence of Exponential Random Variables. *Journal of Statistical Computation and Simulation* 30(4): 285–298.

Hall, P. (1990). Pseudo-Likelihood Theory for Empirical Likelihood. *Annals of Statistics* 18(1): 121–140.

Hall, P., Hyndman, R. J., and Fan, Y. (2004). Nonparametric Confidence Intervals for Receiver Operating Characteristic Curves. *Biometrika* 91(3): 743–750.

Hall, P., and La Scala, B. (1990). Methodology and Algorithms of Empirical Likelihood. *International Statistical Review/Revue Internationale de Statistique* 58(2): 109–127.

Hall, P., and Owen, A. B. (1993). Empirical Likelihood Confidence Bands in Density Estimation. *Journal of Computational and Graphical Statistics* 2(3): 273–289.

Hall, P., Peng, L., and Rau, C. (2001). Local Likelihood Tracking of Fault Lines and Boundaries. *Journal of the Royal Statistical Society: Series B (Statistical Methodology)* 63(3): 569–582.

Hall, P., and Welsh, A. H. (1983). Amendments and Corrections: A Test for Normality Based on the Empirical Characteristic Function. *Biometrika* 71(3): 655.

Hall, P., and Wilson, S. R. (1991). Two Guidelines for Bootstrap Hypothesis Testing. *Biometrics* 47(2): 757–762.

Hall, P., and Zhou, X.-H. (2003). Nonparametric Estimation of Component Distributions in a Multivariate Mixture. *Annals of Statistics* 31(1): 201–224.

Halperin, M., Gilbert, P. R., and Lachin, J. M. (1987). Distribution-Free Confidence Intervals for Pr ($X1 < X2$). *Biometrics* 43(1): 71–80.

Hammersley, J. M., and Handscomb, D. C. (1964). *Monte Carlo Methods.* Springer, New York.

Han, C., and Carlin, B. P. (2001). Markov Chain Monte Carlo Methods for Computing Bayes Factors. *Journal of the American Statistical Association* 96(455): 1122–1132.

Hanfelt, J. J., and Liang, K.-Y. (1995). Approximate Likelihood Ratios for General Estimating Functions. *Biometrika* 82(3): 461–477.

Hanley, J. A., and McNeil, B. J. (1982). The Meaning and Use of the Area under a Receiver Operating Characteristic (ROC) Curve. *Radiology* 143(1): 29–36.

Hans, P., Albert, A., Born, J. D., and Chapelle, J. P. (1985). Derivation of a Bioclinical Prognostic Index in Severe Head Injury. *Intensive Care Medicine* 11(4): 186–191.

Hardell, L. (1981). Relation of Soft-Tissue Sarcoma, Malignant Lymphoma and Colon Cancer to Phenoxy Acids, Chlorophenols and Other Agents. *Scandinavian Journal of Work, Environment and Health* 7(2): 119–130.

Harel, O., Schisterman, E. F., Vexler, A., and Ruopp, M. D. (2008). Monitoring Quality Control: Can We Get Better Data? *Epidemiology (Cambridge, Mass.)* 19(4): 621.

Harrell, F. E., Lee, K. L., and Mark, D. B. (1996). Tutorial in Biostatistics Multivariable Prognostic Models: Issues in Developing Models, Evaluating Assumptions and Adequacy, and Measuring and Reducing Errors. *Statistics in Medicine* 15: 361–387.

Harter, H. L., and Moore, A. H. (1967). Asymptotic Variances and Covariances of Maximum-Likelihood Estimators, from Censored Samples, of the Parameters of Weibull and Gamma Populations. *Annals of Mathematical Statistics* 38(2): 557–570.

Hartigan, J. (1965). The Asymptotically Unbiased Prior Distribution. *Annals of Mathematical Statistics* 36(4): 1137–1152.

Hartigan, J. (1971). Error Analysis by Replaced Samples. *Journal of the Royal Statistical Society: Series B (Methodological)* 33(2): 98–110.

Hartigan, J. (1996). Locally Uniform Prior Distributions. *Annals of Statistics* 24(1): 160–173.

Hartigan, J. A. (1969). Using Subsample Values as Typical Values. *Journal of the American Statistical Association* 64(328): 1303–1317.

Hartigan, J. A. (1975). Necessary and Sufficient Conditions for Asymptotic Joint Normality of a Statistic and Its Subsample Values. *Annals of Statistics* 3(3): 573–580.

Hawkins, D. M. (1981). A New Test for Multivariate Normality and Homoscedasticity. *Technometrics* 23(1): 105–110.

Hawkins, D. M. (2001). Fitting Multiple Change-Point Models to Data. *Computational Statistics and Data Analysis* 37(3): 323–341.

Hawkins, D. M. (2002). Diagnostics for Conformity of Paired Quantitative Measurements. *Statistics in Medicine* 21(13): 1913–1935.

Hawkins, D. M., and Deng, Q. (2010). A Nonparametric Change-Point Control Chart. *Journal of Quality Technology* 42(2): 165–173.

Hawkins, D. M., and Zamba, K. (2005). Statistical Process Control for Shifts in Mean or Variance Using a Changepoint Formulation. *Technometrics* 47(2): 164–173.

Hawkins, K. (2002). *Law as Last Resort: Prosecution Decision-Making in a Regulatory Agency.* Oxford University Press, Oxford.

Hayter, A. J. (1990). A One-Sided Studentized Range Test for Testing against a Simple Ordered Alternative. *Journal of the American Statistical Association* 85(411): 778–785.

He, X., Metz, C. E., Tsui, B. M., Links, J. M., and Frey, E. C. (2006). Three-Class ROC Analysis—A Decision Theoretic Approach under the Ideal Observer Framework. *IEEE Transactions on Medical Imaging* 25(5): 571–581.

Hegazy, Y., and Green, J. (1975). Some New Goodness-of-Fit Tests Using Order Statistics. *Applied Statistics* 24(3): 299–308.

Herring, A. H. (2010). Nonparametric Bayes Shrinkage for Assessing Exposures to Mixtures Subject to Limits of Detection. *Epidemiology (Cambridge, Mass.)* 21(Suppl. 4): S71–S76.

Hettmansperger, T. P., and McKean, J. W. (1978). Statistical Inference Based on Ranks. *Psychometrika* 43(1): 69–79.

Higgins, J., Whitehead, A., and Simmonds, M. (2011). Sequential Methods for Random-Effects Meta-Analysis. *Statistics in Medicine* 30(9): 903–921.

Hilton, J. F. (1996). The Appropriateness of the Wilcoxon Test in Ordinal Data. *Statistics in Medicine* 15(6): 631–645.

Hinkley, D. (1977). Conditional Inference about a Normal Mean with Known Coefficient of Variation. *Biometrika* 64(1): 105–108.

Hirotsu, C. (1997). Two-Way Change-Point Model and Its Application. *Australian Journal of Statistics* 39(2): 205–218.

Hoeffding, W. (1948). A Non-Parametric Test of Independence. *Annals of Mathematical Statistics* 19(4): 546–557.

Hoeffding, W. (1994). *"Optimum" Nonparametric Tests*. Springer, New York.

Hoel, P. G. (1984). *Introduction to Mathematical Statistics*. 5th ed. Wiley, Mississauga, ON.

Hoff, P. (2000). Constrained Nonparametric Maximum Likelihood via Mixtures. *Journal of Computational and Graphical Statistics* 9(4): 633–641.

Hogan, M., and Siegmund, D. (1986). Large Deviations for the Maxima of Some Random Fields. *Advances in Applied Mathematics* 7(1): 2–22.

Hollander, M., Wolfe, D. A., and Chicken, E. (2013). *Nonparametric Statistical Methods*. John Wiley & Sons, Mississauga, ON.

Hommel, G., and Bretz, F. (2008). Aesthetics and Power Considerations in Multiple Testing—A Contradiction? *Biometrical Journal* 50(5): 657–666.

Horváth, L., and Hušková, M. (2005). Testing for Changes Using Permutations of U-Statistics. *Journal of Statistical Planning and Inference* 128(2): 351–371.

Horváth, L., Kokoszka, P., and Steinebach, J. (2000). Approximations for Weighted Bootstrap Processes with an Application. *Statistics and Probability Letters* 48(1): 59–70.

Horváth, L., and Shao, Q.-M. (1996). Limit Theorem for Maximum of Standardized U-Statistics with an Application. *Annals of Statistics* 24(5): 2266–2279.

Hosmer Jr., D. W., and Lemeshow, S. (2004). *Applied Logistic Regression*. John Wiley & Sons, Hoboken, NJ.

Hsieh, F., and Turnbull, B. W. (1996). Nonparametric and Semiparametric Estimation of the Receiver Operating Characteristic Curve. *Annals of Statistics* 24(1): 25–40.

Hsu, J. C., Qiu, P., Hin, L. Y., Mutti, D. O., and Zadnik, K. (2004). Multiple Comparisons with the Best ROC Curve. *Lecture Notes—Monograph Series* 47: 65–75.

Hsu, J. S. (1995). Generalized Laplacian Approximations in Bayesian Inference. *Canadian Journal of Statistics* 23(4): 399–410.

Huang, P., Tilley, B. C., Woolson, R. F., and Lipsitz, S. (2005). Adjusting O'Brien's Test to Control Type I Error for the Generalized Nonparametric Behrens–Fisher Problem. *Biometrics* 61(2): 532–539.

Huber-Carol, C., Balakrishnan, N., Nikulin, M. S., and Mesbah, M. (2002). *Goodness-of-Fit Tests and Model Validity*. Springer Science & Business Media, New York.

Hung, H. J., O'Neill, R. T., Bauer, P., and Kohne, K. (1997). The Behavior of the P-Value When the Alternative Hypothesis Is True. *Biometrics* 53(1): 11–22.

Hunsberger, S., Sorlie, P., and Geller, N. L. (1994). Stochastic Curtailing and Conditional Power in Matched Case-Control Studies. *Statistics in Medicine* 13(5–7): 663–670.

Hušková, M. (1995). Estimators for Epidemic Alternatives. *Commentationes Mathematicae Universitatis Carolinae* 36(2): 279–291.

Hutson, A. D. (2002). A Semi-Parametric Quantile Function Estimator for Use in Bootstrap Estimation Procedures. *Statistics and Computing* 12(4): 331–338.

Hutson, A. D. (2004). A Semiparametric Bootstrap Approach to Correlated Data Analysis Problems. *Computer Methods and Programs in Biomedicine* 73(2): 129–134.

Hutson, A. D. (2007). An 'Exact' Two-Group Median Test with an Extension to Censored Data. *Nonparametric Statistics* 19(2): 103–112.

Hutson, A. D. (2013). Calculation of the Per Hypothesis Error Rate via Sums of Steck's Determinants. *Annals of Biometrics and Biostatistics* 1(2): 1006.

Hutson, A. D., and Ernst, M. D. (2000). The Exact Bootstrap Mean and Variance of an L-Estimator. *Journal of the Royal Statistical Society: Series B (Methodological)* 62: 89–94.

Ignatz, M., Saxonhouse, M., Sola, M., Pastos, K., Hutson, A., Christensen, R., and Rimsza, L. (2002). Reticulated Platelet Percentages in Non-Thrombocytopenic Neonates of Different Post-Conceptional Ages. *Pediatric Research* 51(4): 243A–243A.

Inglot, T., Kallenberg, W. C., and Ledwina, T. (1997). Data Driven Smooth Tests for Composite Hypotheses. *Annals of Statistics* 25(3): 1222–1250.

Irle, A. (1984). Extended Optimality of Sequential Probability Ratio Tests. *Annals of Statistics* 12(1): 380–386.

James, B., James, K. L., and Siegmund, D. (1987). Tests for a Change-Point. *Biometrika* 74(1): 71–83.

James, N. A., and Matteson, D. S. (2013). ecp: An R Package for Nonparametric Multiple Change Point Analysis of Multivariate Data. Technical Report. Cornell University.

James, W., and Stein, C. (1961). *Estimation with Quadratic Loss.* Springer, New York.

Janes, H., and Pepe, M. S. (2009). Adjusting for Covariate Effects on Classification Accuracy Using the Covariate-Adjusted Receiver Operating Characteristic Curve. *Biometrika* 96(2): 371–382.

Janzen, F. J., Tucker, J. K., and Paukstis, G. L. (2000). Experimental Analysis of an Early Life-History Stage: Selection on Size of Hatchling Turtles. *Ecology* 81(8): 2290–2304.

Jeffreys, H. (1935). Some Tests of Significance, Treated by the Theory of Probability. *Mathematical Proceedings of the Cambridge Philosophical Society* 31(2): 203–222.

Jeffreys, H. (1961). *Theory of Probability.* 3rd ed. Oxford University Press, Oxford.

Jeffreys, H. (1998). *Theory of Probability.* 3rd ed. Oxford University Press, Oxford.

Jennison, C. (1987). Efficient Group Sequential Tests with Unpredictable Group Sizes. *Biometrika* 74(1): 155–165.

Jennison, C., and Turnbull, B. W. (2006). Adaptive and Nonadaptive Group Sequential Tests. *Biometrika* 93(1): 1–21.

Jennison, C., and Turnbull, B. W. (2010). *Group Sequential Methods with Applications to Clinical Trials,* CRC Press, Boca Raton, FL.

Jensen, F. V. (1995). *Saddlepoint Approximations.* Clarendon Press, Oxford.

Jewell, E. L., Darcy, K. M., Hutson, A., Lee, P. S., Havrilesky, L. J., Grace, L. A., Berchuck, A., and Secord, A. A. (2009). Association between the N-Terminally Truncated (Δn) P63α (Δnp63α) Isoform and Debulking Status, VEGF Expression and Progression-Free Survival in Previously Untreated, Advanced Stage Epithelial Ovarian Cancer: A Gynecologic Oncology Group Study. *Gynecologic Oncology* 115(3): 424–429.

Jing, B.-Y., and Wood, A. T. (1996). Exponential Empirical Likelihood Is Not Bartlett Correctable. *Annals of Statistics* 24(1): 365–369.

Johnson, M. E. (2013). *Multivariate Statistical Simulation: A Guide to Selecting and Generating Continuous Multivariate Distributions.* John Wiley & Sons, New York.

Johnson, N. J. (1978). Modified T Tests and Confidence Intervals for Asymmetrical Populations. *Journal of the American Statistical Association* 73(363): 536–544.

Johnson, N. L., Kotz, S., and Balakrishnan, N. (2004). *Continuous Multivariate Distributions*, Vol. 1, *Models and Applications.* John Wiley & Sons, New York.

Johnson, R. A. (1970). Asymptotic Expansions Associated with Posterior Distributions. *Annals of Mathematical Statistics* 41(3): 851–864.

Johnson, V. E. (2008). Properties of Bayes Factors Based on Test Statistics. *Scandinavian Journal of Statistics* 35(2): 354–368.

Johnston, J., and DiNardo, J. (1963). *Econometric Methods.* McGraw Hill, New York.

Julious, S. A. (2001). Inference and Estimation in a Changepoint Regression Problem. *Journal of the Royal Statistical Society: Series D (The Statistician)* 50(1): 51–61.

Jupp, P., and Spurr, B. (1985). Sobolev Tests for Independence of Directions. *Annals of Statistics* 13(3): 1140–1155.

Kac, M., Kiefer, J., and Wolfowitz, J. (1955). On Tests of Normality and Other Tests of Goodness of Fit Based on Distance Methods. *Annals of Mathematical Statistics* 26(2): 189–211.

Kai-Tai, F., and Yao-Ting, Z. (1990). *Generalized Multivariate Analysis.* Science Press, Beijing.

Kalbfleisch, J., and Lawless, J. F. (1989). Inference Based on Retrospective Ascertainment: An Analysis of the Data on Transfusion-Related Aids. *Journal of the American Statistical Association* 84(406): 360–372.

Kallenberg, W. C., and Ledwina, T. (1999). Data-Driven Rank Tests for Independence. *Journal of the American Statistical Association* 94(445): 285–301.

Kang, L., and Tian, L. (2013). Estimation of the Volume under the ROC Surface with Three Ordinal Diagnostic Categories. *Computational Statistics and Data Analysis* 62: 39–51.

Kang, L., Vexler, A., Tian, L., Cooney, M., and Louis, G. M. B. (2010). Empirical and Parametric Likelihood Interval Estimation for Populations with Many Zero Values: Application for Assessing Environmental Chemical Concentrations and Reproductive Health. *Epidemiology* 21(4): S58–S63.

Kaplan, E. L., and Meier, P. (1958). Nonparametric Estimation from Incomplete Observations. *Journal of the American Statistical Association* 53(282): 457–481.

Karlin, S., and Rubin, H. (1956). Distributions Possessing a Monotone Likelihood Ratio. *Journal of the American Statistical Association* 51(276): 637–643.

Kass, R. E. (1993). Bayes Factors in Practice. *The Statistician* 42(5): 551–560.

Kass, R. E., and Raftery, A. E. (1995). Bayes Factors. *Journal of the American Statistical Association* 90(430): 773–795.

Kass, R. E., and Steffey, D. (1989). Approximate Bayesian Inference in Conditionally Independent Hierarchical Models (Parametric Empirical Bayes Models). *Journal of the American Statistical Association* 84(407): 717–726.

Kass, R. E., Tierney, L., and Kadane, J. B. (1990). The Validity of Posterior Asymptotic Expansions Based on Laplace's Method. In *Bayesian and Likelihood Methods in Statistics and Econometrics: Essays in Honor of George A. Barnard*, ed. S. Geisser, J. S. Hodges, S. J. Press, and A. Zellner. North-Holland, New York.

Kass, R. E., and Vaidyanathan, S. K. (1992). Approximate Bayes Factors and Orthogonal Parameters, with Application to Testing Equality of Two Binomial Proportions. *Journal of the Royal Statistical Society: Series B (Methodological)* 54(1): 129–144.

Kass, R. E., and Wasserman, L. (1995). A Reference Bayesian Test for Nested Hypotheses and Its Relationship to the Schwarz Criterion. *Journal of the American Statistical Association* 90(431): 928–934.

Kass, R. E., and Wasserman, L. (1996). The Selection of Prior Distributions by Formal Rules. *Journal of the American Statistical Association* 91(435): 1343–1370.

Kendall, M., and Stuart, A. (1961). *The Advanced Theory of Statistics*, Vol. 2, *Inference and Relationship*. Griffin, London.

Kendall, M., and Stuart, A. (1979). *The Advanced Theory of Statistics*, Vol. 2, *Inference and Relationship*. 4th ed. Griffin, London.

Kendall, M. G. (1938). A New Measure of Rank Correlation. *Biometrika* 30(1/2): 81–93.

Kendall, M. G. (1946). *The Advanced Theory of Statistics*. 2nd ed. Griffin, London.

Kendall, M. G. (1948). *Rank Correlation Methods*. Griffin, London.

Kendall, M. G., and Buckland, W. R. (1957). *A Dictionary of Statistical Terms*. Oliver and Boyd, London.

Kent, J. T. (1982). Robust Properties of Likelihood Ratio Tests. *Biometrika* 69(1): 19–27.

Kepner, J. L., and Chang, M. N. (2003). On the Maximum Total Sample Size of a Group Sequential Test about Binomial Proportions. *Statistics and Probability Letters* 62(1): 87–92.

Khan, J., Wei, J. S., Ringner, M., Saal, L. H., Ladanyi, M., Westermann, F., Berthold, F., Schwab, M., Antonescu, C. R., and Peterson, C. (2001). Classification and Diagnostic Prediction of Cancers Using Gene Expression Profiling and Artificial Neural Networks. *Nature Medicine* 7(6): 673–679.

Khurd, P., and Gindi, G. (2005). Decision Strategies That Maximize the Area under the LROC Curve. *IEEE Transactions on Medical Imaging* 24(12): 1626–1636.

Kiefer, J. (1959). K-Sample Analogues of the Kolmogorov-Smirnov and Cramer-V. Mises Tests. *Annals of Mathematical Statistics* 30(2): 420–447.

Killick, R., and Eckley, I. A. (2011). Changepoint: An R Package for Changepoint Analysis. *Journal of Statistical Software* 58(3): 1–19.

Kim, H.-J. (1994). Tests for a Change-Point in Linear Regression. *Lecture Notes—Monograph Series* 23: 170–176.

Kim, H.-J., and Cai, L. (1993). Robustness of the Likelihood Ratio Test for a Change in Simple Linear Regression. *Journal of the American Statistical Association* 88(423): 864–871.

Kim, H.-J., and Siegmund, D. (1989). The Likelihood Ratio Test for a Change-Point in Simple Linear Regression. *Biometrika* 76(3): 409–423.

Kimeldorf, G., and Sampson, A. R. (1989). A Framework for Positive Dependence. *Annals of the Institute of Statistical Mathematics* 41(1): 31–45.

Kirk, J. L., and Fay, M. P. (2014). An Introduction to Practical Sequential Inferences via Single-Arm Binary Response Studies Using the Binseqtest R Package. *American Statistician* 68(4): 230–242.

Kitamura, Y. (1997). Empirical Likelihood Methods with Weakly Dependent Processes. *Annals of Statistics* 25(5): 2084–2102.

Kitamura, Y. (2001). Asymptotic Optimality of Empirical Likelihood for Testing Moment Restrictions. *Econometrica* 69(6): 1661–1672.

Klauer K. Non-exponential families of distributions. *Metrika* 1986; 33(1): 299–305.

Klein, J., and Moeschberger, M. (2003). *Survival Analysis: Statistical Methods for Censored and Truncated Data*. Springer-Verlag, New York.

Kleinbaum, D., and Klein, M. (2005). *Survival Analysis: A Self Learning Approach*. Springer Science Edition. Springer, New York.

Kleiner, A., Talwalkar, A., Sarkar, P., and Jordan, M. I. (2014). A Scalable Bootstrap for Massive Data. *Journal of the Royal Statistical Society: Series B (Statistical Methodology)* 76(4): 795–816.

Kleinman, K., and Horton, N. J. (2009). *SAS and R: Data Management, Statistical Analysis, and Graphics*. Chapman & Hall/CRC, Boca Raton, FL.

Klemelä, J. (2009). *Smoothing of Multivariate Data: Density Estimation and Visualization*. John Wiley & Sons, New York.

Klugkist, I., and Hoijtink, H. (2007). The Bayes Factor for Inequality and about Equality Constrained Models. *Computational Statistics and Data Analysis* 51(12): 6367–6379.

Koch, A. L. (1966). The Logarithm in Biology 1. Mechanisms Generating the Log-Normal Distribution Exactly. *Journal of Theoretical Biology* 12(2): 276–290.

Korn, E. L., Troendle, J. F., McShane, L. M., and Simon, R. (2004). Controlling the Number of False Discoveries: Application to High-Dimensional Genomic Data. *Journal of Statistical Planning and Inference* 124(2): 379–398.

Kotz, S., Lumelskii, Y., and Pensky, M. (2003). *The Stress-Strength Model and Its Generalizations: Theory and Applications*. World Scientific, Singapore.

Koziol, J. A., and Jia, Z. (2009). The Concordance Index C and the Mann–Whitney Parameter $\Pr(X > Y)$ with Randomly Censored Data. *Biometrical Journal* 51(3): 467–474.

Koziol, J. A., Maxwell, D. A., Fukushima, M., Colmerauer, M., and Pilch, Y. H. (1981). A Distribution-Free Test for Tumor-Growth Curve Analyses with Application to an Animal Tumor Immunotherapy Experiment. *Biometrics* 37(2): 383–390.

Kramar, A., Faraggi, D., Fortuné, A., and Reiser, B. (2001). mROC: A Computer Program for Combining Tumour Markers in Predicting Disease States. *Computer Methods and Programs in Biomedicine* 66(2): 199–207.

Krieger, A. M., Pollak, M., and Yakir, B. (2003). Surveillance of a Simple Linear Regression. *Journal of the American Statistical Association* 98(462): 456–469.

Krishnamoorthy, K., Lu, F., and Mathew, T. (2007). A Parametric Bootstrap Approach for ANOVA with Unequal Variances: Fixed and Random Models. *Computational Statistics and Data Analysis* 51(12): 5731–5742.

Kruskal, W. H., and Wallis, W. A. (1952). Use of Ranks in One-Criterion Variance Analysis. *Journal of the American Statistical Association* 47(260): 583–621.

Kuang, S.-Q., Liao, L., Zhang, H., Lee, A. V., O'Malley, B. W., and Xu, J. (2004). Aib1/Src-3 Deficiency Affects Insulin-Like Growth Factor I Signaling Pathway and Suppresses V-Ha-Ras-Induced Breast Cancer Initiation and Progression in Mice. *Cancer Research* 64(5): 1875–1885.

Küchenhoff, H. (1996). An Exact Algorithm for Estimating Breakpoints in Segmented Generalized Linear Models. Collaborative Research Center 386, Discussion Paper 27. Collaborative Research Center.

Küchenhoff, H., and Carroll, R. (1997). Segmented Regression with Errors in Predictors: Semi-Parametric and Parametric Methods. *Statistics in Medicine* 16(2): 169–188.

Küchenhoff, H., and Ulm, K. (1997). Comparison of Statistical Methods for Assessing Threshold Limiting Values in Occupational Epidemiology. *Computational Statistics* 12(2): 249–264.

Kudo, A. (1963). A Multivariate Analogue of the One-Sided Test. *Biometrika* 50(3/4): 403–418.

Kulathinal, S., Kuulasmaa, K., and Gasbarra, D. (2002). Estimation of an Errors-in-Variables Regression Model When the Variances of the Measurement Errors Vary between the Observations. *Statistics in Medicine* 21(8): 1089–1101.

Kuriki, S. (1993). One-Sided Test for the Equality of Two Covariance Matrices. *Annals of Statistics* 21(3): 1379–1384.

Kutner, M. H., Nachtsheim, C. J., Neter, J., and Li, W. (2005). *Applied Linear Statistical Methods.* 5th ed. McGraw Hill, New York.

Lachin, J. M., and Lan, S.-P. (1992). The Lupus Nephritis Collaborative Study Group Termination of a Clinical Trial with No Treatment Group Difference: The Lupus Nephritis Collaborative Study. *Controlled Clinical Trials* 13: 62–79.

Lai, T. L. (1978). Pitman Efficiencies of Sequential Tests and Uniform Limit Theorems in Nonparametric Statistics. *Annals of Statistics* 6(5): 1027–1047.

Lai, T. L. (1995). Sequential Changepoint Detection in Quality Control and Dynamical Systems. *Journal of the Royal Statistical Society: Series B (Methodological)* 57(4): 613–658.

Lai, T. L. (1997). On Optimal Stopping Problems in Sequential Hypothesis Testing. *Statistica Sinica* 7(1): 33–51.

Lai, T. L. (2001). Sequential Analysis: Some Classical Problems and New Challenges. *Statistica Sinica* 11: 303–350.

Lai, T. L. (2004). Likelihood Ratio Identities and Their Applications to Sequential Analysis. *Sequential Analysis* 23(4): 467–497.

Lai, T. L., and Shih, M.-C. (2004). Power, Sample Size and Adaptation Considerations in the Design of Group Sequential Clinical Trials. *Biometrika* 91(3): 507–528.

Lai, T. L., Shih, M.-C., and Su, Z. (2009). Tests and Confidence Intervals for Secondary Endpoints in Sequential Clinical Trials. *Biometrika* 96(4): 903–915.

Lam, F., and Longnecker, M. (1983). A Modified Wilcoxon Rank Sum Test for Paired Data. *Biometrika* 70(2): 510–513.

Lane-Claypon, J. E. (1926). A Further Report on Cancer of the Breast with Special Reference to Its Associated Antecedent Conditions. Reports on Public Health and Medical Subjects 32. Ministry of Health, London.

Lariccia, V. N. (1986). Asymptotically Chi-Squared Distributed Tests of Normality for Type II Censored Samples. *Journal of the American Statistical Association* 81(396): 1026–1031.

Lasko, T. A., Bhagwat, J. G., Zou, K. H., and Ohno-Machado, L. (2005). The Use of Receiver Operating Characteristic Curves in Biomedical Informatics. *Journal of Biomedical Informatics* 38(5): 404–415.

Lauzon, C., and Caffo, B. (2009). Easy Multiplicity Control in Equivalence Testing Using Two One-Sided Tests. *American Statistician* 63(2): 147–154.

Lavine, M., and Schervish, M. J. (1999). Bayes Factors: What They Are and What They Are Not. *American Statistician* 53(2): 119–122.

Lawless, J. F. (2011). *Statistical Models and Methods for Lifetime Data.* John Wiley & Sons, Hoboken, NJ.

Lawson, A. D. (2004). Futility. *Current Anaesthesia and Critical Care* 15(3): 219–223.

Lawson, J. (2010). *Design and Analysis of Experiments with SAS.* CRC Press, Boca Raton, FL.

Lazar, N., and Mykland, P. A. (1998). An Evaluation of the Power and Conditionality Properties of Empirical Likelihood. *Biometrika* 85(3): 523–534.

Lazar, N. A. (2003). Bayesian Empirical Likelihood. *Biometrika* 90(2): 319–326.

Lazar, N. A., and Mykland, P. A. (1999). Empirical Likelihood in the Presence of Nuisance Parameters. *Biometrika* 86(1): 203–211.

Le Cam, L. (1986). *Asymptotic Methods in Statistical Decision Theory.* Springer-Verlag, New York.

Le Cam, L. (1990). Maximum Likelihood: An Introduction. *International Statistical Review/Revue Internationale de Statistique* 58(2): 153–171.

Ledwina, T., and Wyłupek, G. (2012). Two-Sample Test against One-Sided Alternatives. *Scandinavian Journal of Statistics* 39(2): 358–381.

Lee, A. (1990). U-*Statistics*, Vol. 110, *Statistics: Textbooks and Monographs*. Marcel Dekker, New York.

Lee, E. T., and Wang, J. W. (2013). *Statistical Methods for Survival Data Analysis*. John Wiley & Sons, Hoboken, NJ.

Lee, J. W., and DeMets, D. L. (1992). Sequential Rank Tests with Repeated Measurements in Clinical Trials. *Journal of the American Statistical Association* 87(417): 136–142.

Lee, S., and Seo, M. H. (2008). Semiparametric Estimation of a Binary Response Model with a Change-Point due to a Covariate Threshold. *Journal of Econometrics* 144(2): 492–499.

Lee, S., Seo, M. H., and Shin, Y. (2011). Testing for Threshold Effects in Regression Models. *Journal of the American Statistical Association* 106(493): 220–231.

Lee, S. M., and Young, G. A. (1999). Nonparametric Likelihood Ratio Confidence Intervals. *Biometrika* 86(1): 107–118.

Lee, Y. J., and Wolfe, D. A. (1976). A Distribution-Free Test for Stochastic Ordering. *Journal of the American Statistical Association* 71(355): 722–727.

Lehéricy, S., Biondi, A., Sourour, N., Vlaicu, M., Du Montcel, S. T., Cohen, L., Vivas, E., Capelle, L., Faillot, T., and Casasco, A. (2002). Arteriovenous Brain Malformations: Is Functional MR Imaging Reliable for Studying Language Reorganization in Patients? Initial Observations 1. *Radiology* 223(3): 672–682.

Lehmann, E. L. (1959). *Testing Statistical Hypotheses*. Wiley, New York.

Lehmann, E. L. (1966). Some Concepts of Dependence. *Annals of Mathematical Statistics* 37: 1137–1153.

Lehmann, E. L. (1986). *Testing Statistical Hypotheses*. 2nd ed. John Wiley & Sons, New York. Transferred to Wadsorth & Brooks/Cole, 1991.

Lehmann, E. L. (1998). *Elements of Large-Sample Theory*. Springer Verlag, New York.

Lehmann, E. L. (2012). On Likelihood Ratio Tests. *IMS Lecture Notes—Monograph Series 2nd Lehmann Symposium—Optimality* 49: 209–216.

Lehmann, E. L., and Casella, G. (1998). *Theory of Point Estimation*. Springer-Verlag, New York.

Lehmann, E. L., and Romano, J. P. (2006). *Testing Statistical Hypotheses*. Springer-Verlag, New York.

Lehmann, E. L., and Stein, C. (1949). On the Theory of Some Non-Parametric Hypotheses. *Annals of Mathematical Statistics* 20(1): 28–45.

Leisenring, W., and Pepe, M. S. (1998). Regression Modelling of Diagnostic Likelihood Ratios for the Evaluation of Medical Diagnostic Tests. *Biometrics* 54(2): 444–452.

Lemdani, M., and Pons, O. (1999). Likelihood Ratio Tests in Contamination Models. *Bernoulli* 5(4): 705–719.

Leonard, T., Hsu, J. S., and Tsui, K.-W. (1989). Bayesian Marginal Inference. *Journal of the American Statistical Association* 84(408): 1051–1058.

Lesaffre, E., Scheys, I., Frohlich, J., and Bluhmki, E. (1993). Calculation of Power and Sample-Size with Bounded Outcome Scores. *Statistics in Medicine* 12(11): 1063–1078.

Leuraud, K., and Benichou, J. (2001). A Comparison of Several Methods to Test for the Existence of a Monotonic Dose–Response Relationship in Clinical and Epidemiological Studies. *Statistics in Medicine* 20(22): 3335–3351.

Levin, B., and Kline, J. (1985). The Cusum Test of Homogeneity with an Application in Spontaneous Abortion Epidemiology. *Statistics in Medicine* 4(4): 469–488.

Levin, G. P., Emerson, S. C., and Emerson, S. S. (2014). An Evaluation of Inferential Procedures for Adaptive Clinical Trial Designs with Pre-Specified Rules for Modifying the Sample Size. *Biometrics* 70(3): 556–567.

Li, G. (1995). Nonparametric Likelihood Ratio Estimation of Probabilities for Truncated Data. *Journal of the American Statistical Association* 90(431): 997–1003.

Li, G., Hollander, M., McKeague, I. W., and Yang, J. (1996). Nonparametric Likelihood Ratio Confidence Bands for Quantile Functions from Incomplete Survival Data. *Annals of Statistics* 24(2): 628–640.

Li, G., and Wang, Q.-H. (2003). Empirical Likelihood Regression Analysis for Right Censored Data. *Statistica Sinica* 13(1): 51–68.

Li, M., Peng, L., and Qi, Y. (2011). Reduce Computation in Profile Empirical Likelihood Method. *Canadian Journal of Statistics* 39(2): 370–384.

Li, R., and Nie, L. (2008). Efficient Statistical Inference Procedures for Partially Nonlinear Models and Their Applications. *Biometrics* 64(3): 904–911.

Li, X. (2009). A Generalized P-Value Approach for Comparing the Means of Several Log-Normal Populations. *Statistics and Probability Letters* 79(11): 1404–1408.

Liang, H., Wang, S., and Carroll, R. J. (2007). Partially Linear Models with Missing Response Variables and Error-Prone Covariates. *Biometrika* 94(1): 185–198.

Liang, H., Wang, S., Robins, J. M., and Carroll, R. J. (2004). Estimation in Partially Linear Models with Missing Covariates. *Journal of the American Statistical Association* 99(466): 357–367.

Limpert, E., Stahel, W. A., and Abbt, M. (2001). Log-Normal Distributions across the Sciences: Keys and Clues on the Charms of Statistics, and How Mechanical Models Resembling Gambling Machines Offer a Link to a Handy Way to Characterize Log-Normal Distributions, Which Can Provide Deeper Insight into Variability and Probability—Normal or Log-Normal: That Is the Question. *BioScience* 51(5): 341–352.

Lin, C.-C., and Mudholkar, G. S. (1980). A Simple Test for Normality against Asymmetric Alternatives. *Biometrika* 67(2): 455–461.

Lin, D. (1991). Nonparametric Sequential Testing in Clinical Trials with Incomplete Multivariate Observations. *Biometrika* 78(1): 123–131.

Lin, H., Zhou, L., Peng, H., and Zhou, X. H. (2011). Selection and Combination of Biomarkers Using ROC Method for Disease Classification and Prediction. *Canadian Journal of Statistics* 39(2): 324–343.

Lin, J.-J., Chang, C.-H., and Pal, N. (2015). A Revisit to Contingency Table and Tests of Independence: Bootstrap Is Preferred to Chi-Square Approximations as Well as Fisher's Exact Test. *Journal of Biopharmaceutical Statistics* 25(3): 438–458.

Lin, Y., and Shih, W. J. (2004). Adaptive Two-Stage Designs for Single-Arm Phase IIa Cancer Clinical Trials. *Biometrics* 60(2): 482–490.

Lindley, D. V. (1980). Approximate Bayesian Methods. *Trabajos de Estadística y de Investigación Operativa* 31(1): 223–245.

Lindsey, J. (1996). *Parametric Statistical Inference*. Oxford University Press, Oxford.

Littell, R. C. (2006). *SAS for Mixed Models*. SAS Institute, Cary, NC.

Little, R. J., and Rubin, D. B. (2014). *Statistical Analysis with Missing Data*. John Wiley & Sons, Hoboken, NJ.

Liu, A., and Hall, W. (1999). Unbiased Estimation Following a Group Sequential Test. *Biometrika* 86(1): 71–78.

Liu, A., Li, Q., Liu, C., Yu, K., and Yu, K. F. (2010). A Rank-Based Test for Comparison of Multidimensional Outcomes. *Journal of the American Statistical Association* 105(490): 578–587.

Liu, A., Schisterman, E., and Teoh, E. (2004). Sample Size and Power Calculation in Comparing Diagnostic Accuracy of Biomarkers with Pooled Assessments. *Journal of Applied Statistics* 31(1): 49–59.

Liu, A., and Schisterman, E. F. (2003). Comparison of Diagnostic Accuracy of Biomarkers with Pooled Assessments. *Biometrical Journal* 45(5): 631–644.

Liu, A., Schisterman, E. F., and Wu, C. (2006). Multistage Evaluation of Measurement Error in a Reliability Study. *Biometrics* 62(4): 1190–1196.

Liu, A., Schisterman, E. F., and Zhu, Y. (2005). On Linear Combinations of Biomarkers to Improve Diagnostic Accuracy. *Statistics in Medicine* 24(1): 37–47.

Liu, C., Liu, A., and Halabi, S. (2011). A Min–Max Combination of Biomarkers to Improve Diagnostic Accuracy. *Statistics in Medicine* 30(16): 2005–2014.

Liu, J. P., Ma, M. C., Wu, C. Y., and Tai, J. Y. (2006). Tests of Equivalence and Non-Inferiority for Diagnostic Accuracy Based on the Paired Areas under ROC Curves. *Statistics in Medicine* 25(7): 1219–1238.

Liu, L., and Yu, Z. (2008). A Likelihood Reformulation Method in Non-Normal Random Effects Models. *Statistics in Medicine* 27(16): 3105–3124.

Liu, Y., Zou, C., and Zhang, R. (2008). Empirical Likelihood Ratio Test for a Change-Point in Linear Regression Model. *Communications in Statistics—Theory and Methods* 37(16): 2551–2563.

Lloyd, C. J. (1998). Using Smoothed Receiver Operating Characteristic Curves to Summarize and Compare Diagnostic Systems. *Journal of the American Statistical Association* 93(444): 1356–1364.

Lloyd, C. J. (2000). Regression Models for Convex ROC Curves. *Biometrics* 56(3): 862–867.

Lombard, F. (1987). Rank Tests for Changepoint Problems. *Biometrika* 74(3): 615–624.

Looney, S. W., and Gulledge Jr., T. R. (1985). Use of the Correlation Coefficient with Normal Probability Plots. *American Statistician* 39(1): 75–79.

Loschi, R. H., Pontel, J. G., and Cruz, F. R. (2010). Multiple Change-Point Analysis for Linear Regression Models. *Chilean Journal of Statistics* 1: 93–112.

Louis, G. B., Weiner, J., Whitcomb, B., Sperrazza, R., Schisterman, E., Lobdell, D., Crickard, K., Greizerstein, H., and Kostyniak, P. (2005). Environmental PCB Exposure and Risk of Endometriosis. *Human Reproduction* 20(1): 279–285.

Lucito, R., West, J., Reiner, A., Alexander, J., Esposito, D., Mishra, B., Powers, S., Norton, L., and Wigler, M. (2000). Detecting Gene Copy Number Fluctuations in Tumor Cells by Microarray Analysis of Genomic Representations. *Genome Research* 10(11): 1726–1736.

Lusher, J., Roberts, H., Davignon, G., Joist, J., Smith, H., Shapiro, A., Laurian, Y., Kasper, C., and Mannucci, P. (1998). A Randomized, Double-Blind Comparison of Two Dosage Levels of Recombinant Factor VIIa in the Treatment of Joint, Muscle and Mucocutaneous Haemorrhages in Persons with Haemophilia A and B, with and without Inhibitors. *Haemophilia (Oxford)* 4: 790–798.

Lusted, L. B. (1971). Signal Detectability and Medical Decision-Making. *Science* 171(3977): 1217–1219.

Lyle, R. M., Melby, C. L., Hyner, G. C., Edmondson, J. W., Miller, J. Z., and Weinberger, M. H. (1987). Blood Pressure and Metabolic Effects of Calcium Supplementation in Normotensive White and Black Men. *JAMA* 257(13): 1772–1776.

Lyles, R. H., Tang, L., Lin, J., Zhang, Z., and Mukherjee, B. (2012). Likelihood-Based Methods for Regression Analysis with Binary Exposure Status Assessed by Pooling. *Statistics in Medicine* 31(22): 2485–2497.

Ma, C.-X., Vexler, A., Schisterman, E. F., and Tian, L. (2011). Cost-Efficient Designs Based on Linearly Associated Biomarkers. *Journal of Applied Statistics* 38(12): 2739–2750.

Ma, S., and Huang, J. (2005). Regularized ROC Method for Disease Classification and Biomarker Selection with Microarray Data. *Bioinformatics* 21(24): 4356–4362.

Ma, S., and Huang, J. (2007). Combining Multiple Markers for Classification Using ROC. *Biometrics* 63(3): 751–757.

Madure, M., and Greenland, S. (1992). Tests for Trend and Dose Response: Misinterpretations and Alternatives. *American Journal of Epidemiology* 135(1): 96–104.

Magni, P., Bellazzi, R., De Nicolao, G., Poggesi, I., and Rocchetti, M. (2002). Nonparametric AUC Estimation in Population Studies with Incomplete Sampling: A Bayesian Approach. *Journal of Pharmacokinetics and Pharmacodynamics* 29(5–6): 445–471.

Malinovsky, Y., Albert, P. S., and Schisterman, E. F. (2012). Pooling Designs for Outcomes under a Gaussian Random Effects Model. *Biometrics* 68(1): 45–52.

Manski, C. F. (1975). Maximum Score Estimation of the Stochastic Utility Model of Choice. *Journal of Econometrics* 3(3): 205–228.

Manski, C. F. (1985). Semiparametric Analysis of Discrete Response: Asymptotic Properties of the Maximum Score Estimator. *Journal of Econometrics* 27(3): 313–333.

Mantel, N., Bohidar, N. R., and Ciminera, J. L. (1977). Mantel-Haenszel Analyses of Litter-Matched Time-to-Response Data, with Modifications for Recovery of Interlitter Information. *Cancer Research* 37(11): 3863–3868.

Maor, E., and King, J. P. (1994). *E: The Story of a Number*, Oxford University Press, Oxford.

Marden, J. I. (2000). Hypothesis Testing: From P Values to Bayes Factors. *Journal of the American Statistical Association* 95(452): 1316–1320.

Mardia, K. V. (1967). A Non-parametric Test for the Two-sample Location Problem. *Journal of the Royal Statistical Society: Series B* 29: 320–342.

Mardia, K. V. (1968). Small Sample Power of a Non-Parametric Test for the Bivariate Two-Sample Location Problem in the Normal Case. *Journal of the Royal Statistical Society: Series B (Methodological)* 30(1): 83–92.

Mardia, K. V. (1970). *Families of Bivariate Distributions*. Griffin, London.

Martinsek, A. T. (1981). A Note on the Variance and Higher Central Moments of the Stopping Time of an SPRT. *Journal of the American Statistical Association* 76(375): 701–703.

Maurer, W., and Mellein, B. (1988). *On New Multiple Tests Based on Independent P-Values and the Assessment of Their Power*. Springer, Berlin.

May, S., and Bigelow, C. (2005). Modeling Nonlinear Dose-Response Relationships in Epidemiologic Studies: Statistical Approaches and Practical Challenges. *Nonlinearity in Biology, Toxicology, Medicine* 3(4): 474–490.

McCulloch, R., and Rossi, P. E. (1991). A Bayesian Approach to Testing the Arbitrage Pricing Theory. *Journal of Econometrics* 49(1): 141–168.

McIntosh, M. W., and Pepe, M. S. (2002). Combining Several Screening Tests: Optimality of the Risk Score. *Biometrics* 58(3): 657–664.

McLeish, D., and Small, C. G. (1986). Likelihood Methods for the Discrimination Problem. *Biometrika* 73(2): 397–403.

McMahan, C. S., Tebbs, J. M., and Bilder, C. R. (2013). Regression Models for Group Testing Data with Pool Dilution Effects. *Biostatistics* 14(2): 284–298.

McNaughton, L., and Davies, P. (1987). The Effects of a 16 Week Aerobic Conditioning Program on Serum Lipids, Lipoproteins and Coronary Risk Factors. *Journal of Sports Medicine and Physical Fitness* 27(3): 296–302.

Meeker, W. Q., and Escobar, L. A. (1995). Teaching about Approximate Confidence Regions Based on Maximum Likelihood Estimation. *American Statistician* 49(1): 48–53.

Mei, Y. (2006). Sequential Change-Point Detection When Unknown Parameters Are Present in the Pre-Change Distribution. *Annals of Statistics* 34(1): 92–122.

Meng, X.-L., and Wong, W. H. (1996). Simulating Ratios of Normalizing Constants via a Simple Identity: A Theoretical Exploration. *Statistica Sinica* 6(4): 831–860.

Metropolis, N., and Ulam, S. (1949). The Monte Carlo Method. *Journal of the American Statistical Association* 44(247): 335–341.

Metz, C. E., Herman, B. A., and Shen, J. H. (1998). Maximum Likelihood Estimation of Receiver Operating Characteristic (ROC) Curves from Continuously-Distributed Data. *Statistics in Medicine* 17(9): 1033–1053.

Miecznikowski, J. C., Vexler, A., and Shepherd, L. (2013). Dbemplikegof: An R Package for Nonparametric Likelihood Ratio Tests for Goodness-of-Fit and Two Sample Comparisons Based on Sample Entropy. *Journal of Statistical Software* 54(3): 1–19.

Miller, E. G. (2003). A New Class of Entropy Estimators for Multi-Dimensional Densities. Acoustics, Speech, and Signal Processing. In *International Conference on Acoustics, Speech, and Signal Processing*, Vol. 3, pp. 297–300.

Miller, R. G. (1976). Least Squares Regression with Censored Data. *Biometrika* 63(3): 449–464.

Molanes Lopez, E. M., Keilegom, I. V., and Veraverbeke, N. (2009). Empirical Likelihood for Non-Smooth Criterion Functions. *Scandinavian Journal of Statistics* 36(3): 413–432.

Molenberghs, G., and Verbeke, G. (2007). Likelihood Ratio, Score, and Wald Tests in a Constrained Parameter Space. *American Statistician* 61(1): 22–27.

Molodianovitch, K., Faraggi, D., and Reiser, B. (2006). Comparing the Areas under Two Correlated ROC Curves: Parametric and Non-Parametric Approaches. *Biometrical Journal* 48(5): 745–757.

Monahan, J. F., and Boos, D. D. (1992). Proper Likelihoods for Bayesian Analysis. *Biometrika* 79(2): 271–278.

Montgomery, D. C. (1991). *Introduction to Statistical Quality Control*. Wiley, New York.

Moran, P. A. P. (1950). Notes on Continuous Stochastic Phenomena. *Biometrika* 37: 17–23.

Moses, L. E., Shapiro, D., and Littenberg, B. (1993). Combining Independent Studies of a Diagnostic Test into a Summary ROC Curve: Data-Analytic Approaches and Some Additional Considerations. *Statistics in Medicine* 12(14): 1293–1316.

Mosteller, F., and Wallace, D. (1964). *Inference and Disputed Authorship: The Federalist.* Addison-Wesley, Reading, MA.

Moustakides, G. V. (1986). Optimal Stopping Times for Detecting Changes in Distributions. *Annals of Statistics* 14(4): 1379–1387.

Mudholkar, G. S., and Hutson, A. D. (1997). Continuity Corrected Approximations for an 'Exact' Inference with Pearson's X 2. *Journal of Statistical Planning and Inference* 59(1): 61–78.

Mudholkar, G. S., and Tian, L. (2001). On the Null Distributions of the Entropy Tests for the Gaussian and Inverse Gaussian Models. *Communications in Statistics—Theory and Methods* 30(8–9): 1507–1520.

Mudholkar, G. S., and Tian, L. (2002). An Entropy Characterization of the Inverse Gaussian Distribution and Related Goodness-of-Fit Test. *Journal of Statistical Planning and Inference* 102(2): 211–221.

Mudholkar, G. S., and Wilding, G. E. (2003). On the Conventional Wisdom Regarding Two Consistent Tests of Bivariate Independence. *Journal of the Royal Statistical Society: Series D (The Statistician)* 52(1): 41–57.

Muggeo, V. M. (2003). Estimating Regression Models with Unknown Break-Points. *Statistics in Medicine* 22(19): 3055–3071.

Muggeo, V. M. (2008). Segmented: An R Package to Fit Regression Models with Broken-Line Relationships. *R News* 8(1): 20–25.

Mulder, J. (2014). Bayes Factors for Testing Inequality Constrained Hypotheses: Issues with Prior Specification. *British Journal of Mathematical and Statistical Psychology* 67(1): 153–171.

Müller, H. H., and Schäfer, H. (2001). Adaptive Group Sequential Designs for Clinical Trials: Combining the Advantages of Adaptive and of Classical Group Sequential Approaches. *Biometrics* 57(3): 886–891.

Müller, P., and Parmigiani, G. (1995). Optimal Design via Curve Fitting of Monte Carlo Experiments. *Journal of the American Statistical Association* 90(432): 1322–1330.

Mumford, S. L., Schisterman, E. F., Vexler, A., and Liu, A. (2006). Pooling Biospecimens and Limits of Detection: Effects on ROC Curve Analysis. *Biostatistics* 7(4): 585–598.

Murota, K., and Takeuchi, K. (1981). The Studentized Empirical Characteristic Function and Its Application to Test for the Shape of Distribution. *Biometrika* 68(1): 55–65.

Murphy, S. A., and Van der Vaart, A. W. (1997). Semiparametric Likelihood Ratio Inference. *Annals of Statistics* 25(4): 1471–1509.

Murrell, P. (2005). *R Graphics.* CRC Press, Boca Raton, FL.

Murtaugh, P. A. (1995). ROC Curves with Multiple Marker Measurements. *Biometrics* 51(4): 1514–1522.

Mykland, P. A. (1995). Dual Likelihood. *Annals of Statistics* 23(2): 396–421.

Mykland, P. A. (1999). Bartlett Identities and Large Deviations in Likelihood Theory. *Annals of Statistics* 27(3): 1105–1117.

Mykland, P. A. (2001). Likelihood Computations without Bartlett Identities. *Bernoulli* 7(3): 473–485.

Nachar, N. (2008). The Mann-Whitney U: A Test for Assessing Whether Two Independent Samples Come from the Same Distribution. *Tutorials in Quantitative Methods for Psychology* 4(1): 13–20.

Naik-Nimbalkar, U., and Rajarshi, M. (1997). Empirical Likelihood Ratio Test for Equality of K Medians in Censored Data. *Statistics and Probability Letters* 34(3): 267–273.

Nakas, C. T., and Yiannoutsos, C. T. (2004). Ordered Multiple-Class ROC Analysis with Continuous Measurements. *Statistics in Medicine* 23(22): 3437–3449.

Nazarov, A., and Stepanova, N. (2009). On Asymptotic Efficiency of Multivariate Version of Spearman's Rho. *arXiv* preprint: 0906.1059.

Nelder, J., and Lee, Y. (1992). Likelihood, Quasi-Likelihood and Pseudolikelihood: Some Comparisons. *Journal of the Royal Statistical Society: Series B (Methodological)* 51(4): 273–284.

Nelsen, R. B. (1992). On Measures of Association as Measures of Positive Dependence. *Statistics and Probability Letters* 14(4): 269–274.

Neuhäuser, M. (2002). Nonparametric Identification of the Minimum Effective Dose. *Drug Information Journal* 36(4): 881–888.

Neuhäuser, M., Liu, P. Y., and Hothorn, L. A. (1998). Nonparametric Tests for Trend: Jonckheere's Test, a Modification and a Maximum Test. *Biometrical Journal* 40(8): 899–909.

Newton, M. A., and Raftery, A. E. (1994). Approximate Bayesian Inference with the Weighted Likelihood Bootstrap. *Journal of the Royal Statistical Society: Series B (Methodological)* 56(1): 3–48.

Neyman, J., and Pearson, E. S. (1928). On the Use and Interpretation of Certain Test Criteria for Purposes of Statistical Inference. Part II. *Biometrika* 20A(3/4): 263–294.

Neyman, J., and Pearson, E. S. (1933). The Testing of Statistical Hypotheses in Relation to Probabilities A Priori. *Mathematical Proceedings of the Cambridge Philosophical Society* 29(4): 492–510.

Neyman, J., and Pearson, E. S. (1938). Contributions to the Theory of Testing Statistical Hypotheses. *Journal of Statistical Research Memoirs (University of London)* 2: 25–58.

Neyman, J., and Pearson, E. S. (1992). *On the Problem of the Most Efficient Tests of Statistical Hypotheses.* Springer, New York.

Ng, P. Y. B., Donley, M., Hausmann, E., Hutson, A. D., Rossomando, E. F., and Scannapieco, F. A. (2007). Candidate Salivary Biomarkers Associated with Alveolar Bone Loss: Cross-Sectional and In Vitro Studies. *FEMS Immunology and Medical Microbiology* 49(2): 252–260.

Nie, L., Chu, H., Liu, C., Cole, S. R., Vexler, A., and Schisterman, E. F. (2010). Linear Regression with an Independent Variable Subject to a Detection Limit. *Epidemiology (Cambridge, Mass.)* 21(Suppl. 4): S17–S24.

Ning, W. (2012). Empirical Likelihood Ratio Test for a Mean Change Point Model with a Linear Trend Followed by an Abrupt Change. *Journal of Applied Statistics* 39(5): 947–961.

Ning, W., Pailden, J., and Gupta, A. (2012). Empirical Likelihood Ratio Test for the Epidemic Change Model. *Journal of Data Science* 10(1): 107–127.

O'Brien, P. C. (1984). Procedures for Comparing Samples with Multiple Endpoints. *Biometrics* 40(4): 1079–1087.

O'Brien, P. C. (1988). Comparing Two Samples: Extensions of the T, Rank-Sum, and Log-Rank Tests. *Journal of the American Statistical Association* 83(401): 52–61.

O'Brien, P. C., and Fleming, T. R. (1979). A Multiple Testing Procedure for Clinical Trials. *Biometrics* 35(3): 549–556.

Obuchowski, N. A. (1997). Nonparametric Analysis of Clustered ROC Curve Data. *Biometrics* 53(2): 567–578.

Obuchowski, N. A. (2003). Receiver Operating Characteristic Curves and Their Use in Radiology 1. *Radiology* 229(1): 3–8.

O'Hagan, A. (1995). Fractional Bayes Factors for Model Comparison. *Journal of the Royal Statistical Society: Series B (Methodological)* 57(1): 99–138.

Oja, H. (1981). Two Location and Scale-Free Goodness-of-Fit Tests. *Biometrika* 68(3): 637–640.

Oja, H. (1983). New Tests for Normality. *Biometrika* 70(1): 297–299.

Olshen, A. B., Venkatraman, E., Lucito, R., and Wigler, M. (2004). Circular Binary Segmentation for the Analysis of Array-Based DNA Copy Number Data. *Biostatistics* 5(4): 557–572.

O'Malley, A. J., and Zou, K. H. (2006). Bayesian Multivariate Hierarchical Transformation Models for ROC Analysis. *Statistics in Medicine* 25(3): 459–479.

O'Malley, A. J., Zou, K. H., Fielding, J. R., and Tempany, C. (2001). Bayesian Regression Methodology for Estimating a Receiver Operating Characteristic Curve with Two Radiologic Applications: Prostate Biopsy and Spiral CT of Ureteral Stones. *Academic Radiology* 8(8): 713–725.

Orawo, L. A. O., and Christen, J. A. (2009). Bayesian Sequential Analysis for Multiple-Arm Clinical Trials. *Statistics and Computing* 19(1): 99–109.

Owen, A. B. (1988). Empirical Likelihood Ratio Confidence Intervals for a Single Functional. *Biometrika* 75(2): 237–249.

Owen, A. B. (1990). Empirical Likelihood Ratio Confidence Regions. *Annals of Statistics* 18(1): 90–120.

Owen, A. B. (1991). Empirical Likelihood for Linear Models. *Annals of Statistics* 19(4): 1725–1747.

Owen, A. B. (2001). *Empirical Likelihood.* CRC Press, Boca Raton, FL.

Page, E. (1954). Continuous Inspection Schemes. *Biometrika* 41(1/2): 100–115.

Page, E. (1955). A Test for a Change in a Parameter Occurring at an Unknown Point. *Biometrika* 42(3/4): 523–527.

Pal, N., and Berry, J. C. (1992). On Invariance and Maximum Likelihood Estimation. *American Statistician* 46(3): 209–212.

Pampallona, S., and Tsiatis, A. A. (1994). Group Sequential Designs for One-Sided and Two-Sided Hypothesis Testing with Provision for Early Stopping in Favor of the Null Hypothesis. *Journal of Statistical Planning and Inference* 42(1): 19–35.

Park, E., and Chang, Y.-C. I. (2010). Sequential Analysis of Longitudinal Data in a Prospective Nested Case–Control Study. *Biometrics* 66(4): 1034–1042.

Park, E., and Kim, Y. (2004). Analysis of Longitudinal Data in Case-Control Studies. *Biometrika* 91: 321–330.

Park, S. (1999). A Goodness-of-Fit Test for Normality Based on the Sample Entropy of Order Statistics. *Statistics and Probability Letters* 44(4): 359–363.

Pastor, R., and Guallar, E. (1998). Use of Two-Segmented Logistic Regression to Estimate Change-Points in Epidemiologic Studies. *American Journal of Epidemiology* 148(7): 631–642.

Pastor-Barriuso, R., Guallar, E., and Coresh, J. (2003). Transition Models for Change-Point Estimation in Logistic Regression. *Statistics in Medicine* 22(7): 1141–1162.

Pawitan, Y. (2000). A Reminder of the Fallibility of the Wald Statistic: Likelihood Explanation. *American Statistician* 54(1): 54–56.

Pawitan, Y. (2001). *In All Likelihood: Statistical Modelling and Inference Using Likelihood*. Oxford University Press, Oxford.

Pearson, E., and Hartley, H. (1966). *Biometrika Tables for Statisticians*. Vol. I. Cambridge University Press, Cambridge.

Pearson, E. S., and Neyman, J. (1930). *On the Problem of Two Samples*. Imprimerie de l'University, Paris.

Pearson, K. (1920). Notes on the History of Correlation. *Biometrika* 13(1): 25–45.

Peck, C. C., Beal, S. L., Sheiner, L. B., and Nichols, A. I. (1984). Extended Least Squares Nonlinear Regression: A Possible Solution to the "Choice of Weights" Problem in Analysis of Individual Pharmacokinetic Data. *Journal of Pharmacokinetics and Biopharmaceutics* 12(5): 545–558.

Pencina, M. J., D'Agostino, R. B., and Vasan, R. S. (2008). Evaluating the Added Predictive Ability of a New Marker: From Area under the ROC Curve to Reclassification and Beyond. *Statistics in Medicine* 27(2): 157–172.

Peng, L., and Zhou, X.-H. (2004). Local Linear Smoothing of Receiver Operating Characteristic (ROC) Curves. *Journal of Statistical Planning and Inference* 118(1): 129–143.

Pepe, M. S. (1997). A Regression Modelling Framework for Receiver Operating Characteristic Curves in Medical Diagnostic Testing. *Biometrika* 84(3): 595–608.

Pepe, M. S. (2000a). An Interpretation for the ROC Curve and Inference Using GLM Procedures. *Biometrics* 56(2): 352–359.

Pepe, M. S. (2000b). Receiver Operating Characteristic Methodology. *Journal of the American Statistical Association* 95(449): 308–311.

Pepe, M. S. (2003). *The Statistical Evaluation of Medical Tests for Classification and Prediction*. Oxford University Press, Oxford.

Pepe, M. S., Cai, T., and Longton, G. (2006). Combining Predictors for Classification Using the Area under the Receiver Operating Characteristic Curve. *Biometrics* 62(1): 221–229.

Pepe, M. S., and Thompson, M. L. (2000). Combining Diagnostic Test Results to Increase Accuracy. *Biostatistics* 1(2): 123–140.

Perkins, N. J., and Schisterman, E. F. (2005). The Youden Index and the Optimal Cut-Point Corrected for Measurement Error. *Biometrical Journal* 47(4): 428–441.

Perkins, N. J., Schisterman, E. F., and Vexler, A. (2007). Receiver Operating Characteristic Curve Inference from a Sample with a Limit of Detection. *American Journal of Epidemiology* 165(3): 325–333.

Perkins, N. J., Schisterman, E. F., and Vexler, A. (2009). Generalized ROC Curve Inference for a Biomarker Subject to a Limit of Detection and Measurement Error. *Statistics in Medicine* 28(13): 1841–1860.

Perkins, N. J., Schisterman, E. F., and Vexler, A. (2011). ROC Curve Inference for Best Linear Combination of Two Biomarkers Subject to Limits of Detection. *Biometrical Journal* 53(3): 464–476.

Perkins, N. J., Schisterman, E. F., and Vexler, A. (2013). Multivariate Normally Distributed Biomarkers Subject to Limits of Detection and Receiver Operating Characteristic Curve Inference. *Academic Radiology* 20(7): 838–846.

Perlman, M. D. (1969). One-Sided Testing Problems in Multivariate Analysis. *Annals of Mathematical Statistics* 40(2): 549–567.

Perlman, M. D., and Wu, L. (2004). A Note on One-Sided Tests with Multiple Endpoints. *Biometrics* 60(1): 276–280.

Persing, A., Jasra, A., Beskos, A., Balding, D., and De Iorio, M. (2014). A Simulation Approach for Change-Points on Phylogenetic Trees. *Journal of Computational Biology* 22(1): 10–24.

Petrone, S., Rousseau, J., and Scricciolo, C. (2014). Bayes and Empirical Bayes: Do They Merge? *Biometrika* 101(2): 285–302.

Pettitt, A. (1976). Cramér-Von Mises Statistics for Testing Normality with Censored Samples. *Biometrika* 63(3): 475–481.

Pettitt, A. (1977). Testing the Normality of Several Independent Samples Using the Anderson-Darling Statistic. *Applied Statistics* 26(2): 156–161.

Pettitt, A. (1979). A Non-Parametric Approach to the Change-Point Problem. *Applied Statistics* 28(2): 126–135.

Pettitt, A. N., and Stephens, M. A. (1976). Modified Cramer-Von Mises Statistics for Censored Data. *Biometrika* 63(2): 291–298.

Phillips, P. J., Moon, H., Rizvi, S., and Rauss, P. J. (2000). The Feret Evaluation Methodology for Face-Recognition Algorithms. *IEEE Transactions on Pattern Analysis and Machine Intelligence* 22(10): 1090–1104.

Piantadosi, S. (2005). *Clinical Trials: A Methodologic Perspective.* John Wiley & Sons, Hoboken, NJ.

Pierce, D. A., and Gray, R. J. (1982). Testing Normality of Errors in Regression Models. *Biometrika* 69(1): 233–236.

Pierce, D. A., and Kopecky, K. J. (1979). Testing Goodness of Fit for the Distribution of Errors in Regression Models. *Biometrika* 66(1): 1–5.

Pitman, E. J. (1949). *Notes on Non-Parametric Statistical Inference.* Department of Statistics, University of North Carolina, New York.

Platt, R. W., Hanley, J. A., and Yang, H. (2000). Bootstrap Confidence Intervals for the Sensitivity of a Quantitative Diagnostic Test. *Statistics in Medicine* 19(3): 313–322.

Pocock, S. J. (1977). Group Sequential Methods in the Design and Analysis of Clinical Trials. *Biometrika* 64(2): 191–199.

Polansky, A. M. (2000). Stabilizing Bootstrap-T Confidence Intervals for Small Samples. *Canadian Journal of Statistics* 28(3): 501–516.

Pollak, M. (1985). Optimal Detection of a Change in Distribution. *Annals of Statistics* 13: 206–227.

Pollak, M. (1987). Average Run Lengths of an Optimal Method of Detecting a Change in Distribution. *Annals of Statistics* 5(2): 749–779.

Pollak, M., and Tartakovsky, A. G. (2007). On Optimality Properties of the Shiryaev-Roberts Procedure. *Statistica Sinica* 19: 1729–1739.

Posch, M., and Bauer, P. (2000). Interim Analysis and Sample Size Reassessment. *Biometrics* 56(4): 1170–1176.

Posch, M., Bauer, P., and Brannath, W. (2003). Issues in Designing Flexible Trials. *Statistics in Medicine* 22(6): 953–969.

Powers, L. (1936). The Nature of the Interaction of Genes Affecting Four Quantitative Characters in a Cross between *Hordeum deficiens* and *Hordeum vulgare. Genetics* 21(4): 398.

Poynter, J. N., Gruber, S. B., Higgins, P. D., Almog, R., Bonner, J. D., Rennert, H. S., Low, M., Greenson, J. K., and Rennert, G. (2005). Statins and the Risk of Colorectal Cancer. *New England Journal of Medicine* 352(21): 2184–2192.

Praagman, J. (1988). Bahadur Efficiency of Rank Tests for the Change-Point Problem. *Annals of Statistics* 16(1): 198–217.

Prabhakar, S., and Jain, A. K. (2002). Decision-Level Fusion in Fingerprint Verification. *Pattern Recognition* 35(4): 861–874.

Pratt, J. W. (1961). Review of Lehmann's Testing Statistical Hypotheses. *Journal of the American Statistical Association* 56(293): 163–167.

Pratt, J. W. (1962). On the Foundations of Statistical Inference: Discussion. *Journal of the American Statistical Association* 57(298): 307–326.

Preisser, J. S., Sen, P. K., and Offenbacher, S. (2011). Multiple Hypothesis Testing for Experimental Gingivitis Based on Wilcoxon Signed Rank Statistics. *Statistics in Biopharmaceutical Research* 3(2): 372–384.

Prescott, P. (1976). On a Test for Normality Based on Sample Entropy. *Journal of the Royal Statistical Society: Series B (Methodological)* 38(3): 254–256.

Proschan, M. A., and Hunsberger, S. A. (1995). Designed Extension of Studies Based on Conditional Power. *Biometrics* 51(4): 1315–1324.

Provost, F. J., and Fawcett, T. (1997). Analysis and Visualization of Classifier Performance: Comparison under Imprecise Class and Cost Distributions. *KDD* 97: 43–48.

Pyke, R. (1965). Spacings. *Journal of the Royal Statistical Society: Series B (Statistical Methodology)* 27: 395–449.

Qin, G., Davis, A. E., and Jing, B.-Y. (2011). Empirical Likelihood-Based Confidence Intervals for the Sensitivity of a Continuous-Scale Diagnostic Test at a Fixed Level of Specificity. *Statistical Methods in Medical Research* 20(3): 217–231.

Qin, G., and Zhou, X. H. (2006). Empirical Likelihood Inference for the Area under the ROC Curve. *Biometrics* 62(2): 613–622.

Qin, J. (1991). Likelihood and Empirical Likelihood Ratio Confidence Intervals in Two Sample Semi-Parametric Models. Technical Report Series, Stat-91-6. University of Waterloo.

Qin, J. (1993). Empirical Likelihood in Biased Sample Problems. *Annals of Statistics* 21(3): 1182–1196.

Qin, J. (1999). Empirical Likelihood Ratio Based Confidence Intervals for Mixture Proportions. *Annals of Statistics* 27(4): 1368–1384.

Qin, J. (2000). Combining Parametric and Empirical Likelihoods. *Biometrika* 87(2): 484–490.

Qin, J., and Lawless, J. (1994). Empirical Likelihood and General Estimating Equations. *Annals of Statistics* 22(1): 300–325.

Qin, J., and Leung, D. H. (2005). A Semiparametric Two-Component "Compound" Mixture Model and Its Application to Estimating Malaria Attributable Fractions. *Biometrics* 61(2): 456–464.

Qin, J., and Wong, A. (1996). Empirical Likelihood in a Semi-Parametric Model. *Scandinavian Journal of Statistics* 23(2): 209–219.

Qin, J., and Zhang, B. (2003). Using Logistic Regression Procedures for Estimating Receiver Operating Characteristic Curves. *Biometrika* 90(3): 585–596.

Qin, J., and Zhang, B. (2005). Marginal Likelihood, Conditional Likelihood and Empirical Likelihood: Connections and Applications. *Biometrika* 92(2): 251–270.

Qin, J., and Zhang, B. (2007). Empirical-Likelihood-Based Inference in Missing Response Problems and Its Application in Observational Studies. *Journal of the Royal Statistical Society: Series B (Statistical Methodology)* 69(1): 101–122.

Qin, J., and Zhang, B. (2010). Best Combination of Multiple Diagnostic Tests for Screening Purposes. *Statistics in Medicine* 29(28): 2905–2919.

Qin, Y., and Zhang, S. (2008). Empirical Likelihood Confidence Intervals for Differences between Two Datasets with Missing Data. *Pattern Recognition Letters* 29(6): 803–812.

Quandt, R. E. (1960). Tests of the Hypothesis That a Linear Regression System Obeys Two Separate Regimes. *Journal of the American Statistical Association* 55(290): 324–330.

Quesenberry, C., Giesbrecht, F., and Burns, J. (1983). Some Methods for Studying the Validity of Normal Model Assumptions for Multiple Samples. *Biometrics* 39(3): 735–739.

Quesenberry, C., Whitaker, T., and Dickens, J. (1976). On Testing Normality Using Several Samples: An Analysis of Peanut Aflatoxin Data. *Biometrics* 32(4): 753–759.

Quessy, J. F. (2012). Testing for Bivariate Extreme Dependence Using Kendall's Process. *Scandinavian Journal of Statistics* 39(3): 497–514.

R Development Core Team. (2014). *R: A Language and Environment for Statistical Computing.* R Foundation for Statistical Computing, Vienna, Austria.

Račkauskas, A., and Suquet, C. (2006). Testing Epidemic Changes of Infinite Dimensional Parameters. *Statistical Inference for Stochastic Processes* 9(2): 111–134.

Rahman, M. M., and Govindarajulu, Z. (1997). A Modification of the Test of Shapiro and Wilk for Normality. *Journal of Applied Statistics* 24(2): 219–236.

Rakovski, C., Weisenberger, D. J., Marjoram, P., Laird, P. W., and Siegmund, K. D. (2011). Modeling Measurement Error in Tumor Characterization Studies. *BMC Bioinformatics* 12(1): 284.

Ramanayake, A., and Gupta, A. K. (2003). Tests for an Epidemic Change in a Sequence of Exponentially Distributed Random Variables. *Biometrical Journal* 45(8): 946–958.

Rao, P. S., and Dorvlo, A. S. (1985). The Jackknife Procedure for the Probabilities of Misclassification. *Communications in Statistics—Simulation and Computation* 14(4): 779–790.

Razali, N. M., and Wah, Y. B. (2011). Power Comparisons of Shapiro-Wilk, Kolmogorov-Smirnov, Lilliefors and Anderson-Darling Tests. *Journal of Statistical Modeling and Analytics* 2(1): 21–33.

Redelmeier, D. A., and Tibshirani, R. J. (1997). Association between Cellular-Telephone Calls and Motor Vehicle Collisions. *New England Journal of Medicine* 336(7): 453–458.

Regenwetter, M., Dana, J., and Davis-Stober, C. P. (2011). Transitivity of Preferences. *Psychological Review* 118(1): 42.

Reid, N. (1996). Likelihood and Higher-Order Approximations to Tail Areas: A Review and Annotated Bibliography. *Canadian Journal of Statistics* 24(2): 141–166.

Reid, N. (2000). Likelihood. *Journal of the American Statistical Association* 95(452): 1335–1340.

Reid, N. (2003). Asymptotics and the Theory of Inference. *Annals of Statistics* 31(6): 1695–1731.

Reimherr, M., and Nicolae, D. L. (2013). On Quantifying Dependence: A Framework for Developing Interpretable Measures. *Statistical Science* 28(1): 116–130.

Reiser, B. (2001). Confidence Intervals for the Mahalanobis Distance. *Communications in Statistics—Simulation and Computation* 30(1): 37–45.

Reiser, B., and Faraggi, D. (1997). Confidence Intervals for the Generalized ROC Criterion. *Biometrics* 53(2): 644–652.

Rényi, A. (1959). On Measures of Dependence. *Acta Mathematica Hungarica* 10(3–4): 441–451.

Reshef, D. N., Reshef, Y. A., Finucane, H. K., Grossman, S. R., McVean, G., Turnbaugh, P. J., Lander, E. S., Mitzenmacher, M., and Sabeti, P. C. (2011). Detecting Novel Associations in Large Data Sets. *Science* 334(6062): 1518–1524.

Rezaei, S., Tahmasbi, R., and Mahmoodi, M. (2010). Estimation of P [Y < X] for Generalized Pareto Distribution. *Journal of Statistical Planning and Inference* 140(2): 480–494.

Richards, R. J., Hammitt, J. K., and Tsevat, J. (1996). Finding the Optimal Multiple-Test Strategy Using a Method Analogous to Logistic Regression: The Diagnosis of Hepatolenticular Degeneration (Wilson's Disease). *Medical Decision Making* 16(4): 367–375.

Richardson, D. B., and Ciampi, A. (2003). Effects of Exposure Measurement Error When an Exposure Variable Is Constrained by a Lower Limit. *American Journal of Epidemiology* 157(4): 355–363.

Riesz, F. (1930). Sur Une Inegalite Integarale. *Journal of the London Mathematical Society* 1(3): 162–168.

Riffenburgh, R. H. (2012). *Statistics in Medicine*, Third Edition. *Graefe's Archive for Clinical and Experimental Ophthalmology* 251(6): 1661–1662.

Robinson, P. M. (1991). Consistent Nonparametric Entropy-Based Testing. *Review of Economic Studies* 58(3): 437–453.

Rosenbaum, P. R. (2005). An Exact Distribution-Free Test Comparing Two Multivariate Distributions Based on Adjacency. *Journal of the Royal Statistical Society: Series B (Statistical Methodology)* 67(4): 515–530.

Rosenbaum, P. R., and Rubin, D. B. (1984). Sensitivity of Bayes Inference with Data-Dependent Stopping Rules. *American Statistician* 38(2): 106–109.

Rothman, K. J., Greenland, S., and Lash, T. L. (2008). *Modern Epidemiology*. Lippincott Williams & Wilkins, Philadelphia.

Rousseeuw, P. J. (1984). Least Median of Squares Regression. *Journal of the American Statistical Association* 79(388): 871–880.

Rousseeuw, P. J., and Leroy, A. M. (2005). *Robust Regression and Outlier Detection*. John Wiley & Sons, Hoboken, NJ.

Royston, J. (1982). An Extension of Shapiro and Wilk's W Test for Normality to Large Samples. *Applied Statistics* 31: 115–124.

Rubin, D. B., and Schenker, N. (1986). Multiple Imputation for Interval Estimation from Simple Random Samples with Ignorable Nonresponse. *Journal of the American Statistical Association* 81(394): 366–374.

Rubinstein, R. Y., and Kroese, D. P. (2011). *Simulation and the Monte Carlo Method.* John Wiley & Sons, Hoboken, NJ.

Rukhin, A. L., and Osmoukhina, A. (2005). Nonparametric Measures of Dependence for Biometric Data Studies. *Journal of Statistical Planning and Inference* 131(1): 1–18.

Sackrowitz, H., and Samuel-Cahn, E. (1994). Rationality and Unbiasedness in Hypothesis Testing. *Journal of the American Statistical Association* 89(427): 967–971.

Sackrowitz, H., and Samuel-Cahn, E. (1999). P Values as Random Variables—Expected P Values. *American Statistician* 53(4): 326–331.

Sacks, H. S., Chalmers, T. C., Blum, A. L., Berrier, J., and Pagano, D. (1990). Endoscopic Hemostasis: An Effective Therapy for Bleeding Peptic Ulcers. *JAMA* 264(4): 494–499.

Sarkadi, K. (1975). The Consistency of the Shapiro–Francia Test. *Biometrika* 62(2): 445–450.

SAS Institute (2015) *SAS® 9.4 Macro Language: Reference*, Fourth Edition. SAS Institute Inc., Cary, NC.

Sawitzki, G. (1994). Diagnostic Plots for One-Dimensional Data. Computational Statistics. In *Papers Collected on the Occasion of the 25th Conference on Statistical Computing at Schloss Reisensburg* 237–258. Physica-Verlag, Heidelberg.

Scaillet, O. (2005). A Kolmogorov-Smirnov Type Test for Positive Quadrant Dependence. *Canadian Journal of Statistics* 33(3): 415–427.

Scannapieco, F. A., Yu, J., Raghavendran, K., Vacanti, A., Owens, S. I., Wood, K., and Mylotte, J. M. (2009). A Randomized Trial of Chlorhexidine Gluconate on Oral Bacterial Pathogens in Mechanically Ventilated Patients. *Critical Care* 13(4): R117.

Scharfstein, D. O., Tsiatis, A. A., and Robins, J. M. (1997). Semiparametric Efficiency and Its Implication on the Design and Analysis of Group-Sequential Studies. *Journal of the American Statistical Association* 92(440): 1342–1350.

Schatzoff, M. (1966). Sensitivity Comparisons among Tests of the General Linear Hypothesis. *Journal of the American Statistical Association* 61(314): 415–435.

Schechtman, E., and Wolfe, D. A. (1988). Distribution-Free Tests for the Changepoint Problem. *American Journal of Mathematical and Management Sciences* 8(1–2): 93–119.

Schervish, M. J. (1996). P Values: What They Are and What They Are Not. *American Statistician* 50(3): 203–206.

Schisterman, E. (1999). *Lipid Peroxidation and Cardiovascular Disease: An ROC Approach.* Doctoral dissertation, State University of New York at Buffalo.

Schisterman, E. F., Faraggi, D., Browne, R., Freudenheim, J., Dorn, J., Muti, P., Armstrong, D., Reiser, B., and Trevisan, M. (2001). Tbars and Cardiovascular Disease in a Population-Based Sample. *Journal of Cardiovascular Risk* 8(4): 219–225.

Schisterman, E. F., and Little, R. J. (2010). Opening the Black Box of Biomarker Measurement Error. *Epidemiology (Cambridge, Mass.)* 21(Suppl. 4): S1–S3.

Schisterman, E. F., and Vexler, A. (2008). To Pool or Not to Pool, from Whether to When: Applications of Pooling to Biospecimens Subject to a Limit of Detection. *Paediatric and Perinatal Epidemiology* 22(5): 486–496.

Schisterman, E. F., Vexler, A., Mumford, S. L., and Perkins, N. J. (2010). Hybrid Pooled–Unpooled Design for Cost-Efficient Measurement of Biomarkers. *Statistics in Medicine* 29(5): 597–613.

Schisterman, E. F., Vexler, A., Whitcomb, B. W., and Liu, A. (2006). The Limitations Due to Exposure Detection Limits for Regression Models. *American Journal of Epidemiology* 163(4): 374–383.

Schisterman, E. F., Vexler, A., Ye, A., and Perkins, N. J. (2011). A Combined Efficient Design for Biomarker Data Subject to a Limit of Detection Due to Measuring Instrument Sensitivity. *Annals of Applied Statistics* 5(4): 2651–2667.

Schmid, C. H., and Rosner, B. (1993). A Bayesian Approach to Logistic Regression Models Having Measurement Error Following a Mixture Distribution. *Statistics in Medicine* 12(12): 1141–1153.

Schmid, F., and Schmidt, R. (2007). Multivariate Extensions of Spearman's Rho and Related Statistics. *Statistics and Probability Letters* 77(4): 407–416.

Schmitz, N., Duscha, G., Lübbert, J., and Meyerthole, T. (1993). *Optimal Sequentially Planned Decision Procedures*. Springer-Verlag, New York.

Scholz, F. W., and Stephens, M. A. (1987). K-Sample Anderson–Darling Tests. *Journal of the American Statistical Association* 82(399): 918–924.

Schriever, B. F. (1987). An Ordering for Positive Dependence. *Annals of Statistics* 15(3): 1208–1214.

Schuster, E. F. (1975). Estimating the Distribution Function of a Symmetric Distribution. *Biometrika* 62(3): 631–635.

Schwarz, G. (1978). Estimating the Dimension of a Model. *Annals of Statistics* 6(2): 461–464.

Schweder, T., and Hjort, N. L. (2002). Confidence and Likelihood*. *Scandinavian Journal of Statistics* 29(2): 309–332.

Schweizer, B., and Wolff, E. F. (1981). On Nonparametric Measures of Dependence for Random Variables. *Annals of Statistics* 9(4): 879–885.

Searle, S. R., Casella, G., and McCulloch, C. (1992). *Variance Components*. Wiley, New York.

Sellke, T., Bayarri, M., and Berger, J. O. (2001). Calibration of P Values for Testing Precise Null Hypotheses. *American Statistician* 55(1): 62–71.

Sen, A., and Srivastava, M. S. (1975). On Tests for Detecting Change in Mean. *Annals of Statistics* 3(1): 98–108.

Sen, P. K. (1967). A Note on Asymptotically Distribution-Free Confidence Bounds for P {X < Y}, Based on Two Independent Samples. *Sankhyā: The Indian Journal of Statistics: Series A* 29(1): 95–102.

Sen, P. K. (1978). Invariance Principles for Linear Rank Statistics Revisited. *Sankhyā: The Indian Journal of Statistics: Series A* 40(3): 215–236.

Senn, S., and Bretz, F. (2007). Power and Sample Size When Multiple Endpoints Are Considered. *Pharmaceutical Statistics* 6(3): 161–170.

Serfling, R. J. (1980). *Approximation Theorems of Mathematical Statistics*. John Wiley & Sons, Mississauga, ON.

Serfling, R. J. (2009). *Approximation Theorems of Mathematical Statistics*. John Wiley & Sons, Mississauga, ON.

Seshan, V. E., Gönen, M., and Begg, C. B. (2013). Comparing ROC Curves Derived from Regression Models. *Statistics in Medicine* 32(9): 1483–1493.

Severini, T. (2010). Likelihood Ratio Statistics Based on an Integrated Likelihood. *Biometrika* 97(2): 481–496.

Shao, J., and Tu, D. (1995). *The Jackknife and Bootstrap*. Springer Science & Business Media, New York.

Shapiro, D. E. (1999). The Interpretation of Diagnostic Tests. *Statistical Methods in Medical Research* 8(2): 113–134.

Shapiro, S. S., and Francia, R. (1972). An Approximate Analysis of Variance Test for Normality. *Journal of the American Statistical Association* 67(337): 215–216.

Shapiro, S. S., and Wilk, M. B. (1965). An Analysis of Variance Test for Normality (Complete Samples). *Biometrika* 52(3/4): 591–611.

Sheather, S. J., and Marron, J. S. (1990). Kernel Quantile Estimators. *Journal of the American Statistical Association* 85(410): 410–416.

Shirahata, S. (1978). An Approach to a One-Sided Test in the Bivariate Normal Distribution. *Biometrika* 65(1): 61–67.

Shorack, G. R., and Wellner, J. A. (2009). *Empirical Processes with Applications to Statistics*. Society for Industrial and Applied Mathematics, Philadelphia.

Si, Y., and Liu, P. (2013). An Optimal Test with Maximum Average Power While Controlling FDR with Application to RNA-Seq Data. *Biometrics* 69(3): 594–605.

Siegmund, D. (1968). On the Asymptotic Normality of One-Sided Stopping Rules. *Annals of Mathematical Statistics* 39(5): 1493–1497.

Siegmund, D. (1985). *Sequential Analysis: Tests and Confidence Intervals*. Springer Science & Business Media, New York.

Siegmund, D. (1986). Boundary Crossing Probabilities and Statistical Applications. *Annals of Statistics* 14(2): 361–404.

Siegmund, D. (1988). Approximate Tail Probabilities for the Maxima of Some Random Fields. *Annals of Probability* 16(2): 487–501.

Silvapulle, M. J. (1997). A Curious Example Involving the Likelihood Ratio Test against One-Sided Hypotheses. *American Statistician* 51(2): 178–180.

Silverman, B. W. (1986). *Density Estimation for Statistics and Data Analysis*. CRC Press, London.

Simon, N., and Tibshirani, R. (2014). Comment on "Detecting Novel Associations in Large Data Sets" by Reshef et al, *Science* Dec 16, 2011. *arXiv* preprint: 1401.7645.

Simon, R. (1989). Optimal Two-Stage Designs for Phase II Clinical Trials. *Controlled Clinical Trials* 10(1): 1–10.

Simonoff, J. S. (1996). *Smoothing Methods in Statistics*. Springer Science & Business Media, New York.

Singh, K., Xie, M., and Strawderman, W. E. (2005). Combining Information from Independent Sources through Confidence Distributions. *Annals of Statistics* 33(1): 159–183.

Sinharay, S., and Stern, H. (2001). *Bayes Factors for Variance Component Testing in Generalized Linear Mixed Models*. Iowa State University, Ames.

Sinharay, S., and Stern, H. S. (2002). On the Sensitivity of Bayes Factors to the Prior Distributions. *American Statistician* 56(3): 196–201.

Sinnott, E. W. (1937). The Relation of Gene to Character in Quantitative Inheritance. *Proceedings of the National Academy of Sciences of the United States of America* 23(4): 224.

Sklar, R., and Strauss, B. (1980). Role of the uvrE Gene Product and of Inducible O6-Methylguanine Removal in the Induction of Mutations by N-Methyl-N'-Nitro-N-Nitrosoguanidine in *Escherichia coli*. *Journal of Molecular Biology* 143(4): 343–362.

Smirnov, N. V. (1939a). Estimate of Deviation between Empirical Distribution Functions in Two Independent Samples. *Bulletin Moscow University* 2(2): 3–16.

Smirnov, N. V. (1939b). On the Estimation of the Discrepancy between Empirical Curves of Distribution for Two Independent Samples. *Bull. Math. Univ. Moscou* 2(2).

Smith, A. F., and Roberts, G. O. (1993). Bayesian Computation via the Gibbs Sampler and Related Markov Chain Monte Carlo Methods. *Journal of the Royal Statistical Society: Series B (Methodological)* 55(1): 3–23.

Smith, J. B., and Batchelder, W. H. (2008). Assessing Individual Differences in Categorical Data. *Psychonomic Bulletin and Review* 15(4): 713–731.

Smith, R. L. (1989). Extreme Value Analysis of Environmental Time Series: An Application to Trend Detection in Ground-Level Ozone. *Statistical Science* 4(4): 367–377.

Snapinn, S., Chen, M. G., Jiang, Q., and Koutsoukos, T. (2006). Assessment of Futility in Clinical Trials. *Pharmaceutical Statistics* 5(4): 273–281.

Snedecor, G. (1946). *Statistical Methods*. Iowa State University Press, Ames.

Snedecor, G. W., and Cochran, G. C. (1967). *Statistical Methods*. Iowa State University Press, Ames.

Song, H. H. (1997). Analysis of Correlated ROC Areas in Diagnostic Testing. *Biometrics* 53(1): 370–382.

Song, W. (2011). Empirical Likelihood Confidence Intervals for Density Function in Errors-in-Variables Model. *Journal of Statistical Research* 45(2): 95.

Spearman, C. (1904). The Proof and Measurement of Association between Two Things. *American Journal of Psychology* 15(1): 72–101.

Spezzaferri, F., Verdinelli, I., and Zeppieri, M. (2007). Bayes Factors for Goodness of Fit Testing. *Journal of Statistical Planning and Inference* 137(1): 43–56.

Spiegelhalter, D. (1977). A Test for Normality against Symmetric Alternatives. *Biometrika* 64(2): 415–418.

Spokoiny, V. G. (1998). Estimation of a Function with Discontinuities via Local Polynomial Fit with an Adaptive Window Choice. *Annals of Statistics* 26(4): 1356–1378.

Staudenmayer, J., and Spiegelman, D. (2002). Segmented Regression in the Presence of Covariate Measurement Error in Main Study/Validation Study Designs. *Biometrics* 58(4): 871–877.

Stein, C. (1956). Inadmissibility of the Usual Estimator for the Mean of a Multivariate Normal Distribution. *Proceedings of the Third Berkeley Symposium on Mathematical Statistics and Probability* 1: 197–206.

Stephens, M. A. (1974). EDF Statistics for Goodness of Fit and Some Comparisons. *Journal of the American Statistical Association* 69(347): 730–737.

Stigler, S. M. (1977). Do Robust Estimators Work with Real Data? *Annals of Statistics* 5(6): 1055–1098.

Strassburger, K., and Bretz, F. (2008). Compatible Simultaneous Lower Confidence Bounds for the Holm Procedure and Other Bonferroni-Based Closed Tests. *Statistics in Medicine* 27(24): 4914–4927.

Su, J. Q., and Liu, J. S. (1993). Linear Combinations of Multiple Diagnostic Markers. *Journal of the American Statistical Association* 88(424): 1350–1355.

Suchard, M. A., Weiss, R. E., and Sinsheimer, J. S. (2005). Models for Estimating Bayes Factors with Applications to Phylogeny and Tests of Monophyly. *Biometrics* 61(3): 665–673.

Sutton, C. D. (1993). Computer-Intensive Methods for Tests about the Mean of an Asymmetrical Distribution. *Journal of the American Statistical Association* 88(423): 802–810.

Swartz, T. B., Haitovsky, Y., Vexler, A., and Yang, T. Y. (2004). Bayesian Identifiability and Misclassification in Multinomial Data. *Canadian Journal of Statistics* 32(3): 285–302.

Sweeting, T. J. (1995). A Framework for Bayesian and Likelihood Approximations in Statistics. *Biometrika* 82(1): 1–23.

Székely, G. J., and Rizzo, M. L. (2005). A New Test for Multivariate Normality. *Journal of Multivariate Analysis* 93(1): 58–80.

Székely, G. J., and Rizzo, M. L. (2009). Brownian Distance Covariance. *Annals of Applied Statistics* 3(4): 1236–1265.

Tabesh, H., Ayatollahi, S. M. T., and Towhidi, M. (2010). A Simple Powerful Bivariate Test for Two Sample Location Problems in Experimental and Observational Studies. *Theoretical Biology and Medical Modelling* 7(1): 13–13.

Tan, M., Fang, H. B., Tian, G. L., and Houghton, P. J. (2002). Small-Sample Inference for Incomplete Longitudinal Data with Truncation and Censoring in Tumor Xenograft Models. *Biometrics* 58(3): 612–620.

Tang, D.-I. (1994). Uniformly More Powerful Tests in a One-Sided Multivariate Problem. *Journal of the American Statistical Association* 89(427): 1006–1011.

Tang, L., Emerson, S. S., and Zhou, X. H. (2008). Nonparametric and Semiparametric Group Sequential Methods for Comparing Accuracy of Diagnostic Tests. *Biometrics* 64(4): 1137–1145.

Tanizaki, H. (2004). Power Comparison of Empirical Likelihood Ratio Tests: Small Sample Properties through Monte Carlo Studies. *Kobe University Economic Review* 50: 13.

Taplin, R. H. (2005). A Robust Bayes Factor for Linear Models. *Australian and New Zealand Journal of Statistics* 47(4): 449–462.

Tartakovsky, A. G., Polunchenko, A. S., and Moustakides, G. V. (2009). Design and Comparison of Shiryaev–Roberts and Cusum-Type Change-Point Detection Procedures. Presented at Proceedings of the 2nd International Workshop in Sequential Methodologies, Troyes, France.

Taskinen, S., Oja, H., and Randles, R. H. (2005). Multivariate Nonparametric Tests of Independence. *Journal of the American Statistical Association* 100(471): 916–925.

Taylor, J. R., and Thompson, W. (1998). An Introduction to Error Analysis: The Study of Uncertainties in Physical Measurements. *Measurement Science and Technology* 9(6): 1015.

Terry, M. E. (1952). Some Rank Order Tests Which Are Most Powerful against Specific Parametric Alternatives. *Annals of Mathematical Statistics* 23(3): 346–366.

Thall, P. F., Logothetis, C., Pagliaro, L. C., Wen, S., Brown, M. A., Williams, D., and Millikan, R. E. (2007). Adaptive Therapy for Androgen-Independent Prostate Cancer: A Randomized Selection Trial of Four Regimens. *Journal of the National Cancer Institute* 99(21): 1613–1622.

Thomas, D. R., and Grunkemeier, G. L. (1975). Confidence Interval Estimation of Survival Probabilities for Censored Data. *Journal of the American Statistical Association* 70(352): 865–871.

Thompson, M. L. (2003). Assessing the Diagnostic Accuracy of a Sequence of Tests. *Biostatistics* 4(3): 341–351.

Tian, L., Li, X., and Yan, L. (2012). Testing Equality of Generalized Treatment Effects. *Journal of Biopharmaceutical Statistics* 22(3): 582–595.

Tian, L., Vexler, A., Yan, L., and Schisterman, E. F. (2009). Confidence Interval Estimation of the Difference between Paired AUCs Based on Combined Biomarkers. *Journal of Statistical Planning and Inference* 139(10): 3725–3732.

Tierney, L., and Kadane, J. B. (1986). Accurate Approximations for Posterior Moments and Marginal Densities. *Journal of the American Statistical Association* 81(393): 82–86.

Tierney, L., Kass, R. E., and Kadane, J. B. (1989). Fully Exponential Laplace Approximations to Expectations and Variances of Nonpositive Functions. *Journal of the American Statistical Association* 84(407): 710–716.

Todd, S. (2007). A 25-Year Review of Sequential Methodology in Clinical Studies. *Statistics in Medicine* 26(2): 237–252.

Tsai, W., Gurevich, G., and Vexler, A. (2013). Optimal Properties of Parametric Shiryaev-Roberts Statistical Control Procedures. *Operation Research* 17(1): 37–50.

Tsiatis, A. A., and Mehta, C. (2003). On the Inefficiency of the Adaptive Design for Monitoring Clinical Trials. *Biometrika* 90(2): 367–378.

Tsiatis, A. A., Rosner, G. L., and Mehta, C. R. (1984). Exact Confidence Intervals Following a Group Sequential Test. *Biometrics* 40(3): 797–803.

Tucker, H. G. (1959). A Generalization of the Glivenko-Cantelli Theorem. *Annals of Mathematical Statistics* 30(3): 828–830.

Tukey, J. W. (1962). The Future of Data Analysis. *Annals of Mathematical Statistics* 33(1): 1–67.

Tukey, J. W. (1977). *Exploratory Data Analysis*. Addison-Wesley, Reading, MA.

Tukey, J. W. (1986). Sunset Salvo. *American Statistician* 40(1): 72–76.

Tukey, J. W., and Wilk, M. (1966). Data Analysis and Statistics: An Expository Overview. In *Proceedings of the ACM Joint Computer Conference*, November 7–10.

Turnbull, B. W., Brown Jr., B. W., and Hu, M. (1974). Survivorship Analysis of Heart Transplant Data. *Journal of the American Statistical Association* 69(345): 74–80.

Tusnady, G. (1977). On Asymptotically Optimal Tests. *Annals of Statistics* 5(2): 385–393.

Ulm, K. (1991). A Statistical Method for Assessing a Threshold in Epidemiological Studies. *Statistics in Medicine* 10(3): 341–349.

U.S. Department of Health, Education, and Welfare. (1964). *Smoking and Health: Report of the Advisory Committee to the Surgeon General of Public Health Service*. Public Health Service Publications No. 1103. U.S. Department of Health, Education, and Welfare, Washington, DC.

Vaillancourt, C., Shrier, I., Vandal, A., Falk, M., Rossignol, M., Vernec, A., and Somogyi, D. (2004). Acute Compartment Syndrome: How Long before Muscle Necrosis Occurs? *Canadian Journal of Emergency Medicine* 6(3): 147.

Vandal, A. C., Gentleman, R., and Liu, X. (2005). Constrained Estimation and Likelihood Intervals for Censored Data. *Canadian Journal of Statistics* 33(1): 71–83.

van der Laan, M. J., and Pollard, K. S. (2003). A New Algorithm for Hybrid Hierarchical Clustering with Visualization and the Bootstrap. *Journal of Statistical Planning and Inference* 117(2): 275–303.

Van Der Tweel, I., and Van Noord, P. A. (2003). Early Stopping in Clinical Trials and Epidemiologic Studies for "Futility": Conditional Power versus Sequential Analysis. *Journal of Clinical Epidemiology* 56(7): 610–617.

Van Dijk, H. K. (1984). *Posterior Analysis of Econometric Models Using Monte Carlo Integration*. Reproduktie Wondestein, Erasmus University, Rotterdam.

Van Dijk, H. K., Hop, J. P., and Louter, A. S. (1987). An Algorithm for the Computation of Posterior Moments and Densities Using Simple Importance Sampling. *The Statistician* 36(2/3): 83–90.

Van Elteren, P. (1960). On the Combination of Independent Two Sample Tests of Wilcoxon. *Bulletin of International Statistical Institute* 37: 351–361.

Vardi, Y. (1982). Nonparametric Estimation in the Presence of Length Bias. *Annals of Statistics* 10(2): 616–620.

Vasicek, O. (1976). A Test for Normality Based on Sample Entropy. *Journal of the Royal Statistical Society: Series B (Methodological)* 38(1): 54–59.

Venkatraman, E. (2000). A Permutation Test to Compare Receiver Operating Characteristic Curves. *Biometrics* 56(4): 1134–1138.

Venkatraman, E., and Begg, C. B. (1996). A Distribution-Free Procedure for Comparing Receiver Operating Characteristic Curves from a Paired Experiment. *Biometrika* 83(4): 835–848.

Verbeke, G., and Molenberghs, G. (2003). The Use of Score Tests for Inference on Variance Components. *Biometrics* 59(2): 254–262.

Verdonck, A., De Ridder, L., Verbeke, G., Bourguignon, J., Carels, C., Kühn, E., Darras, V., and de Zegher, F. (1998). Comparative Effects of Neonatal and Prepubertal Castration on Craniofacial Growth in Rats. *Archives of Oral Biology* 43(11): 861–871.

Verrill, S., and Johnson, R. A. (1987). The Asymptotic Equivalence of Some Modified Shapiro-Wilk Statistics—Complete and Censored Sample Cases. *Annals of Statistics* 15(1): 413–419.

Verrill, S., and Johnson, R. A. (1988). Tables and Large-Sample Distribution Theory for Censored-Data Correlation Statistics for Testing Normality. *Journal of the American Statistical Association* 83(404): 1192–1197.

Versluis, C. (1996). Comparison of Tests for Bivariate Normality with Unknown Parameters by Transformation to an Univariate Statistic. *Communications in Statistics—Theory and Methods* 25(3): 647–665.

Vexler, A. (2006). Guaranteed Testing for Epidemic Changes of a Linear Regression Model. *Journal of Statistical Planning and Inference* 136(9): 3101–3120.

Vexler, A. (2008). Martingale Type Statistics Applied to Change Points Detection. *Communications in Statistics—Theory and Methods* 37(8): 1207–1224.

Vexler, A., Chen, X., and Hutson, A. (2015a). Dependence and Independence: Structure and Inference. *Statistical Methods in Medical Research*. DOI: 10.1177/0962280215594198.

Vexler, A., Chen, X., and Yu, J. (2014a). Evaluations and Comparisons of Treatment Effects Based on Best Combinations of Biomarkers with Applications to Biomedical Studies. *Journal of Computational Biology* 21(9): 709–721.

Vexler, A., Deng, W., and Wilding, G. E. (2013a). Nonparametric Bayes Factors Based on Empirical Likelihood Ratios. *Journal of Statistical Planning and Inference* 143(3): 611–620.

Vexler, A., and Gurevich, G. (2009). Average Most Powerful Tests for a Segmented Regression. *Communications in Statistics—Theory and Methods* 38(13): 2214–2231.

Vexler, A., and Gurevich, G. (2010a). Density-Based Empirical Likelihood Ratio Change Point Detection Policies. *Communications in Statistics—Simulation and Computation* 39(9): 1709–1725.

Vexler, A., and Gurevich, G. (2010b). Empirical Likelihood Ratios Applied to Goodness-of-Fit Tests Based on Sample Entropy. *Computational Statistics and Data Analysis* 54(2): 531–545.

Vexler, A., and Gurevich, G. (2011). A Note on Optimality of Hypothesis Testing. *Journal MESA* 2(3): 243–250.

Vexler, A., Gurevich, G., and Hutson, A. D. (2013b). An Exact Density-Based Empirical Likelihood Ratio Test for Paired Data. *Journal of Statistical Planning and Inference* 143(2): 334–345.

Vexler, A., Hutson A. D., and Yu, J. (2014f) Empirical Likelihood Methods in Clinical Experiments. *Methods and Applications of Statistics in Clinical Trials*, Vol. 2. Encyclopedia of Clinical Trials, N. Balakrishnan. John Wiley & Sons, Newark, NJ.

Vexler, A., Kim, Y. M., Yu, J., Lazar, N. A., and Hutson, A. D. (2014b). Computing Critical Values of Exact Tests by Incorporating Monte Carlo Simulations Combined with Statistical Tables. *Scandinavian Journal of Statistics* 41(4): 1013–1030.

Vexler, A., Liu, A., Eliseeva, E., and Schisterman, E. F. (2008a). Maximum Likelihood Ratio Tests for Comparing the Discriminatory Ability of Biomarkers Subject to Limit of Detection. *Biometrics* 64(3): 895–903.

Vexler, A., Liu, A., and Schisterman, E. (2010a). Nonparametric Deconvolution of Density Estimation Based on Observed Sums. *Journal of Nonparametric Statistics* 22(1): 23–39.

Vexler, A., Liu, A., and Schisterman, E. F. (2006a). Efficient Design and Analysis of Biospecimens with Measurements Subject to Detection Limit. *Biometrical Journal* 48(5): 780–791.

Vexler, A., Liu, A., Schisterman, E. F., and Wu, C. (2006b). Note on Distribution-Free Estimation of Maximum Linear Separation of Two Multivariate Distributions. *Nonparametric Statistics* 18(2): 145–158.

Vexler, A., Liu, S., Kang, L., and Hutson, A. D. (2009a). Modifications of the Empirical Likelihood Interval Estimation with Improved Coverage Probabilities. *Communications in Statistics—Simulation and Computation* 38(10): 2171–2183.

Vexler, A., Liu, S., and Schisterman, E. F. (2011a). Nonparametric-Likelihood Inference Based on Cost-Effectively-Sampled-Data. *Journal of Applied Statistics* 38(4): 769–783.

Vexler, A., Schisterman, E. F., and Liu, A. (2008b). Estimation of ROC Curves Based on Stably Distributed Biomarkers Subject to Measurement Error and Pooling Mixtures. *Statistics in Medicine* 27(2): 280–296.

Vexler, A., Shan, G., Kim, S., Tsai, W.-M., Tian, L., and Hutson, A. D. (2011b). An Empirical Likelihood Ratio Based Goodness-of-Fit Test for Inverse Gaussian Distributions. *Journal of Statistical Planning and Inference* 141(6): 2128–2140.

Vexler, A., Tanajian, H., and Hutson, A. D. (2014c). Density-Based Empirical Likelihood Procedures for Testing Symmetry of Data Distributions and K-Sample Comparisons. *STATA Journal* 4(2): 304–328.

Vexler, A., Tao, G., and Chen, X. (2015b). A Toolkit for Clinical Statisticians to Fix Problems Based on Biomarker Measurements Subject to Instrumental Limitations: From Repeated Measurement Techniques to a Hybrid Pooled–Unpooled Design. In *Advanced Protocols in Oxidative Stress III*, ed. D. Armstrong, 439–460. Springer, Berlin.

Vexler, A., Tao, G., and Hutson, A. (2014d). Posterior Expectation Based on Empirical Likelihoods. *Biometrika* 101(3): 711–718.

Vexler, A., and Tarima, S. (2011). An Optimal Approach for Hypothesis Testing in the Presence of Incomplete Data. *Annals of the Institute of Statistical Mathematics* 63(6): 1141–1163.

Vexler, A., Tsai, W.-M., and Hutson, A. D. (2014e). A Simple Density-Based Empirical Likelihood Ratio Test for Independence. *American Statistician* 68(3): 158–169.

Vexler, A., Tsai, W. M., Gurevich, G., and Yu, J. (2012a). Two-Sample Density-Based Empirical Likelihood Ratio Tests Based on Paired Data, with Application to a Treatment Study of Attention-Deficit/Hyperactivity Disorder and Severe Mood Dysregulation. *Statistics in Medicine* 31(17): 1821–1837.

Vexler, A., Tsai, W. M., and Malinovsky, Y. (2012b). Estimation and Testing Based on Data Subject to Measurement Errors: From Parametric to Non-Parametric Likelihood Methods. *Statistics in Medicine* 31(22): 2498–2512.

Vexler, A., and Wu, C. (2009). An Optimal Retrospective Change Point Detection Policy. *Scandinavian Journal of Statistics* 36(3): 542–558.

Vexler, A., Wu, C., Liu, A., Whitcomb, B. W., and Schisterman, E. F. (2009b). An Extension of a Change-Point Problem. *Statistics* 43(3): 213–225.

Vexler, A., Wu, C., and Yu, K. F. (2010b). Optimal Hypothesis Testing: From Semi to Fully Bayes Factors. *Metrika* 71(2): 125–138.

Vexler, A., and Yu, J. (2011). Two-Sample Density-Based Empirical Likelihood Tests for Incomplete Data in Application to a Pneumonia Study. *Biometrical Journal* 53(4): 628–651.

Vexler, A., Yu, J., and Hutson, A. D. (2011c). Likelihood Testing Populations Modeled by Autoregressive Process Subject to the Limit of Detection in Applications to Longitudinal Biomedical Data. *Journal of Applied Statistics* 38(7): 1333–1346.

Vexler, A., Yu, J., Tian, L., and Liu, S. (2010c). Two-Sample Nonparametric Likelihood Inference Based on Incomplete Data with an Application to a Pneumonia Study. *Biometrical Journal* 52(3): 348–361.

Vexler A., Zou L., and Hutson, A. (2016). Data-Driven Confidence Interval Estimation Incorporating Prior Information with an Adjustment for Skewed Data. *The American Statistician*. Accepted.

Volodin, I. N., and Novikov, A. A. (1998). Local Asymptotic Efficiency of a Sequential Probability Ratio Test for D-Guarantee Discrimination of Composite Hypotheses. *Teoriya Veroyatnostei i ee Primeneniya* 43(2): 209–225.

Vostrikova, L. (1981). Detection of the Disorder in Multidimensional Random-Processes. *Doklady Akademii Nauk SSSR* 259(2): 270–274.

Wainer, H. (1990). Graphical Visions from William Playfair to John Tukey. *Statistical Science* 5(3): 340–346.

Wald, A. (1947). *Sequential Analysis*. Wiley, New York.

Wald, A., and Wolfowitz, J. (1948). Optimum Character of the Sequential Probability Ratio Test. *Annals of Mathematical Statistics* 19(3): 326–339.

Wallis, W. A. (1942). Compounding Probabilities from Independent Significance Tests. *Econometrica: Journal of the Econometric Society* 10(3/4): 229–248.

Walter, S. (2005). The Partial Area under the Summary ROC Curve. *Statistics in Medicine* 24(13): 2025–2040.

Wand, M. P., and Jones, M. C. (1994). *Kernel Smoothing*. CRC Press, London.

Wang, H.-H., Wu, Y., Fu, Y., and Wang, X. (2012). Data Fusion Using Empirical Likelihood. *Open Journal of Statistics* 2(05): 547.

Wang, J. (2006). Quadratic Artificial Likelihood Functions Using Estimating Functions. *Scandinavian Journal of Statistics* 33(2): 379–390.

Wang, M. C., and Li, S. (2012). Bivariate Marker Measurements and ROC Analysis. *Biometrics* 68(4): 1207–1218.

Wang, Q., and Rao, J. (2002a). Empirical Likelihood-Based Inference under Imputation for Missing Response Data. *Annals of Statistics* 30(3): 896–924.

Wang, Q., and Rao, J. N. (2002b). Empirical Likelihood-Based Inference in Linear Errors-in-Covariables Models with Validation Data. *Biometrika* 89(2): 345–358.

Wang, S., Qian, L., and Carroll, R. J. (2010). Generalized Empirical Likelihood Methods for Analyzing Longitudinal Data. *Biometrika* 97(1): 79–93.

Wang, S. K., and Tsiatis, A. A. (1987). Approximately Optimal One-Parameter Boundaries for Group Sequential Trials. *Biometrics* 43(1): 193–199.

Wang, Y., and McDermott, M. P. (1998). Conditional Likelihood Ratio Test for a Nonnegative Normal Mean Vector. *Journal of the American Statistical Association* 93(441): 380–386.

Wason, J., and Seaman, S. R. (2013). Using Continuous Data on Tumour Measurements to Improve Inference in Phase II Cancer Studies. *Statistics in Medicine* 32(26): 4639–4650.

Wedderburn, R. W. (1974). Quasi-Likelihood Functions, Generalized Linear Models, and the Gauss–Newton Method. *Biometrika* 61(3): 439–447.

Westfall, P. H., Tobias, R. D., and Wolfinger, R. D. (2011). *Multiple Comparisons and Multiple Tests Using SAS*. SAS Institute, Cary, NC.

Wheeler, B. (2009). Suppdists: Supplementary Distributions. R package version 1.1-8. Available at https://cran.r-project.org/web/packages/SuppDists/index.html.

Whitcomb, B. W., Perkins, N. J., Zhang, Z., Ye, A., and Lyles, R. H. (2012). Assessment of Skewed Exposure in Case-Control Studies with Pooling. *Statistics in Medicine* 31(22): 2461–2472.

Whitehead, J. (1986). On the Bias of Maximum Likelihood Estimation Following a Sequential Test. *Biometrika* 73(3): 573–581.

Whitehead, J. (1999). A Unified Theory for Sequential Clinical Trials. *Statistics in Medicine* 18(17–18): 2271–2286.

Whitehead, J., and Jones, D. (1979). The Analysis of Sequential Clinical Trials. *Biometrika* 66(3): 443–452.

Whitehead, J., and Matsushita, T. (2003). Stopping Clinical Trials Because of Treatment Ineffectiveness: A Comparison of a Futility Design with a Method of Stochastic Curtailment. *Statistics in Medicine* 22(5): 677–687.

Wickham, H. (2009). *Ggplot2: Elegant Graphics for Data Analysis*. Springer, New York.

Wieand, S., Gail, M. H., James, B. R., and James, K. L. (1989). A Family of Nonparametric Statistics for Comparing Diagnostic Markers with Paired or Unpaired Data. *Biometrika* 76(3): 585–592.

Wiest, M. C., Thomson, E., Pantoja, J., and Nicolelis, M. A. (2010). Changes in S1 Neural Responses during Tactile Discrimination Learning. *Journal of Neurophysiology* 104(1): 300–312.

Wilcox, R. R. (2001). Detecting Nonlinear Associations, Plus Comments on Testing Hypotheses about the Correlation Coefficient. *Journal of Educational and Behavioral Statistics* 26(1): 73–83.

Wilcox, R. R. (2012). *Introduction to Robust Estimation and Hypothesis Testing*. Academic Press, Boston.

Wilcoxon F. (1945). Individual Comparisons by Ranking Methods. *Biometrics* 1: 80–83.

Wilk, M., and Gnanadesikan, R. (1961). Graphical Analysis of Multi-Response Experimental Data Using Ordered Distances. *Proceedings of the National Academy of Sciences of the United States of America* 47(8): 1209.

Wilk, M., and Gnanadesikan, R. (1964). Graphical Methods for Internal Comparisons in Multiresponse Experiments. *Annals of Mathematical Statistics* 35(2): 613–631.

Wilk, M., Gnanadesikan, R., and Freeny, A. E. (1963a). Estimation of Error Variance from Smallest Ordered Contrasts. *Journal of the American Statistical Association* 58(301): 152–160.

Wilk, M., Gnanadesikan, R., and Huyett, M. J. (1963b). Separate Maximum Likelihood Estimation of Scale or Shape Parameters of the Gamma Distribution Using Order Statistics. *Biometrika* 50(1/2): 217–221.

Wilk, M., Gnanadesikan, R., and Huyett, M. M. (1962a). Probability Plots for the Gamma Distribution. *Technometrics* 4(1): 1–20.

Wilk, M., Gnanadesikan, R., and Lauh, E. (1966). Scale Parameter Estimation from the Order Statistics of Unequal Gamma Components. *Annals of Mathematical Statistics* 37(1): 152–176.

Wilk, M. B., and Gnanadesikan, R. (1968). Probability Plotting Methods for the Analysis of Data. *Biometrika* 55(1): 1–17.

Wilk, M. B., Gnanadesikan, R., and Huyett, M. J. (1962b). Estimation of Parameters of the Gamma Distribution Using Order Statistics. *Biometrika* 49(3/4): 525–545.

Wilk, M. B., and Shapiro, S. (1968). The Joint Assessment of Normality of Several Independent Samples. *Technometrics* 10(4): 825–839.

Wilks, S. S. (1938). The Large-Sample Distribution of the Likelihood Ratio for Testing Composite Hypotheses. *Annals of Mathematical Statistics* 9(1): 60–62.

Williams, E. J., and Williams, E. (1959). *Regression Analysis*. Wiley, New York.

Wolfe, D. A., and Schechtman, E. (1984). Nonparametric Statistical Procedures for the Changepoint Problem. *Journal of Statistical Planning and Inference* 9(3): 389–396.

Wong, W. H. (1983). A Note on the Modified Likelihood for Density Estimation. *Journal of the American Statistical Association* 78(382): 461–463.

Wood, S. N. (2013). A Simple Test for Random Effects in Regression Models. *Biometrika* 100(4): 1005–1010.

Woodworth, G. G. (1966). On the Asymptotic Theory of Tests of Independence Based on Bivariate Layer Ranks. Technical Report 75. Department of Statistics, University of Minnesota.

Wu, C. (2005). Algorithms and R Codes for the Pseudo Empirical Likelihood Method in Survey Sampling. *Survey Methodology* 31(2): 239.

Wu, C., and Zhang, R. (2007). The Asymptotic Distributions of Empirical Likelihood Ratio Statistics in the Presence of Measurement Error. *ACTA Mathematica Scientia* 27(2): 232–242.

Wu, W. B., Woodroofe, M., and Mentz, G. (2001). Isotonic Regression: Another Look at the Changepoint Problem. *Biometrika* 88(3): 793–804.

Wu, X., and Ying, Z. (2011). An Empirical Likelihood Approach to Nonparametric Covariate Adjustment in Randomized Clinical Trials. *arXiv* preprint: 1108.0484.

Xu, W., Hou, Y., Hung, Y., and Zou, Y. (2013). A Comparative Analysis of Spearman's Rho and Kendall's Tau in Normal and Contaminated Normal Models. *Signal Processing* 93(1): 261–276.

Xue, L., and Zhu, L. (2007). Empirical Likelihood Semiparametric Regression Analysis for Longitudinal Data. *Biometrika* 94(4): 921–937.

Yakir, B., Krieger, A. M., and Pollak, M. (1999). Detecting a Change in Regression: First-Order Optimality. *Annals of Statistics* 27(6): 1896–1913.

Yang, D., and Small, D. S. (2013). An R Package and a Study of Methods for Computing Empirical Likelihood. *Journal of Statistical Computation and Simulation* 83(7): 1363–1372.

Yang, S., and Zhao, Y. (2007). Testing Treatment Effect by Combining Weighted Log-Rank Tests and Using Empirical Likelihood. *Statistics and Probability Letters* 77(12): 1385–1393.

Yao, Q. (1989). Large Deviations for Boundary Crossing Probabilities of Some Random Fields. *Journal of Mathematical Research and Exposition* 9: 181–192.

Yao, Q. (1993a). Boundary-Crossing Probabilities of Some Random Fields Related to Likelihood Ratio Tests for Epidemic Alternatives. *Journal of Applied Probability* 30(1): 52–65.

Yao, Q. (1993b). Tests for Change-Points with Epidemic Alternatives. *Biometrika* 80(1): 179–191.

Yi, J., Fang, L., and Su, Z. (2012). Hybridization of Conditional and Predictive Power for Futility Assessment in Sequential Clinical Trials with Time-to-Event Outcomes: A Resampling Approach. *Contemporary Clinical Trials* 33(1): 138–142.

Yoshida, K., and Ogata, N. (1984). 'The Tensile Properties of Yarn Comprising Parallel Filaments', Sen-I Gakkaishi. *Journal of the Society of Fiber Science and Technology* 40(6): 35–42.

You, J., Chen, G., and Zhou, Y. (2006). Block Empirical Likelihood for Longitudinal Partially Linear Regression Models. *Canadian Journal of Statistics* 34(1): 79–96.

Young, G. A. (1994). Bootstrap: More Than a Stab in the Dark? *Statistical Science* 9(3): 382–395.

Yu, B., Zhou, C., and Bandinelli, S. (2011). Combining Multiple Continuous Tests for the Diagnosis of Kidney Impairment in the Absence of a Gold Standard. *Statistics in Medicine* 30(14): 1712–1721.

Yu, J., Vexler, A., Hutson, A. D., and Baumann, H. (2014). Empirical Likelihood Approaches to Two-Group Comparisons of Upper Quantiles Applied to Biomedical Data. *Statistics in Biopharmaceutical Research* 6(1): 30–40.

Yu, J., Vexler, A., Kim, S. E., and Hutson, A. D. (2011). Two-Sample Empirical Likelihood Ratio Tests for Medians in Application to Biomarker Evaluations. *Canadian Journal of Statistics* 39(4): 671–689.

Yu, J., Vexler, A., and Tian, L. (2010). Analyzing Incomplete Data Subject to a Threshold Using Empirical Likelihood Methods: An Application to a Pneumonia Risk Study in an ICU Setting. *Biometrics* 66(1): 123–130.

Yule, G. U. (1919). *An Introduction to the Theory of Statistics*. Griffin, London.

Yule, G. U. (1950). *An Introduction to the Theory of Statistics*, Hafner, New York.

Zaslavsky, B. G. (2013). Bayesian Hypothesis Testing in Two-Arm Trials with Dichotomous Outcomes. *Biometrics* 69(1): 157–163.

Zeileis, A. (2005). A Unified Approach to Structural Change Tests Based on Ml Scores, F Statistics, and OLS Residuals. *Econometric Reviews* 24(4): 445–466.

Zeileis, A. (2006). Implementing a Class of Structural Change Tests: An Econometric Computing Approach. *Computational Statistics and Data Analysis* 50(11): 2987–3008.

Zeileis, A., and Kleiber, C. (2005). Validating Multiple Structural Change Models—A Case Study. *Journal of Applied Econometrics* 20(5): 685–690.

Zeileis, A., Kleiber, C., Krämer, W., and Hornik, K. (2003). Testing and Dating of Structural Changes in Practice. *Computational Statistics and Data Analysis* 44(1): 109–123.

Zeileis, A., Leisch, F., Hornik, K., and Kleiber, C. (2001). Strucchange. An R Package for Testing for Structural Change in Linear Regression Models. *Journal of Statistical Software* 7: 1–38.

Zeileis, A., Shah, A., and Patnaik, I. (2010). Testing, Monitoring, and Dating Structural Changes in Exchange Rate Regimes. *Computational Statistics and Data Analysis* 54(6): 1696–1706.

Zellner, A. (1996). *An Introduction to Bayesian Inference in Econometrics*. Wiley, New York.

Zhang, B. (1997). Empirical Likelihood Confidence Intervals for M-Functionals in the Presence of Auxiliary Information. *Statistics and Probability Letters* 32(1): 87–97.

Zhang, B. (2006). A Semiparametric Hypothesis Testing Procedure for the ROC Curve Area under a Density Ratio Model. *Computational Statistics and Data Analysis* 50(7): 1855–1876.

Zhang, B., and Zhang, Y. (2009). Mann-Whitney U Test and Kruskal-Wallis Test Should Be Used for Comparisons of Differences in Medians, Not Means: Comment on the Article by Van Der Helm-Van Mil et al. *Arthritis and Rheumatism* 60(5): 1565–1565.

Zhang, D., Lin, X., Raz, J., and Sowers, M. (1998). Semiparametric Stochastic Mixed Models for Longitudinal Data. *Journal of the American Statistical Association* 93(442): 710–719.

Zhang, D. D., Zhou, X. H., Freeman, D. H., and Freeman, J. L. (2002). A Non-Parametric Method for the Comparison of Partial Areas under ROC Curves and Its Application to Large Health Care Data Sets. *Statistics in Medicine* 21(5): 701–715.

Zhang, J., and Wu, Y. (2005). Likelihood-Ratio Tests for Normality. *Computational Statistics and Data Analysis* 49(3): 709–721.

Zhang, L., Xu, X., and Chen, G. (2012). The Exact Likelihood Ratio Test for Equality of Two Normal Populations. *American Statistician* 66(3): 180–184.

Zhang, M., Megahed, F. M., and Woodall, W. H. (2014). Exponential Cusum Charts with Estimated Control Limits. *Quality and Reliability Engineering International* 30(2): 275–286.

Zhang, Z. (2008). Quotient Correlation: A Sample Based Alternative to Pearson's Correlation. *Annals of Statistics* 36(2): 1007–1030.

Zhang, Z., and Albert, P. S. (2011). Binary Regression Analysis with Pooled Exposure Measurements: A Regression Calibration Approach. *Biometrics* 67(2): 636–645.

Zhao, Y., Vexler, A., Hutson, A., and Chen, X. (2015). A Statistical Software Procedure for Exact Parametric and Nonparametric Likelihood-Ratio Tests for Two-Sample Comparisons. *Communications in Statistics—Simulation and Computation*. DOI: 10.1080/03610918.2015.1062103.

Zhao, Y., and Wang, H. (2008). Empirical Likelihood Inference for the Regression Model of Mean Quality-Adjusted Lifetime with Censored Data. *Canadian Journal of Statistics* 36(3): 463–478.

Zheng, S., Shi, N.-Z., and Zhang, Z. (2012). Generalized Measures of Correlation for Asymmetry, Nonlinearity, and Beyond. *Journal of the American Statistical Association* 107(499): 1239–1252.

Zhong, B., Chen, J., and Rao, J. N. (2000). Empirical Likelihood Inference in the Presence of Measurement Error. *Canadian Journal of Statistics* 28(4): 841–852.

Zhou, W. (2008). Statistical Inference for P (X < Y). *Statistics in Medicine* 27(2): 257–279.

Zhou, X.-H., and Mcclish, D. K. (2002). *Statistical Methods in Diagnostic Medicine*. Wiley, New York.

Zhou, X.-H., Obuchowski, N. A., and McClish, D. K. (2011). *Statistical Methods in Diagnostic Medicine*. 2nd ed. John Wiley & Sons, Hoboken, NJ.

Zhou, X. H., and Qin, G. (2005). Improved Confidence Intervals for the Sensitivity at a Fixed Level of Specificity of a Continuous-Scale Diagnostic Test. *Statistics in Medicine* 24(3): 465–477.

Zhou, Y., and Liang, H. (2005). Empirical-Likelihood-Based Semiparametric Inference for the Treatment Effect in the Two-Sample Problem with Censoring. *Biometrika* 92(2): 271–282.

Zhu, L.-X., Wong, H. L., and Fang, K.-T. (1995). A Test for Multivariate Normality Based on Sample Entropy and Projection Pursuit. *Journal of Statistical Planning and Inference* 45(3): 373–385.

Zou, C., Liu, Y., Qin, P., and Wang, Z. (2007). Empirical Likelihood Ratio Test for the Change-Point Problem. *Statistics and Probability Letters* 77(4): 374–382.

Zou, C., Zhang, Y., and Wang, Z. (2006). A Control Chart Based on a Change-Point Model for Monitoring Linear Profiles. *IIE Transactions* 38(12): 1093–1103.

Zou, F., and Fine, J. (2002). A Note on a Partial Empirical Likelihood. *Biometrika* 89(4): 958–961.

Zou, F., Fine, J., and Yandell, B. (2002). On Empirical Likelihood for a Semiparametric Mixture Model. *Biometrika* 89(1): 61–75.

Zou, K. H., Hall, W., and Shapiro, D. E. (1997). Smooth Non-Parametric Receiver Operating Characteristic (ROC) Curves for Continuous Diagnostic Tests. *Statistics in Medicine* 16(19): 2143–2156.

Zou, K. H., O'Malley, A. J., and Mauri, L. (2007). Receiver-Operating Characteristic Analysis for Evaluating Diagnostic Tests and Predictive Models. *Circulation* 115(5): 654–657.

Webliographies

1. http://onlinelibrary.wiley.com/doi/10.1002/sim.4467/suppinfo R programs of realization of the two-sample density-based empirical likelihood ratio tests based on paired data.
2. http://cran.r-project.org/web/packages/dbEmpLikeNorm/ The R package "dbEmpLikeNorm": Test for joint assessment of normality.

3. http://cran.r-project.org/web/packages/dbEmpLikeGOF/index.html The R package "dbEmpLikeGOF" for nonparametric density-based likelihood ratio tests for goodness of fit and two-sample comparisons.

4. http://sphhp.buffalo.edu/biostatistics/research-and-facilities/software/stata.html The STATA package entitled "novel and efficient density-based empirical likelihood procedures for symmetry and k-sample comparisons."

5. http://www.sciencedirect.com/science/article/pii/S0167947314002710 The R function for obtaining the empirical likelihood ratio confidence interval estimation of best linear combinations of biomarkers.

Author Index[*]

A

Airola, A., 221
Aitchison, J., 334
Aitkin, M., 174
Akritas, M. G., 133
Albers, W., 14, 15
Albert, A., 220
Albert, P. S., 429, 431, 445, 446, 447
Alfredas, R., 385
Altman, D. G., 12
Aly, E.-E. A. A., 384
Andersen, E. B., 130
Anderson, D. R., 125
Anderson, T. W., 250
Andrews, D. W., 386
Anscombe, F. J., 39, 67
Arizono, I., 333
Armitage, P., 137, 395, 396, 409
Armstrong, D., 312
Aroian, L. A., 409, 469
Ashby, D., 179
Auh, S., 391
Austin, P. C., 15, 422
Ayatollahi, S. M. T., 249
Azzalini, A., 49, 278

B

Baddour, Y., 338, 339
Baggerly, K. A., 127, 130
Bai, J., 392
Bailey, L. B., 583
Bakeman, R., 412
Baker, S. G., 222
Bakir, S. T., 393
Balakrishnan, N., 14, 266, 272, 273, 275, 279, 327
Ball, P., 278
Bamber, D., 191, 274
Bandos, A. I., 218
Banerjee, M., 84
Bantis, L. E., 216
Barbieri, M. M., 178
Bargmann, E., 334
Barlow, R. E., 78
Barnard, F. R., 39

Barnard, G. A., 398
Barnett, V., 67
Barry, D., 387
Bartholomew, D., 86
Bartky, W., 397
Barton, D. E., 45
Basu, A., 178
Batchelder, W. H., 325
Bauer, P., 406, 413, 414
Baum, C. W., 412
Baumgartner, W., 247
Bayarri, M., 9, 10
Bayes, T., 143
Beal, S. L., 282
Beeton, M., 263
Begg, C. B., 212, 213
Bell, C., 319
Bellazzi, R., 178, 217
Bembom, O., 416
Bender, R., 388
Benichou, J., 83, 102, 247
Benjamini, Y., 426
Berger, J. O., 8, 9, 12, 80, 145, 146, 161, 174, 178, 401
Berk, R. H., 402, 409
Bernardo, J. M., 146
Berry, J. C., 80
Berwick, M., 213
Betensky, R. A., 409, 410
Bhagwat, J. G., 187
Bhat, K., 89
Bhattacharya, P., 239
Bhattacharyya, G., 319, 351
Bhuchongkul, S., 318, 319
Bickel, P., 130
Bigelow, C., 264
Biondi, A., 248
Birnbaum, M., 325
Bithell, J., 20
Bland, J. M., 12
Bleistein, N., 153
Blest, D. C., 320
Bloch, D. A., 88
Blum, J. R., 318
Bock, M., 222
Bohidar, N. R., 132

---

[*] The second author of every "et al." reference is included in this index.

633

Boies, J.-C., 264, 272, 274
Bolboaca, S.-D., 322
Boon, P. C., 14, 15
Boos, D. D., 118
Booth, J. G., 480
Borovkov, A. A., 343, 381
Bouzar, N., 384
Bowman, A., 49, 334
Box, G. E., 15, 58, 96, 171, 191, 329, 330
Bradley, E. L., 213
Branscum, A. J., 215
Braun, J. V., 383
Braun, R., 383
Bravo, F., 130
Breiman, L., 267
Bretz, F., 30, 37, 425, 427, 428
Brodsky, E., 369, 385
Brooks, S. P., 175
Brown, B. W., Jr., 173
Brown, R. L., 366
Browne, R. H., 103
Bruce, M. L., 135
Brumback, L. C., 214
Buckland, S. T., 125
Buckland, W. R., 267
Burman, C. F., 415
Buse, A., 79

C

Caffo, B., 89
Cai, L., 386
Cai, T., 225
Campbell, G., 187
Canner, P. L., 235, 242, 359
Cao, R., 132
Capon, J., 319
Carlin, B. P., 119, 122, 153, 155, 156, 174, 175, 176, 434, 435, 437
Carlin, J. B., 162, 171
Carlstein, E., 382
Carpenter, J., 20, 586
Carroll, R., 388, 389, 429, 430
Casella, G., 93, 94, 432
Caussinus, H., 385
Chakraborti, S., 16, 22, 231, 461
Chalmers, T. C., 7, 74, 419
Chan, J. S., 387
Chan, K. C. G., 139
Chan, N. H., 135
Chang, C.-H., 586
Chang, M. N., 398, 411
Chang, Y.-C. I., 418

Chapman, D. G., 319
Charles, S., 385
Chater, N., 85
Chen, C.-H., 69
Chen, C. W., 387
Chen, G., 133, 136
Chen, H., 128
Chen, J., 128, 131, 224, 341, 342, 345, 369, 385
Chen, L., 102, 136
Chen, M. G., 407, 416
Chen, Q., 445
Chen, S. X., 124, 124, 135, 463
Chen, S. Y., 131
Chen, X., 205, 206, 264, 265, 274, 463
Cheng, G., 587
Cheng, J., 135
Chernoff, H., 342
Cheung, K., 417
Cheung, Y. K., 417
Chib, S., 175, 176
Chibishov, D., 130
Choi, S., 81, 210
Christen, J. A., 181
Chrzanowski, M., 222
Chu, C.-S. J., 391
Chu, H., 438, 445
Chuang, C.-S., 571
Chuang-Stein, C., 37
Ciampi, A., 437
Claeskens, G., 105, 218, 327
Clarkson, E., 220
Clayton, D., 442
Clemens, J., 418
Cleveland, W. S., 39
Cochran, G. C., 180
Cochran, W. G., 279
Cody, R., 37
Cohen, J., 103
Coin, D., 331
Cole, B. F., 134
Conigrave, K. M., 224
Conover, W., 251
Cook, N. R., 218
Cook, R. D., 68, 320
Cook, T. D., 413
Cooke, T., 223
Copas, J., 195, 198, 213
Corbett, P., 195, 198, 213
Cordy, C. B., 442
Cox, C. P., 402
Cox, D., 126, 191, 266, 366
Crawley, M. J., 28, 30, 38
Crupi, V., 85

Csörgö, M., 354, 355, 362, 375, 383
Csorgo, S., 332
Cutler, S., 407
Czajkowski, M., 391

D

D'Agostino, R. B., 220
Dalla Valle, A., 278
Dana, J., 325
Daniel, C., 58, 59
Daniels, M. J., 117, 121
Darbellay, G., 335
Darcy, K. M., 315
Darkhovskh, B., 382
Darkhovsky, B. S., 369, 385
Darling, D. A., 250
DasGupta, A., 108
Dass, S. C., 178
David, H. A., 10, 272, 468
David, H. T., 250
Davies, O. L., 329, 333
Davies, P., 322
Davis, A. E., 138
Davis, C. S., 478
Davison, A., 79
Davison, A. C., 21, 472
Dawid, A. P., 179
De Bruijn, N. G., 153
DeGroot, M. H., 148, 396
Delaigle, A., 448
Delampady, M., 8, 9
DeLong, D. M., 211, 217
DeLong, E. R., 211, 217
Delwiche, L. D., 25, 33, 34, 36
DeMets, D. L., 410, 411
Deming, W. E., 10
Dempster, A. P., 10, 11
Deng, Q., 350
Deng, W., 108, 117, 121, 181
Denny, J., 220
De Ridder, L., 248
De Santis, F., 175
Desmond, R. A., 381
Desquilbet, L., 25
Dey, D. K., 172, 176
Diaconis, P., 222
DiCiccio, T. J., 88, 122, 157, 177, 433
DiNardo, J., 279
Ding, A. A., 321
Djogbenou, A., 586
Dmitrienko, A., 37, 396, 422
Dodge, H. F., 397

Doksum, K., 67, 90, 319
Domhof, S., 428
Dong, L. B., 331
Dong, X., 264
Donley, M., 315
Dorvlo, A. S., 213
Drummond, G. B., 69
Dubins, L. E., 220
Duhaney, R. L., 583
Duin, R. P. W., 79
Dumbgen, L., 382
Durbin, J., 323, 366
Duscha, G., 416
Dwass, M., 251

E

Eales, J. D., 415
Eckley, I. A., 385
Eddy, D. M., 221
Edelman, D., 411
Edwards, A. L., 277
Edwards, L. J., 391
Efron, B., 17, 120, 126, 174, 195, 213, 218, 220,
        471, 472, 475, 488, 528, 570, 571
Eilertsen, A., 249
Einmahl, J. H., 113, 130, 264, 270, 312,
        317, 356, 357, 451
Elffers, H., 273
Embrechts, P., 263, 266
Emerson, S. C., 135, 179, 416, 418, 419
Emerson, S. S., 417
Eng, J., 187
Epps, T. W., 332
Ernst, M. D., 18, 570
Escobar, L. A., 81
Evans, M., 153, 176
Everitt, B. S., 396

F

Fagerland, M. W., 102, 249
Fan, J., 76, 84, 105, 133, 454, 456, 457
Fan, J. Q., 447
Fang, H. B., 85, 446
Fang, L., 419
Faraggi, D., 204, 217, 223, 429, 431, 434, 443
Farcomeni, A., 103
Farmen, M., 105, 454, 456, 457
Fawcett, T., 187, 214
Fay, M. P., 419
Fears, T. R., 83
Fellingham, S., 239

Feng, P., 221
Ferger, D., 341
Feuerverger, A., 586
Fieller, E. C., 318
Fienberg, S. E., 68
Fine, J., 130
Finner, H., 427
Fishbein, L., 575
Fisher, L. D., 412
Fisher, M., 417
Fisher, N., 264, 321
Fisher, R. A., 57, 246, 318, 319, 332
Fleming, T. R., 409
Ford, I., 411
Foster, P., 334
Francia, R., 330
Fréchet, M., 275
Fredricks, G. A., 323
Freedman, D., 15, 22
Freeman, H. A., 397
Freidlin, B., 414
Freiman, J. A., 7, 74
Friedman, M., 397
Frömke, C., A., 249
Fu, L., G., 69
Fukumizu, K., 324
Fuller, W. A., 4, 429

G

Gail, M. H., 187, 188, 191, 193, 194, 217, 218, 220, 417
Ganocy, S. J., 384
Gao, F., 225
Gardener, M., 25, 30, 38
Gastwirth, J., 239
Gavit, P., 338, 339
Gelber, R. D., 134
Gelfand, A. E., 172, 176
Gelman, A., 162, 171, 175
Genest, C., 264, 272, 274, 320, 323
Gentleman, R., 85
Genz, A., 156
Geweke, J., 156
Ghitany, M., 221
Ghosh, B., 402
Ghosh, M., 76
Ghosh, S. P., 334
Gibbons, J. D., 10, 16, 22, 231, 461
Giesbrecht, F., 334
Gijbels, I., 457
Gilbert, P. R., 216
Giles, D. E., 331
Gill, R., 126, 391

Gillespie, B. W., 445
Gilovich, T., 173
Gindi, G., 225
Gnanadesikan, R., 57, 59, 60, 67, 264, 328
Gnedenko, B., 249, 250
Godambe, V. P., 81
Gombay, E., 341, 342, 343, 347, 350, 354, 384
Gonçalves, S., 586
Gönen, M., 160, 179, 215
Good, I., 171, 175
Good, P., 571
Goodman, L. A., 326
Goodman, S. N., 8, 177
Gordon, L., 342
Gordon Lan, K., 410
Gössl, C., 388
Govindarajulu, Z., 216, 331
Graubard, B. I., 247
Gray, R. J., 334
Greaney, V., 173
Green, D. M., 187
Green, J., 329
Green, P. J., 172
Greenhouse, S., 407
Greenland, S., 4, 7, 8, 9, 22, 427, 428
Gretton, A., 324
Grimmett, G., 94
Gruber, S. B., 448
Grunkemeier, G. L., 126
Gu, M., 264
Guallar, E., 386, 390
Guan, Z., 341, 360, 362, 363, 374
Guggenberger, P., 132
Gulledge Jr., T. R., 68
Guo, Y., 4, 446, 448
Gupta, A., 430, 436, 439
Gupta, A. K., 341, 342, 345, 363, 369, 383, 385
Gupta, R. C., 221
Gurevich, G., 73, 112, 113, 139, 233, 235, 240, 242, 243, 327, 332, 342, 346, 347, 357, 369, 370, 382
Guttman, I., 176
Györfi, L., 324

H

Habbema, J. D. F., 79
Habibi, R., 382
Haccou, P., 347
Haitovsky, Y., 22, 178
Hall, P., 84, 113, 122, 123, 124, 213, 332, 433, 448, 463, 586
Hall, W., 81, 192, 210, 397, 408

Halperin, M., 216
Hammersley, J. M., 156, 173
Hammitt, J. K., 194
Han, C., 153
Handelsman, R. A., 153
Handscomb, D. C., 156, 173
Hanfelt, J. J., 81
Hanley, J. A., 211, 214, 216
Hans, P., 220
Hardell, L., 182
Härdle, W. K., 69
Harel, O., 393, 445
Harrell, F. E., 264
Harter, H. L., 436, 437
Hartigan, J., 173, 177, 471
Hartigan, J. A., 387
Hartley, H., 453
Hartley, H. O., 318
Hawkins, D. M., 139, 334, 381, 350
Hawkins, K., 139
Hayter, A. J., 86
He, X., 219
Hebbema, J. D. F., 334
Hegazy, Y., 329
Herman, B. A., 191
Hermans, J., 79
Herring, A. H., 445
Hettmansperger, T. P., 230
Higgins, J., 419
Hilton, J. F., 247
Hinkley, D., 88, 266, 366
Hinkley, D. V., 21, 472
Hirotsu, C., 381
Hjort, N. L., 17, 85, 105, 327
Hochberg, Y., 426
Hoeffding, W., 273, 318, 319
Hoel, P. G., 14
Hoff, P., 83
Hogan, J. W., 117, 121
Hogan, M., 364
Hoijtink, H., 180
Hollander, M., 126, 273
Hommel, G., 427
Hop, J. P., 173
Hornik, K., 391
Horton, N. J., 30, 37
Horvath, L., 342, 343, 347, 350, 354, 355,
        362, 375, 381, 382, 383
Hosmer, D. W., Jr., 199
Hothorn, L. A., 249
Hothorn, T., 30, 37, 428
Hou, Y., 325
Hsieh, F., 187, 188, 191

Hsu, J. C., 224
Hsu, J. S., 174
Huang, J., 218, 226
Huang, P., 252, 428
Huber-Carol, C., 327
Hung, H. J., 11
Hunsberger, S., 412, 414
Hunter, W. G., 58, 96
Hušková, M., 369, 378, 383
Hutson, A. D., 18, 423, 424, 451, 570
Hyndman, R. J., 213

I

Ignatz, M., 582
Inglot, T., 268
Irle, A., 410

J

Jain, A. K., 223
James, B., 342, 366, 377
James, K. L., 342, 366, 377
James, N. A., 385
James, W., 120
Janes, H., 215
Jäntschi, L., 322
Janzen, F. J., 168
Jasra, A., 392
Jeffreys, H., 146, 161, 173, 177
Jennison, C., 404, 405, 408, 409, 411, 415, 416
Jensen, F. V., 88
Jewell, E. L., 315
Jia, Z., 220
Jiang, J., 133
Jing, B. Y., 126, 218
Johnson, M. E., 277, 278, 279, 284, 320
Johnson, N. J., 102
Johnson, N. L., 14, 278
Johnson, R. A., 173, 319, 331, 351
Johnson, V. E., 180
Johnson, W. O., 160, 179, 215
Johnston, J., 279
Jones, D., 409
Jones, M. C., 68
Julious, S. A., 379, 386
Jupp, P., 319

K

Kac, M., 329
Kadane, J. B., 153, 173, 175
Kai-Tai, F., 278

Kalbfleisch, J., 125
Kallenberg, W. C., 264, 267, 268, 312
Kang, L., 203
Kaplan, E. L., 556
Karlin, S., 86
Kass, R. E., 146, 147, 153, 154, 155, 156, 157, 161,
       168, 172, 173, 174, 175, 176, 177, 428, 430
Keiding, N., 126
Keilegom, I. V., 135
Kellaghan, T., 173
Kendall, M. G., 263, 267, 319, 329
Kent, J. T., 79
Kepner, J. L., 398
Khan, J., 249
Khurd, P., 225
Kiefer, J., 251, 318, 329
Killick, R., 385
Kim, H.-J., 376, 377, 386
Kim, Y., 418
Kim, Y. M., 451, 452, 454, 455, 456, 461, 464, 470
Kimeldorf, G., 320
King, J. P., 278
Kirk, J. L., 419
Kitamura, Y., 129, 433
Kittelson, J. M., 179, 416
Klauer, 269
Kleiber, C., 392
Klein, J., 22
Klein, M., 22
Kleinbaum, D., 22
Kleiner, A., 587
Kleinman, K., 30, 37
Klemelä, J., 44, 45, 69
Kline, J., 363, 364, 365
Klugkist, I., 180
Koch, A. L., 13
Kohne, K., 406
Kokoszka, P., 381
Kopecky, K. J., 334
Korn, E. L., 247, 414, 426
Korolyuk, V., 250
Kotz, S., 191, 192, 218, 278
Koziol, J. A., 85, 220, 446
Kramar, A., 223
Krieger, A. M., 342, 346
Krishnamoorthy, K., 586
Kroese, D. P., 452
Kruskal, W. H., 244, 326
Kuang, S.-Q., 446
Küchenhoff, H., 388, 389
Kudo, A., 86
Kuechenhoff, H., 388
Kulathinal, S., 282

Kuriki, S., 87
Kutner, M. H., 456
Kuulasmaa, K., 282

L

Lachin, J. M., 414
Lai, C.-D., 266, 272, 273, 275, 279
Lai, T. L., 88, 135, 343, 397, 408, 413, 415, 417, 571
Lam, F., 239
Lan, S.-P., 414
Lane-Claypon, J. E., 395
Langer, F., 428
La Scala, B., 123
Lasko, T. A., 187
Lauzon, C., 89
Lavine, M., 177
Lawless, J., 105, 108, 124, 134, 360
Lawless, J. F., 125, 126
Lawson, A. D., 415
Lawson, J., 37
Lazar, N., 105, 110, 117, 121, 126, 128, 456
Le Cam, L., 80, 81, 151
Ledwina, T., 90, 264, 267, 268, 312
Lee, A., 354
Lee, E. T., 14, 67
Lee, I., 386
Lee, J. W., 411
Lee, K. L., 264
Lee, S., 389
Lee, S. M., 127
Lee, Y., 80
Lee, Y. J., 210, 246
Lehéricy, S., 248
Lehmann, E. L., 6, 7, 8, 11, 22, 75, 90,
       93, 94, 230, 319, 573
Leisch, F., 392
Leisenring, W., 211
Lemdani, M., 83
Lemeshow, S., 199
Leonard, T., 174
Lesaffre, E., 247
Leung, D. H., 116
Leuraud, K., 102, 247
Levin, B., 363, 364, 365
Levin, G. P., 419
Li, G., 125, 126, 131
Li, M., 138
Li, Q., 251, 428
Li, R., 248
Li, S., 226
Li, X., 221
Liang, H., 132, 133, 134

Liang, K.-Y., 81
Liao, L., 446
Limpert, E., 14
Lin, C.-C., 330
Lin, D., 411
Lin, H., 227
Lin, J.-J., 586
Lin, X., 133
Lin, Y., 398
Lindley, D. V., 173
Lindsey, J., 13
Liseo, B., 178
Littell, R. C., 37
Little, R. J., 4, 181, 446, 448
Liu, A., 203, 208, 220, 224, 226, 251, 397, 408, 428, 431, 434, 443
Liu, C., 203
Liu, J. P., 214
Liu, J. S., 204, 207
Liu, P., 182
Liu, P. Y., 247
Liu, S., 105, 106, 136, 431, 433, 434, 447
Liu, Y., 341, 383, 387
Lloyd, C. J., 187, 212
Logothetis, C., 416
Lombard, F., 373, 376
Longnecker, M., 239
Looney, S. W., 68
Loschi, R. H., 387
Louis, G. B., 449
Louis, T. A., 119, 122, 155, 156, 174, 434, 435, 437
Lu, F., 586
Lucito, R., 338
Lumelskii, Y., 191, 192, 218
Lusher, J., 182
Lusted, L. B., 187
Lyle, R. M., 179
Lyles, R. H., 448

M

Ma, C.-X., 447
Ma, S., 218, 226
Magni, P., 178, 217
Malinovsky, Y., 429, 431, 447
Mallows, C. L., 45
Mamdani, M. M., 15, 422
Manski, C. F., 389
Mantel, N., 132
Maor, E., 278
Marden, J. I., 9, 161, 172
Mardia, K. V., 278, 333
Mariotti, F., 25

Marron, J. S., 487
Martin, M. A., 88
Martinsek, A. T., 397, 401, 402, 404
Matsushita, T., 415
Matteson, D. S., 385
Maurer, W., 427
Maxwell, D. A., 85, 446
May, S., 264
Mcclish, D. K., 187
McCulloch, R., 155
McDermott, M. P., 87
McIntosh, M. W., 191, 223
McKeague, I. W., 113, 130, 264, 270, 312, 317, 356, 357, 451
McKean, J. W., 230
McLeish, D., 80
McMahan, C. S., 449
McNaughton, L., 322
McNeil, A., 263
McNeil, B. J., 211, 216
McPherson, C., 409
Meeker, W. Q., 81
Meelis, E., 347
Megahed, F. M., 393
Mehta, C., 414, 416
Mei, Y., 338
Meier, P., 556
Melby, C. L., 179
Mellein, B., 427
Meng, X.-L., 177
Mestre, O., 385
Metropolis, N., 452
Metz, C. E., 191, 219
Miecznikowski, J. C., 114
Miller, E. G., 335
Miller, R. G., 131
Moeschberger, M., 22
Molanes Lopez, E. M., 135
Molenberghs, G., 89, 248, 396
Molodianovitch, K., 217
Monahan, J. F., 118
Montgomery, D. C., 339
Moon, H., 322
Moore, A. H., 436, 437
Moran, P. A. P., 318
Morris, C., 120
Moses, L. E., 212
Mosteller, F., 154, 173
Moustakides, G. V., 342
Mudholkar, G. S., 263, 330, 333, 451
Muggeo, V. M., 390, 391
Mulder, J., 182
Müller, H. H., 412

Müller, P., 175
Mumford, S. L., 431, 443
Murota, K., 331
Murphy, S. A., 82
Murrell, P., 30, 37
Murtaugh, P. A., 210
Mykland, P. A., 81, 82, 85, 105, 110, 126, 128

N

Nachar, N., 215, 248
Nachtsheim, C. J., 456
Nagaraja, H. N., 272, 468
Naik-Nimbalkar, U., 126
Nakas, C. T., 203, 216
Nazarov, A., 324
Nelder, J., 80
Nelsen, R. B., 320, 323
Nešlehová, J., 323
Neuhäuser, M., 247
Newton, M. A., 80, 157
Neyman, J., 73, 101, 398
Ng, P. Y. B., 315
Nicolae, D. L., 326
Nie, L., 248, 438, 445
Ning, W., 372, 373, 383
Novikov, A. A., 413

O

O'Brien, P., 575
O'Brien, P. C., 247, 251, 409, 428
Obuchowski, N. A., 187, 192, 214
O'Hagan, A., 172, 174, 175
Ohta, H., 333
Oja, H., 322, 331
Olshen, A. B., 341
O'Malley, A. J., 187, 214
O'Neill, R. T., 11
Orawo, L. A. O., 181
Osmoukhina, A., 322
Owen, A. B., 105, 106, 107, 113, 123, 124, 129, 135, 360, 374, 433

P

Page, E., 342, 343, 350
Pahikkala, T., 221
Pailden, J., 372, 373
Pal, N., 80
Palmer, C., 396
Pampallona, S., 412
Park, E., 418

Park, S., 333
Parmigiani, G., 175
Pastor, R., 390
Pastor-Barriuso, R., 386
Pawitan, Y., 83
Peake, M., 223
Pearson, E., 453
Pearson, E. S., 73, 101, 398
Pearson, K., 263
Peck, C. C., 282
Pencina, M. J., 220
Peng, L., 84, 138, 211
Pepe, M. S., 187, 188, 191, 194, 203, 211, 212, 214, 215, 222, 223, 225, 430
Pericchi, L. R., 174
Perkins, N. J., 4, 226, 429, 430, 437, 438, 442, 443, 446, 448, 449
Perlman, M. D., 87, 88
Perron, P., 392
Persing, A., 392
Petrone, S., 183
Pettitt, A., 330, 352, 353, 366
Phillips, P. J., 322
Piantadosi, S., 408
Pierce, D. A., 334
Pitman, E. J., 408
Platt, R. W., 214
Pocock, S. J., 406, 409
Polansky, A. M., 586
Pollak, M., 342, 343, 346, 379
Pollard, K. S., 62
Polunchenko, A. S., 343, 346
Pons, O., 83
Pontel, J. G., 387
Posch, M., 413, 414
Powers, L., 14
Poynter, J. N., 448
Praagman, J., 380
Prabhakar, S., 223
Pratt, J. W., 8, 10
Preisser, J. S., 250
Prescott, P., 332
Proschan, M. A., 412
Provost, F. J., 187
Pulley, L. B., 332
Pyke, R., 468

Q

Qian, L., 136
Qin, G., 138, 192, 213, 219
Qin, J., 105, 108, 115, 116, 123, 124, 125, 128, 131, 134, 139, 213, 226, 360, 361

Qin, Y., 134
Qiu, P., 224
Quandt, R. E., 380
Quera, V., 412
Quesenberry, C., 334
Quessy, J. F., 324, 325
Qvigstad, E., 249

R

Račkauskas, A., 379
Raftery, A. E., 80, 147, 153, 154, 155,
    156, 157, 161, 168, 173
Rahman, M. M., 331
Rajarshi, M., 126
Rakovski, C., 264
Ramanayake, A., 363, 369, 383
Rao, J., 129
Rao, K. A., 89
Rao, P. S., 213
Razali, N. M., 327
Redelmeier, D. A., 83
Regenwetter, M., 325
Reid, N., 82, 83
Reimherr, M., 326
Reiser, B., 204, 213, 217, 429, 431, 434, 443
Rényi, A., 319
Reshef, D. N., 264, 272, 273, 277, 284
Reshef, Y. A., 264, 272, 273, 277, 284
Rezaei, S., 221
Richards, R. J., 194
Richardson, D. B., 437
Riesz, F., 220
Riffenburgh, R. H., 22, 98
Rivest, L.-P., 320
Rizzo, M. L., 324, 335
Roberts, G. O., 156, 175
Roberts, H., 182
Robinson, B. F., 412
Robinson, J., 586
Robinson, P. M., 333
Robison, D., 469
Rockette, H. E., 218
Romano, J. P., 6, 7, 22, 75, 230, 573
Romig, H., 397
Roseberry, T. D., 402
Rosenbaum, P. R., 248, 410
Rosner, B., 430
Rosner, B. A., 218
Rosner, G. L., 410
Rossi, P. E., 155
Roters, M., 427
Rothman, K. J., 4, 7, 8, 9, 22, 427

Rousseau, J., 183
Rousseeuw, P. J., 560
Royston, J., 331
Rubin, D. B., 175, 181, 410, 430, 437, 438
Rubin, H., 86
Rubinstein, R. Y., 452
Rudser, K. D., 418
Rukhin, A. L., 322
Ruppert, D., 430

S

Sackrowitz, H., 7, 8, 9, 10, 11, 22
Sacks, H. S., 419
Sampson, A. R., 320, 391
Samuel-Cahn, E., 7, 8, 9, 10, 11, 22
Sandvik, L., 102, 249
Sarkadi, K., 330
Sarkar, S., 480
Savarino, S., 418
Sawitzki, G., 68
Saxonhouse, M., 582
Scaillet, O., 322
Scannapieco, F. A., 138
Schäfer, H., 412
Scharfstein, D. O., 412
Schatzoff, M., 10, 11
Schechtman, E., 341, 353
Schenker, N., 430, 437, 438
Schervish, M. J., 177
Scheys, I., 247
Schisterman, E. F., 4, 71, 203, 215, 224,
    226, 312, 393, 429, 430, 431, 434,
    435, 437, 438, 439, 442, 443, 444,
    446, 449
Schmid, C. H., 430
Schmid, F., 323
Schmidt, R., 323
Schmitz, N., 416
Scholz, F. W., 250
Schriever, B. F., 275, 320
Schuit, E., 222
Schuster, E. F., 241
Schwarz, G., 155
Schweder, T., 17, 85
Schweizer, B., 319
Seaman, S. R., 25
Searle, S. R., 432
Sellke, T., 9, 10, 161
Sen, A., 352
Sen, P. K., 216, 250, 353
Senn, S., 427
Seo, M. H., 389

Serfling, R. J., 192, 255, 258, 259, 354, 451, 461
Seshan, V. E., 215
Severini, T., 90
Shah, A., 392
Shan, G., 235, 327
Shao, J., 472, 474. 485
Shao, Q.-M., 350, 382
Shapiro, D., 212
Shapiro, D. E., 187, 211
Shapiro, S., 334
Shapiro, S. S., 55, 327, 329, 330, 332, 334
Sheather, S. J., 487
Shi, N.-Z., 325
Shih, M.-C., 135, 415, 417
Shih, W. J., 398
Shirahata, S., 86
Shorack, G. R., 376
Shrier, I., 85
Si, Y., 182
Siegmund, D., 364, 365, 367, 377, 378, 386, 401
Sievers, G. L., 67
Silvapulle, M. J., 87
Silverman, B. W., 205
Simon, N., 274
Simon, R., 397, 410
Simonoff, J. S., 321
Singh, K., 17
Sinharay, S., 153, 161, 170
Sinnott, E. W., 14
Skene, A. M., 179
Sklar, R., 173
Slaughter, S. J., 25, 33, 34, 36
Small, C. G., 80
Small, D., 135
Small, D. S., 139
Smirnov, N. V., 231, 247
Smith, A. F., 146, 156
Smith, J. B., 325
Smith, R. J., 132
Smith, R. L., 173
Snapinn, S., 407, 416
Snedecor, G., 180, 329
Snell, E. J., 126
Sonesson, C., 415
Song, H. H., 211
Song, W., 447
Sorlie, P., 414
Spearman, C., 263, 266
Spezzaferri, F., 175, 180
Spiegelhalter, D., 330
Spiegelman, C. H., 429
Spiegelman, D., 390

Spokoiny, V. G., 386
Spurr, B., 319
Srivastava, M. S., 352
Stahel, W. A., 14
Staudenmayer, J., 390
Steffey, D., 428
Stein, C., 120, 319
Stepanova, N., 324
Stephens, M. A., 250, 330, 329
Stern, H., 153, 161, 170
Stewart, P. W., 391
Stigler, S. M., 312
Stirzaker, D., 94
Stoker, D., 239
Strassburger, K., 425
Strauss, B., 173
Stuart, A., 263, 323
Su, J. Q., 204, 207
Suchard, M. A., 176
Suquet, C., 379
Sutton, C. D., 102
Swartz, T., 22, 153, 178
Sweeting, T. J., 177
Swets, J. A., 187
Switzer, P., 264, 321
Székely, G. J., 324, 335

T

Tabesh, H., 250
Tahmasbi, R., 221
Takeuchi, K., 331
Talwalkar, A., 587
Tamhane, A. C., 422
Tan, M., 85, 446
Tanajian, H., 114, 115, 244, 246, 454, 462, 463
Tang, D.-I., 87
Tang, L., 417, 448
Tanizaki, H., 131
Tao, G., 12, 15, 105, 108, 117, 118, 120,
        155, 174, 455, 456
Taplin, R. H., 179
Tarima, S., 73, 181
Tartakovsky, A. G., 343, 346
Taskinen, S., 322
Taylor, J. R., 4
Tebbs, J. M., 449
Ten Have, T. R., 135
Terry, M. E., 319
Thall, P. F., 416
Thomas, D. R., 126, 442
Thompson, M. L., 191, 194, 222, 324

Thompson, W., 4
Thomson, E., 570
Tian, L., 203, 221, 226, 227, 333
Tiao, G. C., 330
Tibshirani, R. J., 83, 274, 472, 528
Tierney, L., 153, 154, 173, 174, 175
Tilley, B. C., 252, 428
Titterington, D., 411
Tobias, R. D., 37, 38, 427
Todd, S., 416
Troendle, J. F., 426
Tsai, W. M., 114, 138, 231, 271, 272, 314,
        317, 328, 347, 369, 430, 431, 432,
        435, 462
Tsiatis, A. A., 410, 412, 414, 416
Tu, D., 472, 474. 485
Tucker, H. G., 46
Tucker, J. K., 168
Tukey, J. W., 39, 46, 66
Turnbull, B. W., 173, 187, 188, 191, 404,
        405, 408, 409, 416
Tusnady, G., 333

U

Ulam, S., 452
Ulm, K., 388

V

Vaidyanathan, S. K., 153–154, 175
Vaillancourt, C., 85
Vajda, I., 335
Vallone, R., 173
Vandal, A. C., 85
van der Laan, M. J., 62, 416
Van Der Tweel, I., 414
Van der Vaart, A. W., 82
Van Dijk, H. K., 173
Van Elteren, P., 246
Van Keilegom, I., 132, 133
Van Noord, P. A., 414
Vardi, Y., 361
Vasicek, O., 235, 253, 332
Veeravalli, V. V., 412
Venkatraman, E., 212, 341
Ventura, L., 103
Verbeke, G., 89, 248
Verdinelli, I., 180
Verdonck, A., 248
Verrill, S., 331
Versluis, C., 335

Vexler, A., 12, 15, 73, 75, 76, 85, 105, 106, 108, 112,
        113, 114, 115, 116, 117, 118, 120, 121, 136,
        137, 138, 139, 155, 168, 172, 174, 181, 205,
        206, 208, 215, 220, 226, 227, 231, 233, 235,
        235, 238, 240, 242, 243, 246, 264, 265, 271,
        272, 274, 314, 317, 327, 328, 332, 341, 342,
        343, 346, 347, 350, 357, 363, 370, 372, 377,
        378, 379, 380, 381, 382, 389, 430, 431, 432,
        433, 434, 435, 436, 437, 438, 439, 444, 447,
        451, 452, 454, 455, 456, 461, 462, 463, 464,
        470, 570
Volodin, I. N., 413
Vostrikova, L., 341
Vowler, S. L., 69

W

Wah, Y. B., 327
Wainer, H., 68
Wald, A., 398, 401, 404, 409
Wallace, D., 154, 173
Wallis, W. A., 244, 246
Walter, S., 219
Wand, M. P., 68
Wang, H., 134
Wang, H.-H., 138
Wang, J., 105
Wang, J. W., 14
Wang, M. C., 226
Wang, Q., 129
Wang, Q.-H., 131
Wang, S., 133, 134, 136
Wang, S. K., 412
Wang, W., 321
Wang, Y., 87
Wang, Y.-G., 69
Ware, J. H., 410
Wason, J., 25
Wasserman, L., 161, 172, 176
Wedderburn, R. W., 105
Wei, J. S., 249
Weiner, J., 449
Weisberg, S., 68
Weisenberger, D. J., 264
Weiss, H. L., 381
Weiss, R. E., 176
Wellner, J. A., 84, 376
Welsh, A. H., 332
West, J., 338
Westfall, P. H., 37, 38, 427
Wheeler, B., 267
Whitaker, T., 334

Whitcomb, B. W., 448
Whitehead, A., 419
Whitehead, J., 406, 408, 409, 415
Wickham, H., 30, 37
Wieand, S., 187, 188, 191, 193, 194, 217, 218, 220, 417
Wiest, M. C., 570
Wilcox, R. R., 16, 22, 321
Wilding, G. E., 263
Wilk, M., 57, 60, 59, 60, 66
Wilk, M. B., 55, 57, 60, 264, 327, 328, 329, 330, 332, 334
Wilks, S. S., 7, 75
Williams, E., 176
Wilson, S. R., 586
Wolfe, D. A., 210, 246, 273, 341, 353
Wolff, E. F., 319
Wolfowitz, J., 404
Wolpert, R. L., 8, 80
Wong, H. L., 335
Wong, W. H., 79, 125, 177
Wood, A. T., 126
Wood, S. N., 282
Woodroofe, M., 390
Woodworth, G. G., 319
Wu, C., 73, 132, 133, 168, 172, 346, 347, 381, 382
Wu, L., 88
Wu, W. B., 390
Wu, X., 137
Wu, Y., 138, 331
Wyłupek, G., 90

X

Xie, M., 17
Xiong, C., 225
Xu, W., 325
Xu, X., 101
Xue, L., 133

Y

Yakir, B., 342
Yang, D., 139
Yang, S., 133
Yao, Q., 363, 365, 366, 367, 368, 378, 379
Yao-Ting, Z., 278

Yates, F., 318, 319
Yi, J., 419
Yiannoutsos, C. T., 203
Ying, Z., 137
You, J., 133, 136
Young, G. A., 127, 471
Yu, B., 226
Yu, J., 75, 85, 105, 113, 116, 137, 138, 139, 233, 430, 433, 436
Yu, Z., 587
Yule, G., 263
Yule, G. U., 332

Z

Zacks, S., 342
Zamba, K., 350
Zaslavsky, B. G., 182
Zeileis, A., 392
Zellner, A., 148
Zhang, B., 115, 131, 134, 139, 213, 219, 226, 249, 360
Zhang, C., 76, 84
Zhang, D., 133
Zhang, D. D., 217
Zhang, J., 331
Zhang, L., 101
Zhang, M., 393
Zhang, R., 133
Zhang, S., 134
Zhang, Y., 249, 393
Zhang, Z., 323, 446
Zhao, H., 341
Zhao, Y., 133, 134, 454, 455, 462
Zheng, S., 325
Zhong, B., 128
Zhou, C., 226
Zhou, L., 227
Zhou, W., 220
Zhou, X. H., 187, 192, 213, 217, 219, 221
Zhou, Y., 132
Zhu, L., 133
Zhu, L.-X., 335
Zou, C., 341, 383, 387, 393
Zou, F., 130
Zou, K. H., 187, 192, 214
Zou, L., 117, 174

Subject Index

A

ABC, *see* Approximate Bayesian computation
Acquired immune deficiency
 syndrome data, 125
Adaptive sequential designs, 406–407
Adaptive smoothing, 334
Adaptive test, 414
Additive errors, 432–436
ADHD, *see* Attention-deficit/hyperactivity
 disorder
AIDS, 125, 411
AIDS dementia complex (ADC), 203
Alternatives, 81, 84, 88, 89, 103, 130, 133, 171, 177,
 212, 218, 246, 247, 251, 319, 322, 325, 330,
 332, 335, 380, 383, 393, 408, 411
AMOC model, *see* At most one change-point
 model
Analysis of variance (ANOVA), 86, 211, 244
Anderson–Darling rank statistic, 250
Anderson–Darling test, 250, 327, 331, 334
Approximate Bayesian computation (ABC), 392
Approximated most average powerful (AMAP)
 test, 182
Archimedean copulas, 320
Area under the Kendall plot (AUK), 274–277
Area under the ROC curve (AUC), 178, 191, 430
ASN, *see* Average sample number
Aspartate aminotransferase (AST), 224
Association, 320, 321, 388, 443, 449, *see also*
  Dependence and independence
  (structures, testing, and measuring)
Asymptotically uniformly most powerful
 (AUMP) tests, 81
Asymptotic optimality, 333, 343, 415, 418
At most one change-point (AMOC) model, 342
Attention-deficit/hyperactivity disorder
 (ADHD), 114, 139
AUC, *see* Area under the ROC curve
AUK, *see* Area under the Kendall plot
Average power, 130, 182
Average sample number (ASN), 400

B

Backward induction (Bayes factor), 181
Bahadur efficiency, 380
Bahadur exact slopes, 380

Bartlett correction, 110, 123, 136, 177
Baumgartner–Weiß–Schindler statistic, 247
Bayes factor–based test statistics, 143–185
 alternative hypothesis, 158
 applied statistics, 173
 approximated most average
  powerful test, 182
 area under the curve, 178
 asymptotic approximations, 153–156
 backward induction, 181
 Bayes factor, 146–170
 Bayes factor–type decision-making
  mechanisms, 145
 combining simulation and asymptotic
  approximations, 157
 computation of Bayes factors, 147–157
 conditional information matrix, 174
 conjugate beta priors, 182
 conjugate prior, 158
 data example, 168–170
 decision-making rules, 161–168
 Dirichlet models, 180
 elicited prior, 158
 false discovery rate, 181
 first-order approximation, 151
 flat prior, 146
 FORTRAN, 173
 frequentist methodology, 143
 Gaussian quadrature, 156
 Hessian matrix, 155, 172
 highly peaked integrand, 148
 honest prior information, 183
 identifiability problems, 178
 importance sampling, 156
 improper distribution, 158
 inequality constrained hypotheses,
  testing of, 182
 integrated most powerful tests, 145–146
 Laplace approximation, 153–155
 Laplace's method, 173
 Lindley paradox, 174
 loss function, 145
 Markov chain Monte Carlo methods, 156, 176
 modal approximation, 151
 Monte Carlo evaluations, 156
 most powerful test in hypothesis testing, 184
 noninformative prior, 158

nuisance parameter, 175
optimality of LRT in simple hypothesis
        testing case, 183–184
permutation-type nonidentifiabilities, 178
predictive distributions, models
        based on, 176
prior distribution, 144
prior information, 145
prior probability distributions, choice of,
        157–161
p-value fallacy, 177
quadrature, 148
receiver operating characteristic curve, 180
representative values, 144–145
RNA-seq technology, 181
robust Bayes factor, 179
Schwarz criterion, 155–156
semi-Bayes approach, 172
sequential stopping rule, 179
simulating from the posterior, 156–157
superiority trial, 182
supplement, 171–183
Bayesian empirical likelihood, 117–118
Bayesian multivariate hierarchical
        transformation model (BMHTM), 214
Bayes information criterion (BIC), 155, 176
Bias-corrected and accelerated (BCa) method,
        214, 527–534
Bias-corrected (BC) method, 522–527
Binomial distribution, 182, 239, 381, 398, 409, 478
Binormal ROC curve, 189
BioCycle study, 429
Biomarker measurements, *see* Clinical trials
        (biomarker measurements in)
Bivariate distribution, 193, 263, 275, 281, 283,
        319, 320
Bivariate normal correlation, 283, 284
Bivariate normal data, 30, 100
Bivariate normal distribution, 169, 266, 277, 318
Body mass index (BMI), 218
Bonferroni adjustment, 424, 428
Bonferroni confidence intervals, 425
Bonferroni correction, 89, 426
Bonferroni procedures, 422, 424
Bootstrap and permutation methods, 471–590
    attributes, 471
    bias-corrected and accelerated method,
        527–534
    bias-corrected method, 522–527
    bias estimation, 488–491
    books, 472
    bootstrap confidence intervals, 501–537
    bootstrap p-values, 540–534

bootstrap-*t* example macro, 587–590
bootstrap-*t* method, 507–514
bootstrap-*t* method via double
        bootstrapping, 519–522
calibration of intervals, 534–537
censored data, 556–559
correlational model, 559
correlation and regression, 582–586
cumulative distribution function, 523
double bootstrap, 491–501
ease of calculation, 475
empirical likelihood and bootstrap
        methodologies, relationship
        between, 570–571
exact tests, 571
first-order bias correction, 486
Glivenko–Cantelli theorem, 474
jackknife method, 471
macro statements, 482
Monte Carlo resampling, 570
MSE estimation, 491–501
nonparametric tilting, 570
outline of permutation theory, 572–574
percentile method, 502–507
permutation tests, 571–586
poor strategy, 487
primary assumption, 473
random binomial variables, 478
repeated measures and clustered data,
        549–556
rerandomization tests, 571
resampling data with replacement in SAS,
        477–485
robust regression, 560
sampled data, 474
SAS macro language for calculating
        bootstrap-*t* intervals, 545–549
SAS macro language for calculating
        percentile intervals, 543–545
simple regression modeling, 559–569
simple two-group comparisons, 537–559
standard deviation, 564
subroutines, 482
summary statistics, 538–540
supplement, 586–587
theoretical quantities of interest, 485–501
two-sample methods, 574–582
variance estimation, 491–501
variance-stabilized bootstrap-*t* method,
        514–519
Bootstrap statistical method, 17–20
    bootstrap confidence intervals, 19–20
    example, 18

Monte Carlo resampling approximations, 19
Pearson correlation coefficient, 19
pivotal methods, 19
sample bias, 18
statistical functional, 17–19
"well-behaved" statistics, 17
Bootstrap tilting, 570
Box–Cox variable transformations, 223
Boxplots, 40–42
Box-and-whisker plot, 40
Breakpoint, 376, 392
Broken line [stick] regression, 376
Brownian bridges, 375, 381
Brownian covariance, 324
Brownian motion, 84, 324, 408
Brunner–Munzel test, 102

C

Carbohydrate antigenic determinant, 138, 218
Carbohydrate-deficient transferrin (CDT), 224
Cartesian coordinates, 42
Cauchy distribution, 277
CDF, *see* Cumulative distribution function
Censored data, 556–559
Central limit theorems (CLTs), 81
Change-point analysis, 337–394
    adaption to two-sided alternative
        hypothesis, 367
    asymptotic distributions under the
        alternative hypothesis, 367–368
    at most one change-point model, 342
    Bahadur exact slopes, 380
    breakpoint, 376, 392
    change in location, 350–353
    common change-point models, 339–341
    control charts, 338
    CUSUM-based techniques, 342–346
    density-based empirical likelihood
        approaches, 357–360
    empirical likelihood–based approach,
        356–357
    epidemic change point problems, 362–376
    epidemiological studies, quantitative risk
        assessment in, 388
    estimation approach, 371
    estimators of the change points, 369
    general case of the problem, 369–372
    general linear model, 389
    jump discontinuities, 387
    Levin and Kline's statistic, 364
    likelihood ratio statistic, 365
    linear regression, 377, 386

log-likelihood ratio statistic, 364
Markov chain Monte Carlo methods, 388
martingale approach, 381
maximization–maximization–posterior, 384
maximizing a posterior, 384
measurement error models, 388
mixture approach, 370
monotonic trends, isotonic
    regression for, 390
null distribution, 342
online (sequential) change-point
    problem, 338
PELT algorithm, 385
phylogenetic trees, change points on, 392
product partition model, 387
recursive residual statistic, 366–367
regression models, problems in, 376, 386–393
scalar values, 378
score-type statistic, 365–366
segmented linear regression, 376, 378–380
segmented regression, 389–391
semilikelihood ratio statistic, 365
semiparametric approaches, 360, 374
Shiryayev–Roberts statistic, 346, 370
simple case of the problem, 363–369
simple change-point model, 342–362, 380
square-wave alternative, 363
statistical inference, 337
statistical quality control schemes, 393
structural change, 391–392
supplement, 380–393
threshold effects, 388–389
U-statistics-based approaches, 353–356
Characteristic function, 135, 318, 332, 444
Chi-squared distribution, 79, 82, 126, 129, 131,
    132, 138, 219, 222, 406, 434
CI, *see* Confidence interval
Clinical experiments, multiple testing problems
    in, 421–428
    Bonferroni procedures, 422, 424
    comparison error rate, 423
    definitions of error rates, 422–427
    discovery hypotheses, 422
    false discovery rate and false discovery
        proportion, 426
    family-wise error rate, 422–425
    power evaluation, 427
    primary hypotheses, 422
    secondary hypotheses, 422
    supplement, 428
Clinical trials (biomarker measurements in),
    429–449
    additive errors, 432–436

areas under the ROC curves, 430
Bayesian-type methods, 434, 437
deconvolution, 442
detection threshold, 444
distribution function, 442
epidemiological studies, 443
failure in biomarker correction, 442
Fisher approximation, 449
Gaussian random effects model, 447
hybrid pooled–unpooled design, 434, 438
Kaplan–Meier estimator, 445
laboratory assays, 448
limit of detection, 436–439
maximum likelihood estimators, 432
measurements of exposures, 443
methods based on maximum likelihood
        methodology, 436–437
Monte Carlo experiments, 439–441
pooling design, 431
pooling methods, 447
population distributions, 445
regression calibration, 446
repeated measurements, 432–434
ROC curves, 444
single and multiple imputation methods,
        437–438
supplement, 442–449
CLTs, *see* Central limit theorems
Clustering calculation, output of, 62
Coefficient of variation (CV), 88
Cohen's effect size, 103
Comparison error rate, 423
Composite hypothesis, 76, 113, 144, 329, 332
Conditional distribution, 88, 162, 164, 438
Conditional expectation, 277, 278, 411, 438
Conditional information matrix, 174
Conditional power, 407, 409, 410, 414
Conditional probability, 194, 212, 221
Conditional tests, 88
Confidence bands, 113, 124, 126, 213, 218
Confidence interval (CI), 134
    construction of, 16–17
    for differences between characteristics of
            populations, 134
    distribution-free (AUC), 216
    for population quantile, 125
Confidence intervals, bootstrap, 19, 501–537
    bias-corrected and accelerated method,
            527–534
    bias-corrected method, 522–527
    bootstrap-*t* method, 507–514
    bootstrap-*t* method via double
            bootstrapping, 519–522

calibration of intervals, 534–537
cumulative distribution function, 523
percentile method, 502–507
variance-stabilized bootstrap-*t* method,
        514–519
Confidence level(s), 21, 448, 553
Confidence sets, 82, 587
Conjugate beta priors, 182
Conjugate distributions, 158
Consistent estimation, 133, 225
Continuous data, means of, 95–103
    asymmetrical distributions, mean of, 102
    Cohen's effect size, 103
    equal variances, 97
    exact LRT for equality of two normal
            populations, 101
    monotonic dose–response relationship, 102
    multivariate *t*-test, 99–101
    one-sample *t*-test, 96
    paired *t*-test, 97–99
    receiver operating characteristic curves, 103
    supplement, 102–103
    t-type tests, 96–101
    two-sample *t*-test, 97
    unequal variances (Welch's *t*-test), 97
    univariate and *p*-dimensional LRTs, 95–96
    Welch U-test, 102
Continuous-scale diagnostic test, 138
Contour plots, 43–45
Contrasts, 38, 87, 102, 143, 216, 223, 246
Control charts, 338
Copula
    Archimedean, 320
    function, 267
Correlation, theory of, 263
Correlation coefficient, 68, 123, 266, 319, 322,
        323, 325, 447
Cramer–von Mises-type statistics, 130, 264, 321,
        330, 357
Cressie–Read power–divergence statistic, 127
Critical values (for exact tests), calculation of,
        451–470
    Bayesian hybrid method, 456
    decision rule, 461
    empirical likelihood, 458
    hybrid method, 455–462
    illustration, 456
    interpolation method, 453–455
    methods of calculating critical values of
            exact tests, 452–462
    Monte Carlo–based method, 452–453
    software packages, 462–463
    supplement, 463–464

Cumulative distribution function (CDF), 9, 523
CUSUM, 392
CV, *see* Coefficient of variation

D

Data, 2–4
    censored, 556–559
    cleaning, 3–4
    collection, 2
    data entry errors, 5
    -driven rank tests, 267–270
    "frozen" data, 2
    limits of detection, 4
    measurement error, 4
    numerical data, 3
    preparation, 3
    qualitative data, 3
    quality, 3
    raw, descriptive plots of, 40–45
    statistical bias, 4
    types, 3
    vigilance, 212
Decision making (experimental), basic
        concepts in, 1–23
    assumptions, 12
    book atlas, 23
    bootstrap confidence intervals, 19–20
    bootstrap percentile interval, 20
    bootstrap statistical method, 17–20
    components for constructing test
        procedures, 11–12
    confidence intervals, 16–17
    cumulative distribution function, 9
    data, 2–4
    data entry errors, 5
    errors related to statistical testing
        mechanism, 5–8
    error Types I and II, 5–6
    essential elements, 1–5
    example of pretest procedures, 14–15
    exchangeable values, 21
    expected p-values, 10–11
    "frozen" data, 2
    large sample approximate tests, 16
    limitations of parametric approaches, 15–16
    limits of detection, 4
    main testing problem, 14
    measurement error, 4
    misinterpretations, 9
    Monte Carlo approximations, 8
    Monte Carlo resampling approximations, 19
    null hypothesis, 8

numerical data, 3
paired data setting, 21
parametric approach and modeling, 12–15
Pearson correlation coefficient, 19
permutation testing versus bootstrap
        methodology, 20–22
pivotal methods, 19
preliminary *F*-test, 14
pretest procedure, 14
p-values, 8–11
qualitative data, 3
quality, 3
rational choice, 8
rationality and unbiasedness in hypothesis
        testing, 7–8
R code, 13
receiver operating curve, 10
sample bias, 18
significance level of test, 6
statistical bias, 4
statistical functional, 17–19
statistical hypotheses, 4–5
Type I error, 21
uniformly most powerful test, 6
uniformly most powerful unbiased test, 7
Welch's *t*-test, 14
"well–behaved" statistics, 17
Decision-making rules, Bayes factor–based,
        161–168
Deconvolution, 442
Delta method, 191, 388, 442, 443
Dendogram, 62, 66
Density-based empirical likelihood (DBEL)
        methods, 112–115
    change-point analysis, 357–360
    entropy-based goodness-of-fit test
        procedures, 113
    Kolmogorov–Smirnov test, 113–114
    medical trials, 113
    multiple-hypothesis tests, 113
    R package, 114
    Wilcoxon signed-rank test, 114
Density-based empirical likelihood ratio tests,
        231–239
    alternative hypotheses, 232
    asymptotic consistency and null
        distributions of tests, 238–239
    based on paired data, 239–244
    composite hypotheses, 236
    decision rule, 237, 238
    empirical constraint, 234, 236
    goodness-of-fit tests, 235
    hypothesis setting and test statistics, 232–238

independence, 271–272
Lagrange multiplier, 235, 236
likelihood ratio test statistic, 233
nonparametric comparisons of distributions,
    231–239
nonparametric test statistic, 233
null hypothesis, 233
power of, 271–272
statistic, 245, 246
Dependence and independence (structures,
    testing, and measuring), 263–326
    Archimedean copulas, 320
    area under the Kendall plot, 274–277
    bivariate distributions, 278
    Brownian distance covariance, 324
    classical measures of dependence, 273–274
    copula function, 267
    data-driven rank tests, 267–270
    data examples, 312–317
    density-based empirical likelihood ratio test,
        271–272
    discussion, 317–318
    electromagnetic radiation, modeling of, 278
    empirical likelihood–based method, 270–271
    error in variables, 279
    Hilbert spaces, 319
    independence, tests of, 265–272
    indices of dependence, 272–277
    Kendall's rank correlation coefficient, 267
    Legendre polynomials, 267
    linear dependence, 277
    logarithmic dependence, 278
    maximal information coefficient, 273–274
    measurement error, 279
    Monte Carlo comparisons of tests of
        independence, 284–312
    multidimensional random variables, 324
    multiplicative noise, 282
    partial ordering, 320
    Pearson correlation coefficient, 266
    periodontal disease, 315
    Pitman tests, 319
    positive quadrant dependent variables, 322
    quadratic dependence, 277
    random effects–type dependence, 279–284
    rank tests, 318
    reciprocal dependence, 278
    Riemannian manifolds, 319
    Spearman's rank correlation coefficient,
        266–267
    Spearman's rho, 323
    structures of dependence, 277–284
    Student's t-test, 321

    study of dependence, 263
    supplement, 318–326
    TBARS, 312–315
    tests of independence, 318
    theory of correlation, 263
    trigonometric dependence, 278
    VEGF expression, 315–317
Detection threshold (DT), 444
Dihydrofolate reductase (DHFR), 322
Dirichlet distribution, 22, 178
Dirichlet models, 180
Discovery hypotheses, 422
Distribution
    binomial, 182, 239, 381, 398, 409, 478
    bivariate normal, 169, 266, 277, 318, 319
    Cauchy, 277
    chi-squared, 79, 82, 126, 129, 131, 132, 138,
        219, 222, 406, 434
    Dirichlet, 22, 178
    double exponential, 51
    exponential, 13, 51, 102, 329, 348
    F, 127, 223
    gamma, 13, 131, 323, 335, 443
    Hotelling's T^2, 100
    inverse Gaussian, 333, 434, 439
    lognormal distribution, 13, 71, 221, 331
    multinomial, 123, 129
    multivariate normal, 207, 222, 223, 225,
        334, 335, 448
    Pareto, 221
    Poisson, 12, 131, 381
    t-, 86, 96, 266, 451, 567
    uniform distribution, 118, 238
    Weibull, 386
    Wishart, 87, 434
DNA
    copy number changes (chromosomal), 338
    repair mechanism, 173
Dosemeci–Benichou test, 102, 247
Dose–response relationship, 102
Double bootstrap, 491
Double exponential distribution, 51
DT, *see* Detection threshold

E

Edgeworth expansions, 124, 220, 384
Electromagnetic radiation, modeling of, 278
ELISA, *see* Enzyme-linked immunosorbent
    assay
EM algorithm, *see* Expectation–maximization
    algorithm
Empirical distribution Function (EDF), 45

Empirical likelihood (EL), 64, 66, 105–142
   Bartlett correction and location
      adjustment, 123
   Bayesian empirical likelihood, 117–118
   Bayesians and empirical likelihood, 116–121
   bootstrap calibration approach, 124
   bootstrap methods, 123
   carbohydrate antigenic determinant, 138
   classical empirical likelihood methods,
      106–108
   combining likelihoods, 115–116
   confidence interval, 134
   continuous bivariate population, 139
   continuous-scale diagnostic test, 138
   Cressie–Read power–divergence
      statistic, 127
   density-based empirical likelihood methods,
      112–115
   "derived sample" in variance estimation, 125
   ELR test, two-sample density-based,
      141–142
   empirical Bayesian posterior, 118–121
   empirical goodness-of-fit test statistics, 130
   empirical likelihood functional, 124
   empirical likelihood ratio test, 106
   entropy-based goodness-of-fit test
      procedures, 113
   exponential empirical likelihood, 126
   Gaussian–Gaussian model, 120
   generalized empirical likelihood, 132
   generalized likelihood ratio statistics, 133
   James–Stein estimation, nonparametric
      analogue of, 120–121
   kernel regression imputation, 129
   Kolmogorov–Smirnov test, 113–114
   Lagrange multipliers, 106
   local power, comparison of, 130
   maximum likelihood estimator, 111
   mean quality-adjusted lifetime with right
      censoring, 134
   measurement error problems, 138
   medical trials, 113
   multiple-hypothesis tests, 113
   Neyman–Pearson criterion, 129
   nonparametric posterior expectations of
      simple functionals, 118–120
   nuisance parameters, 128
   optimization algorithms (R package), 139
   parametric empirical Bayes point
      estimators, 120
   population quantile, confidence intervals
      for, 125
   as practical statistical analysis tool, 121–122

   procedures for executing the two-sample
      density-based ELR test, 141–142
   quasi-likelihood, 127
   randomly truncated data, 125
   results similar to those related to ELR
      evaluations, 140–141
   R package, 114
   sequential clinical trial, 135
   supplement, 122–140
   synthetic data, 131
   techniques for analyzing empirical
      likelihoods, 108–112
   Type I error, 136
   undersmoothing, 125
   ventilator-associated pneumonia study, 137
   Wilcoxon signed-rank test, 114
   within-subject variance–covariance
      matrices, 136
Enterotoxigenic *Escherichia coli* (ETEC), 418
Enzyme-linked immunosorbent assay (ELISA),
   180, 215
Epidemic change point problems, 362–376
   adaption to two-sided alternative
      hypothesis, 367
   asymptotic distributions under the
      alternative hypothesis, 367–368
   estimation approach, 371
   estimators of the change points, 369
   general case of the problem, 369–372
   Levin and Kline's statistic, 364
   likelihood ratio statistic, 365
   log-likelihood ratio statistic, 364
   mixture approach, 370
   nonparametric approaches, 372–373
   parametric approaches, 363–372
   recursive residual statistic, 366–367
   score-type statistic, 365–366
   semilikelihood ratio statistic, 365
   semiparametric approaches, 374–376
   Shiryayev–Roberts statistic, 370
   simple case of the problem, 363–369
   square-wave alternative, 363
EPV, *see* Expected p-value
Error control, 6, 136, 221, 319, 420
ETEC, *see* Enterotoxigenic *Escherichia coli*
Exact tests, calculating critical values and
   p-values for, 451–470
   Bayesian hybrid method, 456
   decision rule, 461
   empirical likelihood, 458
   hybrid method, 455–462
   illustration, 456
   interpolation method, 453–455

methods of calculating critical values of
  exact tests, 452–462
Monte Carlo–based method, 452–453
software packages, 462–463
supplement, 463–464
Exchangeable values, 21, 281, 579
Expectation–maximization (EM) algorithm, 85
Expected p-value (EPV), 10–11
Experimental decision making, basic
  concepts in, 1–23
 assumptions, 12
 book atlas, 23
 bootstrap confidence intervals, 19–20
 bootstrap percentile interval, 20
 bootstrap statistical method, 17–20
 components for constructing test
  procedures, 11–12
 confidence intervals, 16–17
 cumulative distribution function, 9
 data, 2–4
 data entry errors, 5
 errors related to statistical testing
  mechanism, 5–8
 error Types I and II, 5–6
 essential elements, 1–5
 example of pretest procedures, 14–15
 exchangeable values, 21
 expected p-values, 10–11
 "frozen" data, 2
 large sample approximate tests, 16
 limitations of parametric approaches, 15–16
 limits of detection, 4
 main testing problem, 14
 measurement error, 4
 misinterpretations, 9
 Monte Carlo approximations, 8
 Monte Carlo resampling approximations, 19
 null hypothesis, 8
 numerical data, 3
 paired data setting, 21
 parametric approach and modeling, 12–15
 Pearson correlation coefficient, 19
 permutation testing versus bootstrap
  methodology, 20–22
 pivotal methods, 19
 preliminary F-test, 14
 pretest procedure, 14
 p-values, 8–11
 qualitative data, 3
 quality, 3
 rational choice, 8
 rationality and unbiasedness in hypothesis
  testing, 7–8

R code, 13
receiver operating curve, 10
sample bias, 18
significance level of test, 6
statistical bias, 4
statistical functional, 17–19
statistical hypotheses, 4–5
Type I error, 21
uniformly most powerful test, 6
uniformly most powerful unbiased test, 7
Welch's *t*-test, 14
"well–behaved" statistics, 17
Exponential distribution, 13, 51, 102, 329, 348

F

False discovery rate (FDR), 181, 250, 426
Family-wise error rate (FWER), 422–425
F distribution, 127, 223
Fieller's problem, 178
First-order approximation, 151
First-order bias correction, 486
Fisher approximation, 449
Fisher information, 93, 127, 150, 151, 439, 449
Fisher's exact test, 11, 451
Fisher's z-transformation, 323
Flat prior, 146
Forced expiratory volume (FEV1), 88
Forced vital capacity (FVC), 88
FORTRAN, 173
Frequentist methodology, 143
F-test, 14
Functionals, 17–19, 118–120
Fundamental lemma, *see* Neyman–Pearson
  Lemma
Futility analysis (sequential testing methods), 407
FWER, *see* Family-wise error rate

G

Gamma distribution, 13, 131, 323, 335, 443
Gamma-glutamyltransferase (GGT), 224
Gaussian–Gaussian model, 120
Gaussian random effects model, 447
GAUSS software, 390, 392
Generalized empirical likelihood (GEL), 132
Generalized likelihood ratio (GLR)
  statistics, 133
Generalized linear models, 80, 129, 389, 391,
  480, 583
General linear model (GLM), 389
GGT, *see* Gamma-glutamyltransferase
Glivenko–Cantelli theorem, 46, 474

Global Use of Strategies to Open Occluded
Coronary Arteries (GUSTO) I trial, 137
Gold standard (ROC), 210
Goodness-of-fit tests (tests for normality), 327–335
adaptive smoothing, 334
Shapiro–Wilk test for normality, 327–328
supplement, 329–335
test for normality based on sample entropy,
332–333
tests for multivariate normality, 333–335
tests for normality, 329–332
tests for normality based on characteristic
functions, 332
U-test, 333
Z-test, 330
Graphics, 39–69
boxplots, 40–42
color-coding schemes, 62
comparisons of powers, 66
contour plots, 43–45
dendogram, 62, 66
derivatives of probability plots, 55–57
descriptive plots of raw data, 40–45
empirical distribution function plot, 45–49
empirical likelihood, 64, 66
graphical comparisons of statistical tests,
64–66
heat maps, 62–66
high-dimensional plots, 43–45
internal comparison methods, 57, 58–60
Kolmogorov–Smirnov statistic, 55
Monte Carlo technique, 64
output of clustering calculation, 62
perspective plots, 43
P–P plots, 52, 54
probability plots as informal auxiliary
information to inference, 57–61
Q–Q plots, 50, 54
receiver operating characteristic curve, 57
residuals in regression analysis, 60–61
scatterplots, 42–43
supplement, 67–69
total time on test curves, 57
two-sample comparisons, 50–57
whiskers, 40
Group-sequential tests, 404–406

H

HDL cholesterol, *see* High-density lipoprotein
cholesterol
Heat maps, 62–66
color-coding schemes, 62

comparisons of powers, 66
dendogram, 62, 66
empirical likelihood, 64, 66
functions, 63
graphical comparisons of statistical
tests, 64–66
Monte Carlo technique, 64
output of clustering calculation, 62
visualization of data, 62–64
Hessian matrix
Bayes factor, 172
Schwarz criterion, 155
High-density lipoprotein (HDL) cholesterol,
71, 164, 198
High-dimensional plots, 43–45
Higher order, 90, 128, 177, 264, 360, 515
High-performance liquid chromatography
(HPLC), 222
Hilbert spaces, 319
HIV, 125, 203, 391
Honest prior information, 183
Hormone therapy (HT), 249
Hotelling's T^2 distribution, 100
Hotelling's T^2-test, 88, 96, 100, 135, 249, 333
Hybrid pooled–unpooled design, 434, 438
Hypothesis
alternative hypothesis (Bayes factor), 158
composite hypotheses, 236
discovery hypotheses, 422
primary hypotheses, 422
secondary hypotheses, 422
setting, 232–238
statistical hypotheses, 4–5
two-sided alternative hypothesis, 367
Hypothesis testing
inequality constrained hypotheses, 182
most powerful test in hypothesis testing, 184
null hypothesis, 398
optimality of LRT in, 183–184
rationality and unbiasedness in, 7–8

I

Identifiability problems (Bayes factor), 178
IMPACT clinical trial, 221
Importance sampling function, 156
Increasing failure rate average (IFRA)
distributions, 78
Independence, dependence and (structures,
testing, and measuring), 263–326
Archimedean copulas, 320
area under the Kendall plot, 274–277
bivariate distributions, 278

Brownian distance covariance, 324
  data examples, 312–317
  discussion, 317–318
  electromagnetic radiation, modeling of, 278
  empirical likelihood–based method, 270–271
  error in variables, 279
  Hilbert spaces, 319
  independence, tests of, 265–272
  indices of dependence, 272–277
  linear dependence, 277
  logarithmic dependence, 278
  maximal information coefficient, 273–274
  measurement error, 279
  multidimensional random variables, 324
  multiplicative noise, 282
  partial ordering, 320
  periodontal disease, 315
  Pitman tests, 319
  positive quadrant dependent variables, 322
  quadratic dependence, 277
  random effects–type dependence, 279–284
  rank tests, 318
  reciprocal dependence, 278
  Riemannian manifolds, 319
  Spearman's rho, 323
  structures of dependence, 277–284
  Student's *t*-test, 321
  study of dependence, 263
  supplement, 318–326
  TBARS, 312–315
  theory of correlation, 263
  trigonometric dependence, 278
  VEGF expression, 315–317
Independence, tests of, 265–272, 318
  classical methods, 265–267
  copula function, 267
  data-driven rank tests, 267–270
  density-based empirical likelihood ratio test, 271–272
  empirical likelihood–based method, 270–271
  Kendall's rank correlation coefficient, 267
  Legendre polynomials, 267
  Monte Carlo comparisons of, 284–312
  Pearson correlation coefficient, 266
  Spearman's rank correlation coefficient, 266–267
Independent and identically distributed (i.i.d.) measurements, 229
Indicator function, 139, 176, 274, 351, 378, 473, 529
Inequality constrained hypotheses, testing of, 182
Information matrix, 154, 174, 439

Integrated most powerful decision rule, 185
Interaction, 67, 173, 381, 445
Internal comparison methods, 57, 58–60
Interpolation method, 453–455
Intersection-union test (IUT), 88
Invariant tests, 81, 319, 330, 366, 586
Inverse Gaussian distribution, 333, 434, 439

J

Jackknife, 79, 138, 211, 312, 316, 471, 528
James–Stein estimation, 120–121
Jeffrey's noninformative priors, 182
Jump discontinuities (regression models), 387

K

Kaplan–Meier (KM) estimator, 445
Kendall statistic, 267
Kernel function (U-statistics), 353
Kernel regression imputation, 129
Kernel smoothing estimator (ROC curve), 211
Kolmogorov–Smirnov statistic, derivatives of probability plots, 55
Kolmogorov–Smirnov test, 113–114, 231
Kruskal–Wallis one-way analysis of variance, 244–245
Kuiper statistic, 376
Kurtosis, 279, 331, 335

L

Laboratory assays, 448
Lagrange multiplier, 235, 236
Laplace approximation, 153–155
Laplace's method, 173
Large sample tests, 16
LDA, *see* Linear discriminant analysis
Legendre polynomials, 267
Lévy processes, 135
Likelihood, *see also* Maximum likelihood
  Bayesian empirical likelihood, 117–118
  density-based empirical likelihood, 357–360
  empirical likelihood, 570–571
  generalized empirical likelihood, 132
  parametric likelihood, 71–94
  principle (LP), 80
  ratio (LR), 81, 183
  weighted empirical likelihood, 222
Likelihood ratio test (LRT), 86, 183
  biomedical studies, 208–210
  density-based empirical, 231–239

exact (for equality of two normal populations), 101
optimality of (in simple hypothesis testing case), 183–184
statistic, 93
univariate and *p*-dimensional, 95–96
Limits of detection (LOD), 4, 220, 429
Lindley paradox, 174
Linear dependence, 277
Linear discriminant analysis (LDA), 222
Localization ROC (LROC) methodology, 225
Locally most powerful (LMP) tests, 88
Logarithmic dependence, 278
Log-likelihood ratio, 77, 126, 128, 219
Lognormal distribution, 13, 71, 221, 331
Longitudinal growth curve models, 218
Loss function, 145
LP, *see* Likelihood principle
LR, *see* Likelihood ratio
LROC methodology, *see* Localization ROC methodology
LRT, *see* Likelihood ratio test

M

Magnetic resonance angiography (MRA), 214
Mahalanobis distances, 213
Mann–Whitney statistic, 214
Mann–Whitney U-test, 229, 249
Mann–Whitney–Wilcoxon test, 246
Mantel-extension test, 102
Mantel-Haenszel test, 321
Markov chain Monte Carlo (MCMC) methods, 156, 176, 388
Martingale methods, 81, 381
Maximal information coefficient (MIC), 273–274
Maximization–maximization–posterior (MMP), 384
Maximizing a posterior (MAP), 384
Maximum likelihood
local, 456, 463
methodology, 436–437
parametric, 75–78, 108
t-type tests, 96
Maximum likelihood estimator (MLE), 83, 432
Bayes factor, 149
biomarker measurements, 432
empirical likelihoods, 111
of probability, 83
ROC curve, 189
MCB, *see* Multiple comparison with the best
MCMC methods, *see* Markov chain Monte Carlo methods

ME, *see* Measurement error
Means of continuous data, tests on, 95–103
asymmetrical distributions, mean of, 102
Cohen's effect size, 103
equal variances, 97
exact LRT for equality of two normal populations, 101
monotonic dose–response relationship, 102
multivariate *t*-test, 99–101
one-sample *t*-test, 96
paired *t*-test, 97–99
receiver operating characteristic curves, 103
supplement, 102–103
t-type tests, 96–101
two-sample *t*-test, 97
unequal variances (Welch's *t*-test), 97
univariate and *p*-dimensional LRTs, 95–96
Welch U-test, 102
Measurement error (ME), 4
in clinical trials, 429
models, 388
problems, 138
random effects–type dependence, 279
Median, 8, 17, 102, 123, 126, 137, 248, 419, 550
Mesh plot, 43
MI, *see* Myocardial infarction
MIC, *see* Maximal information coefficient
Missing value, 27, 32, 134, 430, 437, 446, 448, 480
Mixed model, 38, 211, 282, 391, 474
MLE, *see* Maximum likelihood estimator
MMP, *see* Maximization–maximization–posterior
Modal approximation (Bayes factor), 151
Model selection, 9, 39, 90, 177, 384, 445
Monotone likelihood ratio, 86
Monte Carlo methods
experiments (biomarker measurements), 439–441
Markov chain (Bayes factor), 156, 176
resampling (bootstrap), 570
simulation (parametric likelihood), 88
Monte Carlo simulation, 88, 125, 137, 211, 221, 248, 331
Most powerful test, 90, 137, 144, 145, 184, 246, 319, 411
MOSUM, 392
MRA, *see* Magnetic resonance angiography
Multinomial distribution, 123, 129
Multiple comparison, 37, 38, 224, 381, 422, 428
Multiple comparison with the best (MCB), 224
Multiple testing problems (in clinical experiments), 421–428
Bonferroni procedures, 422, 424

comparison error rate, 423
definitions of error rates, 422–427
discovery hypotheses, 422
false discovery rate and false discovery
    proportion, 426
family-wise error rate, 422–425
power evaluation, 427
primary hypotheses, 422
secondary hypotheses, 422
supplement, 428
Multivariate normal distribution, 207, 222, 223,
    225, 334, 335, 448
Multivariate t-test, 99–101
Myocardial infarction (MI), 114

N

NaN value, *see* Not a Number value
National Health and Nutrition Examination
    Survey (NHANES) study, 448
Nested hypotheses, 154, 333
Nested models, 13, 168, 176, 215
Neyman–Pearson lemma, 85, 223, 225, 382
Noninformative prior, 158, 174, 182, 434
Nonparametric comparisons of distributions,
    229–261
    alternative hypotheses, 232
    alternative test statistic, 252
    Anderson–Darling rank statistic, 250
    Baumgartner–Weiß–Schindler statistic, 247
    biomedical and dental research, 250
    combination technique, 246
    composite hypotheses, 236
    DBEL procedures for K-sample comparisons,
        245–246
    DBEL ratio based on paired data, 239–244
    DBEL ratio tests, 231–239
    decision rule, 237, 238
    Dosemeci–Benichou test, 247
    empirical constraint, 234, 236
    false discovery rate, 250
    goodness-of-fit tests, 235
    hypothesis setting and test statistics,
        232–238
    independent and identically distributed
        measurements, 229
    Kolmogorov–Smirnov two-sample test, 231
    Kruskal–Wallis one-way analysis of
        variance, 244–245
    K-sample comparison, 250–252
    Lagrange multiplier, 235, 236
    likelihood ratio test statistic, 233
    Mann–Whitney–Wilcoxon test, 246

Monte Carlo power study, 246
Monte Carlo simulations, 243, 251
multiple-group comparison, 244–246
multivariate samples, 251
nonparametric test statistic, 233
null hypothesis, 233
ordinary least-squares test, 251
parametric likelihood ratio statistic, 240
psychological studies, 248
rank-sum tests, 252
R code (two-sample density-based empirical
    likelihood ratio test), 260–261
robust nonparametric test, 244
significance level of proposed test, 242–244
supplement, 246–252
two-sample data, 247
Type I error, 247
Wilcoxon rank-sum test, 229–230
Nonparametric tilting, 570
Normality (goodness-of-fit tests), 327–335
    adaptive smoothing, 334
    Shapiro–Wilk test for normality, 327–328
    supplement, 329–335
    test for normality based on sample entropy,
        332–333
    tests for multivariate normality, 333–335
    tests for normality, 329–332
    tests for normality based on characteristic
        functions, 332
    U-test, 333
    Z-test, 330
Not a Number (NaN) value, 27
Null hypothesis, 8
Nuisance parameter, 128, 175
Numerical data, 3

O

Odds ratio, 222, 419, 449
One-sample t-test, 96
One-sided likelihood, 86–90
One-sided studentized range test (OSRT), 87
Online (sequential) change-point problem, 338
Optimality, 183, 333, 343, 415, 418
Order statistics, 19, 67, 80, 329, 333, 487
Ordinary least-squares test, 251

P

Paired data, 21, 238–243
Paired t-test, 97–99
Parametric empirical Bayes (PEB) point
    estimators, 120

Parametric likelihood, 71–94
  analysis of variance model, 86
  asymptotically uniformly most powerful
     tests, 81
  autoregressive process of outcomes, 85
  Bonferroni correction, 89
  Brownian motion, 84
  central limit theorems, 81
  chi-square distribution, 79
  coefficient of variation, 88
  expectation–maximization algorithm, 85
  histograms, 72
  increasing failure rate average distributions, 78
  intersection-union test, 88
  kernel weights, 84
  likelihood principle, 80
  likelihood ratio property, 92–94
  likelihood ratio test, 86
  likelihood ratio test and its optimality, 73
  likelihood ratio test statistic, 74–75, 93
  locally most powerful tests, 88
  Martingale methods, 81
  maximum likelihood, 75–78
  monotone likelihood ratio, 86
  Monte Carlo simulation, 88
  most powerful test, 90–92
  one-sided likelihood, 86–90
  one-sided studentized range test, 87
  reconsideration of data example, 76–78
  sampling importance resampling
     algorithm, 80
  supplement, 78–90
  two one-sided tests, 89
  Type I error, 90
  uniformly most powerful test, 82
  univariate normal population, 86
  Wald statistic, 83
  Wald test, poorly behaved, 81
  weighted likelihood bootstrap, 80
  Wilks' theorem, 93–94
Pareto distribution, 221
Parkinson's Disease Questionnaire, 412
Particle marginal Metropolis–Hastings
    (PMMH) algorithm, 392
PCB, *see* Polychlorinated biphenyl
Peak expiratory flow rate (PEFR), 88
PEB point estimators, *see* Parametric empirical
    Bayes point estimators
PELT algorithm, 385
Permutation methods, *see* Bootstrap and
    permutation methods
Permutation tests, 571–586
  correlation and regression, 582–586

  exact tests, 571
  Monte Carlo approach, 571
  outline of permutation theory, 572–574
  rerandomization tests, 571
  semiparametric methods, 572
  two-sample methods, 574–582
Permutation-type nonidentifiabilities, 178
Perspective plots, 43
Phylogenetic trees, change points on, 392
Pitman tests, 319
Plots (graphics)
  boxplots, 40–42
  contour plots, 43–45
  derivatives of probability plots, 55–57
  descriptive plots of raw data, 40–45
  empirical distribution function plot, 45–49
  empirical likelihood, 64, 66
  graphical comparisons of statistical tests,
     64–66
  high-dimensional plots, 43–45
  internal comparison methods, 57, 58–60
  Kolmogorov–Smirnov statistic, 55
  Monte Carlo technique, 64
  output of clustering calculation, 62
  perspective plots, 43
  P–P plots, 52, 54
  probability plots as informal auxiliary
     information to inference, 57–61
  Q–Q plots, 50, 54
  receiver operating characteristic curve, 57
  residuals in regression analysis, 60–61
  scatterplots, 42–43
  supplement, 67–69
  three-dimensional, 39
  total time on test curves, 57
  two-sample comparisons, 50–57
  whiskers, 40
PMMH algorithm, *see* Particle marginal
    Metropolis–Hastings algorithm
Poisson distribution, 12, 131, 381
Polychlorinated biphenyl (PCB), 429
Positive quadrant dependent (PQD)
    variables, 322
Pretest procedure, 14
Primary hypotheses, 422
Prior distribution, 144
Probability–probability plots (P–P plots), 52–54
Product partition model (PPM), 387
p-values, 8–11
  bootstrap, 540–534
  cumulative distribution function, 9
  expected p-values, 10–11
  fallacy, 177

misinterpretations, 9
null hypothesis, 8
receiver operating curve, 10
p-values (for exact tests), 451–470
    Bayesian hybrid method, 456
    decision rule, 461
    empirical likelihood, 458
    hybrid method, 455–462
    illustration, 456
    interpolation method, 453–455
    methods of calculating critical values of
        exact tests, 452–462
    Monte Carlo–based method, 452–453
    software packages, 462–463
    supplement, 463–464

Q

Quadratic dependence, 277
Quadrature, 101, 148
Qualitative data, 3
Quantile–quantile plots (Q–Q plots), 50, 54
Quantitative risk assessment (epidemiological
    studies), 388
Quasi-likelihood, 127

R

Radioimmunoassay (RIA), 222
Radiotherapy with adjuvant chemotherapy
    (RTC), 85
Rank-sum tests, 252
Raw data, descriptive plots of, 40–45
    boxplots, 40–42
    contour plots, 43–45
    high-dimensional plots, 43–45
    perspective plots, 43
    scatterplots, 42–43
Receiver operating curve (ROC), 23, 57, 180
    Bayes factor, 180
    binormal, 189
    biomarker measurements, 430, 444
    derivatives of probability plots, 57
    expected p-values and, 10
    sequential testing methods, 417
    tests on means of continuous data, 103
Receiver operating characteristic (ROC) curve
    analyses, fundamentals of, 187–228
    ADC, *see* AIDS dementia complex
    additive measurement errors, 215
    AIDS dementia complex (ADC), 203
    area under the ROC curve, 191–194
    AUC (supplement), 216

best linear combination of markers,
    206–208
binormal ROC curve, 189
bootstrap, 213
Box–Cox variable transformations, 223
combinations of markers, 222–227
covariate-adjusted ROC curve, 215
decision-analytic quantity, 222
decision theory, ROC analysis based on, 219
distribution-free confidence interval, 216
distribution-free testing procedure, 210
expected bias of ROC curve, 196–203
general form of AUC, 227–228
generalized treatment effect, 221
gold standard, 210
high-performance liquid
    chromatography, 222
HIV-related cognitive dysfunction, 203
kernel smoothing estimator, 211
limit of detection, 220
linear discriminant analysis, 222
logistic regression (comparison and
    overestimation), 194–203
longitudinal growth curve models, 218
magnetic resonance angiography, 214
Mahalanobis distances, 213
Mann–Whitney statistic, 214
marker values, 223
maximum likelihood estimators, 189
maximum likelihood ratio tests, 208–210
misdiagnosis, 212
multiple biomarkers, best combinations
    based on values of, 203–206
multiple comparison with the best, 224
novel semiparametric modeling
    framework, 215
numerical calculations, 210
overestimation of AUC, 196–203
population studies, 217
proteomics biomarker study, 225
p-value, TBARS, 199
Q-Q plots, 223
regression models, 212
repeated screening tests, 224
retrospective and prospective ROC, 196
risk prediction model, 222
ROC (supplement), 210
ROC curve inference, 188–191
smoothly clipped absolute deviation
    penalty, 226
stress–strength model, 220
test usefulness, 212
training samples, 195

treatment effects, 206–210
U-statistics, 217
validation samples, 195
vigilance data, 212
volume under the three-class surface, 220
Wald statistics, 219
Wald test, 211
weighted empirical likelihood, 222
Reciprocal dependence, 278
Recursive residual statistic, 366–367
Regression modeling (bootstrap), 559–569
Regression models (change-point analysis),
 376–380
 breakpoint, 376, 392
 broken line [stick] regression, 376
 epidemiological studies, quantitative risk
  assessment in, 388
 general case of the problem, 379–380
 general linear model, 389
 jump discontinuities, 387
 linear regression, 377, 386
 Markov chain Monte Carlo methods, 388
 measurement error models, 388
 monotonic trends, isotonic
  regression for, 390
 phylogenetic trees, change points on, 392
 product partition model, 387
 scalar values, 378
 segmented linear regression, 376, 378, 389
 segmented regression, 389–391
 simple case of the problem, 379
 statistical quality control schemes, 393
 structural change, 391–392
 threshold effects, 388–389
Rerandomization tests, 571
Resampling algorithm, sampling
 importance, 80
Retrospective data collection, 409
RIA, *see* Radioimmunoassay
Riemannian manifolds, 319
Risk prediction model, 222
RNA-seq technology, 181
Robust regression, 560
ROC, *see* Receiver operating curve
R software, 25–30
 binseqtest, 419
 comments in, 26
 el.convex, 139
 for exact tests, 462
 for goodness-of-fit and two-sample
  comparisons, 114
 inputting data in, 26–27
 manipulating data in, 27–29

Not a Number value, 27
 optimization algorithms, 139
 printing data in, 29–30
 rules for names of variables and data sets, 25
 strucchange, 392
RTC, *see* Radiotherapy with adjuvant
  chemotherapy

S

Sampling importance resampling
 algorithm, 80
SAS software, 30–37
 comments in, 31–32
 inputting data in, 32–33
 macro language for calculating bootstrap-*t*
  intervals, 545–549
 macro language for calculating percentile
  intervals, 543–545
 manipulating data in, 33–35
 printing data in, 35–36
 record length, 33
 resampling data with replacement in
  (bootstrap), 477–485
 rules for names of variables and data
  sets, 31
 summarizing data in, 36–37
SBP, *see* Systolic blood pressure
SCAD penalty, *see* Smoothly clipped absolute
  deviation penalty
Scatterplots, 42–43
Schwarz criterion, 155–156, 176
Score-type statistic, 365–366
Secondary hypotheses, 422
Segmented linear regression, 376, 378–380
Semilikelihood ratio statistic, 365
Sequential clinical trial, 135
Sequential probability ratio test (SPRT),
 398–404
 asymptotic properties of stopping time,
  401–404
 error control, 420
 null hypothesis testing, 398
 stopping boundaries, 400
 Wald approximation to average sample
  number, 400–401
Sequential stopping rule, 179, 416
Sequential testing methods, review of,
 395–420
 adaptive design, 414
 adaptive sequential designs, 406–407
 asymptotic properties of stopping time,
  401–404

clinical trial, 417
conditional power procedures, 410
determination of sample sizes based on
          SPRT error control, 420
flexible designs, 415
futility analysis, 397, 407
group-sequential stopping rule, 416
group-sequential tests, 404–406
invariance principles, 408
MSPRT, 412
null hypothesis testing, 398
operating characteristics, 396
Pitman efficiencies, 408
postsequential analysis, 407–408
retrospective data collection, 409
ROC curve, 417
sequential probability ratio test, 398–404
sequential stopping rule, 416
stochastic process, 410
stopping boundaries, 400
supplement, 408–420
two-stage designs, 397–398
Type I error rate, 419
use in clinical trials, 396
Wald approximation to average sample
          number, 400–401
Wald test, 413
Severe mood dysregulation (SMD), 114, 139
Shapiro–Wilk test for normality, 327–328
Significance level of test, 6, 242–243
SIR algorithm, *see* Sampling importance
          resampling algorithm
SK, *see* Streptokinase
Small interfering RNA (siRNA) transfection
          group, 62, 63
Small, round, blue cell tumors (SRBCTs), 249
SMD, *see* Severe mood dysregulation
Smoothly clipped absolute deviation (SCAD)
          penalty, 226
Software, 25–38
    comments, 31–32
    GAUSS, 390, 392
    inputting data, 26, 32
    manipulating data, 27, 33
    Not a Number value, 27
    packages for exact tests, 462–463
    printing data, 29, 35
    record length, 33
    R software, 25–30
    rules for names of variables, 25, 31
    SAS software, 30–37
    STATA, 462
    summarizing data, 36–37

    supplement, 37–38
    VERDIA, 385
SPRT, *see* Sequential probability ratio test
Square-wave alternative, 363
SRBCTs, *see* Small, round, blue cell tumors
srRNA transfection group, *see* Small interfering
          RNA transfection group
Standard deviation, 564
STATA software, 462
Statistical functional, 17–19
Statistical graphics, 39–69
    boxplots, 40–42
    color-coding schemes, 62
    comparisons of powers, 66
    contour plots, 43–45
    dendogram, 62, 66
    derivatives of probability plots, 55–57
    descriptive plots of raw data, 40–45
    empirical distribution function plot, 45–49
    empirical likelihood, 64, 66
    graphical comparisons of statistical tests,
          64–66
    heat maps, 62–66
    high-dimensional plots, 43–45
    internal comparison methods, 57, 58–60
    Kolmogorov–Smirnov statistic, 55
    modifications, extensions, and hybrids of
          Q–Q and P–P plots, 54–55
    Monte Carlo technique, 64
    output of clustering calculation, 62
    perspective plots, 43
    probability plots as informal auxiliary
          information to inference, 57–61
    probability–probability plots, 52–54
    quantile–quantile plots, 50–52
    receiver operating characteristic curve, 57
    residuals in regression analysis, 60–61
    scatterplots, 42–43
    supplement, 67–69
    total time on test curves, 57
    two-sample comparisons, 50–57
    whiskers, 40
Statistical hypotheses, 4–5
Statistical inference, *see* Decision making
          (experimental), basic concepts in
Statistical software, *see* Software
Stopping boundaries, 400
Streptokinase (SK), 137
Stress–strength model, 220
Student's *t*-test, 321
Surface plot, 43
Synthetic data (empirical likelihood), 131
Systolic blood pressure (SBP), 429

T

t-distribution, 86, 96, 266, 451, 567
Testosterone inhibitor, 89
Thiobarbituric acid reactive substances
    (TBARS), 198, 312
Threshold limiting value (TLV), 388, 389
TIE, *see* Type I error
Tissue plasminogen activator (TPA), 137
TOST, *see* Two one-sided tests
Total positivity, 320
Total time on test (TTT) curves, 57
Trigonometric dependence, 278
t-tests, 96–101
    equal variances, 97
    multivariate *t*-test, 99–101
    one-sample *t*-test, 96
    paired *t*-test, 97–99
    Student's *t*-test, 321
    two-sample *t*-test, 97
    unequal variances, 97
    Welch's *t*-test, 14, 97
TTT curves, *see* Total time on test curves
Two one-sided tests (TOST), 89
Two-sample *t*-test, 97
Type I error (TIE), 90, 136

U

Undersmoothing, 125
Unequal variances (Welch's *t*-test), 97
Unified Parkinson's Disease Rating Scale, 412
Uniform distribution, 118, 238
Uniformly most powerful (UMP) test, 6, 82
Uniformly most powerful unbiased (UMPU)
    test, 7
Univariate normal population, 86
U-test
    Mann–Whitney, 229, 248
    Welch, 102

V

Vascular endothelial growth factor (VEGF), 315
Ventilator-associated pneumonia study, 137
VERDIA software, 385
Vigilance data, 212
Volume under the three-class surface
    (VUS), 220
U-statistics, kernel function in, 353
U-test, 333

W

Wald statistic, 83
Wald test
    diagnostic testing, 211
    poorly behaved, 81
    sequential, 413
Weibull distribution, 386
Weighted empirical likelihood (WEL)
    method, 222
Weighted likelihood bootstrap (WLB), 80
Welch's *t*-test, 14, 97
Welch U-test, 102
Whiskers, 40
Wilcoxon–Mann–Whitney (WMW) test, 249
Wilcoxon rank-sum test, 229–230
Wilcoxon signed-rank test, 114
Wilks' theorem, 93–94
Wire mesh surface plot, 43
Wishart distribution, 87, 434
WLB, *see* Weighted likelihood bootstrap

Y

Yuen–Welch test, 102

Z

Z-test, 330